FREE FROM GLUTEN, SUGAR & DAIRY

mila's meals
THE BEGINNING & THE BASICS

BY CATHERINE BARNHOORN

"At last, a wonderfully creative and thoroughly well researched work of immensely helpful and beneficial guidance, for us as parents!

Food and health are inseparable. In today's information age nutritional concepts can be all too confusing, especially when the information is focused on "what" to eat, rather than exploring and understanding the "why".

This book introduces important and comprehensible "why's" of applying food as your medicine, while at the same time, offering truly sumptuous and easy to follow recipes to give our little genetic investments vibrant health and a greater connection to nature, of which we are all an integral part.

Toward healing, awareness and peace! Thank you Catherine."

- Dr Jon Morley (MBChB)

"Catherine has managed to fit a veritable encyclopedia worth of knowledge and wisdom into this beautiful book.

As a mother, I will value this resource for referring to time and again when preparing food for my family. I will turn to it when deciding on the best choices, in terms of personal and environmental health, while shopping and preparing delicious, healthy meals for my loved ones.

Painstaking attention to detail is paid to all things food and health related that we may all have heard of or read about, but are unsure of how to integrate into our daily lives.

The creative and wholesome recipe ideas will continually be an inspiration in my kitchen, and yours, for years to come!"

- Esmé Morley (MoM)

"This well-researched and masterfully created book is a true gift to aware parents who want to give their children the best start to life."

- Dr Hanna Grotepass (MBChB), Homeopath, Synchronization Harmonics practitioner

"Let medicine be thy food and food thy medicine.
Nature itself is the best physician"

- Hippocrates

Mila's Meals

DELICIOUS & NUTRITIOUS

FREE FROM GLUTEN, SUGAR & DAIRY

Mila's Meals - The Beginning & The Basics
A collection of nourishing wholefood recipes and food ideas for baby's first year
(and the rest of the family too!)
Free from gluten, refined sugar, dairy and artificial additives.

All rights reserved. No part of this book may be reproduced in any form or by any electronic or mechanical means, including photocopying and recording, or by any other information storage and retrieval systems, without permission in writing from the author.

For information, contact Catherine Barnhoorn at catherine@milasmeals.co.za

The content of this book is for general instruction only.
Each person's physical, emotional, and spiritual condition is unique. The instruction in this book is not intended to replace or interrupt the reader's relationship with a physician or other professional. Please consult your doctor for matters pertaining to your specific health and diet. The author, publisher and distributor of this book are not held responsible for any adverse effects or consequences resulting from the use or misuse of any information, suggestions or procedures described hereafter.

To contact the author, visit www.milasmeals.co.za

Publishing Copyright © Catherine Barnhoorn 2015
Recipes Copyright © Catherine Barnhoorn 2015
Photography Copyright © Catherine Barnhoorn 2015

Recipes: Catherine Barnhoorn
Writing: Catherine Barnhoorn
Photographer: Alfred Lor, www.shooot.co.za
Stylist: Catherine Barnhoorn
Design & Layout: Catherine Barnhoorn
Editor & Proof Reader: Alix Verrips
Printing & Binding: Quickfox Publishers
(Thank you Maggie Flynn!)

Fonts used: Helvetica Neue (Latinotype), Boho (Latinotype), Baskerville, Liebecook (Liebe Fonts),
The Hand (La Goupil Paris), Harman (Ahmet Altun)

ISBN 978-0-620-68276-3

- chicken puree
- pies
- blend fruit
- bean salad

enchanted adventure @ beach ...therness

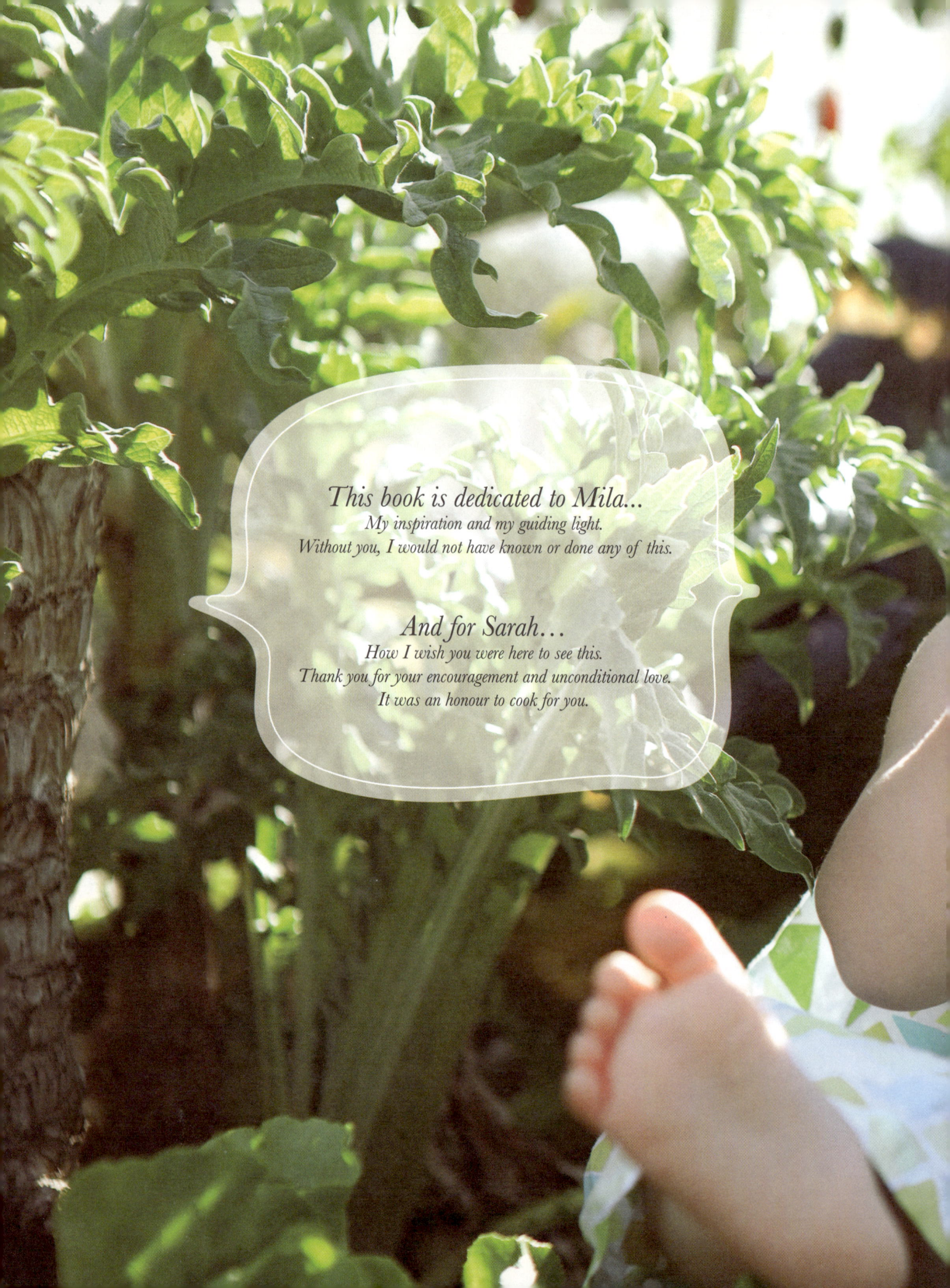

This book is dedicated to Mila…
*My inspiration and my guiding light.
Without you, I would not have known or done any of this.*

And for Sarah…
*How I wish you were here to see this.
Thank you for your encouragement and unconditional love.
It was an honour to cook for you.*

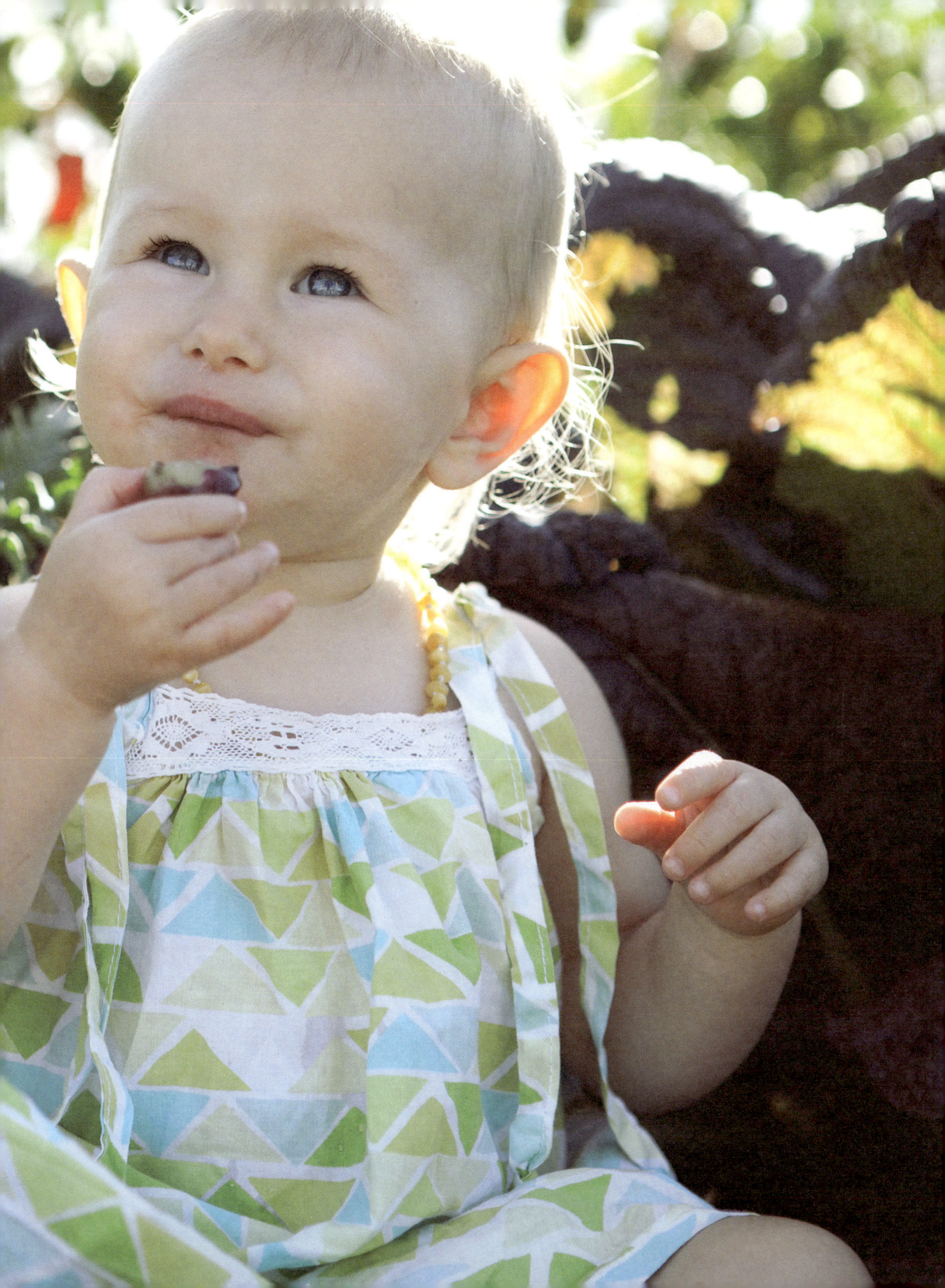

I LOVE YOU

A poem stuck on our fridge – Mila asks me to 'sing' it to her at least once a day.

I AM YOUR PARENT, YOU ARE MY CHILD
I AM YOUR QUIET PLACE, YOU ARE MY WILD
I AM YOUR CALM FACE, YOU ARE MY GIGGLE
I AM YOUR WAIT, YOU ARE MY WIGGLE
I AM YOUR AUDIENCE, YOU ARE MY CLOWN
I AM YOUR LONDON BRIDGE, YOU ARE MY FALLING DOWN
I AM YOUR CARROT STICKS, YOU ARE MY LIQUORICE
I AM YOUR DANDELION, YOU ARE MY FIRST WISH
I AM YOUR WATER WINGS, YOU ARE MY DEEP
I AM YOUR OPEN ARMS, YOU ARE MY RUNNING LEAP
I AM YOUR WAY HOME, YOU ARE MY NEW PATH
I AM YOUR DRY TOWEL, YOU ARE MY WET BATH
I AM YOUR DINNER, YOU ARE MY CHOCOLATE CAKE
I AM YOUR BEDTIME, YOU ARE MY WIDE AWAKE
I AM YOUR FINISH LINE, YOU ARE MY RACE
I AM YOUR PRAYING HANDS, YOU ARE MY SAVING GRACE
I AM YOUR FAVOURITE BOOK, YOU ARE MY NEW LINES
I AM YOUR NIGHTLIGHT, YOU ARE MY SUNSHINE
I AM YOUR LULLABY, YOU ARE MY PEEK-A-BOO
I AM YOUR KISS GOODNIGHT, YOU ARE MY I LOVE YOU."

AUTHOR: MARYANN K CUSIMANO

Acknowledgements

Oh my angel Mila... *I am so blessed to be your mom and infinitely grateful for all you have and continue to teach me. Thank you for being patient with me, for understanding that sometimes I had to work instead of playing with you. Thank you for being a picky eater, for forcing me to get very creative in the kitchen. Thank you for the joy we share in the kitchen as we cook together.*

Mom and Dad... *thank you so very much for the beautiful home in which I can safely raise and nurture my daughter. Thank you too for your generosity and financial support that has allowed me the space and time to pursue my dream.*

Alfred Lor... *creative genius photographer! Thank you so much for your enthusiasm, patience and willingness to work on this project.*

Mona Appels... *I would not have been able to do this without you. Thank you for anticipating my needs in the kitchen and for caring for Mila while I was otherwise occupied.*

Lily & Mathew Barnhoorn... *my brave niece and nephew. Thank you for being the best 'food models' a recipe book author could ask for – not only do you eat all the food, but you look happy while you're doing it! The sauerkraut has been included just for you!*

Sarah Barnhoorn... *Thank you for being my biggest fan and for all your illness, and journey through it, taught me. Thank you for requesting my food, and for the honour of cooking for you when you needed it the most.*

Miemie Bosman, my other mom... *Thank you for the never-ending support, and belief in my vision.*

To my baby-group and other 'mommy' friends... *Thank you for continuously requesting this book – it kept me going! I'm sorry I missed the boat for some of you as your children are now way passed weaning!*

Alix Verrips... *Thank you for showing up to be my editor! It was divine intervention!*

Jaco Bosman (aka Pappa)... *Thank you for all you are and do for Mila.*

Dr. Jon Morley, Dr. Hanna Grotepass and Esmé Morley... *thank you so much for reviewing the book – yes, "reading 400 pages is like studying for an exam!". I really appreciate the time you took and the interest you showed.*

Crowd funders... *thank you for contributing money towards a product that you hadn't seen yet! I am honoured by your faith in me.*

*A special thank you to **Dr. Jon Morley, Dr. Karin Van Niekerk and Megan Franz**, who have supported and guided me on my healing journey and, in doing so, informed various parts of this book.*

To you, *the person who bought this book... I trust it will be an inspiring resource for you. I wish you and your family a long life in good health.*

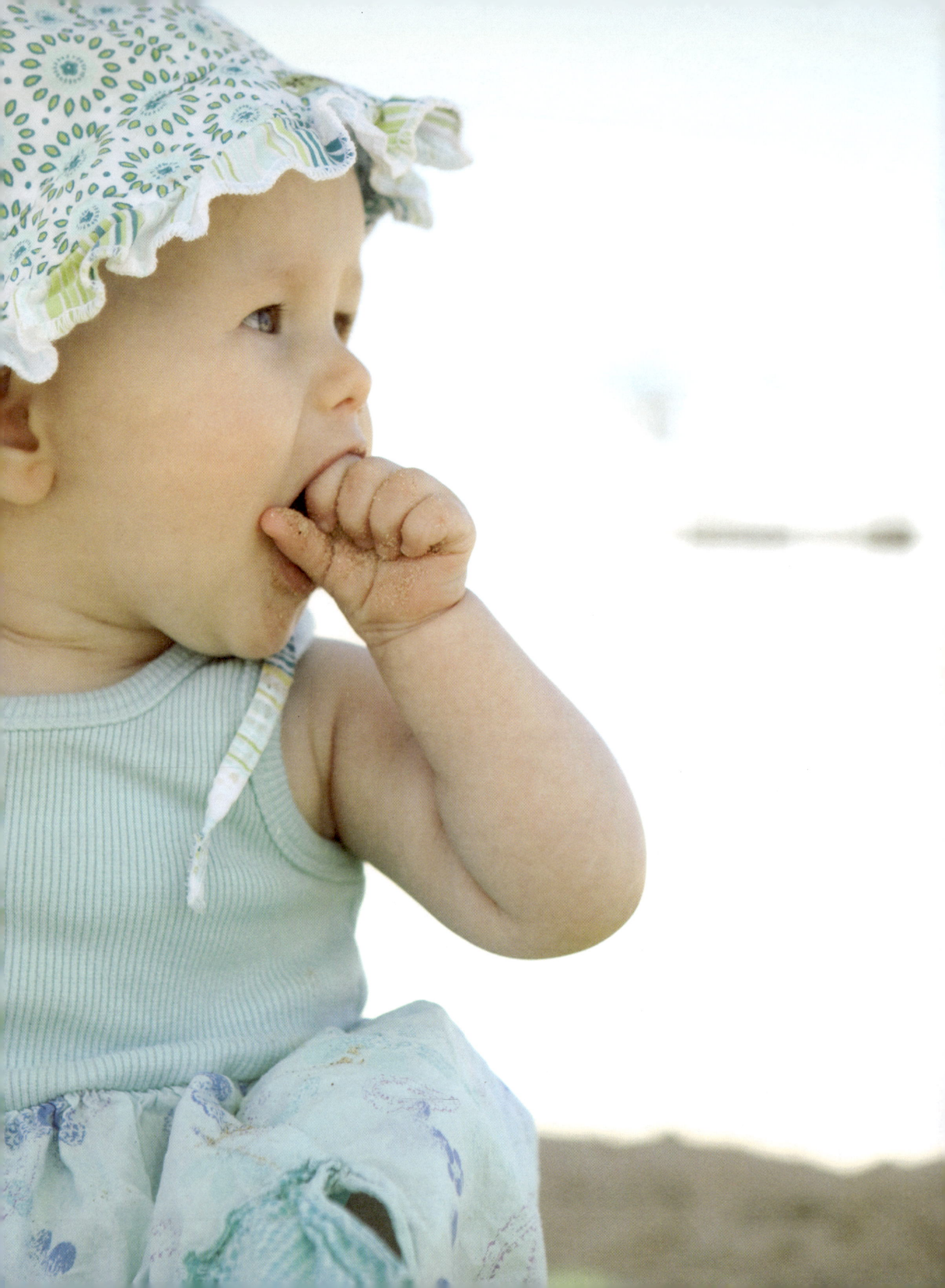

Contents

FOREWARD 13
INTRODUCTION 15

UNLEARN: INFANT FOOD FALLACIES 21
Essential Nutrients 39
What nutrients baby needs and when 39
Essential nutrients, the role they play, and where to find them 39
What to eat when 46

FEEDING WITH AWARENESS 51
Allergens 51
Convenience vs. Conscience 54
Toxins 55
Whole Foods vs. Refined & Processed Foods 62
Chemical Cuisine: Food Additives 66
Raw vs. Cooked... which is better? 72
Eat from the rainbow 74
Enzymes, Nutrients and Anti-nutrients 76
Anti-Nutrients 76
Meat: Organic, Free-Range, Pasture-raised, Grass-fed & GMO. 78
Fruits and Veggies: Organic, Conventional & GMO. 83
Why not Gluten, Dairy and Sugar? 94
What can I eat? Gluten, sugar, & dairy alternatives. 104
Nutrient Enhancers: my kind of food additives! 115
Mess 118
Soul Food 119

FOOD PREPARATION AND STORAGE 131

RECIPES 136
Thirsty 136
Off the spoon 160
Out & About Finger Foods 198
Eating In Finger Foods 232
Dip Dips & Spreads 274
From the Fork (or spoon) 302
Party Food & Something Sweet 318
Pantry Items 348

DON'T JUST EAT FOOD! 381

GLOSSARY OF INGREDIENTS 391

EQUIPMENT 467

CONVERSIONS CHARTS 472

SAY WHO? 474

APPENDIX 478

REFERENCES 486

INDEX 490

RECIPE INDEX 496

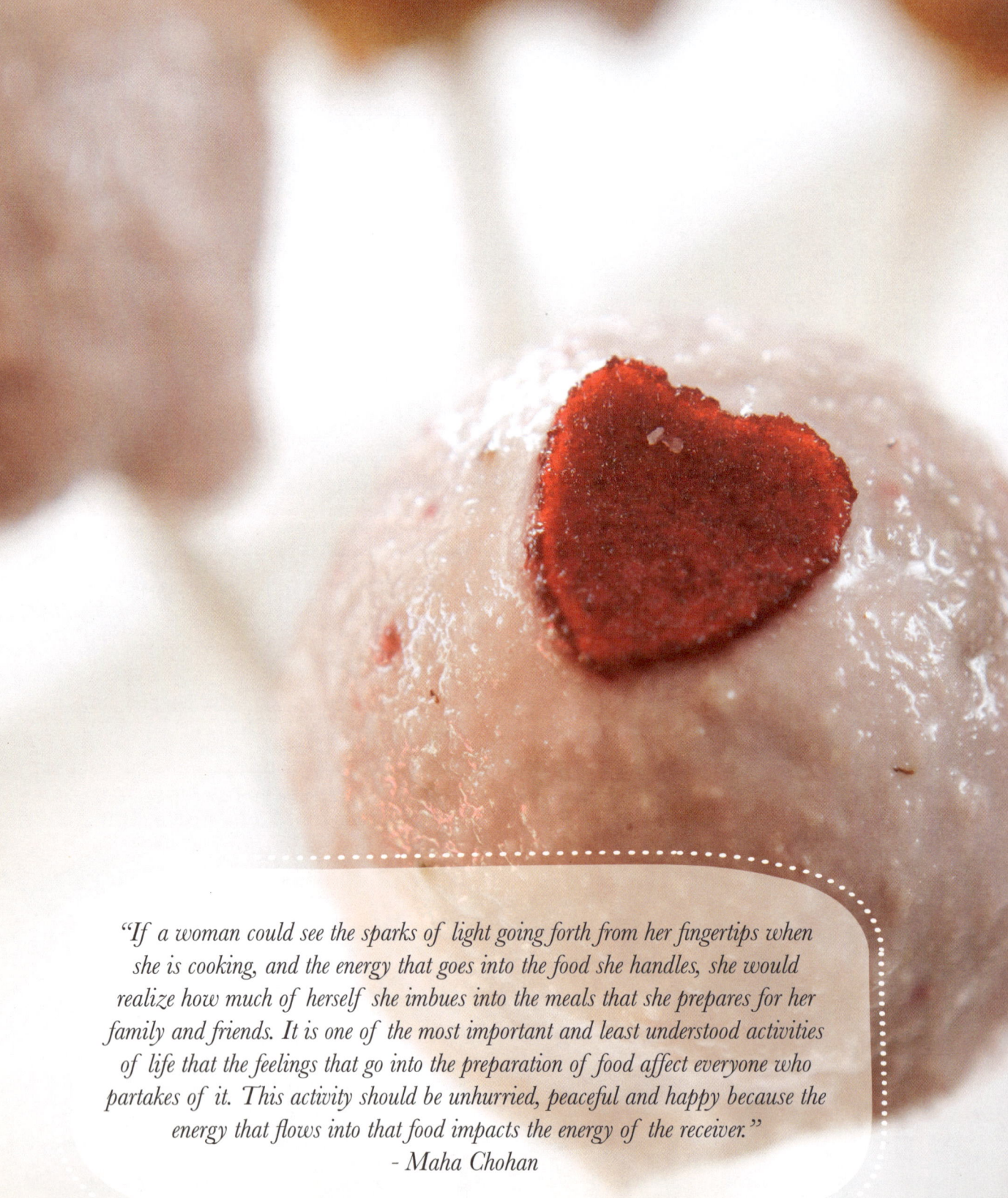

"If a woman could see the sparks of light going forth from her fingertips when she is cooking, and the energy that goes into the food she handles, she would realize how much of herself she imbues into the meals that she prepares for her family and friends. It is one of the most important and least understood activities of life that the feelings that go into the preparation of food affect everyone who partakes of it. This activity should be unhurried, peaceful and happy because the energy that flows into that food impacts the energy of the receiver."
- Maha Chohan

Foreward

Our planet is undergoing great changes and humanity as a whole is being taken to higher levels of consciousness.

Many children born today will become our future leaders and teachers, they are very much part of the great transformation. These children are sensitive, gifted and very aware and need to be treated with respect and special care.

What we expose them to is of the greatest importance, and wholesome nutrition plays a major role in their harmonious development.

Food prepared with reverence and love will feed body, heart and soul.

The acclaimed books and photographs by Professor Masaru Emoto are worth studying to get a better understanding of the workings of energy. His photographs of the structure of water demonstrate the effect thoughts and intentions have on everything in and around us. Love, gratitude and blessing enhance the water structure into diamond-like crystals. Do we fully realise the importance of this for us humans whose bodies consist of seventy percent water?

Catherine weaves these principles into her masterfully created book. This very informative book is crucial to give our special children a healthy start to life.

May it reach far and wide!

Hanna Grotepass

Dr Hanna Grotepass
MBCHB, HOMEOPATH AND ENERGY HEALER

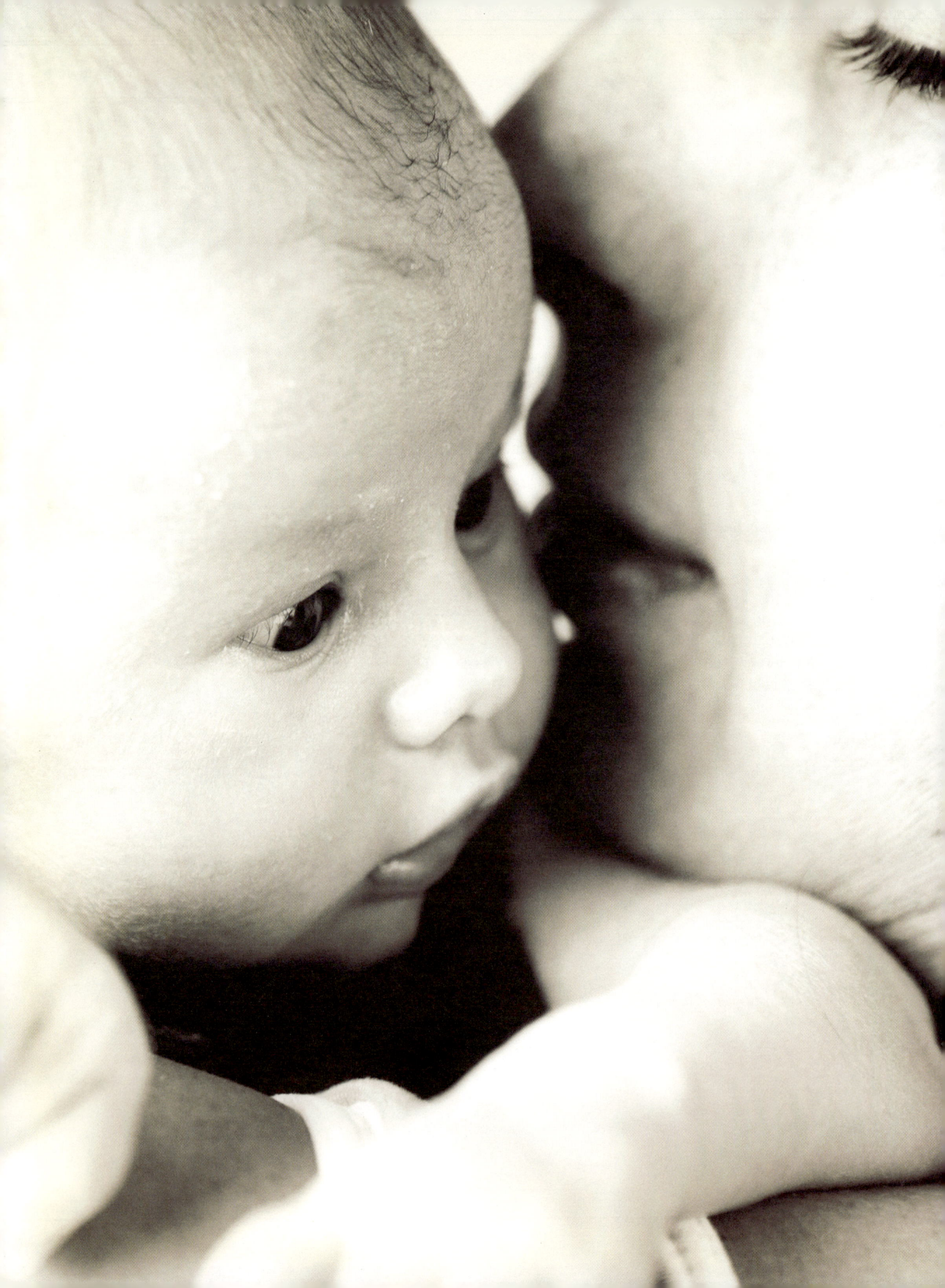

Introduction

This book came about because of green poo – that's right… BRIGHT GREEN BABY POO!

Let me back track a little bit… I was first told I had a candida overgrowth when I was 19 years old. It was long before candida was in mainstream consciousness and after doing a 3 month detox I did not pay it too much attention. A few years later I was diagnosed with endometriosis. While I had always loved preparing my own food, I began to pay extra attention to food and the affect that different foods can have on the body. I learnt about: the connection between Candida and endometriosis; about the affect food preservatives have on the body's hormones; as well as, the impact of conventional cosmetics and body care products. I once again limited my intake of sugar and gluten, and made conscious decisions to only eat homemade wholefood. I also changed to all-natural, organic products – for my body and in the home. I did, however, still go for seven laparoscopies to treat the endometriosis – not believing that there could be a purely natural cure (or reason) for the disease.

Shortly before I got married, and on my sister-in-law's recommendation, I went to see a homeopath in the hope that she could help me fall pregnant (I had been told by my gynaecologist that this may be impossible due to the endometriosis). I was due for another laparoscopy, but I was beginning to doubt the wisdom of this yearly 'quick fix'. Amazingly, two months after I took the homeopathic remedies, I was completely pain-free and pregnant!

It was a complicated pregnancy – I went into premature labour at 26 weeks and was put on bed rest for 10 weeks. As challenging as that was, it gave me a lot of time to bond with my unborn child and to think – about how I had been raised, and about how I wanted my daughter to be raised. With decisions like whether or not to vaccinate having to be made, I once again delved into research on the body and what it needs to be healthy and to fight or prevent disease. With candida, endometriosis and ADHD in my daughter's gene pool, it became clear to me that when I started feeding her, it would be a strictly refined sugar-, preservative-, and additive-free diet of homemade food - so her immune system could reach its full potential and so that those genes would remain dormant. What I did not realise, is that this would have to be my way of eating too!

I became a mom to my beautiful daughter, Mila, in February 2012 – she was born at 41 weeks despite the early scare! I was determined to breastfeed – even after being told I did not have "breastfeeding nipples" and Mila not being able to latch on due to a lip tie (which I only discovered when she was two). We struggled through the first few days, did a happy dance when we discovered nipple shields, and then settled into a routine of what is surely the most magical time in a woman's life.

Mila was a small baby (born at 2,4kg), suffered from colic and needed to be fed every couple of hours for the first nine months. I realise now the reasons for all of this – her imbalanced gut flora

Introduction

inherited during childbirth from my candida overgrowth. If only I had known what I know now. I began to notice that Mila's discomfort was worse after some feeds than after others. My sister-in-law suggested I eliminate certain foods like garlic and onion - two of my favourites! Once again, I began to pay closer attention to food and the effect it has on the body. At the same time, I developed eczema on my hands. Initially I thought it was from compulsive hand washing with Tea Tree soap – but then I noticed it flared up after I ate certain foods – namely gluten, sugar and dairy. You must know that I had eaten a toasted mozzarella, pesto and tomato sandwich on artisan sourdough bread from our local bakery every single day of my pregnancy – actually twice a day towards the end! It was usually followed by a few (or more) pieces of Lindt dark chocolate so the thought that I would have to stop this ritual because of the gluten and dairy was something I resisted. Until I saw the green poo – Mila's that is, not mine.

I was (as a first time mom) completely freaked out when I opened Mila's nappy one day and saw what looked like spinach purée! The homeopath and various other experienced folk told me that it was normal for a breastfed baby to have poo ranging from orange to green. But my instinct had been reawakened, and I knew it was the result of 'something'. Already noticing the physical affects of gluten, sugar and dairy on myself, I quickly realised that when I breastfed Mila after consuming these foods, her colic was worse and a few hours later, her poo would be bright green!

It is amazing how quickly you change something when it is in the best interest of your child! I immediately went on a completely gluten-, sugar-, and dairy-free diet and the result… less colic, no more green poo, less eczema and in six months I lost the 25kg I had gained during my pregnancy.

The whole notion of 'gluten-free foods' was still uncommon then, especially in South Africa. While you did find gluten-free pasta, there was not the extensive range of gluten-free flours, breads, and ready-mixes that you find today. So for me, at that time, being gluten-free simply meant eliminating those types of food from my diet and I was okay with that – there was still plenty else I could (and did) eat. Then came the big curveball… Mila was six months old and needed to start solids! As a (very) anxious first-time mom I immediately ordered some baby food recipe books. I was horrified when I paged through them to find cheese, bread or sugar on every page! I realised that my decision to raise Mila on a free-from diet meant that I was going to have to put in some extra effort. I was acutely aware of the fact that babies have very specific nutritional needs and by eliminating some foods I was going to have to replace their nutrients with other food sources. I also faced a mountain of criticism – like "how can you not feed your child dairy?" Which I had to counter with facts - like "dairy is a difficult-to-digest food and is not the best source of bio-available calcium!". So began my search for recipes and my journey into nutrition.

I developed quite a large collection of free-from recipes on my iPhone - but they were all free from one thing and not the others, so I began to develop my own recipes. With mushy mommy brain I was always losing the pieces of paper I had written my recipes on and forgetting what I had learnt the day before. Also, with lack-of-sleep-blurry-eyes cooking from a recipe on my small screen iPhone became immensely frustrating. I realised that for my own sanity I needed everything I had learnt and created to be in one place – in a folder of sorts. Then it dawned on me - surely I was not the only completely stressed out, sleep deprived new mom wanting to prepare delicious and nutritious whole foods for a new baby in an effortless way – you know, like open the recipe book, see the picture,

Introduction

follow the instructions. And so the idea of writing this book was born!

That was 3 years ago, almost to the day. It has been a long process, with a few pauses in-between when Life presented itself and needed complete attention. I am immensely grateful for each twist and turn (and pause) in this journey – each one has taught me so much, all of which is now included in the book. I did a juice fast with colonics and met David Wolfe, I went on Natasha Campbell-McBride's GAPS diet and learnt about IBS and Leaky Gut, I followed the Body Ecology Diet and learnt about the power of ancient grains and fermented foods, I discovered the Weston A Price Foundation and the concept of traditional, ancestral foods and nutrition and how it affects children and their development, and through my sister-in-law's cancer diagnosis, I learnt how food can both cause and cure cancer and how preparing food for someone is a sacred act of love and a precious gift to give.

As for Mila – she continues to teach me so much everyday. She is a remarkable little girl – intelligent, sensitive, compassionate and just so happy. She seems to withstand all of life's little (and big) knocks with such grace and good humour. As a play therapist told me recently – "how lucky that she was just born with such a happy disposition." Can I see any benefits of raising her as a free-from child? Well, she is now three and a half years old and has only ever taken conventional medication (in the form of antibiotics) once – and after the big life events that occurred before that time, I am not surprised her body could not hold up to the impact of the stress. She has had a sum total of two temper tantrums - both of which lasted for all of 1 minute and which occurred after she had eaten sugar. Yes, she has had coughs and colds - especially during her first winter at school but other than that her biggest health issue currently is constipation (probably due to the antibiotics I mentioned before). She sleeps well, is even tempered, quick witted, has an incredible memory and knows our national anthem off by heart (and it is in four different languages).

This seems like I am boasting – well, I am going to take a moment to pat myself on the back (you need to take a break from the mommy guilt every now and then) – but I mentioned all of this because I want you to know that the effort it takes to prepare all your own food and perhaps even learn a new way of cooking and baking using ingredients you have never heard of before is SO worth it. When people ask me how I can choose to spend so much of my time in the kitchen, my reply is simple – "I would rather spend my time cooking, than spend my time taking care of a frequently sick child or disciplining an unruly child who is acting out because of a sugar rush."

Also, I truly believe in the saying "Do something today that your future self will thank you for". I have no doubt that this nutritious food is benefiting Mila's immune system and development. I am convinced that the effort I am putting in now will benefit her in the future, and my future self, and hers, will thank me for it.

As parents, our children's health is our responsibility – not the doctor's, not the government's, not the supermarket's. I would like to say, "I encourage you to make informed choices about the foods you feed your child", but really, I am begging you! Please, please educate yourself. Explore, discover, and learn. Go beyond the clever marketing, the labels, the government guidelines, and the conventions. Make informed decisions based on information you have sought out, not that which is fed to you by marketers selling a product or pamphlets in a paediatrician's office. Your child and your future self will thank you for it.

Introduction

My food philosophy... "delicious and nutritious".

Like Mila says, food should be "delicious and nutritious" – it should delight the senses as well as the body. I am all for food that is nutrient-dense, free of additives, as close as possible to its natural whole form, and where-ever possible, organically grown and pasture-fed. It should include fruits and vegetables, raw nuts and seeds, healthy fats and naturally fermented foods.

My physical health philosophy... "all disease begins in the gut".

Through my own healing journey and my nutrition studies at the Institute for Integrative Nutrition®, I am fully aligned with the belief that all disease begins in the gut. For this reason, I believe that wholesome, full mind-body nutrition, with an awareness of food intolerances, is imperative for the optimal growth, development and future-health of your little one. Since a newborn's gut is still very permeable (to allow the pre-digested breast milk nutrients through with ease) and with 70% of the immune system located in the gut, it is so very important to take care of it by eating easy-to-digest, age appropriate foods. A strong digestion will allow for greater absorption of nutrients and a stronger immune system.

My holistic health philosophy... "no amount of good food can nourish a starving soul".

Besides the food on your plate, there is a need for Soul Food. At the Institute for Integrative Nutrition® they have developed the concept of Primary Food – essentially, primary food is nourishment that doesn't appear on your dinner plate. The four core primary foods for adults are: exercise, spirituality, career and relationships. The premise is that when these areas of your life are in balance, food is secondary. § (IIN's founder, director and primary teacher), says that, "Healthy relationships, regular physical activity, a fulfilling career, and a spiritual practice can fill your soul and satisfy your hunger for life." They are, essentially soul food.

"The fun, excitement, and love of daily life have the power to feed us so that food becomes secondary." - IIN®

> Introduction

So what would soul food for your little one be? I would venture to say it would be: loving relationships, physical activity, spiritual practise and play.

My 'diet' philosophy... "One man's food is another man's poison".

This is a gluten-free, sugar-free and dairy-free way of eating. I am not saying this is 'The' way to eat, 'The Best' way to eat or 'The only way people should be eating'. This is just what works for me, and what works for my daughter.

I present research findings, which explain why it is working for us. I accept and acknowledge that there is, without a doubt, evidence of why and how another way of eating will be beneficial to many others. That's the thing with the science of nutrition – more so than any other scientific field - there will be two studies that completely contradict each other. This is where intuitive eating comes into play – no one knows your body better than you. You are the best person to know what does and what doesn't work for you. I encourage you to start listening to what your body is telling you. Discover what is poisoning you and what is feeding you, and go with that. As a mom, trust your instinct when it comes to your little one – you are so connected (for the first few years especially). Make use of that, it is a wonderful tool.

On raising a free-from child.

It is quite simple… the benefits far outweigh the costs!

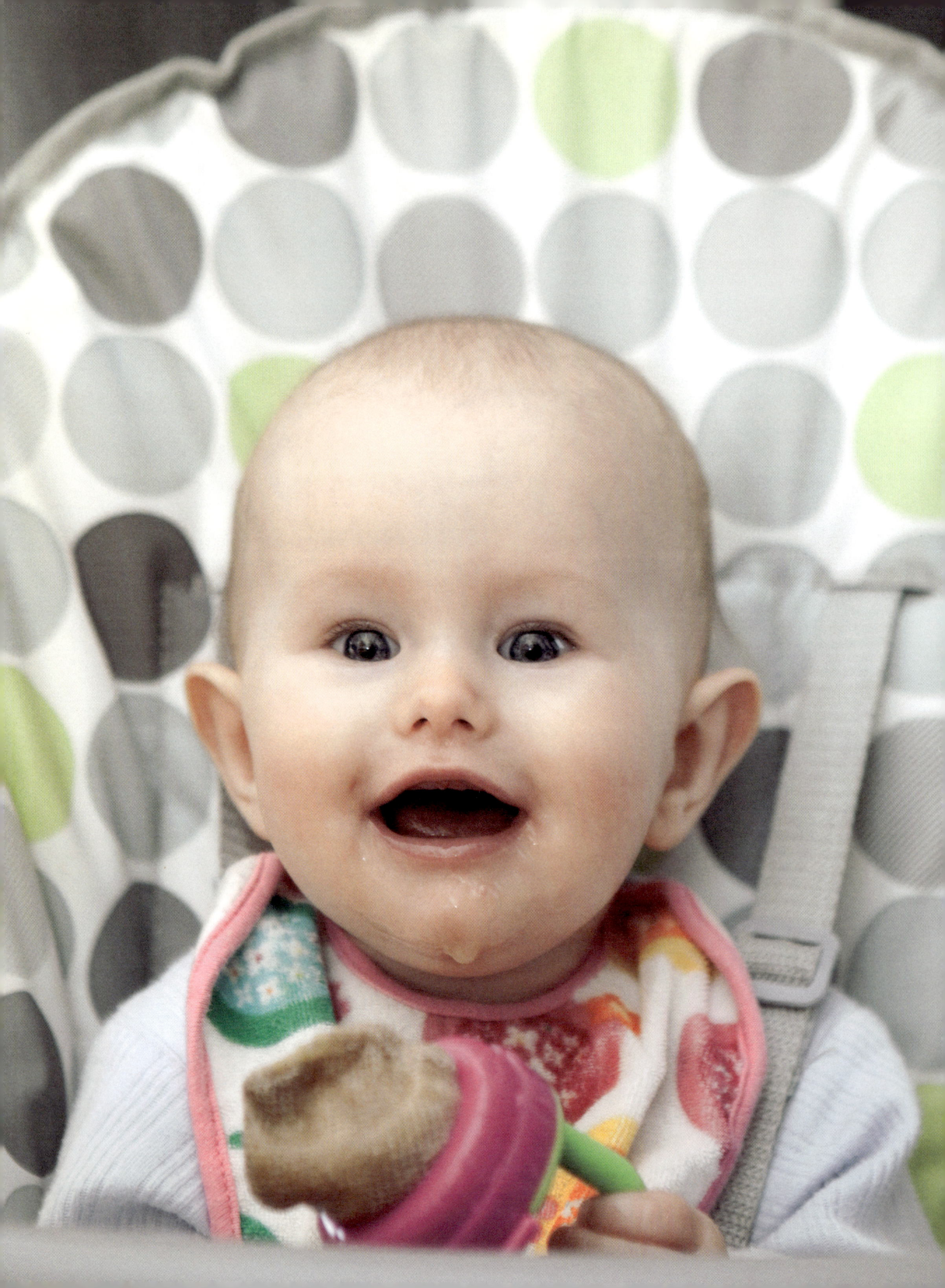

Unlearn

Unlearn: Infant Food Fallacies

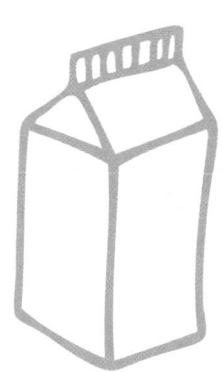

Disclaimer: As with everything concerning food there are two sides to any debate raging around every one of the topics in this section – both sides will be defended with scientific proof, and 'absolute' recommendations. I am merely presenting my beliefs formed by my research and first hand experience of both Mila's, and my own digestive issues. I encourage you to do your own research should anything mentioned here not 'sit well' with you. I am not trying to convince you of anything – I simply hope to provide information, and at the very least prompt you to question what has previously or otherwise been presented as absolute fact and truth.

Unlearn

"Rice cereal is the best first food for baby."

I've got to say I was fooled by this - by the clever marketing of the food companies and by the advice of the clinic sister. Mila had always struggled with constipation, colic and sleeping at night. So when the clinic sister suggested I start feeding her solids at 4 months (to help her sleep better at night), I nervously did. I fed her rice cereal (organic – but that really did not help the situation much). Poor thing! I stopped as quickly as I started (her tummy cramps were too awful after that first meal) and, this is why...

Food has to be broken down into its nutrient components: amino acids, fatty acids, cholesterol, simple sugars, vitamins, minerals, etc. - **our bodies absorb nutrients, not food**. The body produces digestive enzymes that break down our food into nutrients. These nutrients are then absorbed and nourish the body. Digestive enzymes are produced in the pancreas, small intestine, saliva glands and stomach.

Different digestive enzymes are needed to break down different types of food. In order to digest grains, your body uses an enzyme called amylase. Guess what? Pancreatic amylase is not produced by your little one (in sufficient quantities) until they are a year old – sometimes even later. The rule of thumb here is that it is not until your little one's molar teeth are fully developed that they have sufficient quantities of pancreatic amylase to properly digest grains – this can be anywhere from 13 – 24 months of age. Amylase is provided in a mother's breast milk and is produced by your little one's saliva – but these are not sufficient to properly digest grains. Especially processed grains, or grains that have not been prepared properly.

So what happens to this undigested rice cereal (or other grains)? Some undigested food (from other vegetable carbohydrate sources) benefits your little one - fermentation in the colon produces short chain fatty acids, which can improve nutrient absorption, enhance gut health, and even be used as a source of energy for both the microbes and baby. But since grains (especially) cannot be adequately digested, they start rotting. This rotting food matter feeds pathogenic bacteria and fungi (such as Candida) – and this imbalance can lead to food allergies, asthma, eczema, and other autoimmune disorders. Over time, the pathogenic bacteria and fungi (and their toxic by-products) create holes in the gut wall (known as Leaky Gut). A leaky gut allows toxins and partially digested food to spill directly into the blood creating an unpredictable mix of physical, behavioural, emotional and neurological symptoms. This is explained in great detail in Dr. Natasha Campbell-McBride book Gut and Psychology Syndrome.

What else is wrong with commercially available rice cereal?

Rice cereal is processed – meaning it is no longer a whole food. In order for the cereal to have a longer shelf life, the bran and the germ (the most nutritious parts) have been removed, simultaneously stripping the grain of its protein, fibre, nutrients and minerals. Artificial vitamins have to then be added back in – these are far less bio-available to your little one's body and a poor replacement for nature's version.

Rice cereal is an extremely high glycaemic food – that is, it spikes the blood sugar.

Rice cereal contains phytates (the salt form of phytic acid).

Phytic acid is a naturally occurring chemical in grains, nuts and seeds, Phytic acid binds to essential minerals (such as calcium, copper, iron, zinc, and magnesium) in the digestive tract, making them less available to our bodies – and actually flushing them out of our bodies. While the majority of the phytic acid (or phytates) are found in the bran of the rice (which is removed during processing), there will still be some present. So, eating processed rice cereal may actually remove iron, zinc, calcium and magnesium from your little one's body!

Phytates also reduce the digestibility of starches, proteins, and fats.

Please note that simply grinding grains at home and cooking them will result in an even higher amount of phytates in your little one's food. All grains, nuts and seeds must be soaked, sprouted or fermented before cooking in order to break down the phytic acid. Please see the chapter Convenience vs. Conscience: Enzymes, Nutrients and Anti-nutrients for more information on this.

Commercial rice cereal fortified with iron. But surely this is a good thing? A baby is born with sufficient iron reserves to last them until they are 6 months old. While a mother's breast milk is low in iron, the iron that is present is readily absorbed by her little one – as opposed to the artificial sources of iron found in fortified cereals and formula.

While your little one may need additional sources of iron at the age of 6 months, it is far better to provide this from whole foods as opposed to supplemental drops or an additive in a nutrient deficient food. Good sources of additional iron are liver (raw), other cooked meat, blackstrap molasses, avocado and… soil! No, I am not suggesting you feed your little one soil, but the iron from soil **is** absorbed by the body. There is a school of thought that suggests that babies these days may be more prone to iron deficiency because they are not allowed to play in soil as part of an overly hygienic upbringing. Another reason for an increase in infant anaemia may be the practice of immediately clamping the umbilical cord at birth. Waiting even two minutes before clamping the cord after birth allows up to 50% more blood volume to pulse from the placenta to the newborn and has been shown to result in higher total body iron and plasma ferritin (reflecting iron storage) at 6 months of age.

One must question why breast milk is naturally low in iron. It is the perfect food, so perhaps there is a reason for the low amounts of iron. Breast milk actually includes chelators that bind to iron thereby minimizing free iron in the intestines - withholding it from pathogenic bacteria. What is the reason nature designed breast milk this way? There is new research that suggests too much iron, or supplementing with iron when your little one is NOT deficient, may actually be harmful. Too much iron can result in lowered IQ, bacterial infection, cancer and stunted growth.

"No" to cereal, now what?

Some good ideas for baby's first foods:

- ♥ Soft-boiled egg yolk (not the egg white as this contains difficult to digest proteins),
- ♥ Raw liver from pastured animals (frozen for 2 weeks to kill off any parasites which may be present),
- ♥ Non-starchy vegetables (combined with a healthy fat like ghee or coconut oil to add mineral absorption),
- ♥ Soups with homemade bone broth,
- ♥ Mashed banana and avocado.

"Whole grains are good for you."

Whole grains **are good for you and your little one, very good in fact** – but here's the catch – it depends on how you prepare them, when you introduce them and which ones you eat. Eating unprepared grains, introducing them too soon, or eating gluten-containing grains can have negative health effects.

Preparation

Whole grains are the hardest food for the human body to digest, and all grains contain anti-nutrients that must be neutralized before cooking. They all have phytic acid that can block the absorption of calcium, magnesium, copper and zinc as well as enzyme inhibitors that block the digestive enzymes needed to digest it.

In order to unlock a grain's nutritional potential, it is necessary to prepare them in a way that makes them more digestible – such as soaking them for 24 hours, fermenting or sprouting them before cooking.

Preparing grains with a dollop of healthy fat (such as ghee or coconut oil) will help the absorption of calcium, phosphorus, iron, B vitamins and the many other vitamins that grains provide.

When to introduce them

Many traditional cultures have fed their babies grains before their first birthday – as their first food even – but they were all fermented first.

For the reasons mentioned previously, it is best to wait until your little one is a year old before introducing grains. At this age, he/she will have greater quantity of the amalse digestive enzyme that is needed to digest grains.

According to The Nourishing Traditions Book of Baby & Childcare by Sally Fallon Morell and Thomas S. Cowan, if there is a history of celiac disease or gluten intolerance in the family, it is best to wait until your little one's third year before introducing grains.

Which ones to choose

Properly prepared grains are nutritious – they are important sources of many nutrients, including protein, fibre, B vitamins and minerals (iron, magnesium and selenium).

In order to avoid gluten, you need to avoid wheat, barley, rye, spelt and oats (unless they are certified gluten-free). See the chapter Why Not Gluten, Dairy and Sugar? for more on this.

There are many naturally gluten-free grains to choose from including: rice, quinoa, millet, buckwheat, sorghum and amaranth. These grains are nutrient-dense, act as antioxidants and, help the body make serotonin, which improves mood while providing a calming, soothing effect on the nervous system.

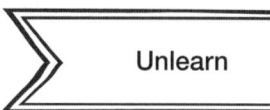

"Raw Milk is dangerous."

This is another very contentious issue.

Many medical professionals and governing bodies will warn you that it is dangerous to consume raw milk. In fact, in many parts of the world it is illegal to sell raw milk - that is, milk that has not been pasteurised.

Milk that is available in grocery stores is pasteurised and homogenised (unless otherwise stated).

Pasteurisation

The process of pasteurisation is named after a French scientist Louis Pasteur who, in 1864, discovered that heating beer and wine just enough to kill most of the bacteria that caused spoilage, prevented these beverages from turning sour (he later extended his studies to prove that milk was the same).

Pasteurisation of milk was instituted in the 1920s to combat TB, infant diarrhoea, undulant fever and other diseases caused by consuming milk sourced from animals who had poor nutrition with dirty production methods.

Modern stainless steel tanks, milking machines, refrigerated trucks and inspection methods make pasteurisation of milk from organic, grass-fed animals unnecessary for public protection in this regard.

However, the current conditions in commercial dairy farms as well as large scale farming methods render it absolutely necessary to pasteurise the milk to 'ensure' the safety of it for human consumption. Today the process of pasteurisation is also used as food preservation method – that is, it extends the shelf life of a product (and increases profits).

Homogenisation

Homogenisation is a process used to make a mixture of two substances that would not otherwise mix. The fat in milk (known as butterfat) normally separates from the water and collects at the top (creating curds and whey). Homogenisation breaks the fat into smaller sizes so it no longer separates. This is accomplished by forcing the milk through a very fine screen at high pressure and allows the sale of non-separating milk at any fat specification – that is, skim milk, low fat or full-cream milk.

There are arguments that this milk then becomes an unnatural food that the body cannot digest as well. The theory goes that the body knows how to deal with fat particles and with liquid proteins but when the fat has been emulsified to that degree, the body doesn't know how to digest it.

The Safety of Raw Milk

Raw milk contains numerous components that assist in naturally killing pathogens which may be present in the milk thus preventing pathogen absorption across the intestinal wall, as well as strengthening the immune system.

Studies show that:

- ♥ Children who consume raw milk have a higher natural resistance to TB than children fed pasteurized milk;
- ♥ Raw milk is very effective in preventing scurvy and protecting against flu, diphtheria and pneumonia;
- ♥ Raw milk prevents tooth decay, even in children who eat a lot of sugar;
- ♥ Raw milk is better than pasteurised milk in promoting growth and calcium absorption;
- ♥ A substance present in raw cream (but not in pasteurised cream) prevents joint stiffness and the pain of arthritis;
- ♥ Children who drink raw milk have fewer allergic skin problems and far less asthma than children who drink pasteurized milk.

Why not pasteurised milk?

Pasteurisation relies on the principle that most harmful bacteria can be killed by heat. It does not, however, always kill the bacteria responsible for Johne's disease (with which most confinement cows are infected) – and which, in turn, is suspected of causing Crohn's disease in humans.

Pasteurisation also destroys enzymes; diminishes vitamin content; denatures fragile milk proteins; destroys vitamins C, B12 and B6; kills beneficial bacteria, and actually promotes the growth of pathogens.

Many studies have linked consumption of pasteurised milk with lactose intolerance, allergies, asthma, frequent ear infections, gastro-intestinal problems, colic, osteoporosis, arthritis, heart disease, cancer, diabetes, autoimmune disease, attention deficit disorder and constipation. Fewer and fewer consumers can tolerate pasteurised (and ultra pasteurised) milk.

*Source: Don't Drink Your Milk, Frank Oski, MD, 1983; Sally Fallon-Morrel, www.realmilk.com

AND REMEMBER... PASTEURISED, HOMOGENISED MILK IS A PROCESSED FOOD.

As with most things, there are two sides to every debate. Having researched this topic, it is my belief that raw, unprocessed, full fat dairy from animals raised organically (outdoors with their natural feed) is a healthy, nutritious food for your little one in moderate amounts. It is, however, imperative to source your milk and dairy products from a farmer who you know and trust and can verify that his animals are disease-free. I choose goat's milk for Mila in order to avoid the casein protein and high concentration of lactose found in cow's milk.

Unlearn

"Liver is dangerous."

As an expecting mom you must have heard the advice to avoid eating liver while pregnant. Conventional dieticians, doctors and governmental health departments also warn against feeding it to your little one. This advice stems from two concerns – the assumption that liver contains many toxins and, the amount of vitamin A that it contains.

The liver and toxins

It is important to clarify that the role of the liver (in both humans and animals) is to neutralise toxins (such as drugs, chemical agents and poisons); but the liver does not store toxins. Poisonous compounds that the body cannot neutralise and eliminate are likely to be stored in the fatty tissues and the nervous system. The liver is not a storage organ for toxins, but it is a storage organ for many important nutrients (vitamins A, D, E, K, B12 and folate, and minerals such as copper and iron). These nutrients provide the body with some of the tools it needs to get rid of toxins.

Of course, we should consume liver from healthy, organically raised animals that spend their lives outdoors and feed on pasture.

Vitamin A

Vitamin A is essential for babies – they need it to develop their eyes, bones, and immune system (to name only a few things). Babies are not good at converting beta-carotene, the precursor to vitamin A found in orange vegetables and fruits, into vitamin A. They need their vitamin A to be preformed – as it is in breast milk.

Liver is high in preformed vitamin A, which is what scares a lot of people away from it. The concerns around vitamin A stem from studies in which moderate doses of **synthetic** preformed vitamin A were found to cause problems and even contribute to birth defects. But the **natural** preformed vitamin A found in liver is an extremely important nutrient for human health and does not cause problems except in extremely large amounts - and moderation of anything, is always important.

Liver is also an excellent source of iron, vitamin C, all the B vitamins, folate, and high quality protein. It is especially beneficial during your little one's weaning stages. Combine liver with healthy probiotic foods, like a bit of sauerkraut, to make it more digestible.

For more nutritional information on liver, please refer to the Glossary chapter.

Unlearn

"Eggs should only be introduced after a year."

I read this piece of advice and heard it often when I was introducing Mila to solid foods. While I didn't have the knowledge I now have, I naturally ignored this advice.

Eggs can be an allergen, but it is important to note that it is the egg whites that contain the difficult-to-digest proteins – they are the ones that are usually responsible for an allergic reaction.

EGGS YOLKS ARE, IN FACT, A PERFECT FIRST FOOD FOR YOUR LITTLE ONE!

Breast milk (nature's most perfect food), and that which your little one has the ability to easily digest, is largely comprised of: fats; proteins; carbohydrates; cholesterol; vitamins and minerals. The nutrient profile in an egg yolk closely resembles this, and as such, it is an easily digestible food for your little one.

Babies need fat, protein and cholesterol for proper brain and nervous system development. Egg yolks from pasture-raised hens provide nutrients as well as choline, amino acids, Omega 3 fatty acids and vitamin A.

For more nutritional information on eggs, please refer to the Glossary chapter.

"Germs are bad for you."

This information is fairly new to many people, and it gets a bit technical - so here are some definitions of words/terms you may not be familiar with:

PROBIOTICS: "GOOD" BACTERIA, A MICRO-ORGANISM WITH BENEFICIAL QUALITIES.
PATHOGENS: BACTERIA, YEASTS, FUNGI THAT CAN CAUSE DIS-EASE ("BAD" IF THEY OUTNUMBER THE GOOD, BUT STILL NECESSARY).
DYSBIOSIS: IMBALANCE IN THE NUMBER OF GOOD BACTERIA TO BAD BACTERIA.
MICROBIOME: THE POPULATION OF BACTERIA, FUNGUS AND YEASTS LIVING IN YOUR INTESTINES.
MICRO-ORGANISM: A MICROSCOPIC ORGANISM, ESPECIALLY A BACTERIA, VIRUS, OR FUNGUS.
GUT: YOUR INTESTINES.

Thanks to the work of Louis Pasteur, many of us have been brought up believing that all bacteria and germs are bad and disease-causing pathogens. As a result we attempt to sterilise ourselves, and our children, into a bubble. Huge strides have been made in science and medicine since Pasteur first proposed the germ theory. We now know that the human body is made up of 10 trillion human cells and… 100 trillion bacteria! We literally have a universe of bacteria within us, known us our microbiome, that has a huge impact on our health, our ability to digest food and more.

Micro-organisms are everywhere. You swallow them, breathe them in, they form invisible colonies on your skin and in your gut. Maintaining the ideal balance of healthy and disease causing microflora (bacteria, yeasts, fungi) forms the foundation for your health—physical, mental and emotional.

In fact, this microscopic zoo in your gut is the first-line defence of your immune system. While a few of these micro-organisms are considered "bad" and can wreak havoc with your system, most of them are considered "good" bacteria or probiotics. All of them are necessary – the good and the bad – but it is important for the balance between them to be maintained.

These bacteria help you digest your food, produce vitamins, absorb minerals, eliminate toxins, keep pathogenic bacteria under control so you stay protected from infections, and even help to prevent autoimmune diseases like asthma, allergies, and diabetes. An imbalance in your gut flora can be a major contributor to many serious illnesses, including autism, Parkinson's and Alzheimer's.

If gut dysbiosis is left uncorrected, pathogens will be able to create holes in the intestinal lining (known as Leaky Gut). This, in turn allows partially digested food particles and pathogenic toxic by-products to be passed into the bloodstream. Depending on the child's particular vulnerability, this can lead to cognitive problems such as ADD and mood disorders, autoimmune disorders and other neurological problems. According to Dr. Campbell McBride, author of Gut & Psychology Syndrome, individuals with autism, dyslexia, dyspraxia, schizophrenia and other disorders all suffer from gut dysbiosis.

This is the terrain Pasteur may have been referring to when he said "the pathogen is nothing; the terrain is everything."*

The body's microbiome is so crucial to health that researchers have compared it to "a newly recognised organ" whose function is so important that you simply cannot be optimally healthy without it. It is also called "The Second Brain" - there are more neurotransmitters made in your gut than are made in your brain. Serotonin (a neurotransmitter associated with mood) is, perhaps, the most striking example. The gut literally has the ability to effect emotions and behaviour independently of 'the' brain. The sayings "gut feeling" and "trust your gut" suddenly have more meaning!

Dysbiosis

About 70% of our immune system is housed in our gut. In a healthy gut, parasites and yeast may be present in small numbers, but don't cause any problems.

However, when enough of the beneficial bacteria are killed (with antibiotics, for example), the bad guys (parasites, yeast and bad bacteria) gain the upper hand, causing dysbiosis - an imbalance that can manifest itself in a variety of unpleasant ways, including:

- ♥ Numerous digestive problems (constipation, colitis, IBS);
- ♥ Skin problems (eczema);
- ♥ Joint problems (arthritis);
- ♥ Altered behaviour patterns and brain function.

In addition to avoiding sugar, genetically modified food, food and environmental toxins, unnecessary antibiotics, and antibacterial soaps, maintaining the gut flora by consuming fermented foods may be

Unlearn

one of the most important steps to take to maintain and improve your health.

A newborn has limited intestinal bacteria prior to birth (some of the mother's is passed on through the amniotic fluid). After passing through the birth canal, contact with the mother's skin, and drinking breast milk, the baby's gut is colonised with the flora which should stay in place for the rest of that child's life. It sets the stage for a healthy immune system and provides the tools necessary for optimum digestion. It must be noted that the baby will inherit whatever colony the mother has – if she has a Candida overgrowth, the baby will inherit this too, as well as all the digestive complaints and symptoms that come with it.

If a healthy gut flora is not established – due to delivery by C-section, an imbalance inherited from the mother, or treatment with antibiotics - it is important for the baby to be given supplemental live bacteria to ensure a healthy gut ecology.

Over sterilisation can also inhibit the development of a healthy gut microbiome in your little one. Let your little one crawl on the floor and eat a handful (or more) of soil from the garden. Actually, this is currently being recommended as one of the best ways to populate your gut – I kid you not! Move over probiotics and fermented foods, we now have SBO's – Soil-Based Organisms!

Bernard (a physiologist and contemporary of Pasteur) believed disease was a condition of imbalance in the internal terrain of body. He emphasized the context or environment in which germs lived and not the germs themselves. On the one hand, if the terrain was balanced (homeostatic), then germs could not flourish. On the other hand, if the terrain were out of balance, then germs would thrive. In short, germs do not cause disease. Instead, they are a sign of the diseased conditions of the terrain and not the cause of those conditions (see Stockton, 2000).

"Colic is normal and some babies just cry all the time."

Colic is not a normal developmental phase! Well, nowadays it may be considered as such – but colic has more to do with nutrition than with your little one's growth and development.

Yes your baby has an immature digestive system – but it should be able to digest breast milk with ease and without the symptoms of colic.

Digestion requires adequate intestinal bacteria colonies. Colic is a digestive distress symptom and is often associated with an inadequate number of probiotics in your little one's digestive tract. When a baby is born via C-section, or naturally to a mother whose microbiome is out of balance, the baby's relatively sterile gut is not populated with sufficient quantities of beneficial bacteria. As such, he/she will struggle with digesting food. A probiotic supplement containing Lactobacillus and Bifidobacterium bacteria may be useful in this situation. The liquid from fermented vegetables can also be fed to your little one in small amounts – simply dip your finger into it and let your little one suck it off.

A breastfeeding mother's diet can also cause colic in a baby that is breastfed. There is a correlation between certain foods that the breastfeeding mother eats and colic in the baby. These include: dairy products; gluten; caffeine-containing foods and drinks (soft drinks, chocolate, coffee, tea, and certain cold remedies); cruciferous vegetables (cabbage, green peppers, broccoli, cauliflower, Brussel sprouts, and onions); spicy foods; garlic; onion; wheat and corn.

A breastfeeding mom you may also want to discover if you have any food sensitivities/intolerances. These can be genetically passed onto your little one. If a food allergy or sensitivity is present, other symptoms will most likely appear, such as gas, bloating, eczema, spitting up, diarrhoea, or bloody or green stools. In my case, as soon as I eliminated gluten, dairy and sugar, Mila's symptoms improved significantly (as did my own health).

In formula fed babies, there can be a colic reaction to the protein or the lactose in cow's milk formula. A lactose-free formula may be beneficial.

The presence of a digestive enzyme called lactase in your little one's digestive system is necessary in order to digest the lactose (found in breast milk and formula). If your little one is insufficient in this enzyme, undigested lactose (milk sugar) will ferment and create lactic acid and hydrogen gas, which can contribute to symptoms of colic. By four months of age, a baby naturally produces more of this enzyme (which is why colic often resolves itself by this time). Adding lactase digestive enzyme drops to your little one's formula or breast milk may help until then.

Once cannot ignore the Brain-Gut connection when talking about colic. Stress affects digestion. A mother's stress can upset an infant enough to interfere with digestion, which can then go on to disrupt intestinal bacteria balance. This can lead to malabsorption and pain, thus more crying.

It is important to realise that colic is not 'normal' and something that you and your little one have to endure . It is a painful condition that will cause your baby much distress. There are logical reasons for it, and practical steps that can be taken to address it.

Once your little one starts solid foods, it is important to start with those that are easy to digest and to include fermented foods as a source of probiotics.

Whatever the cause or trigger, Rooibos tea is known to ease infant colic – it calms nervousness, eases an upset digestive system, induces sound sleep and works as an adaptogen - helping the body adapt to stress.

A homeopathic remedy called Colic Calm was an absolute lifesaver for me! I remember the feeling of relief and joy when I discovered it online at 4am while struggling to breast feed Mila. There was more joy when it was delivered to my door the next day and when it eased Mila's discomfort within minutes!

Unlearn

"Runny snotty noses are normal."

I have to say this is something that causes me a great amount of distress – seeing little kids with snot constantly pouring out of their noses. It's not normal! It's a sign that something is not right within their body.

Permanent snotty noses without other symptoms (such as a fever) are very often a sign of a food allergy or intolerance. The three top offenders in the case of runny noses, nasal congestion, night-time coughing, snot and phlegm are: pasteurised dairy, gluten and sugar. Hence it now affectionately being called 'Milk and Cookie Disease'!

By doing an elimination diet whereby dairy, gluten and sugar are removed from the diet for 7 days, then re-introduced one by one, you can discover if your little one has a food intolerance or allergy.

Even if you are exclusively breastfeeding, your baby might be reacting to these foods through your milk. In this case, you must do the elimination diet.

For better sleep (for you and your little one), better appetivive and overall better mood – finding out if your little one has a food intolerance or sensitivity is well worth it!

For Mila its clear – within 20 minutes of eating dairy or wheat she is full of snot!

"Recurring ear infections are to be expected."

The small eustachian (middle ear to throat) tubes of young children make them particularly prone to ear infections – but that doesn't mean they should always have them!

Colds, bacterial, or viral infections can lead to a blocked eustachian tube and infection. Until recently, most doctors thought bacterial infections were the major cause of ear infections. Research shows, however, that viruses are often the more likely infectious agents, and as such, antibiotics are of no use (antibiotics can only treat bacterial infections).

In such cases, a nutrient-dense diet with probiotic foods will boost the immune system enabling your little one to ward off such infections.

One has to be aware of the fact that ear infections are often preventable, and food allergies or intolerances are the primary modifiable cause. The allergic or food sensitivity reaction can cause the tube connecting the ear to the throat to swell – the inflammation traps fluids (that normally contain bacteria in the throat) inside the middle ear (behind the eardrum). The warm, dark tube in the ear is a perfect place for bacteria to grow. This can cause an ear infection.

Common foods linked to recurrent ear infections are: pasteurised dairy, soy, corn, wheat, egg whites, oranges, sugar and refined carbohydrates.

If your little one suffers from recurrent ear infections, an elimination diet in which the foods mentioned above are avoided can be incredibly useful. If a food allergy or intolerance is the cause, by not feeding your little one the problematic food you could: save him/her a lot of pain and discomfort; avoid antibiotics; avoid repeated use of pain killer medication and/or the need for an operation to insert ear tubes.

Natural remedies for ear infections include: garlic oil ear drops, breast milk ear drops, coconut oil ear drops, garlic rubbed onto the soles of the feet before bed and a warm compress placed on the neck just below the ear. Chiropractic adjustment and homeopathic remedies are also effective.

Mila had her first ear infection when she was 3 and a half years old. She experienced a few infections and colds around that time. It was her first winter at school so I know she was being exposed to more viruses and bacteria than the winters before, but I still looked to food for a cause and a cure. As soon as I removed her one source of dairy (green yoghurt) and her sourdough wheat bread treats, her symptoms disappeared. (Just saying!)

"Eating salt before 1 year is dangerous."

Salt is actually critical for digestion as well as for brain development in your little one. Salt becomes problematic when it in the form of table salt and processed foods.

Pristine white refined 'table salt' is heated to excessive temperatures (some up to 650°C/1200 °F), stripped of all nutrients, and combined with a multitude of undesirable substances, such as aluminium, synthetic iodine, sugar, and anti-caking agents.

Processed foods are a source of large amounts of salt – usually the refined variety too. It is these 'hidden' sources of salt that result in you and your little one consuming more sodium than is good for you. Since your little one's kidneys are immature, they are unable to process large amounts of sodium, but adding a pinch of unrefined sea salt or Himalayan salt to your home cooking is not dangerous and will supply a variety of trace minerals.

"Saturated fats / fats are bad for you."

Fatty foods are often associated with weight issues, obesity, heart disease, and stroke, but this simply is not the case – especially with infants. **BY 'FATTY FOODS', I DO NOT MEAN FRIED FOODS!** We need to distinguish between good fats and bad fats, as eating the good fats provides the body with many health benefits.

The majority of a mother's milk is fat, much of it saturated fat. Your little one needs high levels of fat as it plays an important role in the development of her brain and helps her reach her maximum growth potential. Fat is used in the body as fuel; it is the building block of cell membranes; it is a precursor to the hormonal system and, it helps the body absorb the fat-soluble vitamins, A, D, E, and K.

Unlearn

Types of fat

UNSATURATED FATS include polyunsaturated and monounsaturated fats. They are important for brain, nerve, and eye development in infants.

Great sources of unsaturated fats include salmon, nuts, seeds, olive oil, and avocado.

SATURATED FATS are found mostly in meat and animal products. Saturated fats have had a bad reputation since the 1950's thanks to incomplete science and a fame hungry pathologist named Ancel Keys. They were said to contribute to heart disease, stroke and diabetes. Current research has restored saturated fats' good name – instead, it is transfats, sugar, and refined carbohydrates which have been causing the problems.

The brain is made largely of fat and the majority of the fat in the brain is saturated. The Myelin Sheath that surrounds the nerves in the brain and ensures their proper function is also largely made of saturated fat and cholesterol. As such, consuming saturated fats is extremely important, especially during pregnancy and nursing, as these are times of rapid brain development for babies. So no, you don't have to cut the skin off a roast chicken, or the delicious fatty rind of a lamb chop!

Good sources of saturated fats include coconut oil, pasture raised meat, butter or ghee.

TRANSFATS are the baddies! Also known as partially hydrogenated vegetable oils, they are a processed food. Margarine and canola oil are examples. Transfat increases LDL ('bad') cholesterol levels while decreasing HDL ('good') cholesterol; increases the risk of heart attacks, heart disease and strokes; and, contributes to increased inflammation, diabetes

Sources of transfats include deep-fried fast foods and pre-packaged foods, such as cookies, crackers, and waffles.

Choose a variety of high-fat foods so your little one gets a range of fats, but emphasise the stable saturated fats found in butter, meat and coconut oil, and the monounsaturated fats, found in avocados and olive oil.

"Cholesterol in food is bad for you."

According to Dr. Frank Lipman, "Most of us have been brainwashed into thinking that cholesterol is a harmful foreign substance that should be avoided at all costs. In fact, nothing could be further from the truth.

Cholesterol is an essential component of all cell walls; it is the major building block for your hormones

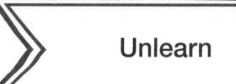

(including sex and adrenal hormones); and, it is vital for the proper functioning of your liver and nervous system. It even helps in the production of vitamin D (in conjunction with sunlight on the skin). The body uses large amounts of cholesterol on a daily basis and it is so important that (with the exception of brain cells), every cell in your body has the ability to make it."

Cholesterol is vital for the insulation of the nerves in the brain and since the brain (and other body systems) are so dependent on it, it is vital to include it in your little ones diet - especially during this time when brain growth is in hyper-speed.

Good sources of cholesterol include egg yolks, liver, and butter (or ghee).

To the mamas and papas who may be concerned about their cholesterol levels, Dr. Lipman has this to say – "a high cholesterol is not necessarily dangerous by itself, although it probably reflects an unhealthy condition or some underlying imbalance. Decreasing the cholesterol will do nothing to improve the underlying problem, which is causing the increased cholesterol. And when you lower the levels too much by taking cholesterol-lowering drugs, the results can actually be detrimental to your health… Contrary to popular belief, the cholesterol in the food you eat has virtually no impact on the cholesterol level of your blood. It's sugar and carbs that trigger production of bad cholesterol in your body."

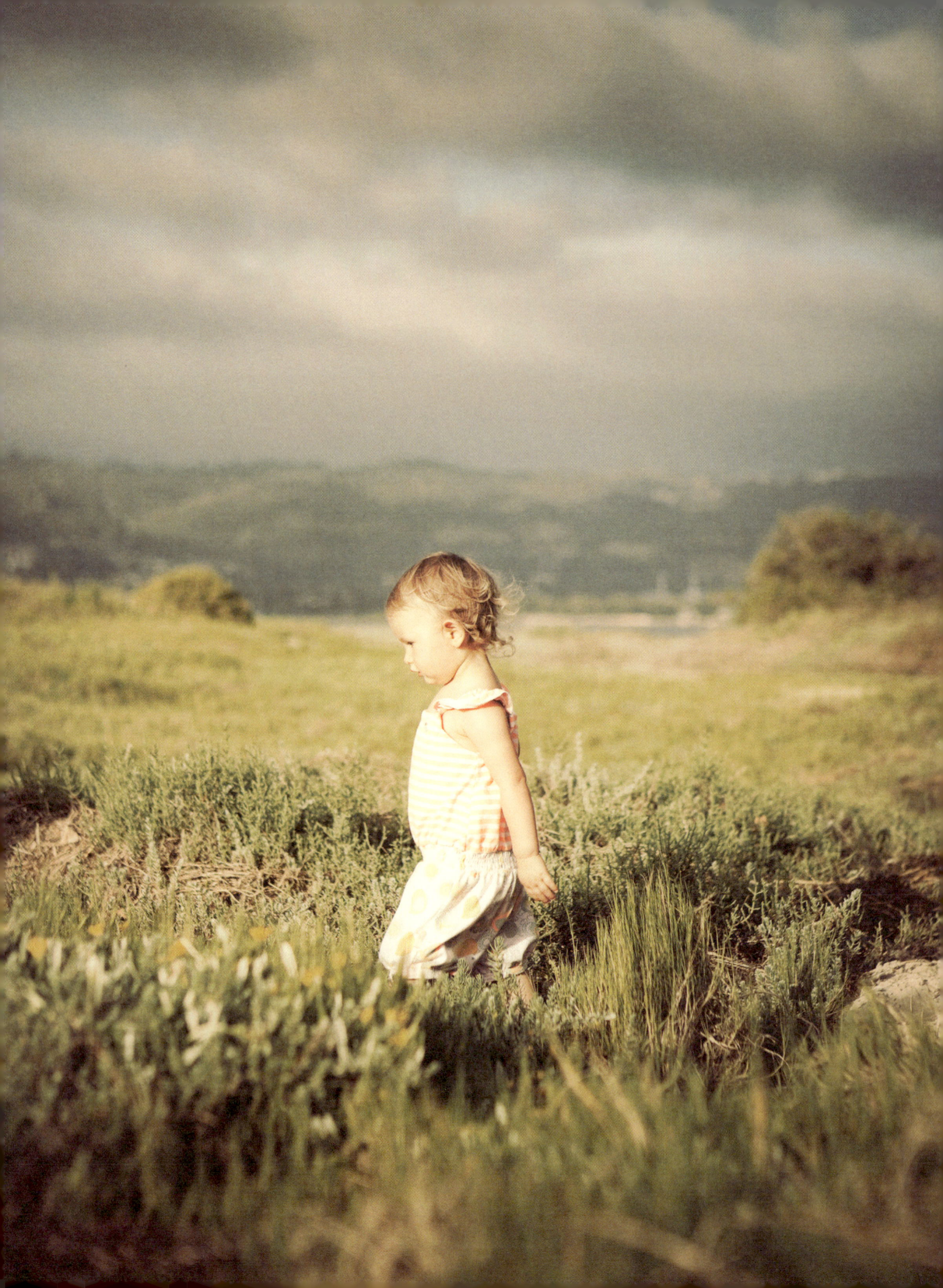

"DO NOT ASK YOUR CHILDREN TO STRIVE FOR EXTRAORDINARY LIVES. SUCH STRIVING MAY SEEM ADMIRABLE, BUT IT IS THE WAY OF FOOLISHNESS. HELP THEM INSTEAD TO FIND THE WONDER AND THE MARVEL OF AN ORDINARY LIFE. SHOW THEM THE JOY OF TASTING TOMATOES, APPLES AND PEARS. SHOW THEM HOW TO CRY WHEN PETS AND PEOPLE DIE. SHOW THEM THE INFINITE PLEASURE IN THE TOUCH OF A HAND. AND MAKE THE ORDINARY COME ALIVE FOR THEM. THE EXTRAORDINARY WILL TAKE CARE OF ITSELF."

- WILLIAM MARTIN, THE PARENT'S TAO TE CHING: ANCIENT ADVICE FOR MODERN PARENTS

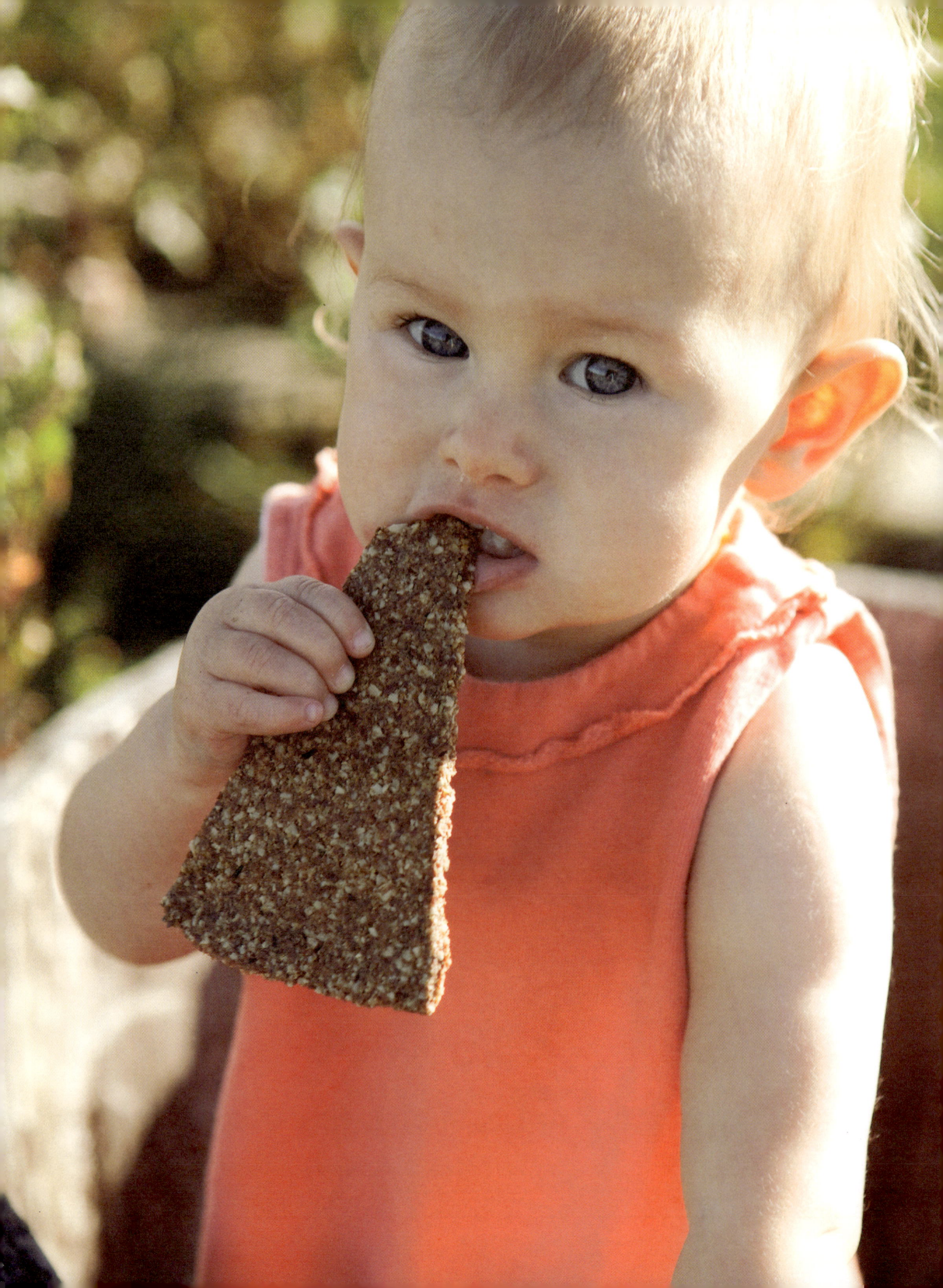

Essential Nutrients
What nutrients baby needs and when

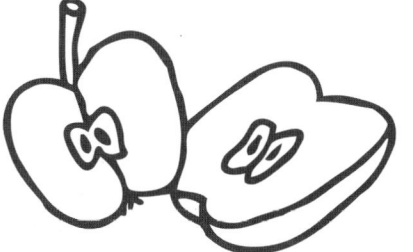

Infant nutrition is critical for ensuring proper physical, emotional, and behavioural development, maximizing learning ability, and preventing illness – both now, and in the future. At no other time in life is nutrition so important – you are literally paving the way for your child's character and immune system. According to Dr. Joel Fuhrman, a high nutrient diet during childhood is the most powerful weapon against developing cancer, cardiovascular disease, and autoimmune disorders in the future. He has also shown (through scientific research) that dietary habits can have a dramatic effect on the occurrences of illness like ear infections, asthma, and allergies. The right foods introduced early in life can even increase your child's IQ.

To ensure that your little one's growth and development proceeds optimally, he/she needs to get adequate amounts (and high-quality forms) of: protein, carbohydrates, cholesterol, essential fatty acids, vitamins, minerals, and other nutrients.

The nutrients that are often in short supply when weaning begins include: protein, zinc, iron and the B-vitamins. Additionally, when following a 'free-from' way of eating, you need to ensure that the nutrients that would have been found in the foods you are avoiding, are replaced by other food sources. For example, when eliminating dairy from your little one's way of eating you will need to ensure she is getting the calcium, fat and protein from one of the many other sources.

Below is a table of all the necessary nutrients and the foods in which you will find them.

Essential nutrients, the role they play, and where to find them

Essential Nutrients

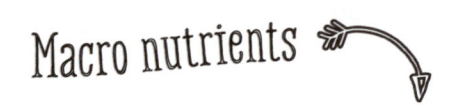

Macro nutrients

Nutrients	Their job	Found in
HEALTHY FATS. **Including Omega 3 (DHA & EPA) & Omega 6**	♡ Supply babies with energy for their liver, brain, and heart, ♡ Provide immunity, ♡ Help the development of the nervous system, ♡ Aid the absorption of vitamins A, D, E, and K, ♡ DHA (docosahexaeonic acid) is a major component of the fats in our brains and plays a critical role in neurological and visual development. *The current recommendation for infants younger than a year is to consume a minimum of 30g/day.* Deficiencies of omega-3s in children are linked to cognitive and psychosocial problems such as: attention-deficit-hyperactivity disorder (ADHD); motor skill dysfunction; depression; and, dyslexia.	Breast milk*, avocado, butter or ghee, walnuts, seeds, olives, meat, sardines, salmon, bone broths, egg yolks, flaxseeds, Brussel sprouts, cauliflower, cod liver oil, avocado oil, hemp seed oil, olive oil, coconut oil, flaxseed oil, raw cacao, moringa, and hemp seeds. Formula milk does not always contain DHA
CHOLESTEROL	♡ Vital for the insulation of the nerves in the brain and the entire central nervous system, ♡ Helps with fat digestion by increasing the formation of bile acids, ♡ Necessary for the production of many hormones. Since the brain is so dependent on cholesterol, it is especially vital during this time when brain growth is in hyper-speed. *The cholesterol in human milk supplies an infant with close to six times the amount most adults consume from food.*	Breast milk*, egg yolk, liver.
CARBOHYDRATES	♡ The primary source of fuel for your little one, ♡ Help the body to utilise fat, ♡ Use protein to build and repair tissue. Complex carbohydrates ensure balanced energy levels that are important for are important for stability of mood, avoiding over-tiredness, difficulties in concentration and interferences with learning. If sufficient amounts are not provided, growth may be stunted (because protein will be used to meet your little one's energy needs instead of being used for growth).	Breast milk* (or formula). Unrefined complex carbohydrates such as: whole grains (oats, brown rice, quinoa, millet, buckwheat), potatoes, sweet potatoes, black beans, green beans, pinto beans, green peas, carrots, beetroot, parsnips. Simple carbohydrates such as: apple, banana, grapes, oranges, pears, and maca.
PROTEIN	♡ Essential for growth and development, ♡ Plays an integral part in nearly all the body's processes, ♡ Responsible for the manufacture of hormones, enzymes, antibodies (infection-fighters), and muscle tissue. Since your little one is growing faster now than he will at any other time in his life, protein requirements are higher per kilogram of weight for babies than for older children and adults.	Breast milk* (or formula), chicken, turkey, beef, lamb, liver, fish, egg, quinoa, buckwheat, millet, rice, oats, beans, lentils, peas, spinach, asparagus, broccoli, cauliflower, nuts, seeds (especially hemp seeds), and sea vegetables (seaweeds), raw cacao, maca, moringa, and hemp seeds.
FIBRE	Promotes optimal gut functioning. Your little one's gut is still developing, which is why cooked foods and purées will be easier to digest, as the fibres are partially digested. Raw fruit skins and other very fibrous vegetables may cause cramps and gas in the first few months of solids.	All natural whole foods are a source of fibre. Particularly good sources are whole grains, legumes, artichokes, chicory, baobab powder, raw cacao, maca, lucuma, and hemp seeds.

Vitamins:
Vitamins are required in small quantities and play a part in a wide variety of body functions.

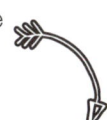

Essential Nutrients

Nutrients	Their job	Found in
VITAMIN A	Required for optimal: ♡ Eyesight, ♡ Skin, ♡ Growth, ♡ Development, ♡ Immune function.	Breast milk* (or formula), meat, egg yolk, liver, orange fruit and veggies, spinach, kale, beetroot leaves, Swiss chard, lucuma, moringa, butter, and ghee.
VITAMIN B1 (THIAMINE)	♡ Helps release energy from foods, so that the nervous system and muscles work properly.	Breast milk* (or formula), sunflower seeds, dried beans, dried peas, green peas, lentils, oats, nuts, broccoli, onions, carrots, kale, tomatoes, Brussels sprouts, cabbage, raw cacao, maca, and moringa.
VITAMIN B2 (RIBOFLAVIN)	♡ Helps break down fats, protein and carbohydrates, ♡ Promotes iron absorption, ♡ Aids other antioxidants.	Breast milk* (or formula), eggs, turkey, chicken, salmon, tuna, meat, nuts, brown rice, raw cacao, lucuma, and moringa.
VITAMIN B3 (NIACIN)	♡ Helps you absorb food, ♡ Promotes growth and energy.	Breast milk* (or formula), eggs, turkey, chicken, salmon, tuna, meat, nuts, brown rice, raw cacao, lucuma, and moringa.
VITAMIN B6	♡ Breaks down protein into energy, ♡ Helps with red blood cell production, ♡ Helps with brain function, ♡ Assists with detoxification of unwanted chemicals from the blood.	Breast milk* (or formula), beef, tuna, salmon, turkey, chicken, sweet potato, potatoes, spinach, banana, sunflower seeds, and moringa.
VITAMIN B12	♡ Helps with red blood cell production, ♡ Help with energy production, ♡ Integral to healthy brain and nervous system development, ♡ Promotes growth, ♡ A co-factor in the production of DNA. ♡ Vitamin B12 deficiency can lead to a form of anaemia. ♡ Vegans can find it hard to get enough vitamin B12 in their diets and might need a supplement.	Breast milk* (or formula), animal foods such as meat, fish, eggs, yoghurt.
VITAMIN C	♡ Well known as an antioxidant that helps you fight infections, ♡ Builds collagen, ♡ Helps absorb iron absorption from food, ♡ Keeps teeth, bones, and gums healthy, ♡ Is necessary to make certain neurotransmitters. These neurotransmitters are the signals that carry thoughts, feelings, and commands around our brains and throughout our nervous system. ♡ Needed to produce serotonin, a hormone that plays a critical role in wide variety of body systems, including the nervous system, endocrine system, immune system, and digestive system.	Breast milk* (or formula), fruits (especially papaya, strawberries, pineapple, oranges, kiwifruit), bell peppers, broccoli, Brussels sprouts, cauliflower, baobab powder, camu camu powder, maca, and moringa.
VITAMIN D	♡ The body uses it to help get calcium into the bones, ♡ Necessary for optimum immunity, ♡ Necessary for blood sugar control. *Children who do not have enough vitamin D in their diet may develop rickets, a painful disease that can cause bones to become unnaturally flexible or misshapen.*	Breast milk* (or formula), sunshine *(before 10am and after 3pm)*, cod liver oil, fish, eggs, liver, butter, ghee, mushrooms, hemp seeds.

41

Essential Nutrients

Minerals are natural substances that are absorbed by your baby's body through food and other supplements. They are necessary for many bodily functions, particularly the growth of your child.

Nutrients	Their job	Found in
VITAMIN E	♡ A powerful antioxidant that boosts your immune system, ♡ Helps with the development of healthy skin, nerves, muscles, circulation, and eyes.	Breast milk* (or formula), butter or ghee, egg yolks, meat, chicken, nuts, avocado, sunflower seeds, almonds, sweet potatoes, dark green leafy vegetables, raw cacao, maca, and hemp seeds.
VITAMIN K	♡ Helps blood to clot, ♡ Plays a role in producing the proteins that keep teeth and bones healthy. Vitamin K2 is made by the bacteria living in your little one's gut - another reason why a healthy gut flora and probiotics are so important.	Kale, spinach, broccoli, Brussels sprouts, green cabbage, beetroot leaves, parsley, egg yolk, cod liver oil, kelp, fermented foods, butter, and ghee.
VITAMIN L	**The Love Vitamin.** "One of the most important nutrients for optimum health is a daily dose (or more) of love… It is necessary for the optimal functioning of all people and all of their cells, tissues, and organs. It is found in a great variety of sources, but must be developed and nurtured to be available." - Elson M. Haas, M.D	In all homemade food!
FOLATE	♡ Helps you absorb protein, ♡ Supports the brain and nervous system, ♡ Supports red blood cell production as well as DNA. *In supplement form it is referred to as folic acid – which is a single form of the folate vitamin.*	Breast milk* (or formula), green leafy vegetables, lentils, beans, broccoli, liver and whole grains.
CHOLINE	♡ Critical for brain development.	Breast milk* (or formula), egg yolk, shrimp, scallops, meat, fish, chicken, turkey, collard greens, broccoli, and moringa.
CALCIUM	♡ Essential for the proper development of bones and teeth, ♡ Important for blood clotting, ♡ Essential for good nerve, muscle, and heart function.	Breast milk* (or formula), salmon, sardines (eaten with bones), almonds, green leafy vegetables, beetroot leaves, baobab powder, sesame seeds, raw cacao, maca, lucuma, moringa, and hemp seeds.
MAGNESIUM	♡ Plays a role in more than 300 enzyme reactions within your body, ♡ Vital for the growth and maintenance of teeth and bones, ♡ Maintains healthy blood sugar levels, ♡ Promotes development and functioning of a healthy heart and nervous system.	Breast milk* (or formula), nuts, pumpkin seeds, sunflower seeds, sesame seeds, spinach, quinoa, blackstrap molasses, green beans, oats, banana, lentils, avocado, baobab, raw cacao, maca, moringa, and hemp seeds. *Protein rich foods aid the absorption of magnesium.*
POTASSIUM	♡ Needed by every cell and organ in the body to work as they should, ♡ Maintains normal blood pressure, ♡ Keeps the heart pumping and the muscles working, ♡ Ensures healthy kidneys.	Breast milk* (or formula), beetroot leaves, bananas, sweet potatoes, potatoes, spinach, avocado, lentils, white beans, baobab powder, raw cacao, and maca.
PHOSPHOROUS	♡ Required for the basic processes of life, from energy storage to the formation of bones and teeth. ♡ Healthy bones and soft tissues require phosphorus to grow and develop throughout life, ♡ Promotes healthy metabolism, ♡ Enables the utilisation of many B-complex vitamins, ♡ Ensures proper muscle and nerve function, ♡ Maintains calcium balance.	Breast milk* (or formula), dried beans, peas, nuts, pumpkin seeds, and hemp seeds.

Trace Minerals:
Called trace minerals because you only need very small amounts of them each day.

Essential Nutrients

Nutrients	Their job	Found in
IRON	♡ Especially important for the brain and blood, ♡ Necessary to support proper metabolism for muscles and other active organs, ♡ It also helps carry oxygen around the body. *Children are at higher risk of iron deficiency, mainly because they need more iron when they go through growth spurts.*	Breast milk* (or formula), lentils, meat, liver, egg yolks, chicken, seafood, dried beans, green leafy vegetables, parsley, olives, whole grains, hemp seeds, sesame seeds, blackstrap molasses, cumin, turmeric, sea vegetables (seaweeds), baobab powder, raw cacao, maca, lucuma, moringa, and hemp seeds
COPPER	♡ Required for normal growth and health, ♡ Plays a role in the formation of connective tissue, ♡ Required for the normal functioning of muscles, and the immune and nervous systems.	Breast milk* (or formula), sesame seeds, sunflower seeds, cashew nuts, walnuts, mushrooms, lentils, beans, avocado and whole grains, raw cacao, moringa, butter, and ghee.
SELENIUM	♡ Essential for many body processes. ♡ One of the most important disease-fighting nutrients in the body, ♡ Assists in the prevention of heart disease, cancer, and inflammatory diseases like rheumatoid arthritis.	Breast milk* (or formula), brazil nuts, seafood, chicken, turkey, lamb, beef, liver, eggs, oats, brown rice, sunflower seeds, sesame seeds, flaxseeds, moringa, broccoli, cabbage, mushrooms, butter, and ghee.
ZINC	♡ Helps with: growth, wound healing, vision, skin health, the male reproductive system and immune system function, ♡ Many of the body's hormones and enzymes depend on zinc to perform their functions, ♡ Zinc is also related to a baby's ability to grow.	Breast milk* (or formula), eggs, beef, lamb, chicken, turkey, seafood, broth, quinoa, oats, lentils, cashew nuts, hemp seeds, sesame seeds, pumpkin seeds, mushrooms, spinach, asparagus, green peas, parsley, Brussels sprouts, sea vegetables, (seaweeds), raw cacao, moringa, hemp seeds, butter, and ghee.
MANGANESE	♡ Vital to many important antioxidant processes in human metabolism, ♡ Important for proper bone formation, ♡ Protects the skin from UV light, ♡ Assists in collagen production for healthy skin, ♡ Helps control blood sugar levels.	Breast milk* (or formula), garlic, basil, peppermint, thyme, dill, parsley, cloves, cinnamon, black pepper, turmeric, oats, quinoa, buckwheat, millet, brown rice, garbanzo beans, spinach, kale, pineapple, raspberries, strawberries, blueberries, pumpkin seeds, sesame seeds, flaxseeds, sea vegetables (seaweeds), moringa, butter, and ghee.
CHROMIUM	♡ Required in only very small amounts, ♡ An essential part of metabolic processes that regulate blood sugar, ♡ Helps insulin transport glucose into cells, where it can be used for energy, ♡ Involved in the metabolism of carbohydrate, fat, and protein.	Breast milk* (or formula), broccoli, oats, green beans, meat, whole grains, Romaine lettuce, ripe tomatoes, black pepper, butter, and ghee.
IODINE	♡ Essential for normal growth and tissue development, ♡ Helps control the ways your cells make energy and use oxygen, ♡ Vital for thyroid health and for the production of the hormones made by the thyroid gland.	Breast milk* (or formula), seafood, sea vegetables (seaweeds), eggs, strawberries, maca, butter, and ghee.

43

Essential Nutrients

Nutrients	Their job	Found in
PROBIOTICS	♡ Complete the digestion process, ♡ Produce vitamins, ♡ Keep pathogenic ('bad') bacteria in check, ♡ Support the immune system.	Breast milk*, all fermented foods: sauerkraut, pickles, kimchi, fermented fruits, yoghurt, kefir, and kombucha.
PREBIOTICS	Prebiotics is a term that refers to all the different kinds of fibre that encourage beneficial species of gut flora (probiotics) to grow. Essentially, prebiotics are the food for the good bacteria.	Baobab powder, artichoke, raw garlic, raw or cooked onion, raw leek, raw asparagus, banana, and chicory.
SODIUM	♡ Plays a critical role in our bodies, ♡ Helps regulate water balance, ♡ Controls muscle and nerve function, ♡ Keeps the circulatory system functioning properly, ♡ Regulates blood pressure, ♡ Protects against unnecessary blood clotting, ♡ Plays a role in the digestive system, helping to metabolise food. *While sodium is necessary, a high intake of sodium through processed salt is not healthy. All processed foods have high levels of salt.*	Breast milk* (or formula), salt (only use Celtic sea salt, or Himalayan salt), eggs, celery, artichokes, almonds, walnuts, green peas, turkey, flaxseeds, seafood, maca, and hemp seeds.
WATER	♡ An essential nutrient that is involved in every function of the body. ♡ Helps transport other nutrients and waste products in and out of cells, ♡ Necessary for healthy digestion, ♡ Enables absorption and excretion processes ♡ Helps regulate body temperature.	Breast milk* (or formula), watermelon, strawberries, grapefruit, melons, pineapple, oranges, blueberries, plums, apples, grapes, cherries, cucumber, lettuce, zucchini, tomato, cauliflower, eggplant, red cabbage, spinach, broccoli, green peas, and of course… water.

*THE QUALITY OF BREAST MILK DEPENDANT UPON THE MOTHER'S DIET - NOT ONLY WITH RESPECT TO MACRONUTRIENTS, BUT ALSO, AND ESPECIALLY TO, VITAMINS, MINERALS, AND PHYTONUTRIENTS. A MOTHER'S MILK CAN ALSO TRANSFER POTENTIALLY PROBLEMATIC FOOD COMPONENTS - ALLERGIC REACTIONS IN A NURSING INFANT, FOR EXAMPLE, CAN OFTEN BE IMPROVED BY CHANGES IN THE MOTHER'S DIET.

**OVER-CONSUMPTION AND EXCESS INTAKE OF MACRONUTRIENTS CAN BE JUST AS PROBLEMATIC FOR INFANTS AS UNDER-CONSUMPTION AND DEFICIENCY.

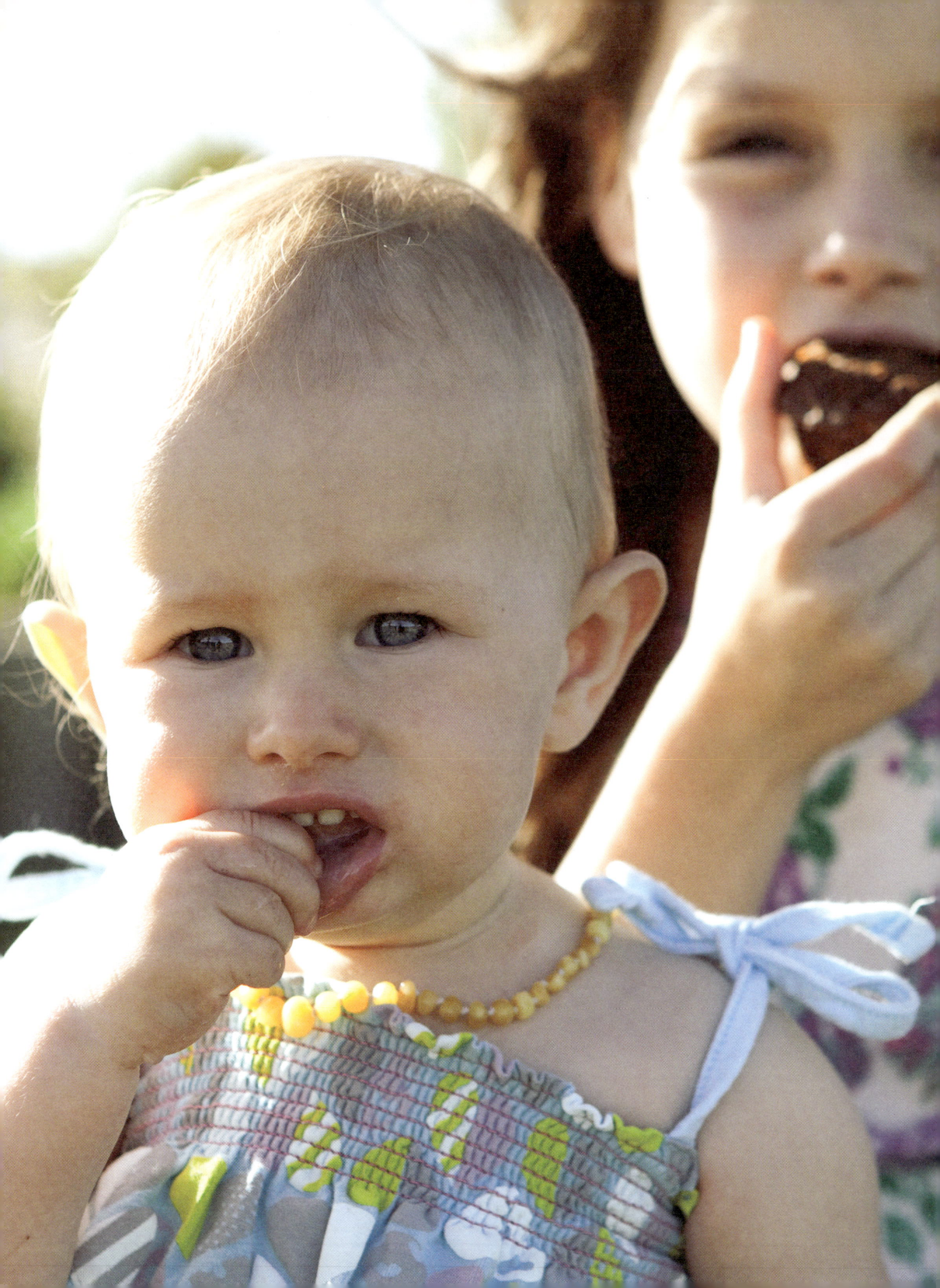

Essential Nutrients

What to eat when

Introducing solid foods can be an exciting but daunting endeavour!

Tips for making food time, happy time:

- **REMEMBER TO USE THE 3-DAY WAIT RULE WHEN INTRODUCING SOLIDS.** For every new food introduced, make sure it is included in your little one's diet for three consecutive days, and don't add any other new food in that time. If there is no negative reaction, this food can now be fed regularly and used as a base for introducing other foods.
- **IT MAY BE USEFUL TO CREATE A FOOD DIARY.** Write a list of all the foods you would like to introduce and then tick them off once you have. You could even draw a smiley face next to the ones that went down well. (The less your "mommy brain" has to remember the better!) This is also a great way of ensuring your little one is introduced to and continues to eat a variety of foods.
- **FOLLOW YOUR LITTLE ONE'S LEAD.** If he/she does not enjoy a particular food, try re-introducing it again in a few weeks time.
- **GO SLOWLY.** This is a completely new experience for your little one and his/her digestive system. Start with small amounts and early in the day – that way you can deal with any unpleasant reactions while your healthcare provider is available and without disrupting your sleep time. Signs of intolerance include redness around the mouth; abdominal bloating, gas and distention; irritability, fussiness, over-activity and awaking throughout the night; constipation and diarrhoea; frequent regurgitation of foods; nasal and/or chest congestion; and red, chapped or inflamed eczema-like skin rash.
- **BREATHE!** Remember your little one will still be getting most of her required nutrients from your breast milk. Initially, introduction to solids is more about flavour and texture than it is about satisfying hunger.

What not to eat

There are certain foods that should be avoided in your little one's first year due to their immature digestive system. They include:

- Cow's milk.
- Honey. Honey may contain Clostridium botulinum spores that can lead to botulism poisoning in a baby's immature intestinal tract.
- Mouldy soft cheeses such as Camembert, Brie, and Stilton.
- Grains*

Essential Nutrients

There are other foods (and food-like substances) that should be avoided in the first year - and for as long as possible after that - because of their negative health consequences. They include:

- ♥ Sugar,
- ♥ Cold drinks and other carbonated drinks, fruit juices, cordials and flavoured milk,
- ♥ High-salt foods: bacon, sausage, and most other processed foods,
- ♥ Commercial fatty foods: fried products, processed meats, chips, chocolates, and pies,
- ♥ Artificial additives: any foods containing preservatives, flavours, flavour enhancers, transfats, sweeteners, colours,
- ♥ Margarine or shortening,
- ♥ Low-fat products.

*This is one of the many highly contentious issues in current nutrition. According to The Weston A. Price Foundation (WAPF), babies have limited digestive enzymes, which are necessary for the digestion of foods. They believe it "takes up to 28 months, just around the time when molar teeth are fully developed, for the big-gun carbohydrate enzymes (namely amylase) to fully kick into gear. Foods like cereals, grains and breads are very challenging for little ones to digest."

By following the nutrient content of breast milk, the WAPF guidelines are that "a baby's earliest solid foods should be mostly animal foods since his digestive system, although immature, is better equipped to supply enzymes for digestion of fats and proteins rather than complex carbohydrates."

Please see the chapter Unlearn: Rice cereal is the best first food for baby for more information, my personal belief, and experience on this matter.

Essential Nutrients

What's for dinner? Food Introduction Chart

FOOD GROUP	FIRST FOODS (6 MONTHS)	7 – 8 MONTHS
DRINKS *water, herbal tea, vegetable juice, fermented drinks*	Breast milk (or formula), small amounts of filtered water	Rooibos tea, Chamomile tea
HEALTHY FATS	Fermented Cod Liver Oil (1/2 teaspoon with food – do not heat)	Organic virgin coconut oil, extra virgin olive oil, ghee, avocado, hemp seed oil.
MEAT / ANIMAL PROTEIN	Soft boiled egg yolks from pasture raised hens, raw liver grated into other food	Chicken or beef broth, organic pasture raised chicken, ostrich, beef, lamb, turkey or fish, liver, venison, coconut milk
DECIDUOUS FRUITS *Apple, pears, plum, peach, apricot, nectarine, cherry, olive*	Avocado, cooked apple and pear	Cooked peach, plum, apricot
TROPICAL FRUITS *Banana, mango, litchi, pineapple, rambotan, durian, papaya, avocado*	Ripe banana (skin must have black spots on it), avocado, papaya	Mango
CITRUS FRUITS *Orange, naartjie, lemon, grapefruit, pomelo, tomato*	Not yet	Lemon
BERRIES *Strawberry, blueberry, blackberry, grape, cranberry*	Not yet	Not yet
ROOT VEGETABLES *Carrot, potato, sweet potato, yam, turnip, parsnip, beetroot*	Steamed and puréed sweet potato, potato, carrots, turnips, parsnips	As before
SQUASH *Butternut, pumpkin, gem squash, baby marrow, patty pans*	Butternut, pumpkin, gem squash, baby marrow, patty pans	As before
BRASSICA *Cabbage, broccoli, cauliflower, Brussel sprouts, kale*	Not yet	Not yet
VEGETABLES FROM FLOWERS *Cucumber, bell pepper, tomato*	Not yet	Cucumber, bell peppers
LEAFY VEGETABLES *Spinach, beetroot leaves, asparagus, chicory*	Not yet	Not yet
FRESH BEANS AND PEAS	Not yet	Not yet
GRAINS, NUTS & SEEDS *Grains: short grain brown rice, quinoa, millet, buckwheat, and oats. Nuts: almonds, cashews, macadamia, coconut Seeds: chia, flax, hemp, pumpkin, sesame, sunflower*	Not yet	Not yet
LEGUMES/PULSES *Dried beans, split peas, lentils and chickpeas*	Not yet	Not yet
SUPERFOODS *Baobab, cacao, green powder, hemp powder, lucuma, maca, moringa*	Baobab, lucuma, maca	Green powder, moringa
FERMENTED FOODS *Sauerkraut and other fermented vegetables, pickles, kefir, beet kvass, fermented fruits*	Fermented apple sauce	Liquid from sauerkraut, fermented carrots

Essential Nutrients

Certain foods, such as spinach, celery, lettuce, radishes, beets, turnips and collard greens, may contain excessive nitrate, which can be converted into nitrite (an undesirable substance) in the stomach. It is best to introduce them closer to your little one's first birthday. When you cook these particular vegetables do not use the cooking water in a purée – as the nitrates will be concentrated in it.

8 – 12 MONTHS	OVER ONE YEAR	IMPORTANT NOTES
Freshly pressed vegetable juices – diluted with water, liquid from sauerkraut	Beet Kvass, undiluted vegetable juices, other herbal teas	*The majority of your little one's liquid intake should be from breast milk or formula until after 1 year.*
As before	As before	
As before	Whole eggs (yolk & whites)	*Shellfish is best avoided until after 1 year.*
Raw apple, raw pears, plum, peach, apricot, nectarine, cherry, olives	As before	*You may want to cook these in the beginning to make them easier to digest.*
Litchi, pineapple, rambotan, durian	As before	*No need to cook these.*
Not yet	Orange, naartjie, grapefruit, pomelo,	*Citrus fruits may be too acidic for your little one – watch for nappy rash as an indication of this.*
Strawberry, blueberry, blackberry, grape, cranberry	As before	*Wash very well!*
Beetroot	As before	*Great veggies to start with.*
As before	As before	*Serve with healthy fats.*
Cabbage, broccoli, cauliflower, Brussel sprouts, kale	As before	*These may cause gas.*
As before	Tomatoes	*Tomatoes can cause nappy rash as they are quite acidic – best left until after 1 year.*
Spinach, beetroot leaves, asparagus, chicory	As before	
Green beans, peas	As before	
Chia seeds	Start with short-grain brown rice, quinoa, oats, and nut butters.	*All grains, nuts, and seeds must be soaked for 12 hours in a salt-water brine.* *Ensure grains are well cooked.*
Not yet	Start with red lentils and split peas (easiest to digest). Then move on to dried beans, lentils, chickpeas.	*All dried legumes and pulses must be soaked for at least 18 hours in an acid medium. Rinse and cook until tender (1 – 3 hours).*
Hemp powder	Cacao	*These are exceptionally nutrient-dense foods – a little goes a long way! Start with an 1/8 teaspoon once a day and gradually increase. It is a good idea to alternate superfood powders daily.*
Sauerkraut, pickles, kefir, fermented berries	Beet Kvass and any other ferments!	*Cultured (fermented) foods are tangy, tart, sour, and salty. They can give your little one a love for flavours beyond sweet.*

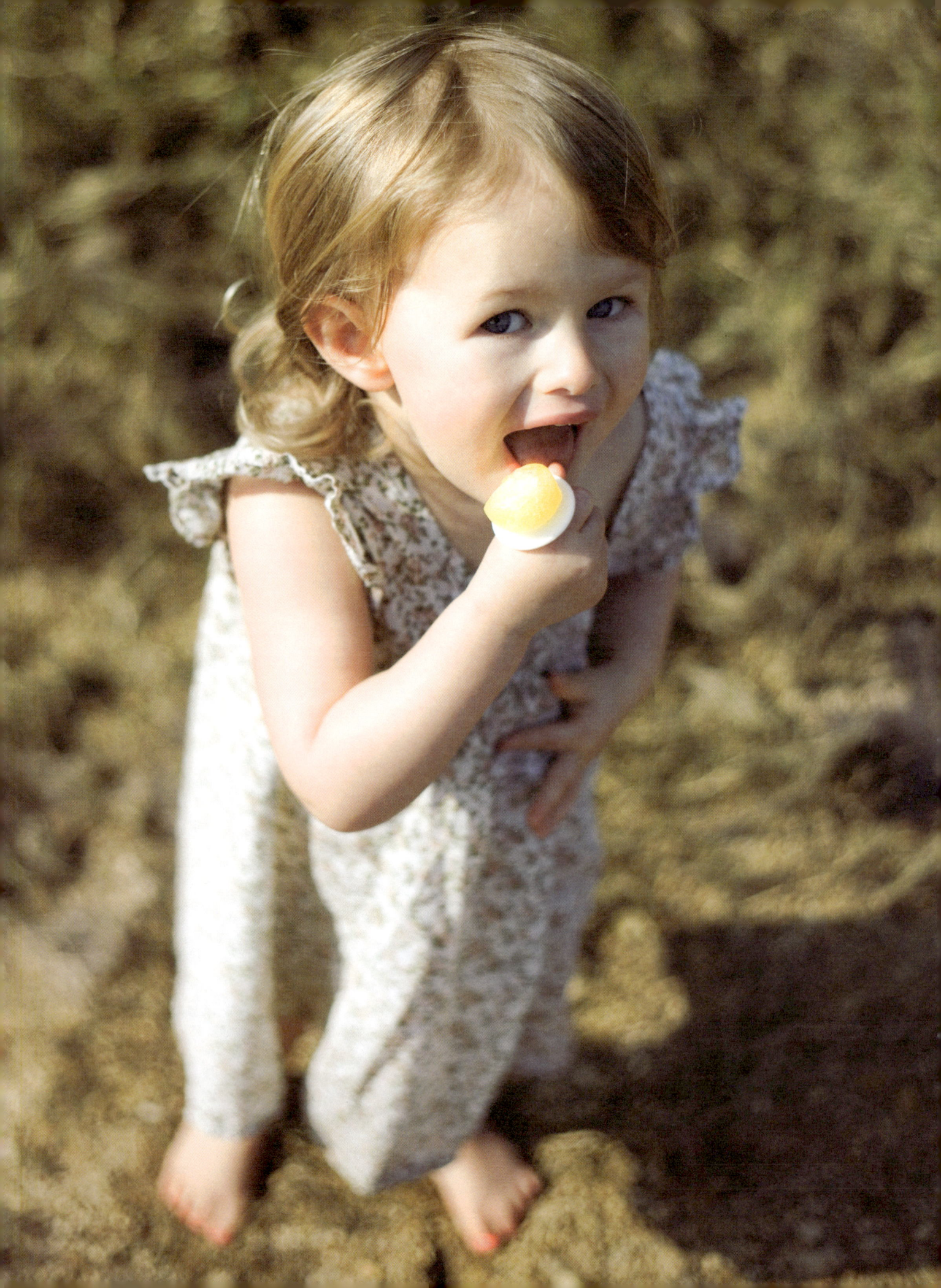

Feeding with Awareness

Allergens

ALLERGY VS. INTOLERANCE

While many new parents are aware of **food allergies** and allergens, with the change in our food production system and food availability, **food intolerances** are now as significant.

A food **allergy** is different from a food **intolerance** and it is important to understand the differences between them. Broadly speaking, a food allergy is a reaction to food proteins involving the immune system, while a food intolerance is a pharmacological reaction (like the side effects of a drug) to the chemicals (natural or synthetic) in foods.

Infants can have a higher incidence of food allergies because their immature and permeable guts allow proteins to pass through more easily. As children mature, they often grow out of these allergies

THE '3-DAY WAIT RULE'

It is useful to follow the three-day wait rule' when introducing your little one to new solid foods - not only if your family has a history of food allergies. It is an excellent opportunity to identify intolerances by discovering how your little one reacts to each particular food and to get to know his/her individual digestive system. While it may seem tedious to have to wait three days in between each new food, it is a far easier (and less stressful) way to identify the culprit (allergen or intolerance) as opposed to having to eliminate a number of foods and then reintroducing them one by one.

Introduce new foods during the morning or early afternoon. This will allow you to deal with any adverse reactions while your paediatrician is in his/her office.

> GLOBALLY, THE EIGHT MOST COMMON ALLERGENS ARE: COW'S MILK, SOY FOODS, HEN'S EGGS, PEANUTS, FISH, CRUSTACEAN SHELLFISH, TREE NUTS (INCLUDING CASHEWS, ALMONDS, WALNUTS, PECANS, PISTACHIOS, BRAZIL NUTS, HAZELNUTS, AND CHESTNUTS), WHEAT.
> SPECIAL MENTION MUST ALSO BE MADE OF: SESAME SEEDS, MUSTARD SEED, CELERY, BUCKWHEAT, AND LUPIN.

Feeding with Awareness

Food Allergy

FAMILY HISTORY OF	Hay fever, eczema or asthma
WHO IS AFFECTED?	♡ Most likely to affect **babies and young children** because of their underdeveloped immune system.
HOW COMMON?	♡ Food allergies are less common than popularly believed - affecting up to 8% of babies under 12 months, 3% of children under five, and less than 1% of adults. **(Source: www.fedup.com)** ♡ According to the Allergy Society of South Africa, it is estimated that only between 2% and 5% of the general population suffers from a definite food allergy.
THE CULPRITS?	♡ An allergy is produced by a combination of inherited susceptibility and frequency or extent of exposure. (So common allergens vary from country to country and culture to culture.) ♡ Globally, **the eight most common allergens are:** cow's milk, soy foods, hen's eggs, peanuts; fish, crustacean shellfish; tree nuts (including cashews, almonds, walnuts, pecans, pistachios, Brazil nuts, hazelnuts, and chestnuts), wheat. ♡ Special mention must also be made of: sesame seed, mustard seed, celery, buckwheat, and lupin. ♡ Allergies to peanut and fish are the most likely to last throughout life and an allergy to peanuts are the most likely to be life-threatening.
TIMING	♡ Allergic reactions can be immediate (within minutes to two hours) or delayed (hours to days after eating the trigger). ♡ Typically they are quick - occurring within 30 minutes and are often easy to identify.
DOSE	Can be to the smallest amount of the particular allergen.
SYMPTOMS	♡ Sudden loose, diarrhoea stools and/or vomiting, ♡ Sudden rashes on the skin and bottom, ♡ Runny nose, ♡ Hives, ♡ Irritability and/or gassiness or colic after a new food/meal, ♡ Breathing or other respiratory troubles after a new food/meal, ♡ Swelling of the face, lips and/or tongue, ♡ Closure or tightening of the throat, ♡ In the most severe of the allergic disorders, anaphylaxis can lead to collapse and death.
DIAGNOSIS	Can be diagnosed with skin prick tests or blood tests.
TREATMENT	Avoidance with regular testing in the case of babies and children who may grow out of it.

Feeding with Awareness

Food Intolerance

FAMILY HISTORY OF	Migraine, irritable bowel symptoms, behaviour problems
WHO IS AFFECTED?	<ul><li>Children (they consume a higher dose of food chemicals per body weight than adults and their digestive and detoxification systems are also underdeveloped).</li><li>Women of childbearing age (hormonal influence).</li><li>Senior citizens (ageing livers and kidneys are slower to eliminate chemicals from the body).</li><li>Any age group exposed to toxic chemicals, pharmaceutical drugs or illness.</li></ul>
HOW COMMON?	<ul><li>Much more common than food allergies and increasingly so (additives continue to increase in our food supply every year). We can expect more and more people to be affected… especially children.</li><li>Affects babies (through breast milk), children, and adults.</li><li>Effects are related to dose (so in theory, everyone will react if the dose is high enough).</li><li>People most likely to be affected by food chemicals are:<ul><li>Those who are most sensitive,</li><li>Those who consume the highest doses.</li></ul></li></ul>
THE CULPRITS?	The food chemicals most likely to cause problems are:<ul><li>Artificial colours,</li><li>Natural colour annatto,</li><li>Preservatives,</li><li>Flavour enhancers,</li><li>Salicylates (naturally occurring in food),</li><li>Amines (naturally occurring in food).</li></ul>
TIMING	Food intolerance reactions can be delayed for up to 48 hours or more, or effects can be cumulative. For instance, children rarely react to the preservative in one slice of commercial bread, but if they eat that bread every day the effects can build up over a month and fluctuate with no obvious cause. This makes intolerance reactions difficult to identify – it's only by the absence of symptoms after the trigger food is removed that one makes the link.
DOSE	Reaction is dose-related with some people being more sensitive than others.
SYMPTOMS	Can be the same as allergy reactions, as well as:<ul><li>Skin - rashes, swelling,</li><li>Airways - asthma, stuffy or runny nose, frequent colds and infections,</li><li>Gastrointestinal tract - irritable bowel symptoms, colic, bloating, diarrhoea, vomiting, frequent mouth ulcers, reflux, bedwetting, 'sneaky poos', 'sticky poos',</li><li>Central nervous system - migraines, headaches, anxiety, depression, lethargy, impairment of memory and concentration, panic attacks, irritability, restlessness, inattention, sleep disturbance, restless legs, mood swings, PMT.</li></ul>Symptoms of food intolerance can come and go and change throughout life.
DIAGNOSIS	No laboratory tests (since the immune system is not involved). The only way to diagnose is by an elimination diet.
TREATMENT	An elimination diet, followed by gradual reintroduction of common trigger foods to identify the culprits, and determine tolerance levels. Avoidance of trigger foods or staying below your personal 'limit'. Healing and sealing the gut lining and repopulating the gut with the ideal bacteria balance to reduce sensitivity.

Feeding with Awareness

Convenience vs. Conscience

Yes, preparing all your little one's food yourself is time-consuming. But you have a decision to make. Does the convenience of store-bought processed food outweigh the costs? The costs aren't immediate – its like loan from a loan shark – one day, he is going to come calling!

If you knew what was in the convenient food, how it had been made, grown or reared, would you still feed it to your little one? Would your conscience outweigh the convenience?

Toxins

"We have a big problem. Our bodies are being invaded by industrial chemicals. We never asked for it. We never approved it. We were never informed about it. In every single blood or human milk sample we find tons of industrial chemicals. You could argue that - and I think particularly that women should argue that - we have the right to know what's inside us. The least society can do is make information available on how much we have accumulated and how much we're sharing with our kids."

- DR. PHILIPPE GRANDJEAN, PROFESSOR OF ENVIRONMENTAL MEDICINE IN DENMARK AND AT HARVARD SCHOOL OF PUBLIC HEALTH.

Reducing your little one's exposure to potentially harmful chemicals may play a significant role in promoting a healthy future for him/her. Due to their smaller size and still developing immune and detoxification systems, the negative effects of these toxins are more significant in children. Some recent research studies have suggested that the exposure we have to carcinogens and toxins in our youth may predispose us to a higher risk of some types of cancers as well as Alzheimer's disease later in life. Maximizing the health potential of your child means minimizing his/her exposure to toxins, such as pesticides, BPA, heavy metals and xenoestrogens.

Pesticides

One of the most common pesticides in use today is Roundup - with an active ingredient known as glyphosate. Crops have been genetically modified in order to withstand this poison which means that it is being used in larger quantities. Its producer, Monsanto, has also encouraged farmers to use Roundup as a desiccant to dry out their crops - so they can harvest them sooner. So Roundup is now routinely sprayed directly on a host of non-GMO crops, including wheat, barley, oats, canola, flax, peas, lentils, soybeans, dry beans and sugar cane. The pesticides cannot be washed – so anytime you eat these crops, or products made from them, you are eating this pesticide. The amount of glyphosate in each product may not be large, but the cumulative effect could be devastating.

Roundup is not only used on food. It is used to kill weeds on roadsides, playgrounds, golf courses, school yards, lawns and home gardens. As with any other toxin, if it comes into contact with your skin, it will be absorbed.

The health consequences of having Roundup and glyphosate in our food, in the water we drink, in the air we breathe and where our children play are numerous. It has been linked to ADHD; autism; birth defects; celiac disease and gluten intolerance; colitis; pregnancy problems (infertility, miscarriages, stillbirths) and brain cancer later in a child's life due to parents being exposed during the two years prior to the child's birth!

Dr. Seneff (a senior research scientist at the MIT Computer Science and Artificial Intelligence Laboratory) has declared, "At today's rate, by 2025, one in two children will be autistic." She has noted that the side effects of autism closely mimic those of glyphosate toxicity, and has presented data showing a remarkably consistent correlation between the use of Roundup on crops (and the creation of Roundup-ready GMO crop seeds) with rising rates of autism. Children with autism have biomarkers indicative of excessive glyphosate, including zinc and iron deficiency, low serum sulphate, seizures, and mitochondrial disorder.

Roundup is only one pesticide – there are many others. A particularly toxic group is the organophosphates. Organophosphate pesticides are used on several crops including corn, apples, pears, grapes, berries, and peaches. Exposure during pregnancy or childhood has been associated with low birth weight, ADHD, behaviour problems and neurodevelopmental deficits in children.

So what can you do?

- ♥ Avoid using synthetic pesticides in your home or garden, or in the form of insect repellent, lice shampoo, pet sprays, or otherwise. There are safe and effective natural alternatives for virtually every pest problem you come across.
- ♥ Ask your little one's school to avoid using pesticides on the school fields. Approach your local municipality and make a case for them not to use it in public areas either.
- ♥ Buy organic produce wherever possible, especially for those fruits and vegetables on the **EWG Dirty Dozen** list, and wash conventional produce in a hydrogen peroxide solution before eating it.

BPA

Bisphenol-A (BPA) is an industrial chemical that is used to make certain plastics. It hardens plastics, and prevents bacteria from contaminating foods and food cans from rusting. It is used to make numerous products, including reusable water bottles, CDs, beverage containers, auto parts, toys, and eyeglasses

It is found in the plastic lining of food cans and is known to leach out of the plastic and into the food that it comes into contact with. BPA is a potent developmental toxin. It mimics the hormone oestrogen and disrupts the natural balance of the endocrine system. It affects the hormones that control the development of the brain, the reproductive system, and the immune system. BPA has been linked: to an increased risk of some cancers; decreased sperm counts and reduced fertility: ADHD; obesity; diabetes; and, the early onset of puberty.

Pregnant women, a developing foetus, infants and young children are the most vulnerable to BPA's

Feeding with Awareness

toxic effects. Unfortunately, they also have the most intense BPA exposure of any age group. BPA used to be found in baby bottles, sippy cups, formula tins, and other infant products. Consumer objection changed that. In 2008 Canada banned the use of BPA in baby bottles and sippy cups. In 2010 they declared BPA toxic, setting the stage for further restrictions on the chemical throughout the world. The European Union, France, the USA, South Africa, China, and Malaysia followed them.

So what can you do?

- Breastfeed your little one if you can. This one step will avoid chemicals in both the bottles and the formula can liners.
- If you bottle-feed, use glass or stainless steel baby bottles, or plastic bottles made from BPA-free plastic which will be labelled "BPA-free".
- Discard baby bottles and sippy cups that turn cloudy or are scratched or cracked. Worn bottles may leach chemicals more easily.
- Avoid putting bottles or sippy cups in the microwave or dishwasher. Studies show that high heat can cause more leaching of all chemicals. To warm the bottle or cup, place it in a bowl of hot water or hold under hot running water.
- When buying plastic, check the bottom of the containers:
- If the bottle has a number 7 and the letters PC or OTHER underneath it, replace it immediately! PC stands for 'polycarbonate'. BPA is a basic constituent of polycarbonate plastic, which means it can never be "BPA free".
- If the bottle has the number 7 and a T, PA or PES underneath it, it is a BPA free plastic and is fine.
- If it has a 5 and the letters PP underneath it, the bottle is made of polypropylene and is BPA free and safe.
- Those labelled with a number 3, may contain phthalates, so you'll want to keep clear of items with that number, too.
- Keep in mind that while containers coded 1, 2, 4, 5, or 6 may not contain BPA or phthalates, the chemicals used in these plastics haven't been studied well enough to determine their safety.
- Avoid canned food (most canned goods have a BPA liner).
- Use alternatives such as glass, porcelain or stainless steel containers for hot foods and liquids instead of plastic containers.

Heavy Metals

Heavy metal toxicity is not uncommon in children and can seriously impair normal development. Lead accounts for most cases of paediatric heavy metal toxicity, but other metals that can significantly harm a child's health include mercury, cadmium, arsenic, and iron. Heavy metals have been linked to autism, ADHD, learning disabilities, low IQ and behaviour problems.

Heavy metals are released into the blood stream during pregnancy and breastfeeding so expectant mothers should be aware that their own toxic exposure may result in toxic effects in their unborn or newborn child. Avoiding neurotoxins before and during pregnancy is one of the greatest gifts you can give your baby.

Children are further exposed to heavy metals through normal hand-to-mouth activity: mouthing objects; playing outside; not washing their hands before eating; as well as the active eating of objects such as keys, cell phones etc. Heavy metals can also be inhaled – they are present in the air around industrial sites, areas of pesticide use, and in cigarette smoke. Fruits and vegetables grown on farms which use chemical fertilisers and pesticides will also be a source of heavy metals.

While these heavy metals are naturally occurring substances, their use in industry and modern day products has radically increased our exposure. It is this high exposure which has toxic effects.

Lead

Lead is found in cosmetics (like lipstick), paint, small appliances, drinking water (from old lead water pipes) and garden soil.

Symptoms of lead toxicity include: learning disabilities; memory loss; poor academic performance; difficulty understanding directions; hyperactivity; aggression; hearing loss; reduced eye-hand coordination; anaemia; abdominal pains; constipation; vomiting; decreased appetite; and weight loss.

Cadmium

Cadmium is a by-product of lead and zinc mining. It is found in batteries, paint, plastics, chemical fertilisers, sewage sludge (used on food crops), irrigation water from galvanised zinc pipes, non-stick cookware and shellfish.

Cadmium is a carcinogen and suspected endocrine disruptor that can accumulate in the body over time with repeated exposure. Children are most likely to be exposed to cadmium through food, water, and secondary tobacco smoke.

Arsenic

Arsenic is found in water, seafood, factory farmed chicken, rice, pesticides, herbicides, and CCA treated wood. It is released into the air during the manufacturing of chemicals and glass.

Arsenic is extremely toxic when ingested or absorbed through the skin. It is a suspected endocrine disruptor and has also been linked to diabetes, hypertension cardiovascular disease. High levels cause nausea, vomiting, diarrhoea, decreased blood cell production, abnormal heart rhythm, and blood vessel damage. It may also increase the risk of many cancers.

Mercury

Mercury is released into the air through the natural degassing of Earth's crust and volcanic emissions. It is also a by-product of mining and the burning of coal and natural gas. The paper industry is responsible for large emissions of mercury. Mercury is also found in: vaccines; food products made with high fructose corn syrup; various items in our medicine cabinets (like Mercurochrome); fish; dental amalgam fillings; thermometers, and thermostats.

Mercury is extremely dangerous – it is the second most toxic substance known to man. The toxic impact of just trace amounts of this metal are multiplied many times when lead is also present in the body. Mercury has been linked to autism, mental illness, and a long list of autoimmune diseases.

So what can you do?

- ♥ Choose organic produce and meat.
- ♥ Purchase fish that are lowest in contaminants. Opt for species that are small in size, low in fat, and do not live on the bottom of waterways. Safe (or at least safer) fish include: herring, mackerel (N. Atlantic, Chub), anchovies, sardines, clams, Wild Alaskan salmon, shrimp, and black sea bass.
- ♥ Only use natural and organic household cleaning products and personal care products.
- ♥ Only use organic, natural cosmetics – especially the ones your little one with be playing with!
- ♥ Avoid the use of pesticides and chemical fertilisers in your garden.
- ♥ Avoid using CCA treated wood around your home.
- ♥ Choose lead-free paint for your home.
- ♥ Only drink filtered or spring water.

Xenoestrogens (in the form of Parabens)

Parabens are synthetic preservatives used to prevent bacteria growth in cosmetics and personal care products (such as shampoos, conditioners, hair styling gels, nail creams, foundations, facial masks, skin creams, and deodorants). They are often an ingredient in baby lotions, shampoos, and other personal care products for children. Parabens from these products are absorbed through the skin and are stored in the body. Methyl and propyl parabens are also allowed to be used in food as a preservative.

Parabens are xenoestrogens – that is, they mimic oestrogen in the body thereby disrupting the delicate balance of the body's natural hormonal system. Our hormones need to remain in balance - excess oestrogen (natural or environmental) is toxic.

Parabens are linked to cancer, endometriosis, endocrine disruption, reproductive toxicity, immunotoxicity, neurotoxicity and skin irritation.

Parabens are not the only environmental oestrogens we are exposed to, but the big difference between them and other xenoestrogens is that we apply parabens to the skin (through which they are absorbed) and we eat them.

So what can you do?

♥ Read labels (even on 'natural' products). Avoid any product that has the ingredients butyl paraben, ethyl paraben, methyl paraben, or propyl paraben on ingredient listings on personal care products.

There are more...

Special mention must be made of the toxins which are found in many personal care and household cleaning products.

These chemicals are linked to allergies, chest pain, chronic fatigue, depression, dizziness, ear infections, headaches, joint pain, and difficulties sleeping. They can trigger asthma, weaken the immune system, disrupt the endocrine and central nervous system and cause cancer.

They are absorbed by you and your little one through the skin or inhaled, and can have as much of a damaging effect as any toxin that is found in, or on, food. I encourage you to do further research on them, and to avoid products which contain them. Read the ingredient list on all products and do your best to avoid these ones:

DEA (Diethanolamine), MEA (Monoethanolamine), **TEA (Triethanolamine)** (shampoos, soaps, bubble baths, and facial cleansers), **Phthalates** (preservative in cosmetics), **FD&C Color Pigments, Fragrance** (shampoos, deodorants, sunscreens, skincare and body care products), **Imidazolidinyl Urea and DMDM Hydantoin** (skin, body and hair products, antiperspirants, and nail polish), **Quaternium-15** (skin and hair products), **Isopropyl Alcohol** (hand lotion), **Mineral Oil** (baby oil), **PEG** (Polyethylene Glycol: hair and skin products), **Propylene Glycol** (makeup, toothpaste, and deodorant), **Sodium Lauryl Sulfate and Sodium Laureth Sulfate** (make-up, shampoo, conditioner, toothpaste), **Triclosan** (antibacterial soaps), **Talc** (baby powder and foundation), **Petrolatum** (petroleum jelly).

So what can you do?

The easiest way to avoid all of these is to only use natural, organic personal care and household cleaning products.

"I didn't know this before, now what?"

You and your little one can eat foods that are known to purify the body from these toxins such as: fermented vegetables; beetroots; sea vegetables; algae (including chlorella, blue-green algae and spirulina); sprouts; broccoli; coriander and turmeric. Drink lots of pure water and add Epsom salts or bicarbonate of soda to your bath water to create a 'detox' bath. Most importantly - avoid further exposure!

For more information on toxins I highly recommend the **Environmental Working Group (EWG)** website: **Healthy Child, Healthy World www.healthychild.org**

Feeding with Awareness

Whole Foods vs. Refined & Processed Foods

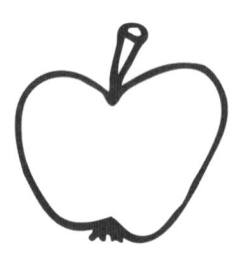

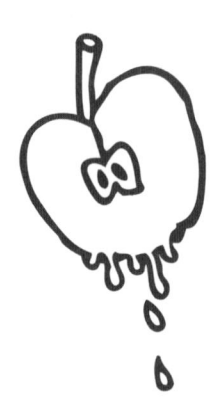

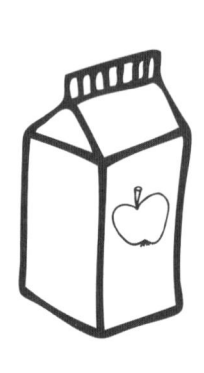

THE GOOD   THE BAD   THE UGLY

	Whole Food	Refined Food	Processed Food
EXAMPLES	**Unrefined grains, beans, nuts, seeds, fruits and vegetables.**	**White rice, white flour, white sugar, fruit juice.**	**Crackers, cereals, fruit juices, soda's, sweets, chips, polony, cold cuts, canned fruits, fish fingers, chicken nuggets, hot dogs.**
	An orange	Freshly squeezed orange juice.	Pasteurised orange juice in a carton (usually with preservatives, colourants, flavour enhancers and added synthetic Vitamin C – "enriched")
	♡ Butter, coconut oil, olive oil, sesame oil and flaxseed oil. Are extracted by slow-moving stone presses or rollers. They are referred to as "expeller expressed" or "cold pressed." These gentle approaches preserve the integrity of the fat molecules and the natural preservatives many oils contain, which preserve their stability. These are unrefined oils.	♡ Sunflower oil, canola oil. Most commercial oils are refined and processed by crushing the oil-bearing seeds and exposing them to extreme heat (often up to 230ºC / 450ºF). In addition to excessive temperatures, the oils are also exposed to high pressure, light, oxygen, and solvents (usually hexane). This process creates free radicals and destroys any of the health benefits of the original seed. When the oils are heated for cooking, more rancid free radicals are formed.	

Feeding with Awareness

Whole Food	Refined Food	Processed Food
Whole foods are a rich source of all the nutritional building blocks - protein, essential fats, complex carbohydrates, and a full complement of vitamins and minerals in their natural form.	Refined foods are processed foods that lack many of the nutrients they once had. They generally add a lot of calories to your diet, when compared to the amount of nutrients they contribute.	Processed foods have had many (if not most) nutrients stripped or cooked out of them. The food industry has to replace these lost nutrients in what is known as "enriching". This is often with synthetic versions of the missing nutrient. *Enriching processed food by adding back some vitamins and minerals (as some white breads and most children's cereals do), does not make the food whole again. Many other elements have been removed and lost through processing. Enriched foods do not supply, and in some cases, rob your child's body of essential nutrition.*
They are nutrient dense foods.	They are nutrient deprived foods.	They are nutrient deficient foods.
Whole foods provide a wealth of protective compounds (antioxidants, phytochemicals, digestive enzymes, probiotics etc.) that can help prevent disease.	The refining process removes many of the most important parts of a whole food, including vitamins, minerals and dietary fibre.	In addition to going through many complex processing steps often involving high heat which changes the molecular structure of certain proteins forming new (toxic) compounds that are foreign to the human body, processed foods usually contain harmful additives, artificial flavourings and other chemical ingredients.
Nature created whole foods with nutrients and protective compounds that work together synergistically to provide all our body needs - in a way that our body is able to effectively use. These nutrients are 'bio-available' – that is they are easily absorbed and used by our bodies.	The food industry has isolated compounds or elements from whole foods and when used (or eaten) on their own they have negative effects on the body.	
An apple (as does any fruit) contains fructose (a natural sugar). But, whole apples also have fibre, water, antioxidants, enzymes and synergistic compounds. For this reason, an apple (like most whole fruits) takes a while to eat and digest, meaning that the fructose is delivered to the liver slowly. The natural enzymes and antioxidants also assist the body in detoxing the sugars. Naturally sweet foods are linked together with the vitamins, minerals, and enzymes needed for their digestion and assimilation by the body.	Refined or processed apple juice has had all the fibre (bulk), enzymes and antioxidants removed or pasteurised out of it. The sugars now exist separately from the nutrients. These 'skeletonised' sugars work quite differently in the body, providing nothing but empty calories that drain the body's nutrient reserves. What is left is a high concentration of fructose – one glass of apple juice will deliver far more fructose than one apple. Fruit juices may even have additional High Fructose Corn Syrup (HFCS), flavourings, colorants and preservatives added to them. The lack of fibre means the fructose enters the bloodstream very quickly, spiking the blood sugar levels. The lack of enzymes and antioxidants mean your body has to do a lot more work to detoxify the sugar.	

An example of fructose:

NUTRITIONAL IMPLICATIONS

63

Feeding with Awareness

An example of grains:

Whole Food	Refined Food	Processed Food
A grain is whole and unrefined if the entire kernel is left unaltered and intact. There are three parts to a whole grain – the endosperm, germ and bran. The endosperm contains mostly starch and protein. The germ is rich in unsaturated fats, protein, carbohydrates, vitamin E, B-complex vitamins and minerals. The bran provides a large concentration of fibre and also contains minerals and B vitamins. Example: Brown Rice	Through the process of refining, the germ and bran are both removed, leaving only the endosperm - which has most of the grain's carbohydrates and protein, but only a small portion of its vitamins and minerals. This process strips the grain of most of its nutritional value, including precious compounds and plant sterols that are important in preventing disease. Example: White rice	Refined grains are then processed to create another food – crackers, for example. These are cooked at high heat. They also may have harmful additives such as flavourings, sweeteners and transfats.
Your child's body relies on the nutrients from these foods for proper growth as well as mental and physical vitality.	Your child's appetite may be satiated after eating these foods, but the nutrient requirements have not been met. A diet high in processed foods, effectively leaves your little one's body malnourished.	
Advantages of eating whole foods: - Reduced risk of diseases such as: cardiovascular disease; many types of cancer; type 2 diabetes, - They keep blood sugar stable, - A strong immune system, - A strong digestive system, - Superior brain function, - Good sleep, - Strong bones, - A calm mind, - While whole foods may be more expensive than their processed counterparts, you will be rewarded in the long run with fewer illnesses, positive emotions, reduced medical bills, no medications, better productivity at work.	Disadvantages of eating refined foods: - They cause blood sugar to spike and then crash, - The lack of fibre may lead to slow and difficult digestion, constipation, compromised gut health, which in turn affects the immune system, - The body lacks vital nutrients, - You need more in order to fill you up, leaving you hungry soon after.	Disadvantages of eating processed foods: - Food additives have been linked to behavioural problems in children (such as ADHD), - Processed foods have been linked with lower IQ's and learning disabilities, - Processed foods increase inflammation in the body which in turn can lead to serious diseases, - Food additives have been linked with cancer, diabetes and other diseases, - Processed foods compromise the immune system, - They contribute towards obesity due to increased sugar consumption, - Leads to bodies that are full, but malnourished.

EFFECTS

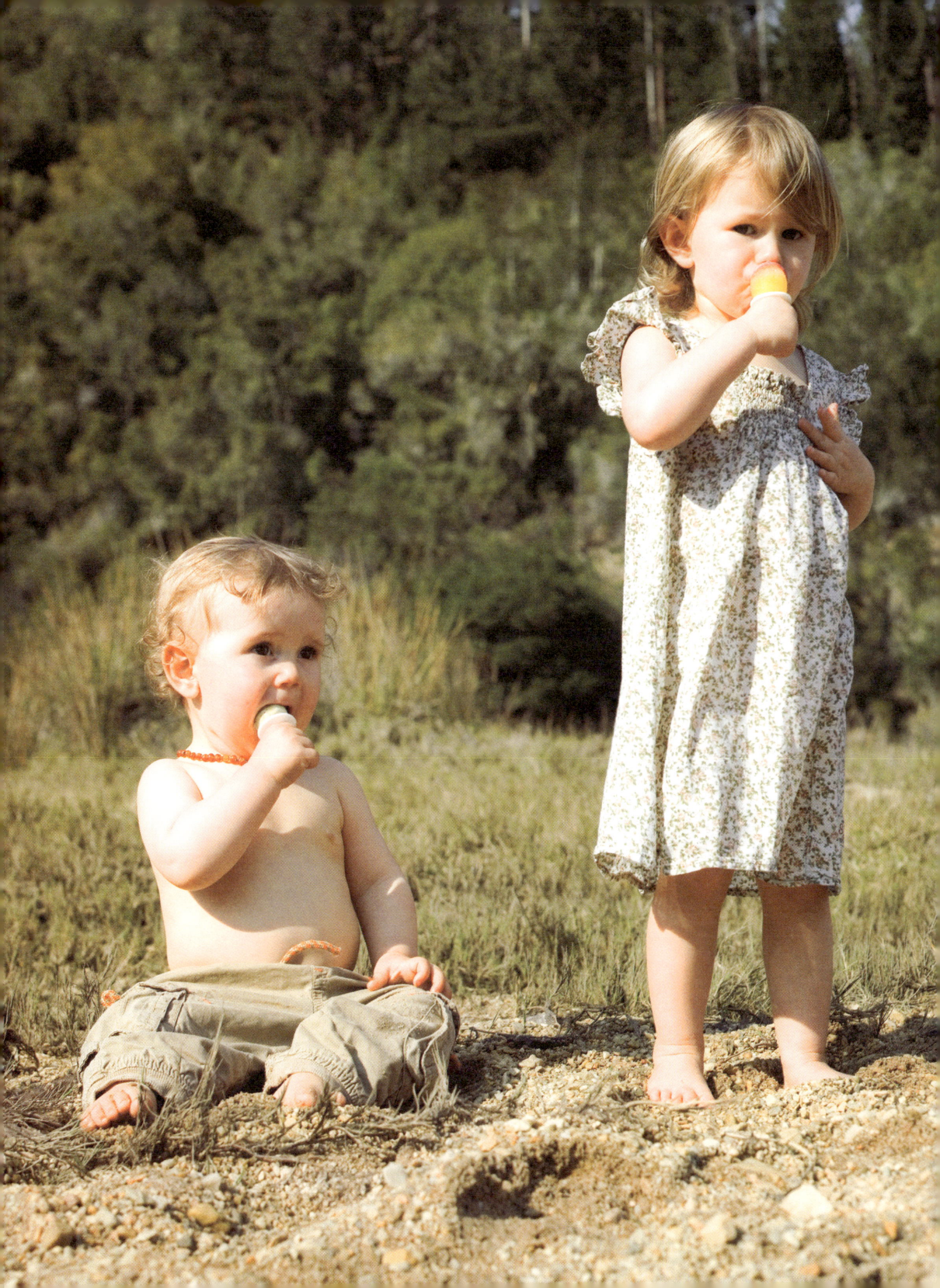

Feeding with Awareness

Chemical Cuisine: Food Additives

ADDITIVES ARE THE COLOURS, PRESERVATIVES, ANTIOXIDANTS, FLAVOUR ENHANCERS, ARTIFICIAL FLAVOURS, ARTIFICIAL SWEETENERS AND TRANS FATS THAT ARE PRESENT IN MANY PROCESSED FOODS.

Some additives have been used for centuries and are harmless - for example, vinegar has been used to preserve vegetables by way of pickling them, and salt and vinegar have been used to preserve meat (for example, biltong or jerky).

With the advent of industrialisation, advanced technology, a global 'big business' food industry, and a consumer that is disassociated from real food, there has been a great increase in the use of food additives (both natural and artificial) with varying levels of safety.

They are used to: improve shelf life, increase transportation or storage time; make food convenient and easy to prepare (think microwave popcorn); increase the nutritional value after the processing has stripped the original nutrients from the ingredients (think enriched fruit juices); provide nutrition to consumers who are not eating a wide variety of natural foods (think iodated salt), improve the look and taste of otherwise unappealing processed foods (think polony); and, enhance the attractiveness or marketability of food products (think artificially brightly coloured fruit leather to attract the kids), and improve consumer acceptance (milk that doesn't separate).

Quite simply – food is big business. It's all about marketing, sales and profits. Its not about what nourishes you, or is needed to nourish you.

There are approximately **3000 FOOD ADDITIVES** approved for use in the food industry today! Some are **natural compounds** (but may be from genetically modified plants), some are **nature-identical** (that is, the chemical composition of a natural substance has been copied), and **nearly 300 additives are completely synthetic**.

While governments and organisations such as Codex* assure us that the additives in our food are thoroughly tested and safe for consumption, there are approved additives that have been shown in subsequent independent studies to be harmful to our health. Also, while additives may have been approved on an individual basis, we are routinely exposed to a combination of them, and it's simply not known what their combined effect on the body may be.

Some artificial food additives have been linked to cancer, digestive problems, neurological conditions, ADHD, heart disease and obesity. Natural additives may be similarly harmful or, be the cause of allergic reactions in certain individuals, since they are isolated compounds – not the whole food.

---

* *Codex - The Codex Alimentarius is a collection of internationally recognized standards, codes of practice, guidelines and other recommendations relating to foods, food production and food safety. Its texts are developed and maintained by the Codex Alimentarius Commission, a body that was established in early November 1961 by the Food and Agriculture Organization of the United Nations (FAO) and joined by the World Health Organization (WHO) in June 1962.*

Symptoms of reactions to additives include:

- Irritability, restlessness, difficulty falling asleep;
- Mood swings, anxiety, depression, panic attacks;
- Inattention, difficulty concentrating or debilitating fatigue;
- Speech delay, learning difficulties;
- Eczema, itchy skin rashes, swelling of the lips;
- Reflux, colic, stomach aches, bloating, and other irritable bowel symptoms including constipation and/or diarrhoea, sneaky poos, sticky poos, bedwetting;
- Headaches or migraines;
- Frequent colds, flu, bronchitis, tonsillitis, sinusitis; stuffy or runny nose, constant throat clearing, cough or asthma;
- Joint pain, arthritis, heart palpitations, racing heartbeat.

Eeeeeeeeee!

Additives have a scientific name as well as an E-number code. These E-Numbers have been formulated by the European Economic Community (EEC) and are universally adopted by the food industry worldwide.

THE E-NUMBERS ARE CATEGORISED AS FOLLOWS:

	E100-199	food colours
	E200-299	preservatives
	E300-399	antioxidants, acidity regulators
	E400-499	thickeners, emulsifiers, stabilizers, vegetable gums
	E500-599	mineral salts, acidity regulators and anti-caking agents
	E600-699	flavour enhancers
	E900-999	glazing agents and sweeteners
	E1000-1399	miscellaneous additives
	E1400-1499	starch derivatives

It is important to note that **not all E numbers are bad** – just as not all additives are bad. Natural substances like vitamin C (E300), paprika (E160c) and even oxygen (E948) are considered to be additives and each have an E number assigned to them, as do many other naturally occurring substances.

In today's world where the toxic load on your little one's tiny body is already high due to environmental toxins such as pesticides, herbicides, air pollution, BPA, electromagnetic radiation (from cell phones, cell towers, Wi-Fi, power lines etc.), avoiding chemical cuisine is one way you can actively lighten the burden.

> WHILE BUYING READY-MADE FOOD FROM A SUPERMARKET MAY BE CONVENIENT AND CERTAINLY LESS TIME-CONSUMING THAN PREPARING ALL THE FOOD FROM SCRATCH, YOU NEED TO ASK YOURSELF - WOULD YOU RATHER SPEND TIME BEING CREATIVE IN THE KITCHEN OR DISCIPLINING YOUR CHILDREN AND SPENDING TIME NURSING THEM BACK TO HEALTH FROM FREQUENT INFECTIONS?

Feeding with Awareness

Food additives to avoid
(AS OF AUGUST 2015)

Much of the information for this section comes from **The Food Intolerance Network (www.fedup.com.au)** which is an Australian based network run by Sue Dengate. In my search for local South African regulations I was presented with legislation that, in some cases, was 40 years old! In needing less outdated regulations, the South African food industry apparently follows the Codex General Standard for Food Additives (*GSFA, Codex STAN 192-1995*). Initially I was comforted to know that there were some current guidelines to follow but, after reviewing the **'General Standard for Food Additives'** document, I felt overwhelming despair… the list of food additives (and what foods they are allowed in) spans some 396 pages! Fair enough, some additives may be of completely natural origin – but many of the additives that are mentioned below (as ones to avoid) are, according to Codex, permitted in a large number of foods, even the ones that have been banned in other countries.

Be a food detective!

It is vitally important to read the labels of any products you buy. Something which you may think of as a healthy food, may have mutated into something quite different due to the additives thrown in during the manufacturing process. Dried fruit and fruit leather is an excellent example of this, as is hummus. They are both really nutritious foods when made at home – but the versions you buy in the supermarkets are full of hydrogenated fats, GMO vegetable oils, preservatives, sugar and colorants. It is truly frightening when you start looking at labels and realise what 'they' are trying to pass off as healthy food. Please remember that the food industry is big business – its primary concern, in my opinion, is its profits – not the health and well being of you and your family. As Michael Pollan mentions in his book In Defence of Food, "the food available today is not anything our ancestors would recognise, it is, rather, an edible food-like substance."

Some good rules of thumb when buying food are: do not buy anything with an ingredient listed which you cannot pronounce; do not buy anything with more than five ingredients listed; and, do not buy anything that will not eventually rot.

Symptoms of additive intolerance

According to Sue Dengate and the Food Intolerance Network, the following symptoms of food intolerance can be helped by a change in diet (that is, by eliminating the culprits):

- **AIRWAYS:** asthma, stuffy blocked or runny nose/ nasal polyps, frequent nose bleeds, catarrh, chronic throat-clearing, sinusitis, frequent ear infections, frequent tonsillitis, frequent colds and flu, symptoms of Samter's Triad, hay fever, allergic rhinitis.
- **SKIN:** eczema, urticaria (hives), cradle cap, other skin rashes, angioedema (swollen lips, eyes, tongue), geographic tongue, pruritus (itching), rosacea, allergic shiners (dark circles under eyes),

IT MAY BE A USEFUL EXERCISE TO PRINT THIS LIST AND CIRCLE WHAT, IF ANY, SYMPTOMS YOU OR YOUR LITTLE ONE HAVE – PERHAPS THEY CAN BE LINKED TO A FOOD INTOLERANCE.

pallor (pale skin), flushing, excessive sweating, body odour, sore vagina in children, alopecia (patchy baldness).

- **DIGESTIVE SYSTEM:** irritable bowel symptoms (IBS), recurrent mouth ulcers, indigestion, nausea, bad breath, vomiting, diarrhoea, stomach ache, bloating, reflux in babies, adults, constipation, colic in babies, sluggish bowel syndrome (feeling of 'more to come'), encopresis, soiling (sneaky poos), dairy intolerance, gluten and wheat intolerance, eating disorders, anorexia nervosa, bulimia nervosa, binge eating disorder (BED).
- **BLADDER:** bedwetting, daytime incontinence, urinary urgency, recurrent inflammation (cystitis).
- **SKELETAL:** growing pains, arthritis.
- **EYES:** nystagmus (involuntary movement), blurred vision.
- **MUSCLES:** low muscle tone, myalgia (muscle pain), tics (involuntary movement), tremor.
- **HEART:** rapid heart beat, heart palpitations, cardiac arrhythmias, pseudo heart attack (feeling of impending doom, chest pressure, pain down arm), tachycardia (fast heart beat), angina-type pain, HHT.
- **CENTRAL NERVOUS SYSTEM:** headaches or migraines, unexplained tiredness, chronic fatigue, feeling 'hung-over', confusion, dizziness, agitation, tinnitus (noises in ear), hyperacusis, auditory sensory processing disorder (ASPD), paraesthesia (pins and needles), dysaesthesia (numbness), hypoglycaemia, salicylate-induced hypoglycaemia, epileptic seizures, fits, sensory symptoms of multiple sclerosis, symptoms of lupus.
- **ANXIETY:** panic attacks, depression, obsessive ruminations (repetitively focusing on bad feelings and experiences from the past), self harm, suicidal thoughts, actions, teeth grinding (bruxism).
- **IMPAIRED MEMORY:** vague or forgetful, unable to concentrate, won't persevere, unmotivated, disorganised, easily distracted, difficulty reading and writing.
- **SPEECH:** loud voice (no volume control), speech hard to understand, speech delay, selective mutism, stuttering, repetitive noises, talks too much (empty chatter).
- **CO-ORDINATION:** poor handwriting, poor coordination, frequent accidents.
- **SLEEP:** difficulty falling asleep, restless legs syndrome (RLS), persistent night waking, insomnia, nightmares/night terrors/sleepwalking, sleep apnoea.
- **MOOD:** brain snaps, mood swings, premenstrual tension, grizzly or unhappy, cries easily or often, irritable, uncooperative.
- **OPPOSITIONAL DEFIANCE:** odd, loses temper, argumentative, refuses requests, defies rules, deliberately annoys others, blames others for own mistakes, touchy, easily annoyed, angry, resentful.
- **OTHER BEHAVIOUR:** ADHD, ADD, autism, Asperger's, inattentive, easily bored, unmotivated, 'unable to entertain himself', restless, fidgety or over-active, head banging, hyperactivity, fights with siblings, difficulty making friends, destructive, aggressive, unreasonable, tantrums, demanding, never satisfied, disruptive, discipline is ineffective, pervasive development disorder.

This extensive list pertains not only to intolerances to additives, dairy and gluten but to the natural food chemicals salicylates and amines as well.

Feeding with Awareness

The Worst Offenders

BELOW IS A TABLE OF THE ADDITIVES YOU WANT TO MAKE EVERY EFFORT TO AVOID. PRINT IT AND KEEP IT IN YOUR WALLET FOR QUICK REFERENCE WHILE YOU ARE GROCERY SHOPPING.

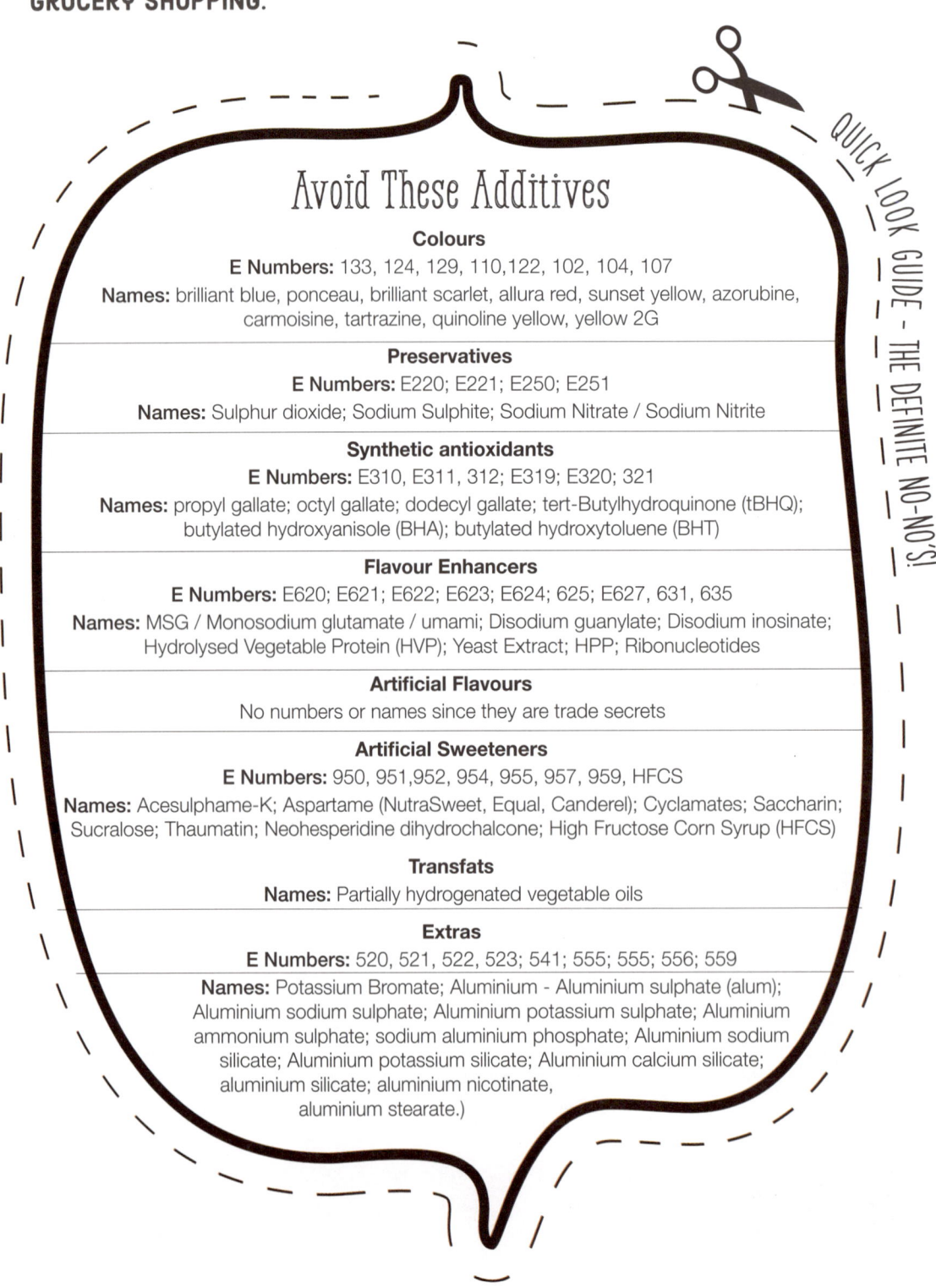

QUICK LOOK GUIDE - THE DEFINITE NO-NO'S!

Avoid These Additives

Colours
E Numbers: 133, 124, 129, 110, 122, 102, 104, 107
Names: brilliant blue, ponceau, brilliant scarlet, allura red, sunset yellow, azorubine, carmoisine, tartrazine, quinoline yellow, yellow 2G

Preservatives
E Numbers: E220; E221; E250; E251
Names: Sulphur dioxide; Sodium Sulphite; Sodium Nitrate / Sodium Nitrite

Synthetic antioxidants
E Numbers: E310, E311, 312; E319; E320; 321
Names: propyl gallate; octyl gallate; dodecyl gallate; tert-Butylhydroquinone (tBHQ); butylated hydroxyanisole (BHA); butylated hydroxytoluene (BHT)

Flavour Enhancers
E Numbers: E620; E621; E622; E623; E624; 625; E627, 631, 635
Names: MSG / Monosodium glutamate / umami; Disodium guanylate; Disodium inosinate; Hydrolysed Vegetable Protein (HVP); Yeast Extract; HPP; Ribonucleotides

Artificial Flavours
No numbers or names since they are trade secrets

Artificial Sweeteners
E Numbers: 950, 951, 952, 954, 955, 957, 959, HFCS
Names: Acesulphame-K; Aspartame (NutraSweet, Equal, Canderel); Cyclamates; Saccharin; Sucralose; Thaumatin; Neohesperidine dihydrochalcone; High Fructose Corn Syrup (HFCS)

Transfats
Names: Partially hydrogenated vegetable oils

Extras
E Numbers: 520, 521, 522, 523; 541; 555; 555; 556; 559
Names: Potassium Bromate; Aluminium - Aluminium sulphate (alum); Aluminium sodium sulphate; Aluminium potassium sulphate; Aluminium ammonium sulphate; sodium aluminium phosphate; Aluminium sodium silicate; Aluminium potassium silicate; Aluminium calcium silicate; aluminium silicate; aluminium nicotinate, aluminium stearate.)

Please see the Appendix for a detailed list of Food Additives and their associated health affects.

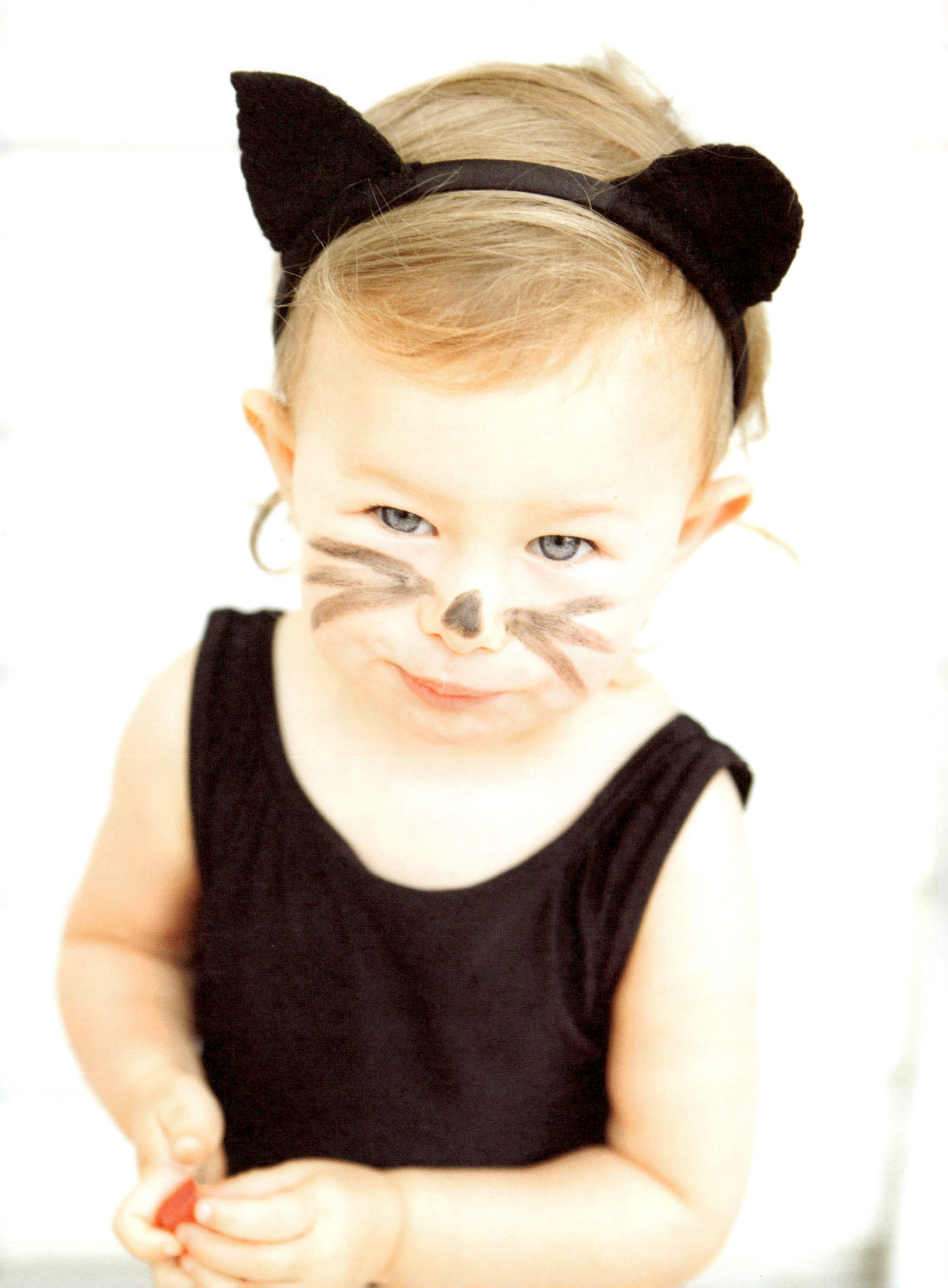

Raw vs. Cooked... which is better?

While I was writing this book and learning how to feed Mila, I was introduced to the Raw Food Movement. I attended a lecture by David Wolfe, and I was sold! I was convinced that children should be raised on a raw food diet, I did a 7-day juice fast and I started incorporating a lot more raw food into my and Mila's diet. A couple of months later I suffered from terrible digestive issues. I was then advised to follow the GAPS diet - basically the complete opposite of raw food whereby you only eat cooked food for a few months! I have since learnt that there is a time and place for everything and, what works for one person may not work for another person. As for feeding a child – I feel a middle ground is the best approach.

The main benefit of raw food is that raw and living foods contain nutrients and digestive enzymes that are destroyed when food is heated. These digestive enzymes are needed to digest the food. Your body does produce them, but we are born with a limited amount. By eating nutrient-rich living foods containing digestive enzymes you can boost your immune system, increase your energy levels and have better digestion – that is, however, if your digestive system is not damaged, or immature.

Even with the digestive enzymes, raw food is more difficult to digest than cooked food. This is due to the fibres remaining intact. If your digestive system is damaged (as mine was), or if it is immature (as your little one's is), 100% raw food is probably not a great idea.

That being said, there are ways of 'pre-digesting' raw food to make it easier for your little one to digest such as: puréeing, juicing and fermenting. The blending process used to make a purée effectively breaks down the fibres, making the food easier to digest. Juicing raw vegetables removes the difficult-to-digest fibres. Fermenting is another way of 'predigesting' or partially digesting raw food before feeding it to your little one – with the added benefit of probiotics that will help the digestion process. I would definitely recommend all of these, as I believe it is important to have raw foods in one's diet.

THERE ARE SOME FOODS THAT ARE, HOWEVER, MORE NUTRITIOUS WHEN THEY ARE COOKED:

- ♥ Carrots can be constipating if eaten raw and more beta carotene is absorbed from cooked carrots than raw ones.
- ♥ Some green veggies contain a chemical called oxalic acid. Oxalic acid is a very irritating substance to the mouth and intestinal tract. It also blocks iron and calcium absorption and may contribute to the formation of kidney stones. Oxalic acid is reduced by a light steaming or cooking. Veggies containing oxalic acid include spinach, chard, parsley, chives, and beet greens.
- ♥ Raw potatoes contain hemaglutinins that disrupt red blood cell function – they should always be eaten well cooked.
- ♥ Raw cruciferous vegetables contain substances called goitrogens which interfere with iodine absorption thereby suppressing your thyroid's hormone production, resulting in fatigue, coldness in your body and a slowing of your metabolism. Cruciferous vegetables include broccoli, Brussels

sprouts, cabbage, cauliflower, kale, mustard greens, radishes, rutabagas and turnips. Fermenting these vegetables reduces the thyroid-suppressing effect and maximises nutrition.
♥ Heating foods which have high amounts of the antioxidant lycopene (tomatoes and red fruits) for 15 minutes breaks down the cell walls in these foods, making the lycopene more available for absorption. Puréeing these foods has the same effect.

Obviously the way in which you cook your vegetables will affect their nutritional value – I recommend baking, simmering, sautéing or lightly steaming them.

Feeding with Awareness

Eat from the rainbow

Eating a variety of food with all the colours of the rainbow represented ensures your little one is getting a complete range of nutrients.

What does it mean to eat a rainbow?

- ♥ Choosing a variety of different-coloured whole foods throughout the day and week.
- ♥ The more naturally occurring colours on your little one's plate at each meal or snack, the better.
- ♥ It does not mean making a rainbow with artificially coloured foods (gummy snacks, soda, popsicles, etc.)!

Rainbow nutrition:

Phytonutrients are natural chemical compounds found in all plants. They protect against diseases and promote health. The phytonutrients in fruits and vegetables give them their different colours with each colour group providing a unique set of vitamins, minerals and nutrients. Using the rainbow as a guide is a great way to ensure your little one is eating the widest range of phytonutrients.

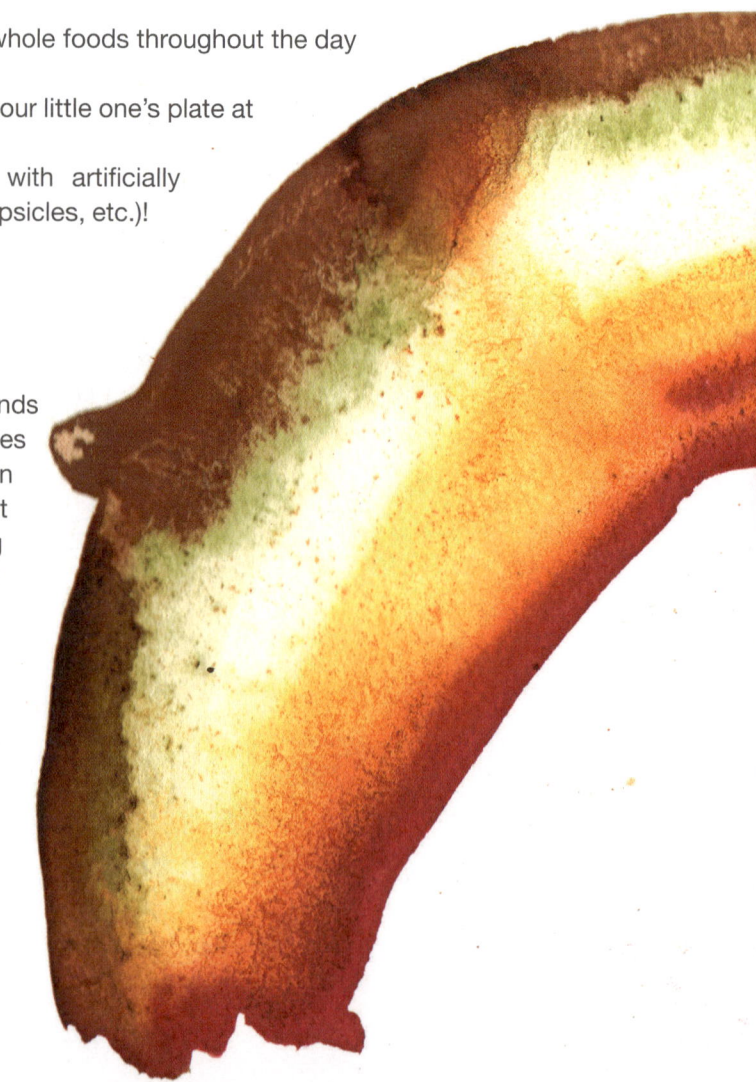

Feeding with Awareness

Colour	Foods	Nutrients	Supports
RED	Red cabbage, red onion, red peppers, kidney beans, red lentils, radishes, tomatoes, strawberries, cherries, watermelon, raspberries, red grapes, guavas, pink grapefruit, plums.	Flavonoids, lycopene, vitamin C, folate, potassium, beta-carotene, anthocyanins, quercetin.	Heart health, memory, reduce symptoms of asthma.
ORANGE	Carrots, butternut, pumpkin, sweet potatoes, orange bell pepper, mangoes, gooseberries, apricots, papaya, peaches, loquats, mandarins, naartjies, nectarines.	Vitamin C, potassium, carotenoids, flavonoids, liminoids, terpenes.	Healthy eyes, heart health, immune function.
YELLOW	Patty pans, lemons, sweet potatoes, yellow peppers, yellow squash, bananas, pineapples, yellow plums.	Beta-carotene, vitamin A, vitamin C, potassium, flavonoids, terpenes, quercetin.	Healthy eyes, heart health, immune function, healthy digestive system and skin, anti-inflammatory.
GREEN	Asparagus, bok choy, broccoli, cabbage, kale, spinach, green beans, peas, zucchini, Brussel sprouts, lettuce, apples, kiwi fruit, cucumbers, grapes, avocado, herbs.	Vitamins C, K and folate, calcium, potassium, iron, carotenoids, flavonoids, indoles, saponins, sulforaphane, omega-3 fatty acids.	Good for the whole body, strengthens the immune system, healthy bones, blood, lungs, teeth and eyes.
BLUE / PURPLE	Dark beans, eggplant, beetroot, blueberries, blackberries, figs, prunes.	Anthocyanin, vitamin C, chlorogenic acid, quercetin.	Memory and healthy aging.
WHITE	Ginger, onions, mushrooms, garlic, potatoes, cauliflower, fennel, leeks, parsnip, white beans, litchis, white nectarines, white peaches.	Flavonoids, starch and protein, B group vitamins, potassium, indoles, isothiocyanates, anthoxanthins.	Heart health, good cholesterol levels, good for energy and growth.

Feeding with Awareness

Enzymes, Nutrients and Anti-nutrients

DIGESTIVE ENZYMES are primarily produced in the pancreas and small intestine. They break down our food into nutrients so that our bodies can absorb them.

A **NUTRIENT** is a substance that provides nourishment essential for growth and the maintenance of life.

So what then are **ANTI-NUTRIENTS**?

Anti-Nutrients

As scientific research methods develop, new information on nutrition comes to light that challenges what we have previously held to be true about our food. One of these new pieces of information is that of 'anti-nutrients'.

Anti-nutrients interfere with the absorption of nutrients and digestion and, irritate the intestinal tract. Whole grains, nuts, seeds and legumes are all high in anti-nutrients. But these foods are meant to be good for you – right? Well yes – if they are correctly prepared, in a way that reduces the anti-nutrients.

Anti-nutrients are part of a seed's natural system of preservation. Nature has ensured that seeds won't sprout until the perfect growing conditions exist. Two of these anti-nutrients worth mentioning are Phytic Acid and Enzyme Inhibitors.

Phytic Acid

Phytic Acid is the storage form of phosphorous – that is, seeds store phosphorus as phytic acid. Grains, nuts and legumes are all seeds and have high levels of phytic acid. So do other edible seeds such as pumpkin and sunflower seeds.

When phytic acid is bound to a mineral in the seed, it's known as phytate.

Phytic acid is an anti-nutrient because it binds to essential minerals (such as calcium, copper, iron, zinc, and magnesium) in the digestive tract, making them less available to our bodies. Phytates also reduce the digestibility of starches, proteins, and fats.

Enzyme Inhibitors

Enzyme inhibitors are present in seeds to prevent them from developing (sprouting) until there are suitable growing conditions. Unfortunately eating seeds with enzyme inhibitors negatively affects our digestive and metabolic enzymes.

It is not necessary to avoid foods containing phytic acid or enzyme inhibitors, but it is important to prepare them correctly – as our ancestors did. Correct preparation reduces the phytic acid, neutralises the enzyme inhibitors and increases the bio-availability of the nutrients.

SOAKING NUTS, GRAINS, SEEDS AND LEGUMES

Soaking and fermenting nuts, grains, seeds and legumes is something our grannies (or granny's granny) did and for good reason. It mimics nature's 'perfect sprouting' conditions by providing moisture, warmth, time and slight acidity. As the seed begins to germinate while soaking, phytic acid is reduced, enzyme inhibitors are neutralised and the production of numerous beneficial enzymes begins. The action of these enzymes increases the amount of vitamins, especially B vitamins. Difficult-to-digest proteins are partially broken down into simpler components that are more readily available for absorption.

HOW TO SOAK GRAINS AND LEGUMES.

Cover with warm water and add one of the following acids: lemon juice, apple cider vinegar, buttermilk, yoghurt, kefir or whey. The ratio of grain to acid should be 2 tablespoons of acid for every 1 cup of grains. Soak for 7 to 24 hours in a warm place. Drain, rinse and cook as usual. Cooking time will be reduced due to the soaking.

HOW TO SOAK NUTS AND SEEDS.

Cover the nuts or seeds with warm water and add sea salt. The ratio of nuts or seeds to salt should be a ½ tablespoon salt for every 2 cups of nuts or seeds. Soak for six to eight hours (or overnight), then drain, rinse and dehydrate or roast.

Dehydrate by placing in a warm oven (no warmer than 65°C/150°F) or dehydrator for 12-24 hours.

Feeding with Awareness

Meat: Organic, Free-Range, Pasture-raised, Grass-fed & GMO... what's the difference and does it matter?

There are so many labels on foods these days - it is important to know what they mean so you can make informed choices. It is also important to know what the absence of any of these labels means.

Factory Farms

One label you wont see on animal products is 'Factory Farmed'. If products aren't organic or free-range, they are raised 'conventionally' – that is, conventional by industrial standards, not traditional or moral ones.

Conventionally raised animals are 'farmed' in what are known as 'factory farms' or 'feedlots' using intensive farming methods. A factory farm is a large, industrial operation that mass produces animals for food. Factory farms pack animals into spaces so tight that most can barely move. The animals or birds have no access to the outdoors, spending their lives on warehouse floors, or housed in cages or pens. Without the room to engage in natural behaviours, confined animals experience severe physical and mental distress.

Standard Factory Farming Practices

- **Unclean air:** Waste piles up in the animal sheds, creating ammonia and dust. The ammonia irritates and can even burn animals' eyes, skin and throats.
- **Unnatural lighting:** Factory farms simulate unnatural day lengths to promote fast growth and desired behaviours.
- **Unnatural growth:** Fast and disproportionate growth and production due to selective breeding and the use of growth hormones causes ailments including chronic pain, heart problems, and in the case of chickens, bodies that are too heavy and big for their legs to carry.
- **Unnatural food:** Animals in factory farms are fed an unnatural diet – usually genetically modified corn or soy and, or "by-product feedstuff". By that I mean – municipal garbage, stale cookies, poultry manure, chicken feathers, bubble gum, and restaurant waste! Until 1997, cattle were even being fed beef off-cuts. This unnatural practice is believed to be the underlying cause of mad cow disease. This unnatural diet leads to health problems, which are then treated with antibiotics.
- **Non-therapeutic medicating:** So that the animals can survive the filthy conditions and grow even faster, they are fed routine and continual antibiotics and/or hormones.

- **Unnatural reproduction:** Many female farm animals spend virtually their entire lives pregnant, putting their bodies under chronic strain.
- **Surgical mutilations:** Many farm animals undergo painful mutilations to their tails, testicles, horns, toes or beaks, without painkillers, to make their behaviour more manageable.
- **Shortened lives:** Factory farmed animals are generally slaughtered at 'market weight' well before the end of their natural life spans. In fact, most are still babies.

Damage to the Environment and Human Health

Waste runoff from factory farms pollutes the water, land and air in neighbouring communities, compromising both human health and quality of life. At the same time, these businesses consume massive quantities of precious, finite resources including water and fossil fuels (growing the corn used to feed livestock uses vast quantities of chemical fertiliser, which in turn requires vast quantities of oil/fossil fuels).

Factory farms also endanger consumer health. Farms that are not properly maintained can be breeding grounds for salmonella and E. coli, which are passed onto humans through the meat, dairy and eggs from these animals. Antibiotic abuse to deal with these infections creates the potential for dangerous, new drug-resistant strains of bacteria to develop and spread amongst people.

Inferior nutrition

Changing an animal's natural diet of grasses to grains lowers the nutritional value of their meat and dairy products. Compared with grass-fed meat, grain-fed meat contains more total fat, saturated fat, and calories (and don't forget the growth hormones and antibiotic residue!). It also has less vitamin E, beta-carotene, and the two health-promoting fats: omega-3 fatty acids and conjugated linoleic acid, or CLA. The milk from dairy cows raised in confinement is similarly low in these nutrients.

Cage-free

Cage-free eggs are eggs from birds that are not raised in cages, but in floor systems usually in an open barn. The hens have bedding material such as pine shavings on the floor, and they are allowed perches and nest boxes to lay their eggs.

Free-range

Free-range indicates that the animal or bird was provided shelter in a building, room, or area with unlimited access to food, fresh water, and continuous access to the outdoors during their production cycle. In some cases, this can mean access only through a 'pop hole', with no full-body access to the outdoors and no minimum space requirement. The outdoor area may or may not be fenced and/or covered with netting-like material. Free-range animals and birds only eat plant-based foods (no animal by-products).

All organic animals are free-range; however all free-range animals are not necessarily organic.

Organic (meat)

As for organic meat, regulations require that: the animals must be raised in living conditions accommodating their natural behaviours (like access to the outdoors and the ability to graze on pasture); they must be fed 100% organic feed and forage; and they must not be administered antibiotics or hormones.

Grass-fed

Grass-fed animals receive a majority of their nutrients from grass throughout their life, while organic animals' pasture diet may be supplemented with grain. The grass-fed label does not limit the use of antibiotics, hormones, or pesticides.

A product may say "grass-fed" on the packaging, but the cow might have been 'finished' on grain, meaning it ate grain during the last 2 or 3 months of its life. Choose products labelled "100% grass-fed".

Pigs and chickens cannot survive only on grass, they need some grain, so you will never see a "grass-fed" pork or chicken label.

Note: a grass-fed cow may live indoors!

Pasture-raised

Although 'pasture-raised' does not have any current regulations, it is being used by sustainable farmers to mean chickens or pigs raised in the outdoors... in the pasture. The hens must be outdoors year-round with mobile or fixed housing where the they can go inside at night to protect themselves from predators. They are only permitted to be indoors for up to two weeks out of the year, due only to very bad weather.

Note: a pasture-raised chicken or pig may be fed GMO grain!

Feeding with Awareness

*So your healthiest choice when it comes to meat is **'organic + 100% grass-fed'** meat (lamb, beef, goat), and for pork, poultry or eggs it is **'organic + pasture-raised'**.*

Oh South Africa!

Identifying authentic free-range and organic produce in South Africa can be tricky, as there is no official legislation or regulation in place for free-range or organic farming. At present the South African law governing organic farming is still in draft form.

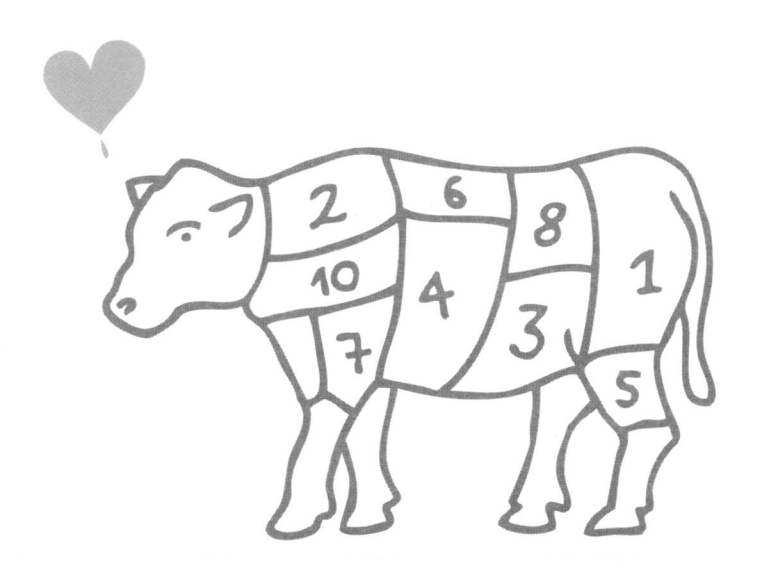

A MILA AND MAMA BEDTIME CONVERSATION

MILA: "NO-ONE IS LOOKING AFTER OUR SEA."

MAMA: "WHAT DO YOU MEAN ANGEL?"

MILA: "WELL ALL THE BOATS DRIVING AROUND, AND PEOPLE THROWING THEIR RUBBISH IN THE WATER"

MAMA: "YES, YOU RIGHT MY ANGEL. AND THEY ARE NOT BEING KIND TO THE FISH."

MILA: "WHAT DO YOU MEAN?"

MAMA: "WELL, THEY TAKING A LOT OF FISH OUT OF THE SEAS."

MILA: "WHY?"

MAMA: "TO EAT."

MILA: "OH NO! THAT'S NOT GOOD. I MUST TALK TO THEM, HEY MAMA?"

MAMA: "YES, MY ANGEL."

MILA: "IN A STRONG VOICE I'M GOING TO SAY 'NO! YOU CAN'T EAT ALL THE FISH AND DON'T THROW YOUR RUBBISH IN THE WATER!'"

MAMA: "GOOD MY ANGEL. YOU ARE GOING TO HELP LOOK AFTER THE EARTH, HEY?"

MILA: "AND THE SEAS. AND I AM GOING TO PROTECT THE FISHIES."

MAMA: "GOOD MY ANGEL." *(With a big glowing heart.)*

Feeding with Awareness

Fruits and Veggies: Organic, Conventional & GMO... what's the difference and does it matter?

What's a GMO?

"A GMO (genetically modified organism) is the result of a laboratory process of taking genes from one species and inserting them into another in an attempt to obtain a desired trait or characteristic." – Institute for Responsible Technology.

What kinds of traits have been added to food crops?

There are currently two types of genetic modifications: herbicide resistant and pesticide producing.

Herbicide resistant crops (known as Roundup ready crops) are able to withstand huge amounts of weed-killer (typically Roundup) being sprayed onto them without dying.

Pesticide producing crops (such as Bt cotton and Bt corn) have had the Bacillus thuringiensis (Bt) bacteria inserted into their genes. This bacterium produces a toxic protein that kills the corn borer and other insects which eat the plant by rupturing their stomachs - saving the farmer from having to spray pesticides. Essentially, the plant is the insecticide. These modifications have no health benefit, only economic benefit.

When you eat a genetically modified crop, or any of its derivatives, you are also eating the pesticides, which were liberally sprayed onto it, as well as the Bt toxin. Since Bt is a bacteria, it doesn't all pass out of your body with the unused remnants of the food it entered with. It joins the other bacteria living in your microbiome, and continues to have the same effect as it does on the insects - harming your digestive system by attacking normal gut cells and burning holes in the intestines. The Bt toxin used in GMO corn, for example, was recently detected in the blood of pregnant women and their babies!

Genetic roulette

When foreign genes are inserted into a plant, dormant genes may be activated or the functioning of genes altered, creating new or unknown proteins, or increasing or decreasing the output of existing proteins inside the plant. The effects of consuming these new combinations of proteins are unknown.

What foods are GM?

Globally the most common GM crops are corn (maize), soy (soya), canola, alfalfa and cotton.

Current commercialised GM crops in the U.S. include soy (94%), cotton (90%), canola (90%), sugar beets (95%), corn (88%), Hawaiian papaya (more than 50%), zucchini and yellow squash.

In South Africa current GM crops include: white Maize (80%); yellow Maize (55%); Soya (90%) and Cotton (100%).

Many other GM crops are currently in field trials and recent approvals include six different varieties of potato, two varieties of apple and one rice variety. In South Africa, numerous field trials have been approved for additional forms of GM maize, GM soya and GM cotton, as well as for GM sugar-cane, GM potato and GM cassava, amongst others.

What are other sources of GMOs?

All products made from the crops listed above, or foods made from any of their isolated compounds, have the genetically modified enzymes. The list of affected products is endless but to give you some idea here are some GM corn products: fresh corn, popcorn, mielie meal (pap), corn tortillas, grits, polenta, masa (corn dough), corn syrup, corn fructose (high fructose corn syrup), corn starch, corn dextrose, corn oil, corn flour, cornmeal.

Processed foods containing GM corn include anything with high fructose corn syrup (which is in almost everything!) and: corn chips, cookies, candies, gum, bread, cereals, pickles, margarine, beer and other alcohol, soft drinks, spritzers, fruit drinks, enriched flours, pastas, salad dressings, infant formula, vitamin C tablets!

GMOS CAN ALSO BE FOUND IN:

- Meat, eggs, and dairy products from animals that have eaten GM feed (and the majority of the GM corn and soy is used for animal feed);
- Dairy products from cows injected with rbGH (a GM growth hormone);
- Food additives, enzymes, flavourings, and processing agents, including the sweetener aspartame (NutraSweet) and rennet used to make hard cheeses;
- Honey and bee pollen that may have GM sources of pollen.
- Wheat is not currently genetically modified but most of the commercial bread (in South Africa) has genetically modified soy added to it.

What are the potential dangers of eating GM foods?

There are a number of dangers that broadly fall into the categories of potential toxins, allergens, carcinogens, new diseases, antibiotic resistant diseases, and nutritional problems.

Hasn't research shown GM foods to be safe?

The biotech industry and governments who approve GMOs will have you believe so by saying GMO crops have been scientifically studied and proven to be safe. Industry funded studies, however, are only conducted for 90 days – which is convenient for the GMO producers since the negative effects seen in independent studies were only found after 120 days.

The only feeding study done with humans showed that GMOs survived inside the stomach of the people eating GMO food. No follow-up studies were done.

Independent feeding studies in animals have shown potentially pre-cancerous cell growth, damaged immune systems, smaller brains, livers, and testicles, partial atrophy or increased density of the liver, odd shaped cell nuclei and other unexplained anomalies, false pregnancies and higher death rates.

The FDA (Food and Drug Administration in America) does not even require safety studies, let alone conduct their own. Instead, if the makers of the GM foods claim that they are safe, the agency approves them.

In both the United States and South Africa, food safety tests do not need to be conducted for GM soya because it is considered to be substantially the same as natural soya. South African regulatory authorities adopted the principle without hesitation, and no subsequent studies have been conducted despite evidence that it does impact on both human and animal health. This means that approximately 70% of South Africa's major food staple (bread) is now genetically modified, without it having been tested for potential health effects. These health effects would include allergenicity, damage to internal organs, antibiotic resistance, and horizontal gene-transfer. These will be added to the impact of the toxic pesticide Round-up which many GM crops are engineered to be used in conjunction with.

Why are children particularly susceptible to the effects of GM foods?

Children face the greatest risk from the potential dangers of GM foods for the same reasons that they also face the greatest risk from other hazards like pesticides and radiation - young, fast-developing bodies are less resilient and influenced most.

Reasons to avoid GMOs:

- Without long term studies on their health effects, eating GM foods is effectively **an experiment**.
- **GMOs contaminate - forever.** GMOs cross-pollinate and their seeds can travel. It is impossible to fully clean up the contaminated gene pool.
- **GMOs increase herbicide use.** GM foods contain higher residues of toxic herbicides which are damaging to your health. The pesticide Roundup (with Glyphosate as its active ingredient), for example, is linked with sterility, hormone disruption, birth defects, and cancer.

- **GMOs harm the environment.** GM crops and their associated herbicides harm bees, birds, insects, amphibians, marine ecosystems, and soil organisms.
- **GMO seeds concentrate power** in the hands of a few biotech corporations and marginalise small farmers. GMO seeds are patented products – you have to pay to have the right to use them. It is a traditional right for farmers to save their seed for replanting, or to exchange with other farmers. However, GMO seed patents effectively put an end to these age-old practices. The control and ownership of seeds passes entirely to multinational corporations that hold the patents, like Monsanto, Syngenta and Pioneer. This undermines farmers' rights, and places control of the food outside the country it is grown in.
- By avoiding GMOs, you contribute to the coming tipping point of consumer rejection, which is the only way to force them out of our food supply. If even a small percentage of us start rejecting brands that contain genetically modified ingredients, GM foods will become a business liability. Recent South African examples of consumer success in rejecting GMO foods and forcing the manufacturers to use non-GMO ingredients include Futurelife cereal and Nestlé infant formula and cereals.

Oh South Africa!

The production of GM crops is supported by the South African government. In 1999 the Genetically Modified Organisms (GMO) Act of 1997 came into force paving the way for the growth of the industry. The first GM crops were planted in 1998. 17 years later South Africa is the 8th largest producer of GMOs in the world. In 2013 alone South Africa produced 2.9 million hectares of GM crops.

South Africa is the **only country in the world** that has allowed its staple foods to be genetically modified (GM). The majority of South Africans are eating genetically modified food in the form of Mielie Meal (pap) or bread everyday, without their knowledge or consent and, in the case of mielie meal, without any other non-GM options. While wheat itself has not been genetically modified, most commercial breads in South Africa are made with the addition of GM soya flour.

South Africa is better off than some other countries in the fact that by law, foods containing GMOs' are required to be labelled as such. In 2011 the Consumer Protection Act came into force requiring that all foods containing 5% or more GMOs content must be labelled.

However, several unintended loopholes created by vague wording in the Consumer Protection Act have allowed food producers to avoid the labelling requirements. Until the Consumer Protection Act is revised, food producers are hiding behind the label "May be genetically modified" – or, not labelling at all.

There is hope

While the rules of the World Trade Organisation (which South Africa and 150 other countries are members of) explicitly prohibits countries from banning GM products, as of August 2015 the following countries have made the decision to ban genetically modified crops: Germany, Scotland, Wales,

Greece, Latvia, Russia, Bulgaria, Poland, Italy, Hungary, Austria, France, Luxembourg, Portugal, Spain, Australia, Kenya, Namibia, Uganda, and Mexico.

There are significant restrictions on GMOs in about sixty other countries.

How to avoid GMO's

In the USA you can use **www.NonGMOShoppingGuide.com**. There are over 27,000 products verified as non-GMO listed. Alternatively, only buy products that have the non-GMO label.

Alternatively, use the **EWG's Shopper's Guide to Avoiding GMOs** and **EWG's Food Scores Database** available on their website **www.ewg.org**.

If you do not see a non-GMO label or live in a country that does not have such labels, you can still avoid GMOs by avoiding products that contain anything that is derived from GMO food crops and ideally from the milk, meat, and eggs of animals that have been fed GMOs. In South Africa this would mean only buying organic milk, meat and eggs.

Alternatively – only shop at natural food stores and buy products that are organic.

If you would like to find out more about GMO's I highly recommend Jeffrey Smith's comprehensive book *Genetic Roulette: The Documented Health Risks of Genetically Engineered Foods*.

What is Organic?

Organic food is produced by farmers who emphasise the use of renewable resources and the conservation of soil and water to enhance environmental quality for future generations. Organic food is produced without using synthetic pesticides; fertilisers made with synthetic ingredients or sewage sludge; bio-engineering (GMOs); or ionising radiation (irradiation).

Why should I choose organic food?

Aside from the fact that organic and biodynamic food are non-GMO and contain higher levels of vital nutrients, organic foods are also lower in contaminants that are detrimental to you and your little one's health. These contaminants may include not only growth hormones, antibiotics and pesticides - many of which have been classified as potential cancer-causing agents - but also heavy metals such as lead and mercury, and solvents like benzene and toluene. Heavy metals can damage nerve function, contributing to diseases such as multiple sclerosis. Solvents can damage white blood cell function and lower the immune system's ability to resist infections. Pesticides have been linked to developmental problems in children (in both the brain and the nervous system); act as carcinogens and, disrupt the endocrine system - according to the U.S. Environmental Protection Agency. They are also highly toxic to honey bees and other pollinators – the creatures responsible for pollinating the plants that produce our food.

When it comes to feeding your little one it is important to remember that infants are more at risk for pesticide toxicity than older children and adults because their underdeveloped systems are less able to detoxify these chemicals. Also, children eat more fruits and vegetables than adults (relative to their body weight) so the negative affects will be more pronounced.

RECENT RESEARCH REVEALS:
- A clear link between a mother's exposure to insecticides during pregnancy and deficits to children's learning and memory that persisted through ages 6 to 9. (*Rauh 2001; Lu 2008, 2010; Engel 2011; Bouchard 2011*)
- An increased risk for ADHD among children exposed to typical levels of pesticides. (*Bouchard 2010*)
- Children with high exposures to pesticides were at greater risks of impaired intelligence and neurological problems.
- Eating organic food lowers your and your family's pesticide exposure within days. Studies led by Chensheng (Alex) Lu of Emory University found that just five days after switching to an all-organic diet, school-age children were essentially pesticide-free (*Lu 2006, 2008*).

By choosing to buy organic produce wherever possible, you are protecting the health of your family and sending a message to food producers that you support environmentally-friendly farming practices that minimise soil erosion, safeguard workers and protect water quality and wildlife.

The Dirty Dozen

The American based non-profit advocacy agency The Environmental Working Group (EWG) helps consumers make the healthiest choices by releasing a 'Shoppers Guide to Pesticides in Produce list' every year. While it comes out of America, fruit and vegetables imported from the rest of the world are included in the testing, and since conventional farming methods are similar across the globe, we can assume that this list will be applicable in your country too.

The Shopper's Guide™ includes **The Dirty Dozen** list (produce with the highest levels of pesticide residue) and **The Clean Fifteen** (produce with the least amount of pesticide residue). Because organic foods tend to be more expensive than conventional produce, these lists will help you make informed choices in order to minimise pesticide consumption while keeping your budget in check!

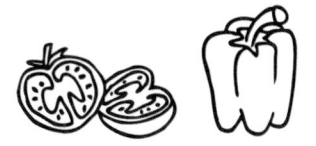

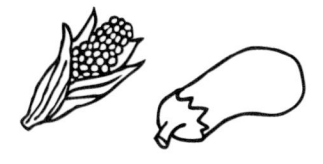

Dirty Dozen PLUS™	The Clean Fifteen™
APPLES	AVOCADOS
PEACHES	SWEET CORN *(but likely to be GMO)*
NECTARINES	PINEAPPLES
STRAWBERRIES	CABBAGE
GRAPES	SWEET PEAS FROZEN
CELERY	ONIONS
SPINACH	ASPARAGUS
SWEET BELL PEPPERS	MANGOES
CUCUMBERS	PAPAYA
CHERRY TOMATOES	KIWI
SNAP PEAS	EGGPLANT (AUBERGINE)
POTATOES	CANTALOUPE (SPANSPEK)
+ HOT CHILLI PEPPERS	CAULIFLOWER
+ KALE / COLLARD GREENS	SWEET POTATOES

+ do not meet traditional Dirty Dozen™ ranking criteria but they contain trace levels of highly hazardous pesticides known to be toxic to the human nervous system. EWG recommends that people who eat a lot of these foods buy organic instead.

Feeding with Awareness

What about washing or peeling the fruits and vegetables?

The data used to create the Shopper's Guide™ is from produce tested as it is typically eaten. This means washed and, when applicable, peeled – so washing a fruit or vegetable would not change its ranking in the EWG's Shopper's Guide™. Also, bare in mind that the pesticides don't just live on the skin of the fruit or vegetable – they are absorbed from the soil through the root system into the flesh.

Fruit and vegetable wash

Not washing your fruits and vegetables certainly increases your exposure to pesticides! In order to wash off as much of the surface pesticide residue as possible use one of the following washes:

HYDROGEN PEROXIDE:
Use 1 tablespoon of 35% hydrogen peroxide solution in a sink full of water. Soak fruits and vegetables for 20 minutes then rinse and scrub.

VINEGAR AND WATER:
Use equal parts white vinegar and water and allow the fruits and vegetables to soak for 20 minutes. Scrub and rinse well.

What if I don't have access to organic fruits and vegetables?

To help your body detoxify pesticides and other contaminants, include fermented vegetables in your diet - the lactic acid bacteria formed during the fermentation of vegetables will help your body break down pesticides.

Plant your own organic veggie garden! This is very rewarding both spiritually and physically. Also, getting your little ones involved in the growing of their own food is not only a fun activity, but a great way to get them interested in food they may otherwise not want to try and, to learn about where food really comes from. Even if you don't have a big garden, or any garden at all – planting herbs in pots on a windowsill, or having some sprouting jars is a great start. The only time Mila will eat peas is when she can pop them out of the pods in our garden!

FOR MORE INFORMATION ON ENVIRONMENTAL AND TOXINS IN OR ON FOOD, PLEASE VISIT THE ENVIRONMENTAL WORKING GROUP WEBSITE: WWW.EWG.ORG

While you may want to avoid eating food contaminated with pesticides, remember that fresh fruits and vegetables (even if they are conventionally grown) are always a healthier choice than processed foods.

A SIDE NOTE – CHILDREN ARE NOT ONLY EXPOSED TO PESTICIDES THROUGH THE FOOD THEY EAT. YOU MAY WANT TO ASK THE SCHOOL THEY ATTEND WHAT THEY ARE SPRAYING ON THEIR PLAYGROUNDS AND SPORTS FIELDS! CHEMICALS ARE ABSORBED THROUGH THE SKIN, AND RUNNING AROUND BAREFOOT ON A GRASSY PATCH THAT HAS BEEN SPRAYED WILL RESULT IN YOUR LITTLE ONE ABSORBING THOSE CHEMICALS.

Irradiation

Irradiation is a food preservation and food safety measure used by the food industry in which foods are treated with radiation from radioactive elements, X-rays, or high energy electron beams. *That's right… radiation… on your food!*

The American Food and Drug Administration (FDA) websites states "Like pasteurising milk and canning fruits and vegetables, irradiation can make food safer for the consumer." *Seriously? I wish I hadn't gone to that website – it makes my blood boil.*

From the same website you can read that irradiation preserves the food by destroying the organisms on natural foods which cause decomposition (think 'good bacteria and probiotics'); delays ripening and sprouting (think 'kills the digestive enzymes in the food') and sterilises the food – essentially, irradiation delivers dead food!

When food is irradiated, some nutrients are destroyed and untested compounds, referred to as URPs (unique radiolytic products), are created.. These products are free radicals, which set off chain reactions in the body that destroy antioxidants, tear apart cell membranes, and make the body more susceptible to cancer, diabetes, heart disease, liver damage, muscular breakdown, and other serious health problems.

No long-term studies have been done on the consumption of irradiated food. The scientific studies which led to the irradiation process being legalised do not meet modern scientific protocols.

Irradiation destroys vitamins, nutrients and essential fatty acids, including up to 95 percent of vitamin A in chicken and 86 percent of vitamin B in oats.

So what foods are commonly irradiated?

MEAT, FRUITS, VEGETABLES, GRAINS, LEGUMES, HERBS, SPICES.

I came to know about irradiation through spices. When I started purchasing organic spices I noticed the labels said, "non irradiated". I compared those to conventional bottles of spices and found that non-organic labels said, "irradiated". I found this very upsetting - I strongly believe in the healing properties of herbs and spices and had been using them accordingly, only to discover that most of the valuable, even medicinal, qualities are purged during the irradiation process. Not only were the healing qualities removed but disease-causing ones had been added.

While you may believe that irradiated foods are safer due to the anti-bacterial action of irradiation, it is important to bare in mind that much of the factory farmed, public slaughter-house meat, and conventionally farmed and produced fruits and vegetables contain food pathogens due to the unsavoury farming practices in which they are created. By purchasing pasture-raised, organic food and following simple food storage and preparation methods, you can reduce your risk of food pathogens.

Also, going back to the spices... two of the main functions of spices and herbs, besides adding flavour to food, are anti-viral and anti-bacterial. They are natural bug inhibitors!

Note to self: *Always buy herbs and spices with labels that say "non-irradiated".*

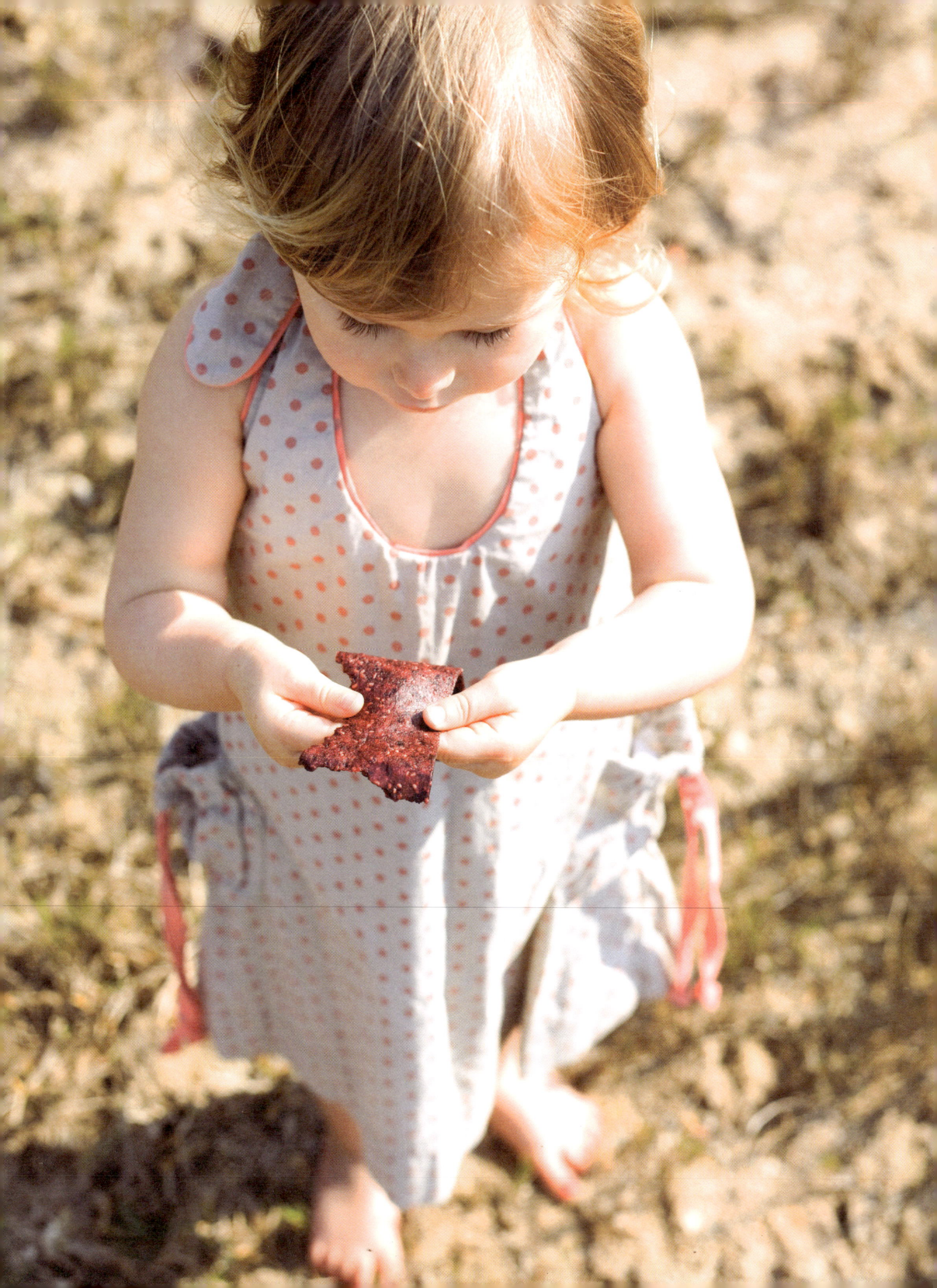

Feeding with Awareness

Why not Gluten, Dairy and Sugar?

"One man's food is another man's poison."

Gluten

Gluten is a difficult-to-digest protein found in the following grains: wheat, barley, rye, spelt and oats*. "Gluten" comes from the Latin word for glue, and its these glue-like properties that hold bread and cake together. But these same properties interfere with the breakdown and absorption of nutrients, including the nutrients from other foods in the same meal.

Gluten triggers inflammatory reactions in people with celiac disease or gluten sensitivity.

SYMPTOMS INCLUDE:

- **Digestive issues** such as gas, bloating, diarrhoea, constipation (particularly in gluten-sensitive children) and diverticulitis,
- **Keratosis Pilaris** (also known as 'chicken skin' on the back of your arms). This tends be as a result of a fatty acid deficiency and vitamin A deficiency secondary to fat-malabsorption caused by gluten damaging the gut,
- **Fatigue, brain fog or feeling tired** after eating a meal that contains gluten,
- **Autoimmune disease** such as Hashimoto's thyroiditis, Rheumatoid arthritis, Ulcerative colitis, Chrohn's Disease, Lupus, Psoriasis, Scleroderma or Multiple sclerosis,
- **Neurologic symptoms** such as dizziness or feeling off balance,
- **Hormone imbalances** such as PMS, PCOS or unexplained infertility,
- **Migraine headaches,**
- **Fibromyalgia,**
- **Inflammation,** swelling or pain in your joints such as fingers, knees or hips,
- **Mood and behavioural issues** such as anxiety, depression, mood swings and ADD.

More than 55 diseases have been linked to gluten and it is also estimated that as much as 15% of the US population is gluten intolerant.

*Oats are technically gluten-free – but since they are often processed in the same facilities as gluten grains, there is the risk of cross-contamination. You can find certified gluten-free oats.

How gluten works *(or doesn't work)* in your system:

As a starting point, it is important to realise that **it is not your stomach that digests food – it is your intestines (or gut)**. It is the stomach's job to break down the food into microscopic particles which can then be effectively digested (by enzymes and the bacteria in your gut) and then, absorbed into the bloodstream through the lining in your intestines.

So, just as gluten holds the ingredients of bread together it also holds together the other food you have eaten with it. This creates a difficult-to-digest 'lump' in your stomach, which is then passed on as only 'partially digested' food to your gut. Partially digested means there are bigger particles of food than can be effectively absorbed by the intestines. The big particles of partially digested gluten are seen as foreign invaders by your immune system, which in turn triggers inflammation of the gut lining in an attempt to protect your body from these 'invaders'. These partially digested food particles also spend longer in the gut than they should, causing them to 'rot'. All this can cause symptoms like diarrhoea or constipation, nausea, and abdominal pain.

The undigested gluten particles irritate your gut and flatten the microvilli (tiny 'hairs') along the small intestine wall. Without those microvilli, you have considerably less surface area with which to absorb the nutrients from your food.

What's the difference between wheat allergy, celiac disease, gluten intolerance, and non-celiac gluten sensitivity?

Gluten intolerance is used when referring to the entire category of gluten issues: celiac disease, non-celiac gluten sensitivity and wheat allergy.

A **wheat allergy** causes the immune system to respond to a food protein because it considers it dangerous to the body. This immune response is often time-limited and does not cause lasting harm to body tissues.

Celiac disease is an autoimmune disorder that affects the digestive process of the small intestine. Essentially it is an allergic reaction to gluten and is characterised by an immune response and intestinal tissue damage. It can be detected via a biopsy. Currently, the only treatment for celiac disease is lifelong adherence to a strict gluten-free diet.

Non-celiac gluten sensitivity (what many call "gluten intolerance") causes the body to mount a stress response (not an immune response). It isn't a food allergy – it's a physical condition in your gut. This may be due to an imbalance in the microflora of your gut, an already damaged gut lining or, a genetic predisposition.

If you remove gluten from the diet, repopulate the microflora and, seal the damaged gut lining, the gut heals and the symptoms disappear. Depending on the level and degree of the intolerance it may be possible to eventually re-introduce properly prepared grains into the diet.

Feeding with Awareness

> *"Waiting until after infancy to introduce grains into a child's diet, raising children on nutrient-dense diets that include liberal amounts of fat-soluble vitamins (especially vitamin A), and keeping good care of intestinal flora may all help prevent celiac disease and non-celiac gluten intolerance in those who are genetically susceptible."*
>
> – CHRIS MASTERJOHN

It must be noted that sugar, antibiotics, environmental toxins, and other allergens (like GMO's, synthetic food additives, transfats etc.) all contribute to imbalanced intestinal flora which can lead to gluten-intolerance (see the Why Not Sugar section next).

I am gluten intolerant (due to a damaged gut lining and gut dysbiosis), which is why I follow a gluten-free diet. As mentioned in the introduction of this book, Mila's 'green poo' alerted me to the fact that she might be too. Whether this is a genetic predisposition inherited from me, or because her microflora was out of balance from birth (again, thanks to me), I chose to feed her a gluten-free diet. I also strongly believe that anything which can potentially damage the digestive system and negatively affect the immune system should be avoided, full stop. Why burden the body unnecessarily? Especially in children, whose digestive and immune systems are still developing.

And besides, gluten just is not necessary.

Dairy

"There is no other food that is as difficult to digest as milk"

– HIROMI SHINYA, M.D

Dairy (from cows) in the form of raw and pasteurised commercial milk and milk products, are a difficult-to-digest food for two reasons:

1. IT CONTAINS A PROTEIN CALLED CASEIN.

Casein makes up nearly 80% of the proteins in cow's milk.

It is a powerful binder – so much so, that it is used to make plastics and furniture glue. It immediately clumps together once it enters the stomach, making digestion very difficult.

Casein is also an allergen – the one responsible for dairy allergies, and the reason why you are advised to only give your little one cow's milk after their first birthday.

When the casein protein is not properly digested, it enters the bloodstream and the immune system reacts, causing inflammation – just as it does with the gluten protein.

Research has also shown that casein stimulates cancer development.

Yes, breast milk does contain casein – but in far lower levels than cow's milk and in a different ratio to milk's other protein - whey. Breast milk also contains an abundance of digestive enzymes, probiotics and other components which will help your little one digest the casein in your milk.

2. IT CONTAINS A SUGAR CALLED LACTOSE.

Lactose intolerance is a non-allergic food sensitivity, and comes from a lack of the enzyme lactase (which is required to digest the lactose). The undigested lactose remains in the digestive tract where the microflora consumes it. As a consequence, there can be bowel urgency, cramps, diarrhoea, and gas.

Our bodies just weren't made to digest milk on a regular basis. The majority of humans naturally stop producing significant amounts of lactase sometime between the ages of two and five. In fact, for most mammals, the normal condition is to stop producing the enzymes needed to properly digest and metabolise milk after they have been weaned. As such, lactose intolerance is considered the normal state for most adults on a worldwide scale and is not typically considered to be a disease condition.

There is another problem with milk too - commercial milk is an unnatural processed 'dead' food. It contains antibiotics, growth hormones and GMO residue to name but a few undesirable components.

IT IS IMPORTANT TO REALISE THAT YOU CAN GET CALCIUM, POTASSIUM, PROTEIN, AND FATS FROM OTHER FOOD SOURCES, LIKE WHOLE PLANT FOODS – VEGETABLES, FRUITS, BEANS, WHOLE GRAINS, NUTS, SEEDS, AND SEAWEED.

Symptoms of Dairy Intolerance:

Classic symptoms are **mucus** (snotty noses, sinusitis, congested ears, ear infections), **respiratory problems** (night-time coughing, asthma), **digestive problems** (such as gas, bloating, diarrhoea, or constipation), **fatigue, joint pains,** and **skin problems** from rashes to acne.

Dairy has been linked to **a range of diseases and conditions** including: cardiovascular diseases; autoimmune diseases; cancer; allergies; asthma; digestive diseases; thyroid problems, and neurological diseases. New research shows that casein may be a factor in autism spectrum disorders (ASD) as well as other physical and mental disorders including chronic fatigue syndrome, fibromyalgia and depression.

According to Hiromi Shinya, commercial pasteurised milk "not only lacks precious enzymes, but the fat is oxidised and the quality of the proteins is changed due to the high temperature." He believes it damages the gut, increasing the amount of bad bacteria and destroying the balance of micro flora.

Herein lies my reason for not feeding dairy to Mila – I want to feed her food that will nourish her, food that is easy to digest, with nutrients that are easy to assimilate into the body. Food that does not have the potential to cause her digestive or immune system any harm and, dairy is not essential or necessary – the nutrients it contains can be sourced from other foods. This decision was also prompted by her 'green poo' and by the fact that I am dairy intolerant. After weaning Mila at 16 months, I did supplement her with homemade goat's milk formula. She did also eat goat's cheese and cow's milk yoghurt for a while. Since the age of 3 she has been completely dairy free – from both cow's milk and goats' milk and their products.

"The 'Calcium myth'- The nurses and doctors will stress that dairy products are the only source of calcium. Did you know that only around 30% of the calcium in animal milk is properly absorbed? Compare this with the 60% of total calcium content of hemp, or plant-based type seeds that is absorbed."

— WH FOODS

Is butter dairy?

Butter is a dairy product, but since it is the lactose and proteins in dairy products that cause digestive issues, butter (which has far less of them than milk) is better tolerated. Butter is about 80-82% fat, 17% water and only about 1% milk solids (proteins). There are only trace amounts of lactose in butter.

If the small percentage of milk proteins in butter still present you or your little one with problems, ghee is a wonderful option.

Ghee is clarified butter. Butter is melted at a low temperature which separates the remaining milk solids (proteins) from the fat. The milk solids (proteins) are then scooped off and all that remains is the fat. There might be minute amounts of lactose in ghee, but they are unlikely to be enough to have an effect on those who are lactose intolerant.

BUTTER / GHEE HAVE MANY NUTRITIONAL BENEFITS:

- They are rich in the most easily absorbed form of Vitamin A - necessary for thyroid and adrenal health,
- Contain lauric acid - important in treating fungal infections and candida,
- Contain lecithin - essential for cholesterol metabolism,
- Contain anti-oxidants that protect against free radical damage,
- A great source of Vitamins E and K,
- A very rich source of the vital mineral selenium,
- Saturated fats in butter and ghee have strong anti-tumour and anti-cancer properties,
- Butter contains conjugated linoleic acid, which is a potent anti-cancer agent, muscle builder, and immunity booster,
- Contain Vitamin D which is essential to absorption of calcium,
- Protect against tooth decay,
- The anti-stiffness factor in butter also prevents hardening of the arteries, cataracts, and calcification of the pineal gland,
- Are a source of Activator X, which helps your body absorb minerals,
- Are a source of iodine in a highly absorbable form,
- Cholesterol found in butterfat is essential to children's brain and nervous system development,
- Contains Arachidonic Acid (AA) which plays a role in brain function and is a vital component of cell membranes,
- Protects against gastrointestinal infections in the very young or the elderly.

Sugar

By sugar, I mean processed sugar - white sugar, corn syrup, high fructose corn syrup, sucrose, dextrose, fructose, and ALL artificial sweeteners.

There are too many bad effects of processed sugar (and any other artificial or processed sweetener) to list here! The one you commonly come across in relation to babies and children is tooth decay. That is merely the tip of the iceberg when it comes to sugar's devastating effects on the body. Its effects are even more pronounced in babies and young children.

With ADD and Candida in Mila's genes, it was a priority for me to avoid sugar in her diet. Research has shown that sugar suppresses the immune system; feeds candida and other pathogens; and, causes a rapid rise of adrenaline, hyperactivity, anxiety, difficulty concentrating, and crankiness in children. According to Dr Sarah Anne Rothman (ND at Pacifica Naturopathic Medicine) **one teaspoon of sugar suppresses your child's immune function by 50% for 24-48 hours!**

According to Nancy Appleton (doctor and author of the book *"Lick the Sugar Habit"*) some of the other negative consequences of sugar include:

- Upsets the mineral relationships in your body: causes chromium and copper deficiencies and, interferes with absorption of calcium and magnesium.
- Feeds cancer cells and has been connected with the development of cancer of the breast, ovaries, prostate, rectum, pancreas, biliary tract, lung, gallbladder and stomach.
- Can cause many problems with the gastrointestinal tract including: an acidic digestive tract; indigestion; malabsorption in patients with functional bowel disease; increased risk of Chrohn's disease; and, ulcerative colitis.
- Greatly promotes the uncontrolled growth of Candida Albicans (yeast infections).
- Can interfere with the absorption of protein.
- Causes food allergies.
- Contributes to eczema in children.
- Can impair the structure of DNA.
- Lowers the ability of enzymes to function.
- Reduces learning capacity, adversely affecting school children's grades and cause learning disorders.
- Worsens the symptoms of children with ADHD.
- In juvenile rehabilitation camps, when children were put on a low sugar diet, there was a 44 percent drop in antisocial behaviour.
- Increases the risk of Polio.
- Dehydrates newborns.
- Contributes to obesity.
- Can cause a decrease in your insulin sensitivity thereby causing an abnormally high insulin levels and eventually diabetes.
- Sugar is addictive.

For the full list of the ways sugar harms your health, I recommend reading "*Lick The Sugar Habit*" by Nancy Appleton.

Besides the negative physical effects sugar has on a child's body, my persistence in not letting Mila have it has a lot to do with the behavioural issues it creates. Clinical research has proven that destructive, aggressive and restless behaviour is significantly correlated with the amount of sugar that is consumed.

I will never forget the first time Mila had (processed) sugar – she was just over 2 years old and at a friend's Tinkerbelle birthday party. It was a fantastic party – décor, dress-up, and treasure hunts! Guess what the treasure was? Gold chocolate coins! Now how could I tell Mila she couldn't have them? I took her aside, sat her on a chair and opened the coins – three of them. I wanted her to be fully aware of the moment. She was mesmerised! The rest of the party didn't exist! She ate her three gold coins, and didn't ask for more. "Oh… that went well", I thought to myself. Twenty minutes later… I came face to face with a little girl that looked like a crack addict! Eyes going in different directions, jaw grinding and wildly racing around the room. I was horrified! I quickly put her in the car, took her home and fed her fried eggs and probiotic capsules! But she was 'difficult' for the rest of that day. We had been in the 'terrible two's' for some time, but there had never been a temper tantrum – not so much as a sulk or shout, until that day. To this day (she is now three and a half years old), Mila has only ever had one other temper tantrum – and that was a couple hours after she had some (very) sugary sweets with her cousin.

This is my choice – I would rather spend time in the kitchen preparing whole free-from foods than spending time caring for a sick child, or disciplining a badly behaved one.

What is life without a little sweetness?

I believe whole, unprocessed natural sweeteners are fine in moderation – one cannot escape the fact that joy is a nutrient too! And sweetness feeds your little one with joy! Healthier sweeteners include: pure maple syrup, molasses, stevia, and raw unfiltered honey.

But what about the parties?

Your child will go to sugar-laden parties and she will want the brightly coloured cake that all her friends are eating. So what do you do?

In choosing to raise Mila as a 'free-from' child it has been very important to me that she never feels 'less than' the other kids – by that I mean, I didn't want her to feel like she was missing out, different, deprived or that there is something wrong with her. That is why I work so hard to create and prepare

Feeding with Awareness

delicious alternatives. I offered these alternatives to Mila at her friends' parties until she was two years old. She did not notice that she was not getting what everyone else was – she was completely satisfied with what I was offering her. In fact, most times her friends wanted some of what she was having!

But there comes a time when mom's free-from chocolate fudge just isn't going to cut it! This is when you have to look at nutrition as more than just food and nutrients. In my studies at the Institute of Integrative Nutrition I have learnt about the power of Primary Foods™. The idea is that as adults, we are nourished by things such as spirituality, exercise, relationships and career. An extension of this is that love is a nutrient – it feeds you - as does joy.

With this in mind, and with my desire for Mila to not feel 'less than', I now let her have the artificially coloured sugary birthday cake. And the result? Mila is fed a healthy dose of Pure Joy! She sings Happy Birthday the loudest, she waits patiently in line to get her slice of cake, then she sits on the side and savours it (often not finishing the whole slice). Does she run around like that crack addict I mentioned earlier? No… but that is because of what happens before the party!

Healthy fats slow down the blood sugar rise caused by the absorption of the sugar into the bloodstream and **probiotics** use the sugar as its food, reducing the amount that gets absorbed into the bloodstream. Eating both fat and probiotics before, or with, sugar in any form, reduces the negative effects of sugar on the body. So, before Mila and I go to a party I feed her a high protein, high fat snack and give her a probiotic supplement! This also helps because she is not hungry at the party – which means she doesn't eat all the other 'less than desirable' food that is on offer. I give her another probiotic supplement when we get home – and ta da… no tantrums, no crazy eyes and, no issues going to sleep at bed time.

> **TREATS NOT SWEETS!**
>
> WHY DO PEOPLE THINK TREATING A CHILD ALWAYS HAS TO INVOLVE SWEETS? HOW ABOUT NEW PAINTS, AN OUTING OR EXPERIENCE, OR ICE LOLLIES FROM FRESHLY MADE JUICE?

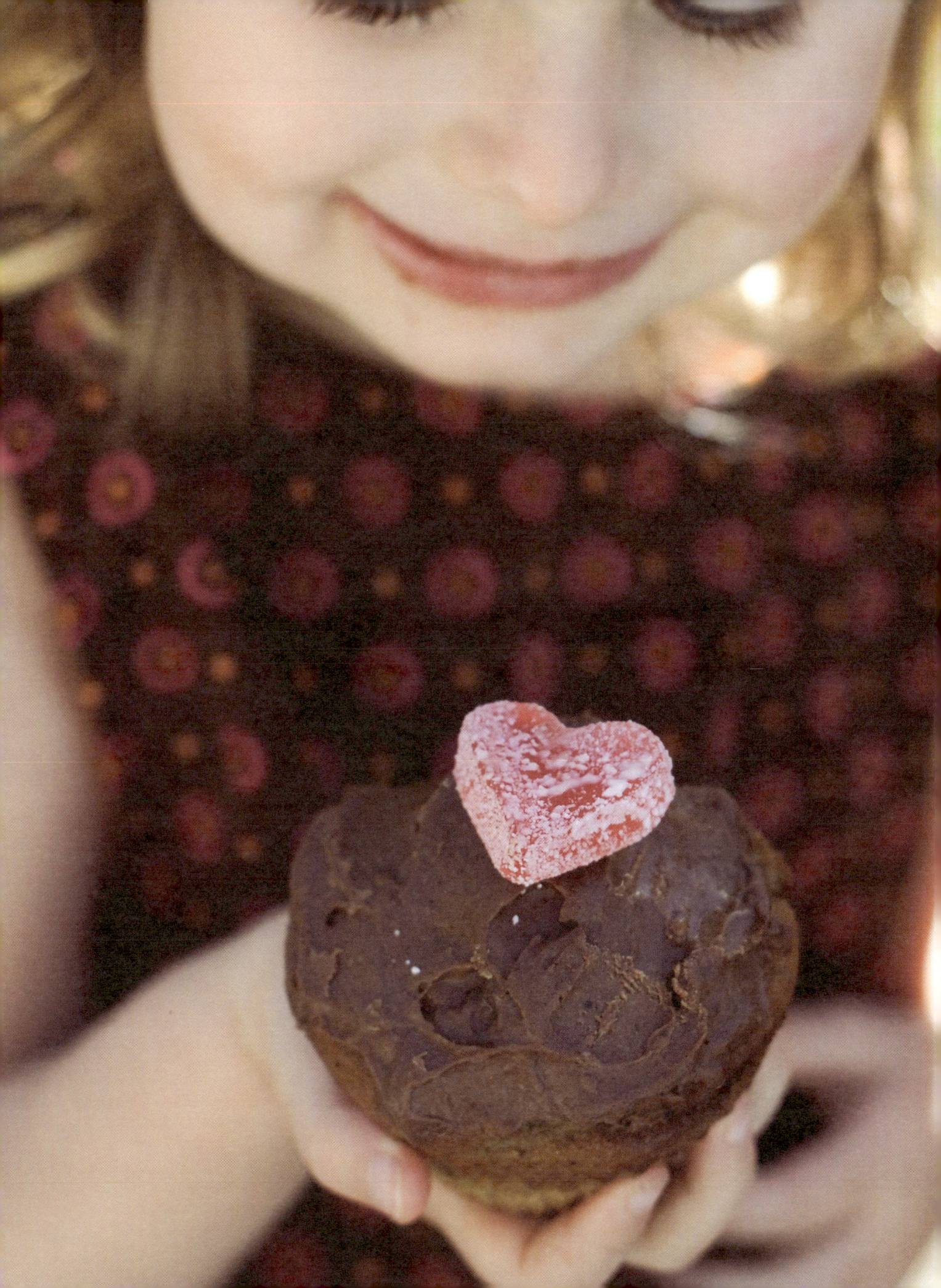

Feeding with Awareness

What can I eat? Gluten, sugar, & dairy alternatives.

I must say, when I realised that I shouldn't eat gluten, dairy and sugar I was left wondering what was left for me to eat! In western culture, we are so accustomed to eating these three things everyday, often many times a day, that when we are asked not to, it seems like an impossible request! But there are so many alternatives… delicious and nutritious ones too! Gluten-free, sugar-free and dairy-free cooking and baking is as rewarding, if not more so, because there is no discomfort after you have eaten the meal!

Gluten-free

The real difficulty in avoiding gluten is when it comes to breads and other baked goods. I'll be honest, I have yet to find a gluten-free bread that is as good in terms of taste and texture as the artisan fermented sourdough bread I used to get from our local baker. It is not really possible to mimic the flexible nature of gluten with gluten-free flours. That being said, Mila enjoys the gluten-free breads I make her, and as for me… well, I've let go of the whole bread attachment. If you get your head around the fact that gluten-free bread is not going to be the same as bread made from wheat flour, you will find that it is as enjoyable – "same same but different", Mila says.

As for the cakes, cupcakes, muffins and cookies – I find gluten-free ones to be much better than wheat-based ones!

The key to gluten-free baking is to use a mix of gluten-free flours in one recipe. No one flour has all the attributes to ensure the baked goods rise and have flexibility. Bags of ready-mixed flours are readily available nowadays.

It is always necessary to add a binding agent such as xanthum gum, guar gum, psyllium husk, chia seeds or flaxseeds to the flour mix for the 'glue-effect' that gluten usually gives. (Ready mixes usually have xanthum gum or guar gum included.)

Another very important thing to know before you begin your gluten-free baking is never, EVER taste the uncooked batter. It just doesn't taste good – ever! (Although Mila eats it by the spoonful – but then again, she doesn't know what she's missing!) The taste of the uncooked gluten-free bread dough or cookie batter is not an indication of what your masterpiece is going to taste like.

The great thing about gluten-free baking is that each of the flours are highly nutritious. Bread is usually just a filler, or base for nutritious toppings. With gluten-free bread, the base itself is nutritious. This gave me great comfort during Mila's 'Toastie' stage – when literally all she wanted to eat was toast!

Gluten-free flour

Almond Flour

Almond flour is, simply, blanched almonds ground into a meal. It is high in protein, heart-healthy fats, and vitamin E. When baking, use almond flour in dense baked goods. You can also use almond flour as a replacement for breadcrumbs, or as coating for chicken or fish.

The trick when baking with almond flour is to beat it with the liquid ingredients from your recipe for a full 2 minutes before adding other ingredients or putting the mixture in the oven. This gives the rather dry flour time to soften and absorb the liquid before it starts cooking. If you do not do this, your baked goods will be incredibly dry and crumbly. (Thanks Justine for this tip which transformed my baking – I am sure Mila and her friends thank you too!)

Rice Flour

Rice flour is made from finely milled rice, and comes in both white and brown varieties. It is a great substitute for wheat flour from a textural perspective so it can be used in traditional baked goods like breads. It is also commonly used in Japanese cuisine to make rice noodles and traditional Japanese desserts.

Amaranth Flour

Amaranth is often considered a grain, but it is actually a seed that dates back 8,000 years. It is made by grinding the seeds into a dust that is rich in fibre and is also a complete protein. It has a slightly earthy, nutty taste and can be used in cookie recipes; however, it may produce a drier batter. You can add some extra water, oil, or applesauce to counteract this effect and get the batter to the desired consistency.

Potato Flour

Potato flour is ground from dehydrated potatoes and is a natural source of B vitamins and fibre. Since potato flour attracts and holds water, it is great for producing moist baked goods such as breads, pancakes, and waffles. It also makes a great thickening agent for sauces and soups.

This flour should not be confused with potato starch flour. Potato flour has a strong potato flavour and is a heavy flour so a little goes a long way.

Buckwheat Flour

Buckwheat is a whole grain and grinding it produces buckwheat flour that is dark in colour and has a strong rich, nutty flavour. It is high in fibre and a good source of calcium and protein. The distinctive flavour makes it great in bread or muffin recipes.

Chickpea Flour

Chickpea flour is a great source of protein, fibre, and iron. It is commonly used in Middle Eastern and Indian cooking to make things like socca (flatbread) and falafel. Since it does have a noticeable chickpea flavour, use it in baked goods that have strong flavours. It is also great in savoury baked items like pizza crust.

Sorghum flour

Sorghum flour is ground from the sorghum grain, which is similar to millet. It is an important staple food in Africa and India. The flour is used to make porridge or flat unleavened breads. I also find it works very well as part of a gluten-free flour mix for muffins and breads. It has high levels of unsaturated fats, protein, fibre, and minerals like phosphorus, potassium, calcium, and iron. It has more antioxidants than blueberries and pomegranates. Some early research suggests is may help reduce the risk of colon and skin cancer.

Quinoa flour *(pronounced 'keen wa')*

Quinoa is related to the plant family of spinach and beets. It has been used for over 5,000 years as a cereal, and the Incas called it "the mother seed". Quinoa provides a good source of vegetable protein and it is the seeds of the quinoa plant that are ground to make flour.

Tapioca flour

Tapioca flour is made from the root of the cassava plant. Once ground, it takes the form of a light, soft, fine white flour. Tapioca flour adds chewiness to baking and is a good thickener. Tapioca flour is an excellent addition to any gluten-free kitchen.

SOME GLUTEN-FREE BLENDS WHICH HAVE WORKED WELL FOR ME:

¾ cup tapioca flour + ¾ cup brown rice flour + ½ cup sorghum flour + 1t. guar gum
1 cup brown rice flour + ½ cup potato flour + ¼ cup tapioca flour + 1t. guar gum

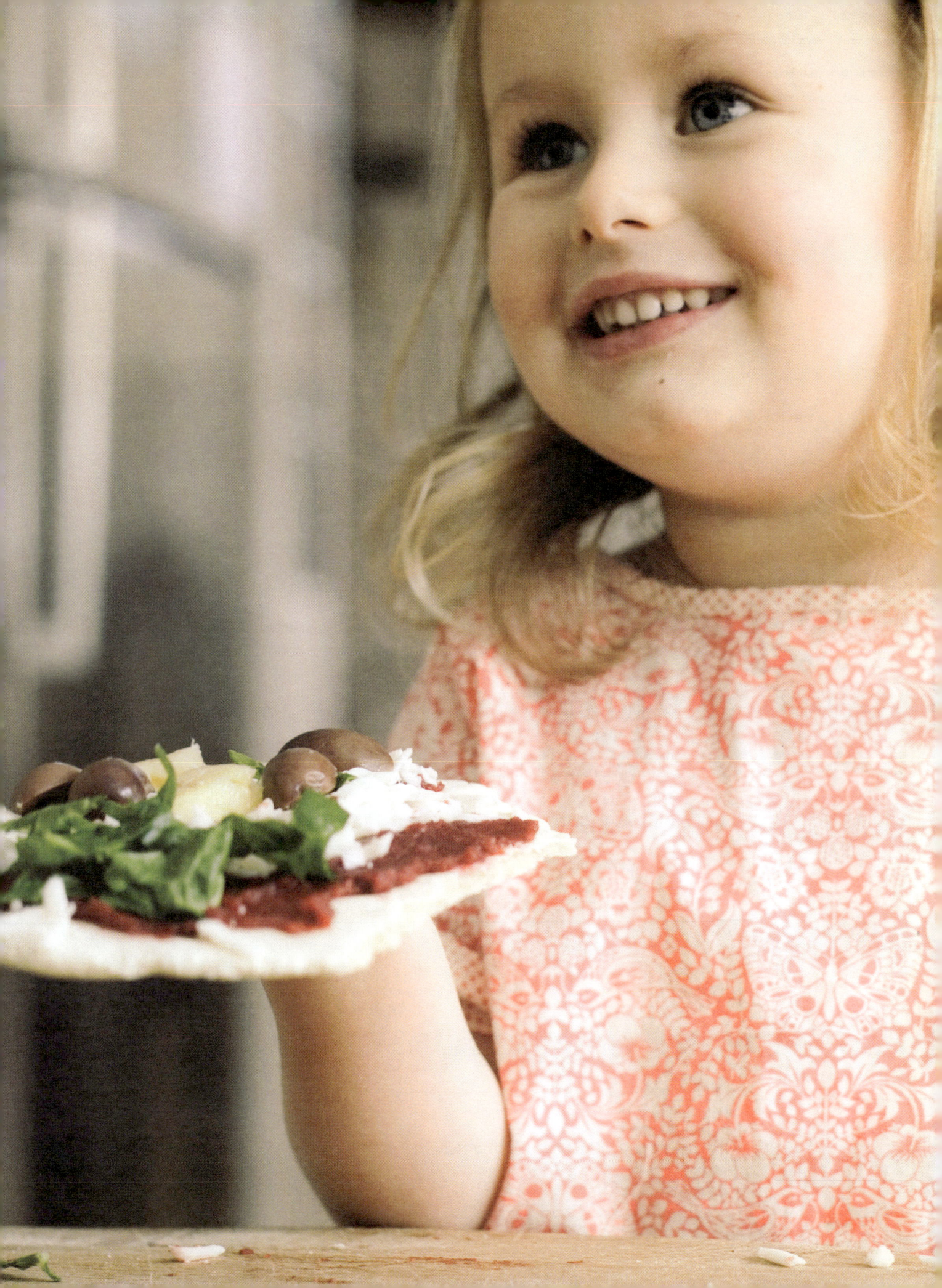

> Feeding with Awareness

Dairy-free

In feeding Mila and for the purpose of this book, 'dairy-free' means free from cow's dairy. I did use goat's milk to make Mila's homemade formula, and I fed her cheese made from goat's milk, and here's why...

Goat's Milk

Goat's milk is generally better tolerated and easier to digest than cow's milk for the following reasons:

- ♥ It is naturally homogenised – the fat globules in goat's milk do not cluster together (which means it does not separate as cow's milk does) making them easier to digest. Cow's milk undergoes a process called homogenisation in order to prevent the milk from separating. This process creates free radicals and makes the milk difficult to digest.
- ♥ It has smaller fat globules as well as higher levels of medium chain fatty acids. These are easier and quicker for intestinal enzymes to digest.
- ♥ Goat milk protein forms a softer curd (the term given to the protein clumps that are formed by the action of your stomach acid on the protein), which allows the body to digest the protein more smoothly and completely. This more rapid transit through the stomach could be an advantage to infants and children who regurgitate cow's milk.
- ♥ It contains only trace amounts of the allergenic casein protein, alpha-S1, found in cow's milk. Goat's milk casein is more similar to that found in human milk.
- ♥ It contains only slightly lower levels of lactose than cow's milk (4.1 percent versus 4.7 percent in cow's milk), but it is said to be better tolerated by people with lactose intolerance. It has been hypothesised that since goat's milk is more easily digested and better absorbed, there is no 'leftover' or undigested lactose which causes the painful and uncomfortable effects of lactose intolerance.
- ♥ Although the mineral content of goat's milk and cow's milk is generally similar, goat's milk contains more calcium, vitamin B-6, vitamin A, potassium, and niacin.
- ♥ The extensive amount of potassium in goat's milk causes it to react in an alkaline way within the body (which is conducive to calcium absorption and retention) whereas cow's milk is lacking in potassium and ends up reacting in an acidic way.
- ♥ Cow's milk is designed to take a 45kg (100 pound) calf and transform it into a 540kg (1200 pound) cow. Goat's milk and human milk were both designed and created for transforming a 3-4kg (7-9 pound) baby/kid into an average adult/goat of anywhere between 45-90kg (100-200 pounds).
- ♥ It is also less likely to be contaminated with antibiotics and growth hormones.

Cow's milk is higher in vitamin B12 and folate, so if you choose to use goat's milk, you need to ensure that these nutrients are being supplied by other foods.

It is my firm belief that once a baby is completely weaned (from breast milk or formula), there is no need for dairy of any kind. The calcium, fats and proteins the milk industry claims we need to get from dairy can all be found in other foods – in a form that is usually more bio-available and more readily absorbed than those from dairy. For example, only about 30% of calcium from dairy sources is absorbed, whereas about 60% of calcium from dark leafy greens is. You can't get your little one to eat her greens? No problem, use baobab powder (twice has much calcium as milk), moringa powder (17 times more calcium than milk), or tahini to get the calcium in.

Okay no goat's milk either – what do I put in my muesli?

There are many dairy-free milks available today but, being dairy-free does not necessarily mean they are healthy!

Soy Milk

Soy milk is made with soybeans, water and a host of other gums, starches and fillers. As with any other unfermented soy product or food, it contains high levels of oestrogen. Due to the fact that soy is a GMO crop and, unless it is fermented, it is a source of anti-nutrients, I avoid it like the plague (in all forms).

Rice Milk

Commercial rice milk is made from soaking and blending rice with water and a host of other ingredients, including GM oils and synthetic vitamins. It is not a suitable substitute for breast milk or formula as it is nutrient deficient.

If you really enjoy rice milk as your dairy alternative, you can easily make your own rice milk to avoid the added ingredients in commercial rice milk:

Place 1 cup cooked rice into a blender and add 4 cups of filtered water. Blend until smooth. Strain through cheesecloth or nut milk bag. Store in the refrigerator and enjoy cold; shake before using. You can add a pinch of vanilla powder or cinnamon for extra flavour, and a date or two for sweetness.

Almond Milk

Almond milk is slightly better than rice and soy milk, though to avoid fillers and added sugars, I suggest making it yourself - which is also be a much cheaper option. If you opt for the store bought versions, choose an unsweetened one.

Feeding with Awareness

A quick almond milk:

Blend 1 cup soaked almonds with 3 cups water, then strain through cheesecloth or nut milk bag. Store in the fridge for up to 3 days. You can sweeten the milk by adding 4 pitted dates to the mix, and flavour with vanilla powder, cinnamon or raw cacao.

Hemp Milk

Do not be confused: although hemp and marijuana/ cannabis come from the same plant, you will not feel any narcotic effects when drinking hemp milk! Hemp does not contain the levels of the active component THC (tetrahydrocannabinol) found in marijuana, and therefore it has no narcotic effect.

Hemp milk has a creamy texture and mild nutty flavour. It is easy to digest and a good source of omega 3 & 6 fatty acids.

Check for added sugars and emulsifiers in commercially available ones. Alternatively, make your own:

Blend 1 cup hemp seeds and 1 tablespoon coconut oil with 3 cups warm water, then strain through cheesecloth or nut milk bag. Store in the fridge for up to 3 days. You can sweeten the milk by adding 4 pitted dates to the mix, and flavour with vanilla powder, cinnamon or raw cacao.

Quinoa Milk

Quinoa milk is made from quinoa grains and water although it may have rice or other grains as part of the mix. It is more nutritious than rice milk and a good source of protein.

Check for added sugars and emulsifiers in store bought ones or make your own:

Blend ½ cup cooked white quinoa with 2 cups water, then strain through cheesecloth or nut milk bag. Store in the fridge for up to 1 week. You can sweeten the milk by adding 4 pitted dates to the blender mix, and flavour with vanilla powder, cinnamon or raw cacao.

Coconut Milk

This is, in my opinion, the best alternative to dairy milk. Coconut milk is made from a blend of coconut fats and fibres and water. Healthy saturated fats and medium chain fatty acids are present in coconut milk. It is a good choice for children because it contains good amounts of fat. Be sure to choose preservative-free, sugar-free and gum-free coconut milk if buying from the shops!

And, if you want to avoid the BPA present in canned milk, make your own:

Blend 1 cup of unsweetened, dried coconut flakes with 2 cups of boiling water, then strain. Store in the fridge for up to 1 week.

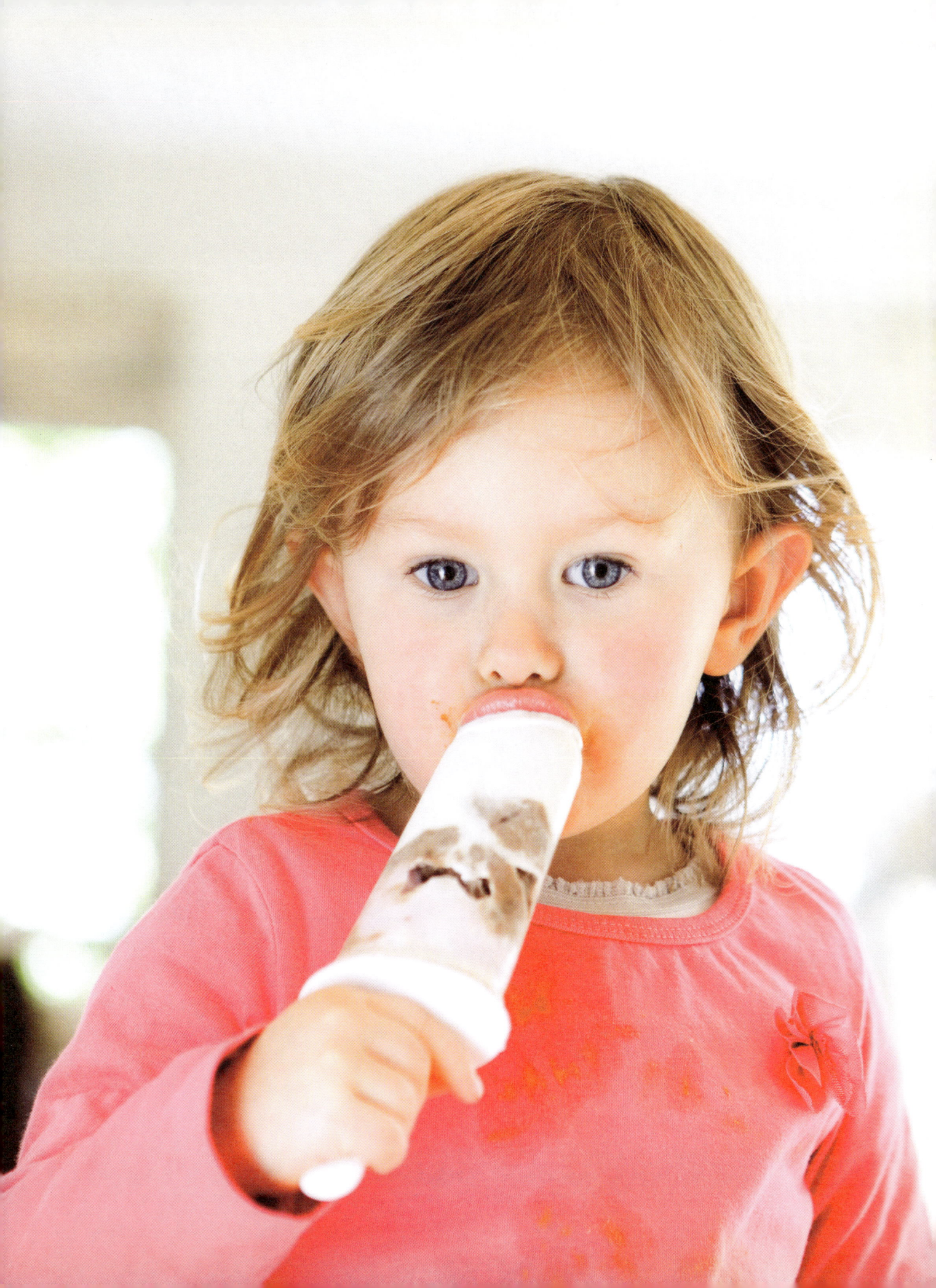

Sugar-free
By 'sugar-free', I mean free-from processed / refined white sugar.

Here is my list of favourite natural sweeteners:

Maple Syrup

Maple syrup is rich in trace minerals and imparts a wonderful flavour to baked goods, cream-based desserts and of course, pancakes and waffles. Be sure to find organic Grade B maple syrup, which is darker and richer in minerals and flavour than Grade A maple syrup. Grade B is also sometimes less expensive than Grade A. "B" stands for "Better" when it comes to maple syrup!

Sucanat

Sucanat is simply dehydrated cane sugar juice and has been used for thousands of year by the people of India. It is available in health food stores.

Blackstrap Molasses

A beneficial by-product from the production of white sugar, molasses has a very strong taste and contains many minerals including iron, calcium, zinc, copper, and especially chromium which is important for the maintenance of healthy blood sugar levels. Be sure to find the unsulphured one.

Raw Honey

Raw honey is loaded with beneficial digestive enzymes and is a great prebiotic.

NOT TO BE GIVEN TO BABIES YOUNGER THAN 1 YEARS OLD.

Stevia

Stevia is a sweet powder made from a South American herb. It is many times sweeter than sugar, so just a pinch of the green stevia powder (or a drop of the liquid) is all that is needed to replace an entire spoonful of sugar. Stevia does not work very well in baked goods.

The strange thing about stevia is that some people perceive the taste as bitter instead of sweet. This is thought to be due to genetic differences.

Coconut Sugar

Coconut sugar is produced from the sap of cut flower buds of the coconut palm. Coconut sugar has been used as a traditional sweetener for thousands of years in the South and South-East Asian regions where the coconut palm is in abundant supply. Coconut sugar has a caramel colour and a taste that is similar to that of brown sugar. It can be substituted for cane sugar in most recipes.

While processed sugar does not contain any vital nutrients and is therefore a source of 'empty' calories, coconut sugar does retain quite a lot of the nutrients found in the coconut palm (such as iron, zinc, calcium and potassium, along with some short chain fatty acids, polyphenols and antioxidants). It is a low glycaemic sugar alternative.

Dates

One of my favourite ways of sweetening Mila's food is by using whole dates. Dates are a source of good fibre, carbohydrate, protein, vitamin B6, potassium, copper, manganese, iron and magnesium. By using the whole food (with the fibre) the sugars are released into the body slowly, so you avoid the 'sugar-spike' effect.

Xylitol

Xylitol is a naturally occurring alcohol found in most plant material, including many fruits and vegetables. It is widely used in natural toothpastes and as a sugar substitute in sugar-free sweets. It can be used as a sugar-free sweetener for diabetics since it has a low glycaemic index and is slowly absorbed and metabolised - independently of insulin. Xylitol can, however, cause diarrhoea and intestinal gas when eaten in large amounts by sensitive individuals or children.

While xylitol can be sourced from the fibres of birch and beech trees, rice, oat, wheat and cotton husks, the main source of xylitol for commercial use is corn cobs – and there is a high chance these are genetically modified.

Xylitol is a highly processed sugar; it is not a whole food (like honey, maple syrup or stevia); and, it is far from natural. I use it occasionally in 'treats', but I prefer to use wholefood sweeteners like dates or honey.

XYLITOL IS HIGHLY TOXIC TO DOGS. So if you own a dog, then keep xylitol out of reach (or out of your house altogether). If you believe your dog has eaten xylitol accidentally, take it to the vet immediately.

But not this...

Agave Nectar

*Fructose in fruit and in cane sugar is bonded to other sugars/carbohydrates, which results in a decrease in its toxicity. The fructose in HFCS and agave is in its 'free' form and not attached to any other carbs, which magnifies its negative effects on the body.

Agave nectar, which has become very popular in alternative health circles, is actually a highly processed sweetener manufactured in a manner similar to high fructose corn syrup (HFCS) and it has an even higher fructose content than HFCS (refined fructose in large doses is more harmful than processed sugar*).

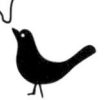

Agave syrup, falsely advertised as "natural," is typically HIGHLY processed and is usually 80 percent fructose. The end product does not even remotely resemble the original agave plant. I would avoid agave nectar at all costs.

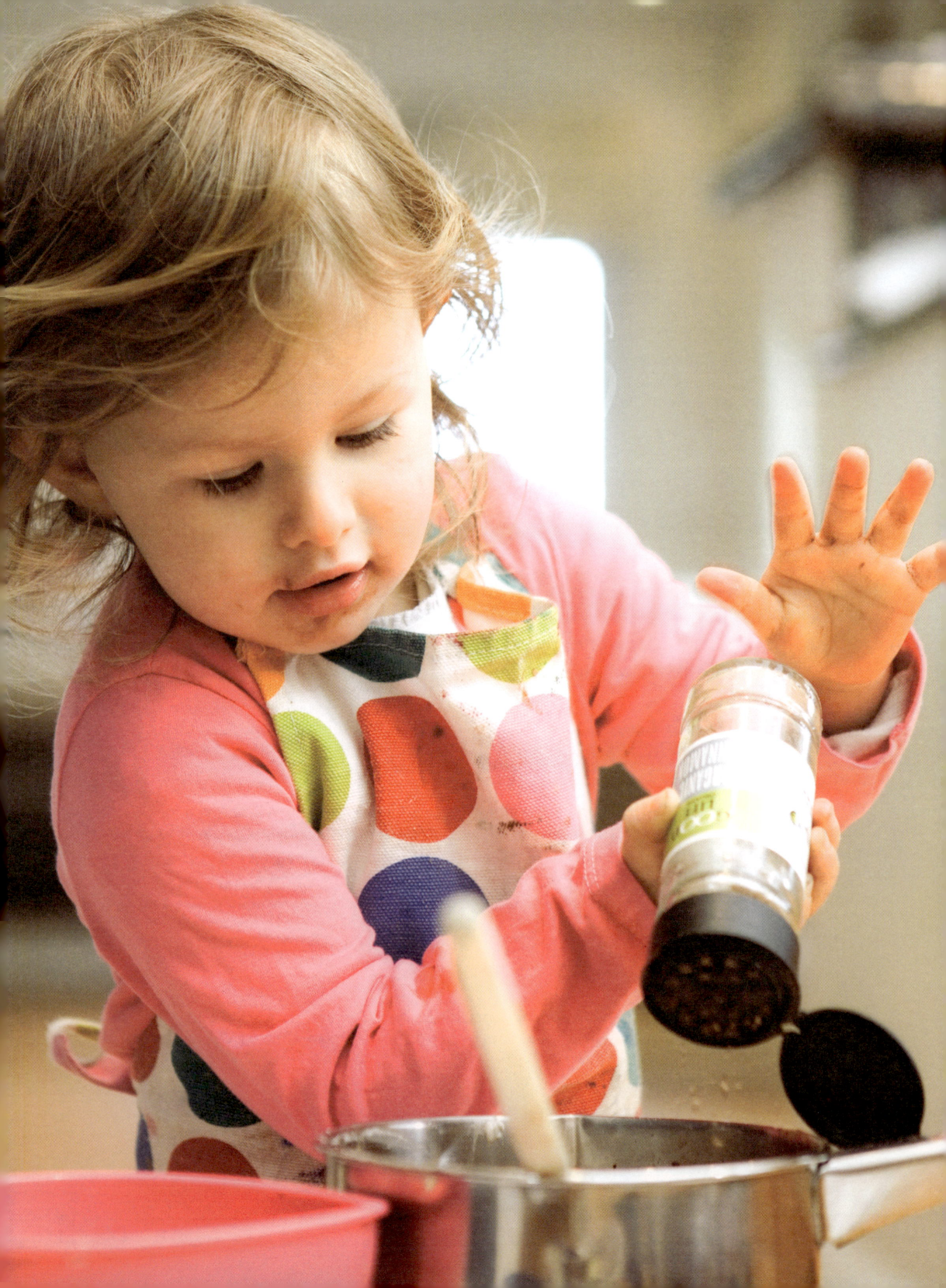

Feeding with Awareness

Nutrient Enhancers: my kind of food additives!

Egg yolk, ghee, flaxseed oil, coconut oil, hemp seed oil, olive oil, sauerkraut liquid, kefir, cinnamon, nutmeg, clove, vanilla, ginger, cardamom, all spice, turmeric, broth, dulse, liver, blackstrap molasses, baobab, cacao, hemp, lucuma, maca, moringa.

It was important for me to make every mouthful of food that Mila swallowed as nutritious as possible because: good nutrition is so important at this stage of life; only a small amount of food is going to go in (at the beginning for some, or forever like with Mila); and, because a lot of food is going to be turned away or spat out when the toddler emerges…

So I developed a list of 'nutrient enhancers' – nutrient dense foods which can be added to almost any purée or meal without significantly changing the taste, texture or appearance… because trust me… there is no greater food detective than an 18 month old!

An excellent example of where nutrient enhancers shine their bright light is in the preparation of plain noodles. "Plain noodles?" I can hear you exclaim! Trust me, there will come a time when your toddler will only want to eat plain noodles, repeatedly, for months on end – and you will make them for her… because you need to choose your battles wisely, because it is the end of a long day, because you have another baby to take care of, or because you are tired!

So this is as plain as Mila's plain noodles got:
I cooked the gluten-free noodles in bone broth with some seaweed (wakame or kombu). Once cooked, I stirred in a raw egg yolk, some coconut oil, a pinch of Himalayan salt and a sprinkle of dulse. Ta da! Plain noodles… that were eaten with glee!

Get creative… there is no end to how sneaky you can be!

Feeding with Awareness

My kind of food additives!

EGG YOLK	♡ Eggs are a source of high-quality protein and have all the B vitamins (including vitamins B1, B2, B3, B5, B6, B12), as well as choline, biotin, folate and cholesterol, selenium, iodine, omega-3 fatty acids, vitamins A, D and E. ♡ Avoid the egg whites for your little one's first year as these contain difficult-to-digest proteins and are what usually cause an allergic reaction. Egg yolks should be softly cooked in the beginning, but from 1 year of age you can add them in raw. They can be blended into all plant-based purées to add fat and protein.
GHEE **FLAXSEED OIL** **COCONUT OIL** **HEMP SEED OIL** **OLIVE OIL**	♡ Adding some healthy fats to your little one's plant-based purées and meals will aid the absorption of vitamins A, D, E and K. ♡ Healthy fats are essential for your little one's brain development
SAUERKRAUT LIQUID **KEFIR**	♡ These will supply probiotics - vital friendly gut bacteria that complete the digestion process, produce vitamins, keep pathogenic ('bad') bacteria in check, and support the immune system.
CINNAMON **NUTMEG** **CLOVE** **VANILLA** **GINGER** **CARDAMOM** **ALL SPICE** **TURMERIC**	Spices are a great way to develop your little one's flavour palette. They also have medicinal qualities and are a source of nutrients. ♡ **Cinnamon** is a great source of manganese, fibre, calcium, potassium, iron, zinc, magnesium and vitamin A. It is known to have antioxidant, anti-diabetic, antiseptic, local aesthetic, anti-inflammatory, warming, and anti-flatulent properties. ♡ **Nutmeg** is a good source of potassium, calcium, iron, manganese, vitamins A, B's and C. It is a useful remedy for: insomnia; anxiety; nausea and vomiting; indigestion (gas) and diarrhoea as well as being an anti-inflammatory and anti-bacterial. ♡ **Cloves** are a great source of manganese, vitamin K, dietary fibre, iron, magnesium, and calcium. They are well known for their ability to relieve tooth and gum pain, aid digestion and provide relief from asthma and bronchitis. ♡ **Vanilla** has antioxidant, anti-depressant and anti-inflammatory properties. ♡ **Ginger** is a good source of vitamin C, magnesium, potassium, copper and manganese. It is a remedy for headaches, motion sickness, nausea, indigestion, wind, colic, cold, flu, bronchitis. Ginger tea is a useful remedy for morning sickness. It boosts the immune system and protects against bacteria and fungi. ♡ **Cardamom** is a great source of iron, manganese, potassium, calcium, magnesium, dietary fibre, riboflavin, niacin, and Vitamin C. It is used as an antiseptic, antispasmodic, carminative, digestive, diuretic, expectorant, stimulant and tonic. It is a remedy for sore throats, constipation, indigestion, and colic. ♡ **Allspice** has a good amounts of potassium, manganese, iron, copper, selenium, magnesium, vitamin A, vitamin B6, riboflavin, niacin and vitamin C. It has anti-inflammatory, warming and soothing and anti-flatulent properties and is known to aid digestion. ♡ **Turmeric** is a powerful anti-inflammatory and anti-oxidant and an excellent source of iron, manganese, vitamin B6, dietary fibre, potassium, Vitamin C and magnesium.
BROTH	♡ Instead of using water to thin a purée or to cook the vegetables in, use bone broth. ♡ Bone broth builds a healthy gut and digestion; aids muscle repair and growth; fights inflammation; creates a balanced nervous system and a strong immune system; inhibits infection caused by cold and flu viruses; helps protein and mineral absorption; promotes strong, healthy bones. ♡ It is a source calcium, magnesium, phosphorous, sulphur, boron, zinc, peptides (healing amino acids and natural antibiotics), collagen, omega-9s, iron, vitamin B6 and B12. All the nutrients are easily absorbed by your little one's body (bio-available).

My kind of food additives!

DULSE	♡ Dulse is an excellent source of calcium, potassium and vitamin B12 - making it a useful addition to any dairy-free or vegan diet. It is also a great source of protein, vitamin B6 and A, iron, phosphorus, manganese, and iodine. ♡ Sprinkle dulse flakes into purées, or other meals.
LIVER	♡ Liver is an excellent source of high quality protein, omega 3 fatty acids, vitamin B complex (including choline, B12 and folate), a highly bio-available form of iron, vitamin D, vitamin E, pre-formed vitamin A (retinol), vitamin K2, various amino acids and trace minerals such as copper, zinc, chromium and cholesterol. ♡ A small amount (1 teaspoon) of raw liver can be grated into any purée. The liver must be frozen for 2 weeks before using it raw (fourteen days will ensure the elimination of pathogens and parasites). Alternatively add some Chicken Liver pâté into purées of other meals.
BLACKSTRAP MOLASSES	♡ Blackstrap molasses is one way to boost your little one's iron intake. Its other nutrients include manganese, copper, calcium, potassium, magnesium, vitamin B6, and selenium. It can be useful in alleviating constipation (but too much will cause diarrhoea). ♡ Mila often had molasses added to her purées and many of her muffins and cookies. It is also an ingredient in the homemade formula.
BAOBAB **CACAO** **HEMP** **LUCUMA** **MACA** **MORINGA**	The superfoods are a blessing to any new mom stressing about getting enough nutrients into her little one! Granted, they are expensive, but a little goes a long way so they are not something you will need to add to your shopping list every month. Mila (now age 3) is an exceptionally picky eater – she will not eat anything that looks like a vegetable. She actually stopped eating chips (homemade in coconut oil!) when she found out they were made from potatoes! Superfoods have been my saving grace. While I do hide vegetables in all of Mila's food, I am secure in the knowledge that any nutrient shortfall is being covered by these easy-to-hide, and in most cases delicious, powders. ♡ **Baobab** contains six times more vitamin C than an orange, twice as much calcium as a glass of milk and more iron than a steak, three times more anti-oxidants than blueberries and six times more potassium than a banana! It is also a good source of magnesium, potassium, and B vitamins. Due to its easily digestible calcium content it is an excellent addition to your little one's diet if you are avoiding dairy. Baobab protects against free radical damage, builds strong bones, boosts the immune system and soothes tummy upsets. ♡ **Cacao** is the food with the highest levels of antioxidants of any food on Earth. It also contains high amounts of iron and magnesium as well as Vitamin C, fibre, calcium, protein potassium, phosphorus, copper, and zinc. The most important healing benefit of cacao is… pure joy! ♡ **Hemp** is an excellent source of healthy fats, protein, fibre, carbohydrates, iron, zinc, copper, calcium, magnesium, potassium, carotene, vitamins B1, B2, B6 and E. Hemp improves the functioning of the immune system; supports brain health; regulates blood sugar; and soothes eczema and psoriasis. ♡ **Lucuma** is an excellent source of carbohydrates, fibre, protein, beta-carotene, niacin and vitamin C. It a good source of minerals such as calcium, phosphorus, zinc, and it has remarkable concentrations of iron. Lucuma has antibiotic, antimicrobial, and antifungal benefits. It can help stabilise blood sugar, boost the immune system and speed up the healing process. ♡ **Maca** is a complete protein and has over 20 amino acids. It an excellent source of vitamins B, C, and E, calcium, zinc, iron, magnesium, phosphorous, potassium, sulphur, copper, selenium and fatty acids. ♡ **Moringa** is an excellent source of vitamins A, B, and C, calcium, iron, potassium and it is a complete protein. Moringa leaves are also one of the few plant sources of omega 3 fatty acids. Moringa boosts the immune system and can benefit condition such as anaemia, asthma, constipation, and diarrhoea.

MESS

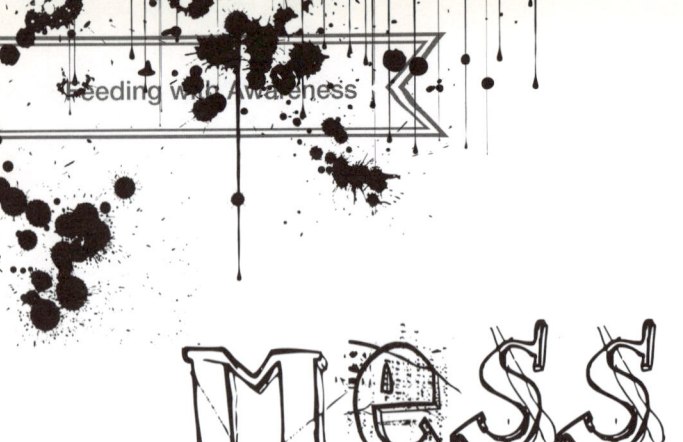

Mess is good!

Meal time with your little ones is about so much more than getting full and being well nourished. Besides learning all sorts of social and cultural norms, it is some of their first active (and rewarding) sensory play experience. Allowing your little ones to play with their food and to eat with their hands, gives them a tactile connection with their food. Eating can (and should) employ all the senses; sight, smell, sound, taste and touch. It is then mindful eating – an important ritual for your little one to carry through life, and for us as adults to relearn.

Playing with food, or eating 'finger foods', plays a very important part in digestion too. In Indian culture, where traditionally they eat with their hands, there is a saying that, *"eating food with your hands, feeds not only the body but also the mind and the spirit"*. As the Indians have known for centuries, and as science is now showing us, digestion begins before the food enters your mouth. Allowing your little one (and yourself) direct hand contact with the food is a great way to improve digestion. When you touch the food with your hands, your brain signals your stomach that you are about to eat. This in turn, releases digestive enzymes and readies your stomach to digest the food it will receive, resulting in better digestion.

The food smearing, throwing and spitting are not signs that your little ones do not approve of your cooking! These antics all serve an important developmental purpose. By smearing the food all over and by getting some off their hands and into their mouths, they are: creating a mental map of where their mouths are; learning that they can feed themselves; realising that the hand can act upon an object; developing manual dexterity; and, developing hand-eye co-ordination. While they will start smearing with their whole hand, at about 9 months old, they will only smear with their index finger. This is the beginning of 'finger isolation' - the ability to move each finger one at a time – which is an essential activity needed to complete countless daily task later in life. These are just some of the many things your little ones are learning with each little mouthful.

With so much going on at a mealtime, you should expect it to take some time – and allow for it.

By allowing the mess (and the learning) you are helping to send the signal that mealtime is safe, fun, and an opportunity to try new things – as well as being delicious and nutritious! Soul Food

Feeding with Awareness

Soul Food

At the Institute for Integrative Nutrition®, where I am currently completing my studies to be a Holistic Health Coach, they have developed the concept of Primary Food. Essentially, primary food is nourishment that doesn't appear on your dinner plate. Joshua Rosenthal (IIN®'s founder, director and primary teacher), says that, "Healthy relationships, regular physical activity, a fulfilling career, and a spiritual practice can fill your soul and satisfy your hunger for life." The premise is that when these areas of your life are in balance, food is secondary. They are, essentially soul food.

"The fun, excitement, and love of daily life have the power to feed us so that food becomes secondary." - IIN®

So what would soul food for your little one be? I would venture to say they would be: **loving relationships, physical activity, spiritual practise and play.**

Love

"Feelings are for the soul what food is for the body." - RUDOLF STEINER

Besides your little one's basic needs (such as food, sleep and shelter), love is the most important 'food' for a young baby. Scientific evidence shows that love, attention, and affection in the first years of life have a direct and measurable impact on a child's physical, mental, and emotional development. Love and touch actually cause your child's brain to grow, according to Marian Diamond, a neuroscientist and author of *'Magic Trees of the Mind: How to Nurture Your Child's Intelligence, Creativity, and Healthy Emotions From Birth Through Adolescence'*.

There really is no such thing as 'spoiling' a newborn. Show your love through: feeding on demand; touch; verbal and non-verbal communication; eye contact; responsiveness (quickly responding to their needs, distress and crying); and, carrying your little one often as you can.

"Children who live in an atmosphere of love and warmth, and who have around them truly good examples to imitate, are living in their proper element." - RUDOLF STEINER, 'THE EDUCATION OF A CHILD'.

Love is essential not only for your little one's growth and development, but for her future health as well. According to Dr. David Hamilton "Some research suggests that a parent's love can have health

Feeding with Awareness

effects later in life. This makes sense, especially if part of the brain's growth is laid down in early infanthood. Thus, the way the child (and eventually, adult) responds to life situations, particularly stressful ones, will be linked with this. It seems like emotional deprivation as an infant can leave the adult less able to deal with stress, like love is the vital nutrient required to build parts of the nervous system. Love in early childhood seemed to confer some sort of resistance to these typically lifestyle associated conditions. Love aids the building of healthy biology."

Food is love

From the moment you start life as a newborn, being fed is an act of **receiving love**. As a new mother, the very intimate act of breastfeeding is the most incredible **gift of love**.

Providing a meal for your family is one of the most basic ways to express love and caring, and putting time and effort into food preparation makes this love and caring apparent. Food is often the medium through which we demonstrate our love and concern for our children – if they are sick, we make chicken soup; if it is their birthday, we prepare their favourite meal. This is also the reason why, when your little one refuses your food, it tends to hurt – we perceive it as rejection.

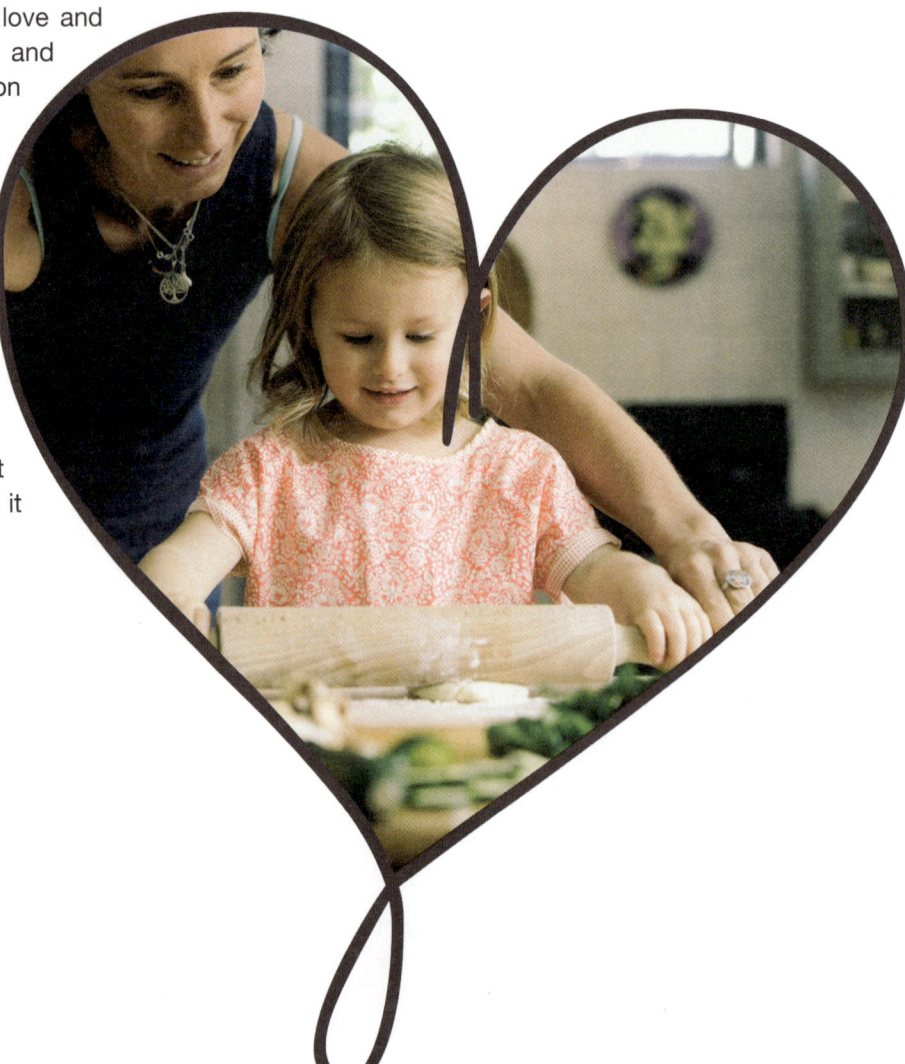

Physical activity

As adults we all know the many benefits of exercise and physical movement. But children it has far greater implications than simply muscle strength, fitness and the release of serotonin, for example. Your little ones' neural pathways and connections are developed through movement. As they learn to reach, roll, sit up, crawl, pull up and walk they are actually developing their brain. The simple act of swopping your little ones from the right breast to the left during breastfeeding, stimulates different areas of their brain!

Infant body movement leads to the development of:

- Fine and gross motor skills,
- Hand-eye coordination,
- Balance,
- Emotional stability and control,
- Visual perception,
- Auditory processing,
- Speech and language abilities,
- Body awareness,
- Self-regulation,
- Regulate muscle tone,
- Improve memory,
- Concentration,
- Organisation,
- Vestibular sensitivity,
- Comprehension.

Research has shown that it is a child's activity level and active playtime that determines his or her ultimate brain development and the extent of adult capabilities (*Carla Hannaford, 2005*).

Early movement and physical development aside, as your little one gets older exercise and physical activity are crucial. They increase the flow of blood to the brain; build new brain cells which leads to your child's openness to learning and greater capacity for knowledge; increase the ability of the brain to shift thinking and produce creative, original thoughts; creates spatial awareness and mental alertness; reduce stress; improve confidence, teamwork and leadership; and, the more children move, the more information they are gathering about the their environment and themselves.

Physical activity and food

Growing your own food is a wonderful opportunity for fun physical activity for you and your little one. In fact, it is one activity that incorporates all the Primary Foods (love, spiritual practice, fun and physical activity) as well as secondary food in the form of delicious and nutritious food.

Spiritual practice

First... What is spirituality?

Spirituality has to do with the spirit. No not as in ghosts, but as in the essence of being human — your **soul** or your **inner life**.

Spirituality is often connected to a formal religion, but it does not have to be. Besides prayer, or attending church, spirituality may be practicing yoga or meditation, or nurturing your spirit by spending time in nature. **Religions usually have defined beliefs, rituals, and guidelines; spirituality is more individual.**

> *"From the day your baby is born, you are a teacher of spirit. Look upon spirituality as a skill in living, since that is what it is. I believe in imparting these skills as early as possible by whatever means a child can understand."*
>
> – DEEPAK CHOPRA

We all need direction and guidance on life's journey, and that is what a spiritual practice gives us - a sense of belonging, peace, joy, hope, ritual, connectedness, protection... And confidence.

The idea that **'we are spiritual beings having a physical experience'** is an important one. While many adults attempt to reconnect with spirit, children are born connected to it. This connection must be acknowledged and nurtured.

"Every child has a spiritual life already. This is because every child is born into the field of infinite creativity and pure awareness that is spirit. But not every child knows that this is true. Spirit must be cultivated; it must be nourished and encouraged. A child raised with spiritual skills… will be able to practice non-judgment, acceptance, and truth, which will be free from fear and anxiety about the meaning of life. When kids understand the way the world works from a spiritual point of view, it makes it easier for them to navigate through life with joy, love, and happiness." – Deepak Chopra

A spiritual practice can be (and usually is) different for each person or family – but essentially, it is **any act that connects you to Spirit**.

For you and your little one it could be: spending time in nature; yoga; meditation; music; dance; prayer; greeting the day; family meals and gatherings; celebrations such as Christmas or Passover; baptisms and christenings. According to psychologist Lisa J Miller, author of the book *The Spiritual Child*, "Regular practice as a family paves a pathway for the child that endures a lifetime. It will be there for your child in times of developmental change and challenge."

As with many things, the best way to introduce spirituality to your child is by example. When they see you living your values, they will take that in more deeply than any preaching or teaching could do.

Feeding with Awareness

I believe for children, spending time in nature is an ideal spiritual practice because, to be a spiritual person is to be a participant in the process of life. And nature shows this so perfectly – from the new leaves in spring, to a flower that grows, wilts and dies.

Spiritual lessons we can learn from nature

- **Nurture.** If you water a plant it will grow, if you don't it will die.
- **Acceptance and non-resistance.** The seasons change no matter what, each brings its own joy.
- **Unconditional love.** The uninhibited, unreserved and forgiving love given by a pet, for example (even a pet that is sat on and pulled around by the tail!).
- **Connectedness.** The flowers create pollen, which the bees use to make honey, which will soothe your little one's sore throat. It is a universal oneness that teaches one to respect and develop loving relationships with nature and animals.
- **Transience.** Nothing is permanent, the day always follows the dark night.
- **Faith in tomorrow.** We plant seeds today, nourish them with love and attention with the faith that our labour will reap fruit in the future.
- **Compassion.** For example, removing spiders from the house instead of squashing them.
- **Gratitude.** Being grateful for the harvest from your vegetable garden, which will feed you tonight.
- **Non-discrimination.** Flowers don't grow for some people and not for others. Nature is available to all.
- **The life cycle and change.** No better example exists than that of a butterfly. Don't resist change. Some of the most beautiful wisdom and changes occur as you grow older and transform from a caterpillar to a butterfly. Appreciate each phase of your life before you transform to a new cycle.
- **Belief that there is something greater than yourself.** The whole rhythm of nature is a wonder. In many ways it is inexplicable.

Whether it be a formal religion, or spending time in nature, incorporate your spiritual practice into your little one's daily life from the beginning so that it becomes instinctive and second nature - not something he/she has to 'learn' at a later stage.

Other ways to nurture spirituality:

- **Use daily events** to teach spirituality. For Mila I did little things – like opening the curtains very morning and greeting the new day with a "Morning beautiful day." When she started talking, she started saying this with me.
- **Tell stories** from how the world was created, to why people sometimes do bad things. Introduce your child to the notion that different people have different beliefs, myths, and traditions by drawing from the Bible, Hindu mythology or Jewish folktales, for example.
- **Build on family traditions** as a way of connecting to the past and to each other. Acknowledging and embracing family life as sacred, gives your child a spiritual place to live in everyday.
- **Make it fun.** Gospel music may not be your music of choice – but little ones love to dance to it!
- **Practicing silence** gives your little one time to collect themselves, connect to the world around them, as well as to their inner voice. What begins as a moment of silence, can lead to a longer meditation.
- **Pray.** I introduced Mila to prayer as a way of practising gratitude. Too often it is all about wants

and needs. Each night we take turns to give thanks for a something that has happened in the day and for the family and friends that love us. It is an amazing chance for reflection and appreciation – and now that Mila is three, the things she says give real insight into who she is and where she is at.
- **Add the spirit back to the holidays** by balancing the commercialism of the holiday seasons with activities that underscore its deeper meaning - such as volunteering at a charity, or donating unused clothes and toys to those in need. Make your own decorations and gifts.

> *"I feel that spiritual parenting will have the most lasting effect if it builds a foundation in the self rather than focusing on principles."*
>
> – DEEPAK CHOPRA

Food is sacred

Rituals centred on food appear in many faiths including Christianity, Judaism, Islam, Hinduism and Buddhism:

- Blessing food has been an important part of the eating experience. People have been **saying blessings, grace, or prayers of thanksgiving** over food as far back as the first human cultures. Today we are discovering that besides being a spiritual act, blessing food creates molecular and physiological changes in yourself as with as in your food (as shown in the studies by Masuro Emoto).
- Some Catholic and Orthodox Christians observe several **feast and fast days** during the year. For example, they may fast or avoid meat on Fridays, during Lent or on Good Friday. Some eat fish instead.
- The ritual of communion is regularly celebrated by many Christians. This involves **eating bread and drinking wine** (or substitutes) to represent the body and blood of Jesus Christ.
- Food forms an integral part a daily Jewish spiritual practice. **Kosher** means that a food is 'fit' or permitted. Foods such as pork and shellfish are strictly forbidden.
- **Ritualised fasting** is also included in Judaism. For example, Yom Kippur – the Day of Atonement – is a Jewish fast that lasts from approximately dusk till dusk.
- Jewish **feast days** include Rosh Hashanah and Passover.
- Moderation in all things (including eating and dietary habits) is central to the Muslim way of life. When done according to the way of Allah, **daily acts like eating are considered a form of worship**.
- The list of **Halal foods** excludes pork, alcohol and any products that contain emulsifiers made from animal fats, particularly margarines.
- Hindus believe in the interdependence of life. People who practice the Hinduism **refrain from eating meat or any food that has involved the taking of a life**. They also avoid foods that may have caused pain to animals during its manufacture. 'Karma' is believed to be the spiritual load we accumulate or relieve ourselves of during our lifetime. If a Hindu consumes animal flesh, they accumulate the Karma of that act, which will then need to be balanced through good actions and learning in this life, or the next.
- In his multiple lives on Earth, Buddha cycled through various animal forms before attaining the form of a human being. Most Buddhists choose to **vegetarianism** in order to avoid killing animals.
- Buddhist monks and nuns are not allowed to cultivate, store or cook their own food - instead, they must rely on **'alms'**, which are donations from believers. This sometimes includes meat, as monks and nuns are not allowed to ask for specific foods.
- All these faiths practice fasting at certain times of the year as a way to promote spiritual growth.

Saying grace

Blessing and giving thanks for your food brings the sacred into your everyday life. When you get into the habit of infusing your food with light and blessings before each meal, you acknowledge the sacred nature of this very important aspect of life.

Saying grace before a meal changes you physiologically - salivation increases, digestive enzymes are released, breathing and brain patterns shift to a receptive mood ready to enjoy. It also changes the food's vibrational energy. Taking this moment before beginning to eat, makes you more mindful of eating which in turn makes it easier for your body to assimilate nutrients.

Saying grace is a wonderful way to bring spirituality into everyday life for your little one. Here are some of my favourites...

Thank you Father,
Thank you Father,
For our Food,
For our Food
And our many blessings,
And our many blessings,
Amen,
Amen.

For our friends,
for our families,
for our meal,
we are thankful.
For life,
for healing,
for joy,
we are thankful.

Thanks to the earth
for the soil.
Thanks to the sky
for the rains.
Thanks to the farmers
for the food.
Thanks to our friends
for the love.

Spiritually symbolic foods

- **Baklava:** in Greece, it is supposed to be made with 33 dough layers, referring to the years of Christ's life.
- **Easter eggs:** associated with Easter, as a symbol of new life.
- **Hot cross buns:** traditionally eaten on Good Friday, to break the fast required of Christians on that day.
- **Pancakes:** traditionally eaten by Christians on Shrove Tuesday to symbolise the end of rich eating before Lent (which begins the following day).
- **Pretzel:** created in Southern France in 610 AD by monks who baked thin strips of dough into the shape of a child's arms folded in prayer.
- **Apples and honey:** eaten on Rosh Hashanah, to symbolise a sweet new year in the Jewish faith.
- **Maror:** a bitter herb eaten at the Jewish Passover Seder to remind followers of the bitterness of slavery.
- **Matzo:** a type of unleavened bread eaten at the Passover Seder (and the following week), symbolically recalling the Jews leaving Egypt in too much haste to allow their bread to rise in the ovens.
- **Dates:** traditionally dates are eaten at the Iftar meal to break the fast of Ramadan, symbolically recalling the tradition that the prophet Muhammad broke his fast by eating three dates.
- **Ghee:** sacred food of the Devas. Burnt in the Hindu ritual of Aarti, offered to gods, and used as libation or anointment ritual.

> *"Spirituality is a way of living, an experiential space. It is a lived reality, so it is a way of being with hardship. It is a way of being with joy. Spirituality is a way of being in the world that informs every moment."*
> Lisa J Miller.

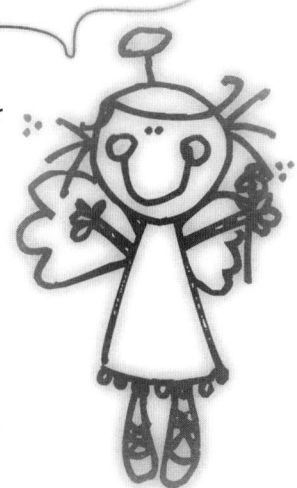

Feeding with Awareness

Feeding with Awareness

Play

Do you remember, as a child, how secondary food was to play? How when your mom called you in from the beach for dinner, your reply was simply that you weren't hungry? How often you simply had a few bites, went out to play again and fell into bed for a long peaceful sleep without the need for a midnight snack? As children, we all lived on primary food, and play is a very important one.

'Play' is to children as 'career' is to adults – it facilitates physical, emotional, cognitive, social, and moral development and self-expression.

Play is an integral part of childhood development. Participating in **early play** with textures, shapes and colours your little one develops cognitive thinking, social and psychomotor skills.

Later, **imaginative and fantasy play** becomes important for emotional development as it allows children to explore their world and express their innermost thoughts and feelings, hopes and fears, likes and dislikes. Through play, decisions are made without threat or fear of failure.

Play allows children to gain control of their thoughts, feelings, actions, and helps them to achieve self-confidence.

Food is the perfect toy!

How many times were you told to stop playing with your food? Well, research has found that toddlers who play with their food are more likely to be better learners! Messy eaters who constantly poke, prod, touch, feel, and even throw their food are simply engaging in active learning strategies.

Your little ones explore their world, and learn, by using their senses. Dinnertime is a perfect time to do this as food appeals to all the senses simultaneously. Exploring the smell, shape, colour, taste, temperature and texture of food helps children learn about their world.

Let your child play with their food. When they are ready, serve food that varies in texture, colour and smell – they will get to practice their pincer grasp and explore their senses. Allowing meal times to be fun, will also allow your little one to develop a healthy relationship with food and will encourage better digestion.

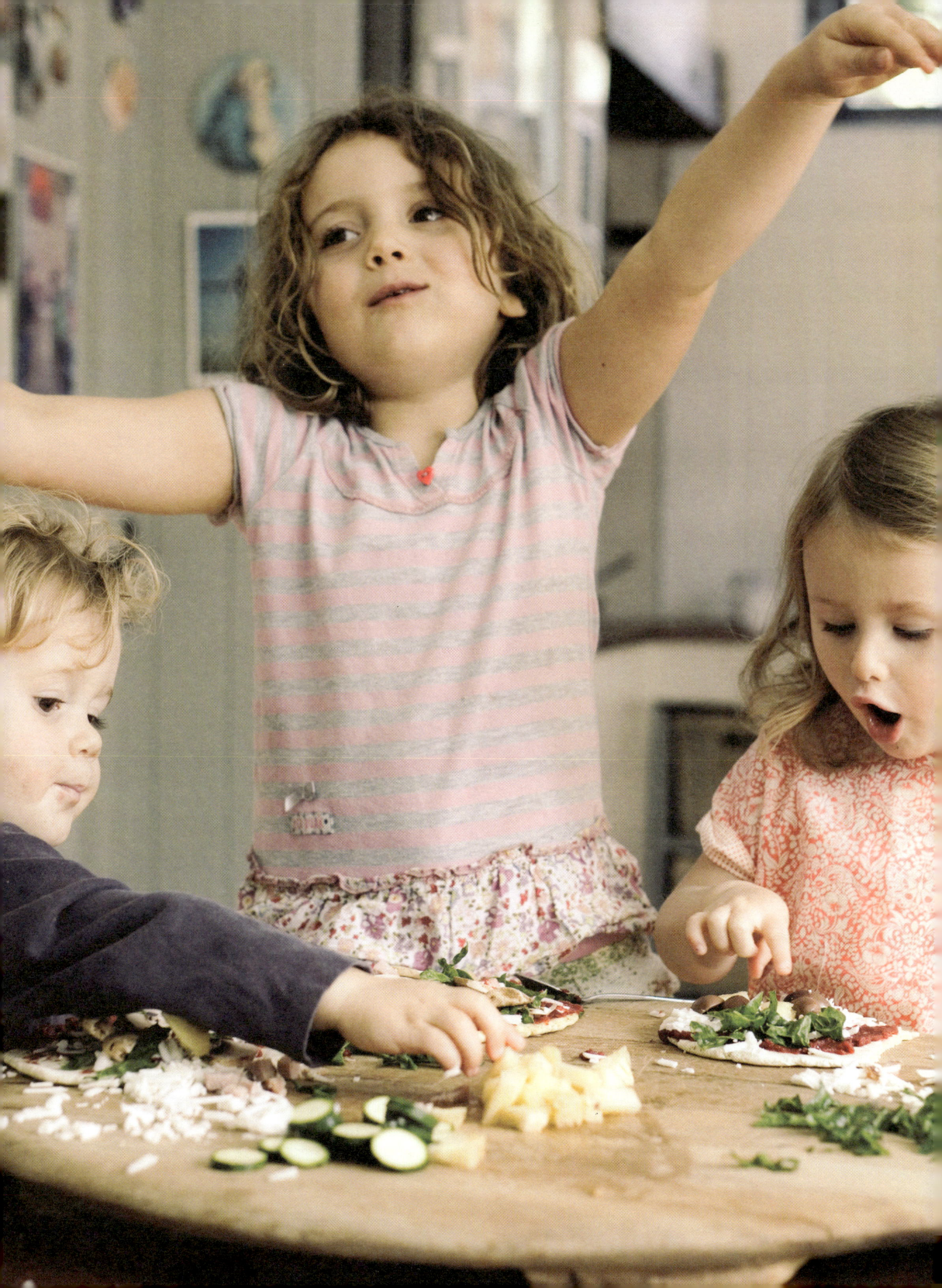

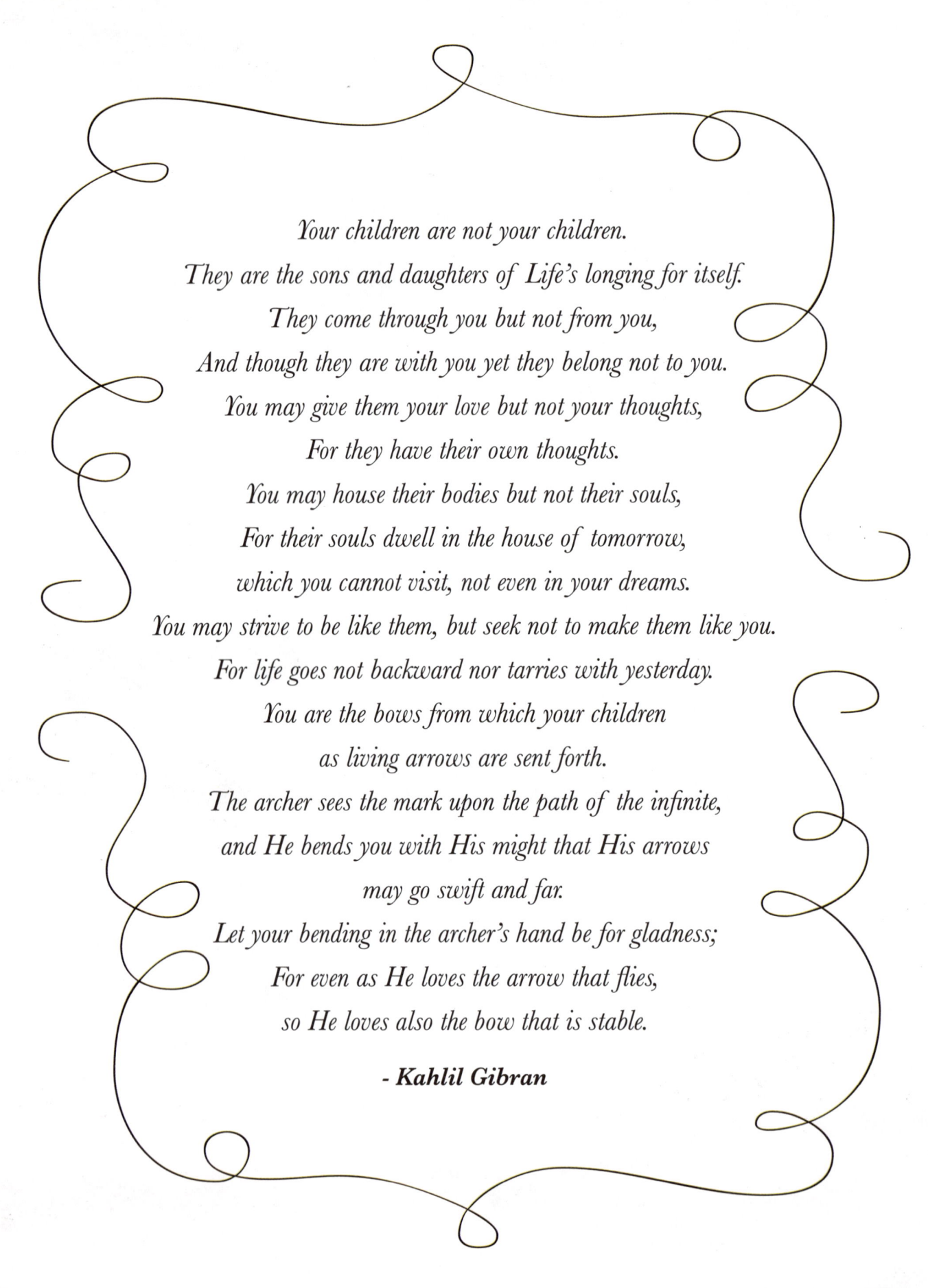

Your children are not your children.

They are the sons and daughters of Life's longing for itself.

They come through you but not from you,

And though they are with you yet they belong not to you.

You may give them your love but not your thoughts,

For they have their own thoughts.

You may house their bodies but not their souls,

For their souls dwell in the house of tomorrow,

which you cannot visit, not even in your dreams.

You may strive to be like them, but seek not to make them like you.

For life goes not backward nor tarries with yesterday.

You are the bows from which your children

as living arrows are sent forth.

The archer sees the mark upon the path of the infinite,

and He bends you with His might that His arrows

may go swift and far.

Let your bending in the archer's hand be for gladness;

For even as He loves the arrow that flies,

so He loves also the bow that is stable.

- Kahlil Gibran

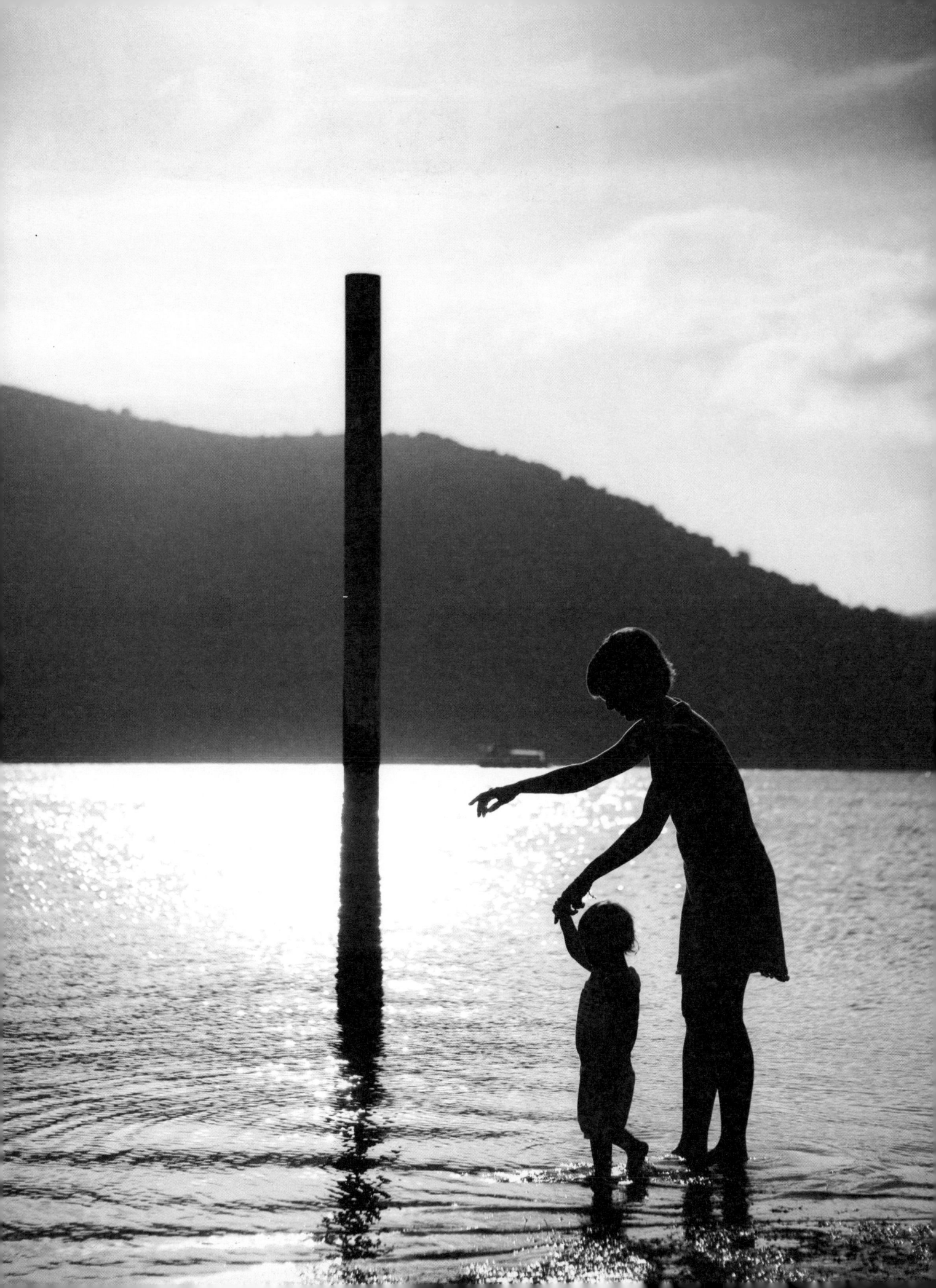

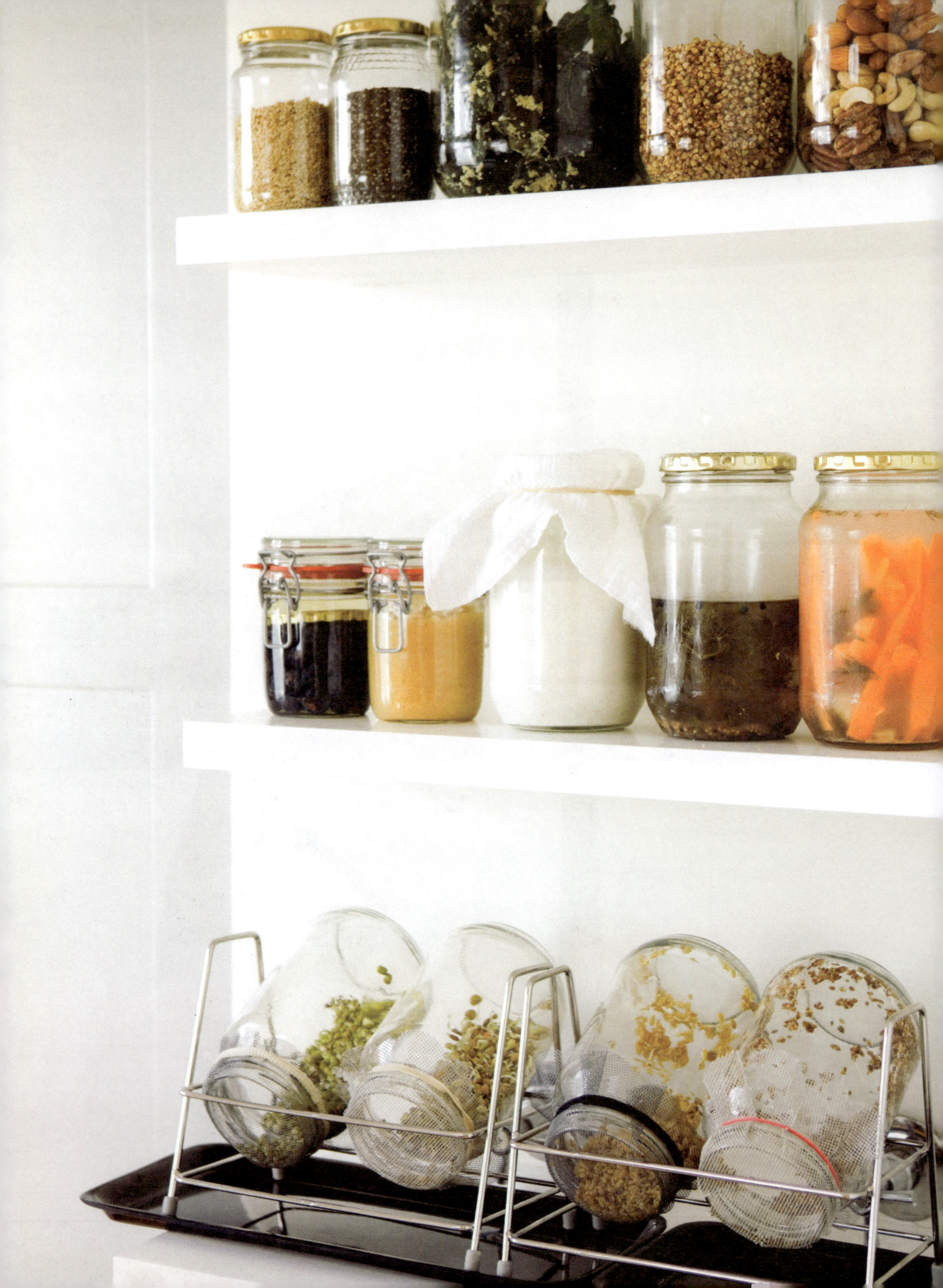

Food Preparation & Storage

Food preparation and storage

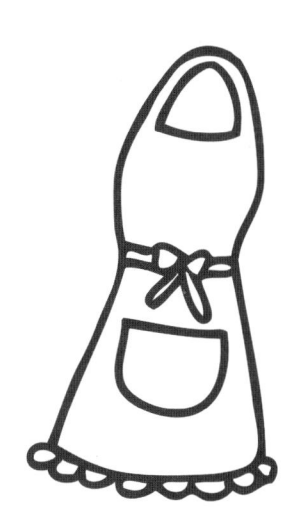

Food preparation and storage guidelines are stricter for infants and young children as their under-developed systems will be more vulnerable to food-borne illnesses.

Preparing food

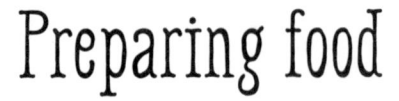

Cleanliness

There are pathogenic bacteria that can be transmitted to your little one through food. It is essential to: wash your hands before preparing food; maintain a clean kitchen; and, ensure that all utensils used for food preparation are kept very clean.

Undercooked food, particularly meat, should be avoided at all times.

Organisation

Ensuring your sanity is a vital step in maintaining a diet of homemade food. Preparing all your little one's food is not difficult, or overly time consuming, if you are organised and plan ahead. Remember, making homemade food does not have to happen on a daily basis – **all the recipes in this book are suitable for freezing.** You can schedule one morning every week as a 'batch cooking morning', leaving the rest of the week open for soul food!

When it comes to making purées, cook and freeze each prepared food separately. I only made the mistake of cooking a large batch of mixed purée from a recipe once. After all the time to prepare it and all the ingredients used, Mila hated the taste of it – and there were 6 trays of it in my freezer! To make up a meal, you can mix and match individual purées from your frozen food supply, and create a healthy, balanced and variable meal. If your little one does not like that particular combination, not much food is wasted and you can simply try another combination next time.

Freezing Food

In many ways freezing food (as opposed to refrigerating it) is a much better way of preserving nutritional content and ensuring that food does not expire.

After blending individual food purées, allow them to cool, scoop into ice cube trays, seal in a Ziploc bag and freeze. Do not forget to label the bags – all food looks pretty much the same when it is frozen, and with 'mushy mommy brain' you simply won't remember what is what. It is also worth writing the date you made it on the bag so you can avoid using food that may have been in the freezer for too long.

Once the purées are frozen you can break them out of the ice trays and into the Ziploc bags and return to the freezer. This frees up your ice trays for the next batch.

For other food, freeze in portion sizes and **label the bags**!

Food is best thawed in the fridge. Before you go to bed at night, choose what you will be feeding your little one the next day. Place it in a container in the fridge so it is thawed and ready to reheat when you need it the next day.

Reheating Food

If you have a microwave, sell it and use the gap on your kitchen shelf to stack your recipe books! Definitely never use it for heating or cooking your little one's food.

The radiation from microwave cooking destroys and deforms food molecules and creates new compounds completely unknown in nature – in a similar way (and with the same effects) as the irradiation process.

While most controversy about microwaves centres around this radiation issue, there are other negative consequences of microwave use too.

Unlike conventional heating which heats and cooks the food from the outside to the inside, microwave ovens heat internally by creating violent friction in the water molecules within the food. This friction tears apart the water molecules and this damage on a molecular level extends to the food particles themselves. The structure of the fats and proteins are changed, causing assimilation issues for the person who consumes the food. Swiss studies have shown that microwave heating causes unfavourable changes in vitamin content and the availability of these nutrients for absorption in the gut.

Dr. Hans Hertel is a Swiss food scientist who carried out a small but high-quality study on the effects of microwaved food on humans. His conclusions were clear: microwave cooking significantly altered the food's nutrients enough so that changes occurred in the participants' blood.

The changes included:
- Increased cholesterol levels,
- Decreased numbers of white blood cells, suggestive of poisoning,
- Decreased numbers of red blood cells,
- Production of radiolytic compounds (compounds unknown in nature),
- Decreased haemoglobin levels, which could indicate anaemic tendencies.

Using plastic or paper containers or covers in a microwave is particularly problematic. Carcinogenic toxins can leach out of the plastic and paper containers/covers, and into your food.

If you have gone to all the trouble of preparing nutritious home-made food for your little one, it would be really counter-productive to then heat this food in a microwave.

Reheat food by placing the container of food (either glass or ceramic) in a bowl of hot water or place the food directly in a suitable container on the stove top and heat over low heat. Both methods will ensure optimal nutrient retention.

It is preferable to prepare smaller portions and then prepare more if your little one is still hungry. If there is leftover food in the bowl which has been used to serve the food to your little one it is best thrown out – leftover food is contaminated by spoons, dirty fingers or other sources of bacteria.

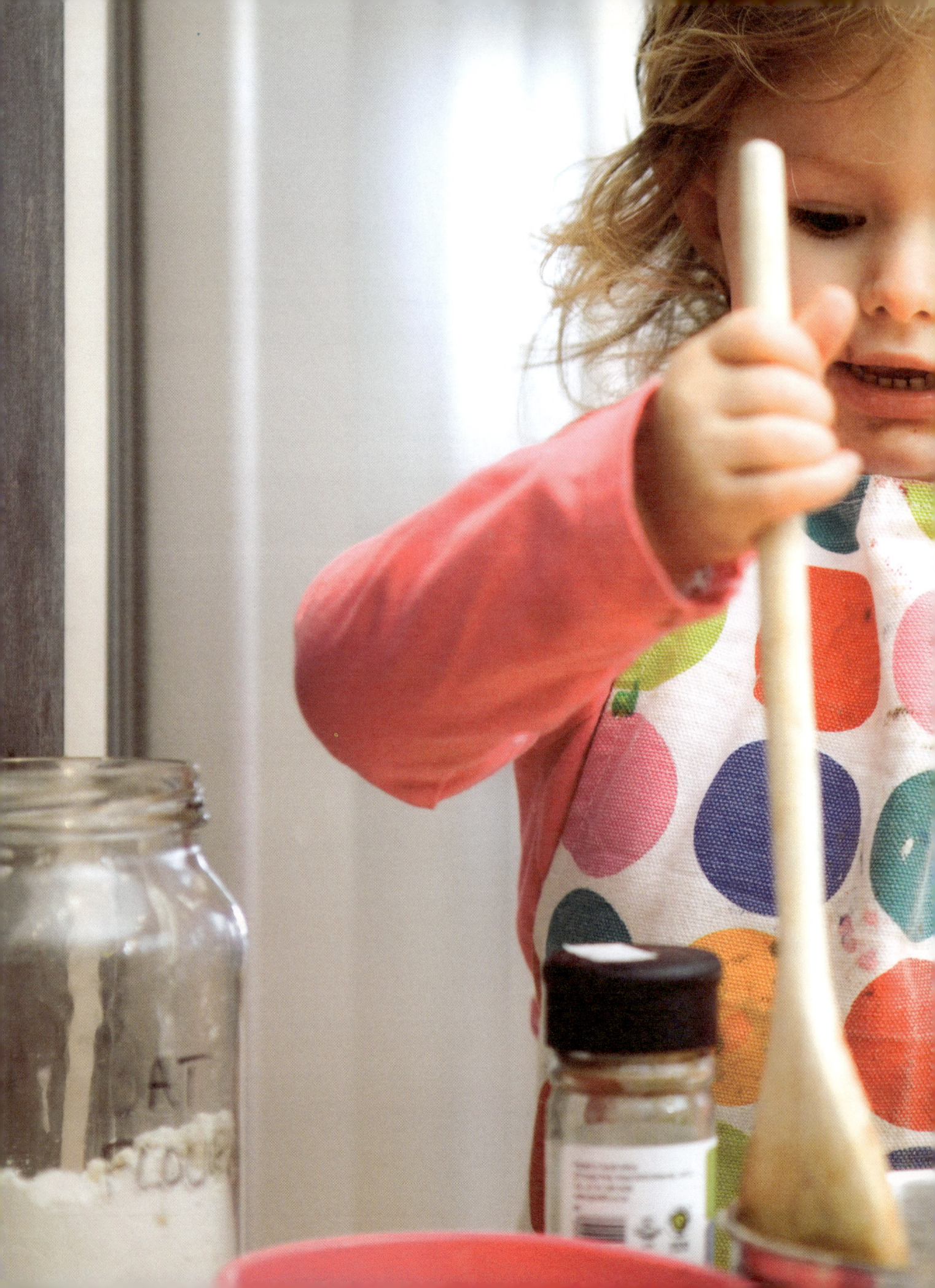

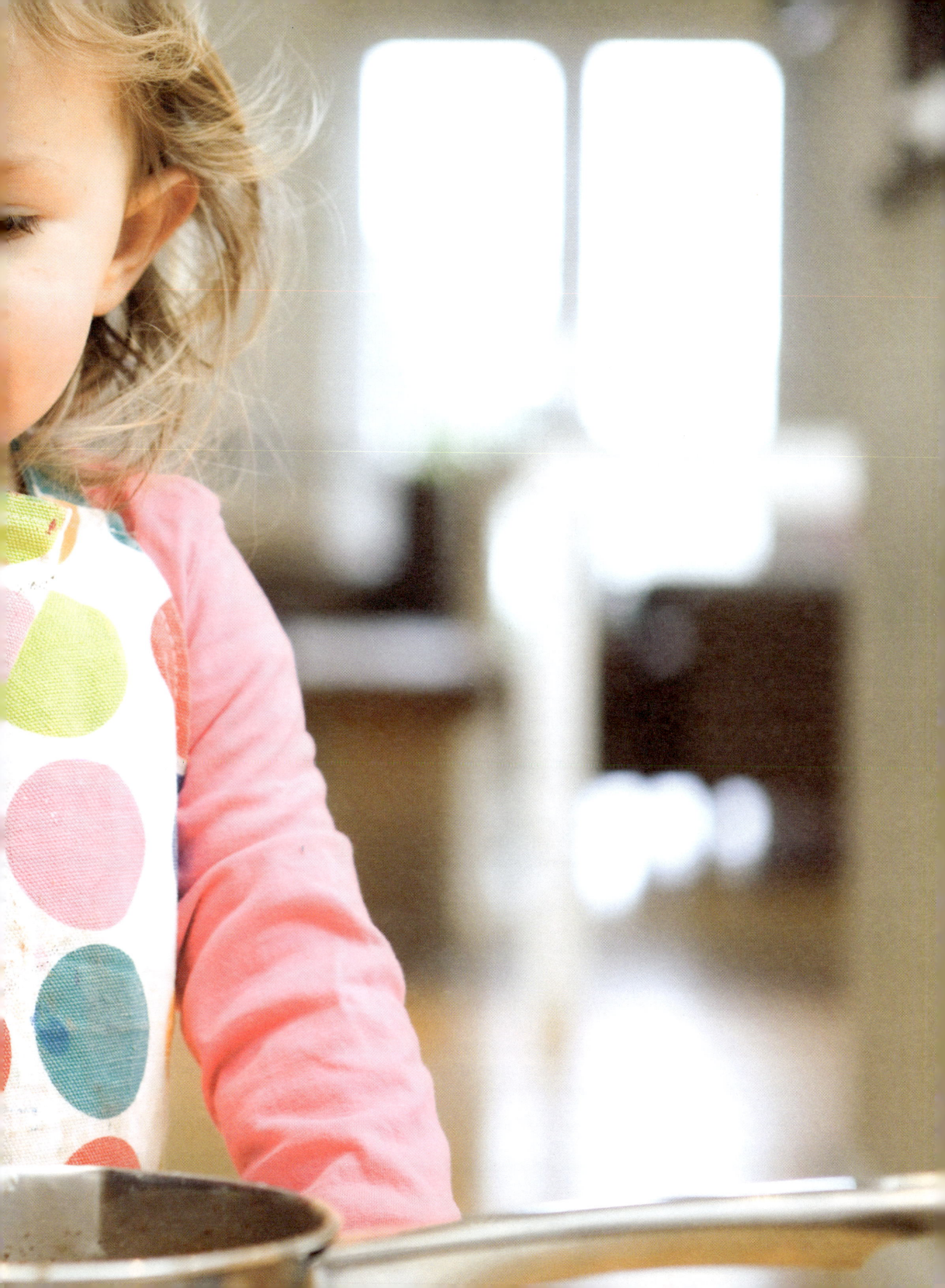

Recipes: Thirsty

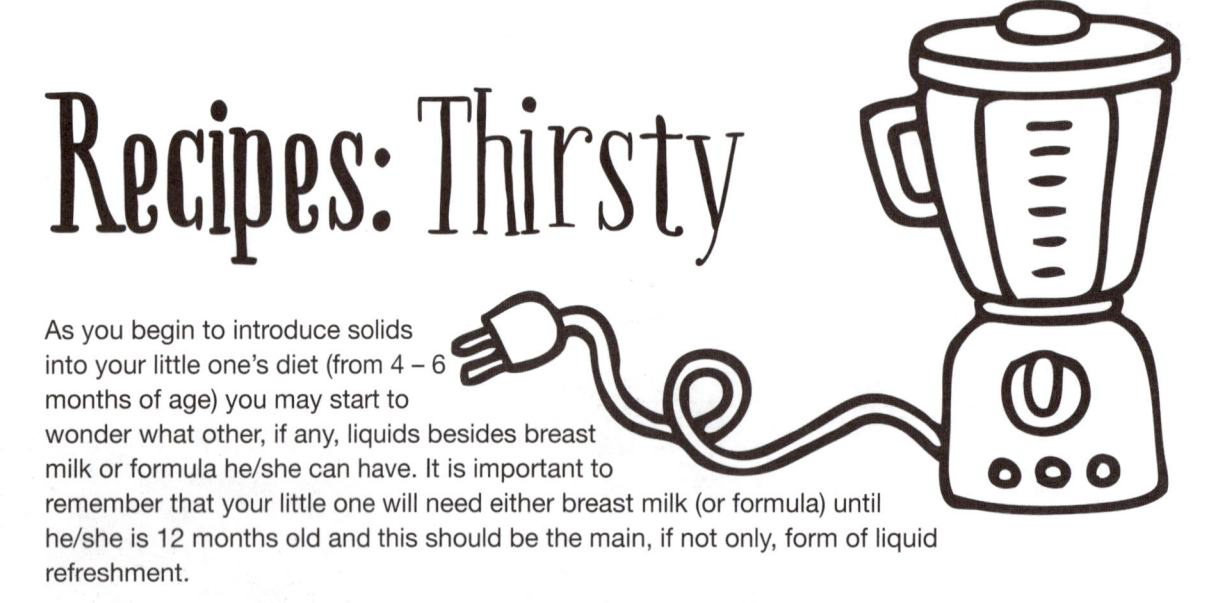

As you begin to introduce solids into your little one's diet (from 4 – 6 months of age) you may start to wonder what other, if any, liquids besides breast milk or formula he/she can have. It is important to remember that your little one will need either breast milk (or formula) until he/she is 12 months old and this should be the main, if not only, form of liquid refreshment.

Mila was exclusively breastfed until she was 14 months old, which is when I started supplementing with **Homemade Goat's Milk Formula** (recipe in this book) due to a low milk supply. I started introducing solids very slowly when she was 6 months old and she was completely weaned when she was 16 months old.

I continued to feed Mila the **Homemade Goats Milk Formula** until she was 18 months old. I believed she still needed a bottle before bed in order for her to sleep through the night. When she started waking up at 3:30 am everyday and having nightmares, I did some research and was very surprised to learn that the milk before bed was actually interfering with her sleep! According to the information I found, the high protein content was too heavy on her digestive system. Instead of resting and repairing, her body was spending the night trying to digest all this milk. Once I replaced the bedtime bottle of milk with Rooibos tea or water, she slept peacefully though the night again.

It was at this time that I stopped all 'Num Num' – Mila's name for milk bottles. At the same time as the night waking restarted, Mila had developed a nappy rash and a snotty nose – two things she had never suffered from before. Removing the goat's milk from her diet resolved both these issues in couple of days. **It was another reminder to listen and watch her body very carefully – it was telling me that the time for milk was over!**

From 18 months, Mila got her liquids from a freshly made vegetable juice after breakfast and then water and Rooibos tea for the rest of the day.

Recipes: Thirsty

BOO BOO SMOOTHIE ↣ 142
HOMEMADE FORMULA ↣ 144

JUICES
BEGINNER'S JUICE ↣ 146
WATERMELON COOLER ↣ 146
EVERYDAY VEGGIE JUICE ↣ 148
WEEKEND BREAK ↣ 148

SMOOTHIES
SUPER SMOOTH ↣ 150
BERRY BLAZE ↣ 1152
GRASS GREEN ↣ 154
CREATE-YOUR-OWN SMOOTHIE FORMULA ↣ 1154

ICED TEA ↣ 156
NUT MILK ↣ 158

Recipes: Thirsty

WATER

Exclusively breastfed babies do not need any other liquids in their diet even if there are extreme circumstances such as very hot weather, diarrhoea or constipation – although, in these situations your little one must be allowed to nurse as often as he/she would like.

According to Dr. Sears, "Breastfeeding babies do not need extra water, though formula-fed babies often do. Your breast milk contains enough water for your baby, even in hot, dry climates. Formula contains higher concentrations of salts and minerals than breast milk does, so that extra water is often necessary for the kidneys to excrete the extra salt. Also, because of less efficient metabolism, formula-fed infants lose more water. "

Water can be introduced from 6 months of age although your little one should not have more than 60 - 125ml (2 – 4 ounces) per day. You do not want your little one to fill up on water instead of nutrient dense breast milk, formula or food. It is, therefore, best to offer the water after a meal.

A word of warning: infants who drink too much water may develop Water Intoxication – this is when too much water dilutes a baby's normal sodium levels and can lead to seizures, coma, brain damage and in extreme cases, death. For children under a year old - and especially during the first nine months of life - drinking too much water may be dangerous.

Some medical professionals recommend boiling tap water until baby is a year old, whereas others feel that, after 6 months, this kind of 'over-sterilisation' is contributing to the current rise in eczema and other allergies.

TAP WATER

According to Dr. Mercola "most tap water is contaminated with a host of pollutants that increase your risk of serious health problems". These can include arsenic, aluminium, chlorine, fluoride, prescription and over-the-counter drugs and disinfection by-products.

BOTTLED WATER

Don't be fooled by the clever marketing of the bottled water industry - a large percentage of bottled water is in fact tap water! Not only that, but the plastic bottles contain a chemical called Bisphenol A (or BPA) which leaches into the water. BPA is a synthetic hormone disruptor that has been linked to serious health problems such as: learning and behavioural problems; altered immune system function; prostate and breast cancer; early puberty in both genders.

FILTERED WATER

This is the most economical and environmentally sound choice. Although water filters are initially expensive to purchase, they are more cost effective than bottled water and the water is far healthier.

LIVING WATER

Living water, like 'living food', is in its raw, natural state the way nature intended. Mountain spring water has an ideal PH range making it some of the healthiest water on earth. If you are fortunate enough to live close to a natural mountain spring, this is by far the best source of water. Be sure to collect your water in glass containers.

TEA

Once your little one is older than 6 months it is considered safe to offer them the occasional drink of caffeine-free herbal tea. Chamomile and Rooibos are two of the most popular choices.

If your little one is older than a year, you can sweeten the tea with a little bit of honey. Alternatively chop some sweet fruit into it while it is brewing and allow the fruit flavours to seep into the tea for some added sweetness.

CHAMOMILE TEA

Chamomile tea has been used for centuries to soothe colicky babies as well as promote peaceful sleep (as it is a mild sedative).

To prepare simply steep the chamomile teabag in boiling water for 5 minutes, cool to room temperature and serve. If your little one is 6 months old, start with 30-60ml (1-2 oz.) and gradually increase as he/she gets older.

Chamomile tea can cause an allergic reaction in children who are allergic to ragweed (a plant similar to chamomile). As with the introduction of any new food, if your little one develops a rash after drinking the tea, stop giving it to him/her.

ROOIBOS TEA

Rooibos tea – pronounced *roy-boss* – is indigenous to South Africa where it has been used by the indigenous Bushman for hundreds of years.

It is rich in anti-oxidants and is a natural calmative. Its naturally sweet, deep, earthy taste makes it a perfect caffeine-free alternative to black tea. Rooibos is well known for soothing colic, tummy troubles, and food allergies and for encouraging peaceful sleep in babies. It also assists with alleviating nausea, diarrhoea and vomiting. (Please see the glossary for more information on Rooibos.)

Recipes: Thirsty

Other teas, which are suitable for older babies and toddlers, include:
- Lemon balm,
- Lemongrass,
- Ginger,
- Mint,
- Red teas with rosehip and hibiscus,
- Honey bush,
- Tulsi.

Teas to avoid include:
- Comfrey,
- St. John's Wort,
- Senna,
- All black teas *(they contain polyphenols, which can reduce iron absorption, and tannins, which may interfere with the digestive process in the very young)*,
- All teas with caffeine.

JUICE

Once your little one is weaned, water is by far the most important liquid for him/her to drink but I am a big believer in juicing. I make a fresh fruit and vegetable juice first thing every morning and Mila has been enjoying them with me since she was 16 months old. I started by diluting hers with water (50% juice, 50% water) and gradually reduced the amount of water.

There are many publicised concerns around giving juice to your little one. One centres around the high concentration of sugars (which can lead to dental decay and raised blood sugar levels). While this may be true of store bought fruit juices, the juice I make for Mila is 90% vegetable juice – I only add half an apple to sweeten it.

Another concern is that your little one will satisfy his/her hunger with the juice and since store bought juices are considered empty calories, this will leave them malnourished. This is not true of a homemade vegetable juices – they are nutrient dense liquids. I also only give Mila her juice after she has eaten breakfast, and she only gets that one. For the rest of the day she drinks water or iced rooibos tea. Since Mila is not too keen on eating vegetables, I rest assured that she is getting the vitamins, minerals, antioxidants, enzymes and phytochemicals she needs from the juice.

A word of warning: store bought fruit juices bear little nutritional resemblance to the fruit from which they are made and they have a lot of other ingredients such as preservatives, sugars and unnatural substances added to them. They are definitely not something you want to add to your little one's diet.

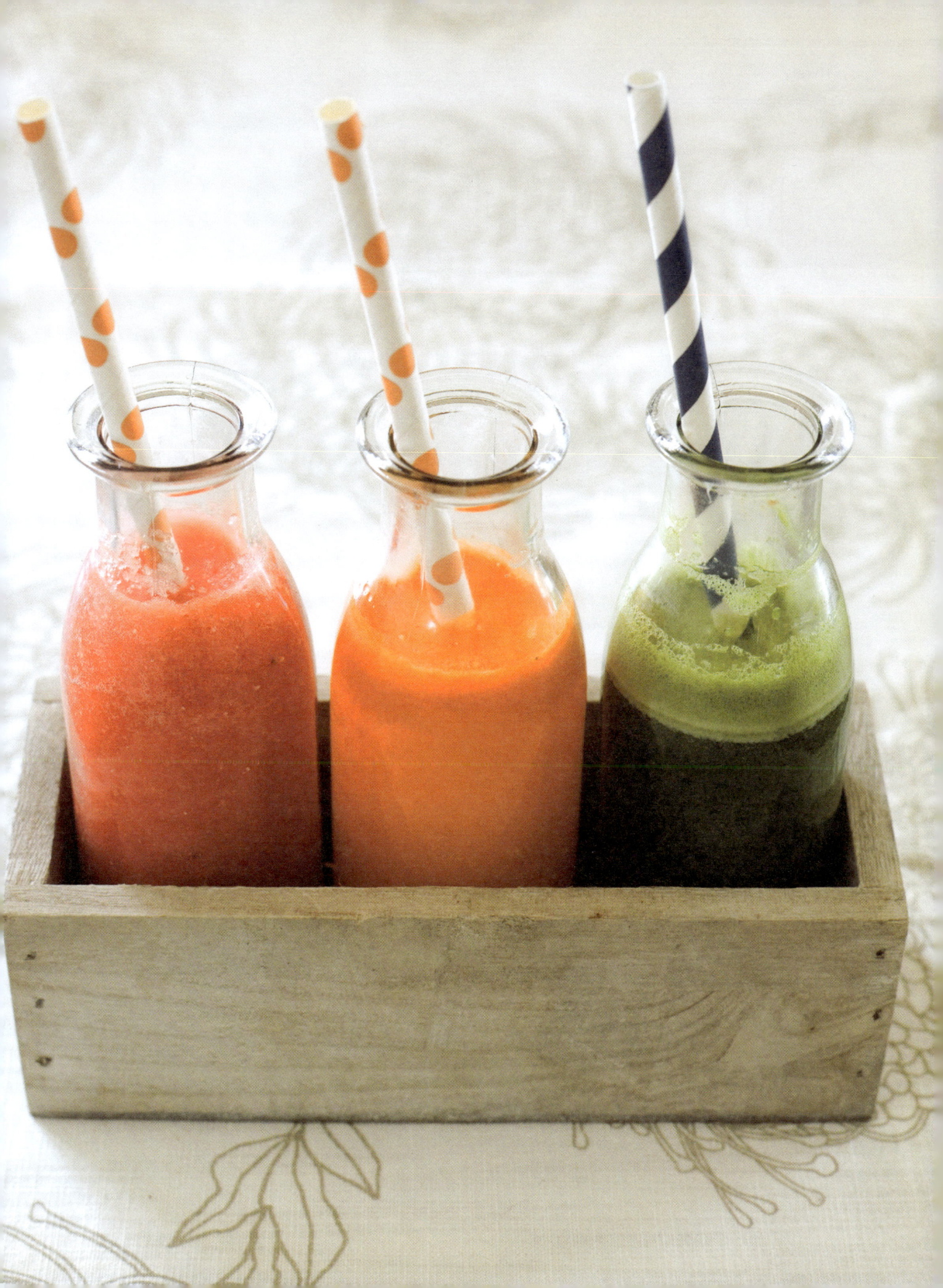

Recipes: Thirsty

BOO BOO SMOOTHIE

raw; superfood; vegetarian; egg-free

Makes 2 cups

....

I couldn't **NOT** *dedicate a page to breast milk or* "Boo Boo" *as Mila called it!*

It was a great reassurance to me as I started weaning Mila and navigating my way through what she could and could not eat (or would and would not eat), that she was still getting most of the nutrients she needed from my breast milk.

Breast milk is nature's perfect blend of proteins, fats, carbohydrates and vitamins… not to mention the antibodies, living cells, enzymes and hormones.

So this recipe is actually one for the Mama's – a smoothie to boost your milk supply!

This is an incredibly nutrient dense recipe - please read the glossary for nutrient information on each ingredient. Briefly: the moringa powder, flaxseeds and oats are lactogenic foods; the kefir (or Greek yoghurt) adds essential probiotics; the seeds add Omega oils; the maca powder balances your hormones; the green powder is full of amino acids (and is a quick way to get your greens in); the baobab powder is a concentrated source of calcium and alkalising on your system; and the honey… well its sweet and yummy!

....

1 banana (very ripe)
4 dates, soaked and pitted
¼ cup almonds, raw and activated *(or 2 T. raw almond nut butter)*
¼ cup goat's milk kefir or coconut milk *(or double fat Greek yoghurt if you are not avoiding dairy)*
¼ cup oats, soaked
2 T. coconut oil
1 T. flax seeds
1 T. sunflower seeds, activated
1 T. sesame seeds, activated
1 T. chia seeds
1 t. moringa powder
1 t. maca powder
1 t. green powder *(optional)*
1 t. baobab powder *(optional)*
2 T. raw honey *(optional)*
water or ice

Place all the ingredients in a blender and blend until smooth.

Add water or ice to achieve your desired consistency.

Serve immediately or store in a sealed glass jar in the fridge to snack on during the day.

Variation:
- *You can replace the banana with half an avocado.*

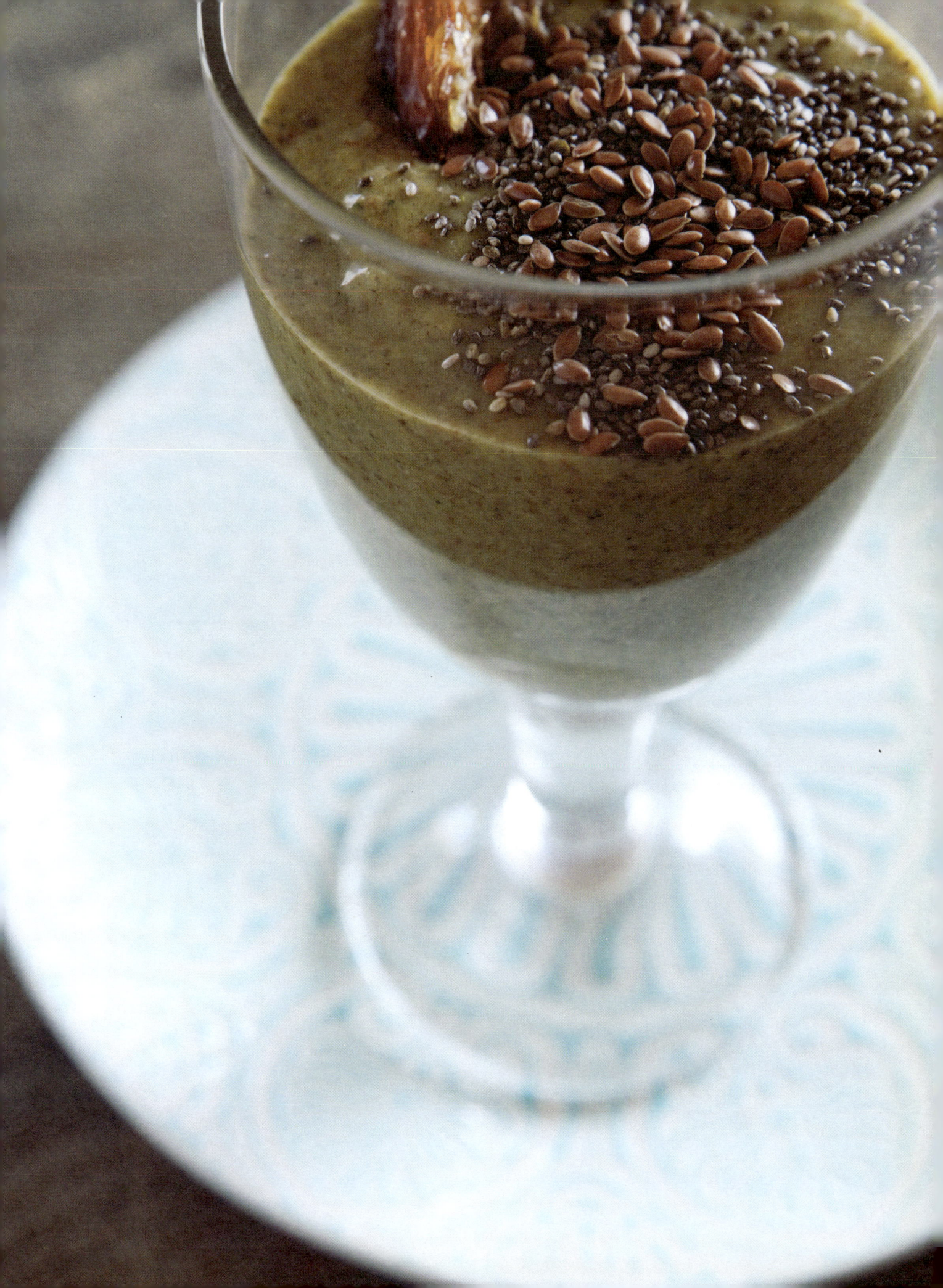

Recipes: Thirsty

HOMEMADE FORMULA

vegetarian; egg-free; grain-free

Makes 1 cup

• •

This recipe was created by Joe Stout, M.S.*, from Mt. Capra. He kindly agreed to let me reprint it in this book.

I cannot tell you how happy I was to find this recipe! While Mila was exclusively breastfed until she was 14 months old, and as such probably didn't need a breast milk replacement, I felt that she still needed a comforting drink and one that was full of nutrients. I am completely against tinned formulas, which have been shown to have high levels of GM ingredients, as well as high quantities of sugar. I did consider using the organic formulas – but I just could not get my head around feeding Mila such a processed food.

This recipe for homemade formula made so much sense to me, and Mila loved it! Please read the full explanation of why all these ingredients are included by visiting the Mt. Capra website at the following link: www.mtcapra.com

A note from Mt. Capra: The Food and Drug Administration have not evaluated this recipe. These products are not intended to diagnose, treat, cure, or prevent any disease. Please consult your doctor before starting your little one on a new formula program.

*Joe Stout is the President of Mt. Capra and holds a Bachelors of Science degree in Human Nutrition and Food Science and a Masters of Science degree in Clinical Human Nutrition. You can read more about the origins of this recipe on his website.

---

1 T. goat milk powder

1 t. organic coconut oil

1 tsp organic olive oil

1 T. organic maple syrup or organic raw turbinado sugar

1/8 t. unsulphured blackstrap molasses

1/8 t. infant probiotic powder or liquid – only needed in one bottle per day Vitamin drops *(follow daily dosage on product insert)* – only needed in one bottle per day.

Fill the bottle with 150ml (5 oz.) very hot water (50ºC or 120ºF).

Add the coconut oil and wait for it to melt.

Add the olive oil, molasses, maple syrup or turbinado sugar, and vitamin drops.

Shake the bottle well.

When all the contents are mixed, add the milk powder and cold water so that the total volume is 240ml (8 oz.).

Shake well.

Lastly add the probiotics (to ensure their viability) and shake well.

Notes:
- *You can use fresh goat's milk instead of powdered milk. Use 170ml hot water and add 170 ml fresh goat's milk instead of the milk powder and cold water.*
- *You can keep a ready-made mixture using powdered milk for up to 4 days (in the fridge). Add the probiotics just before serving.*
- *The formula using powdered milk can be frozen. Again, add the probiotics just before serving.*
- *Once Mila was well over a year old, I swopped the maple syrup for honey.*

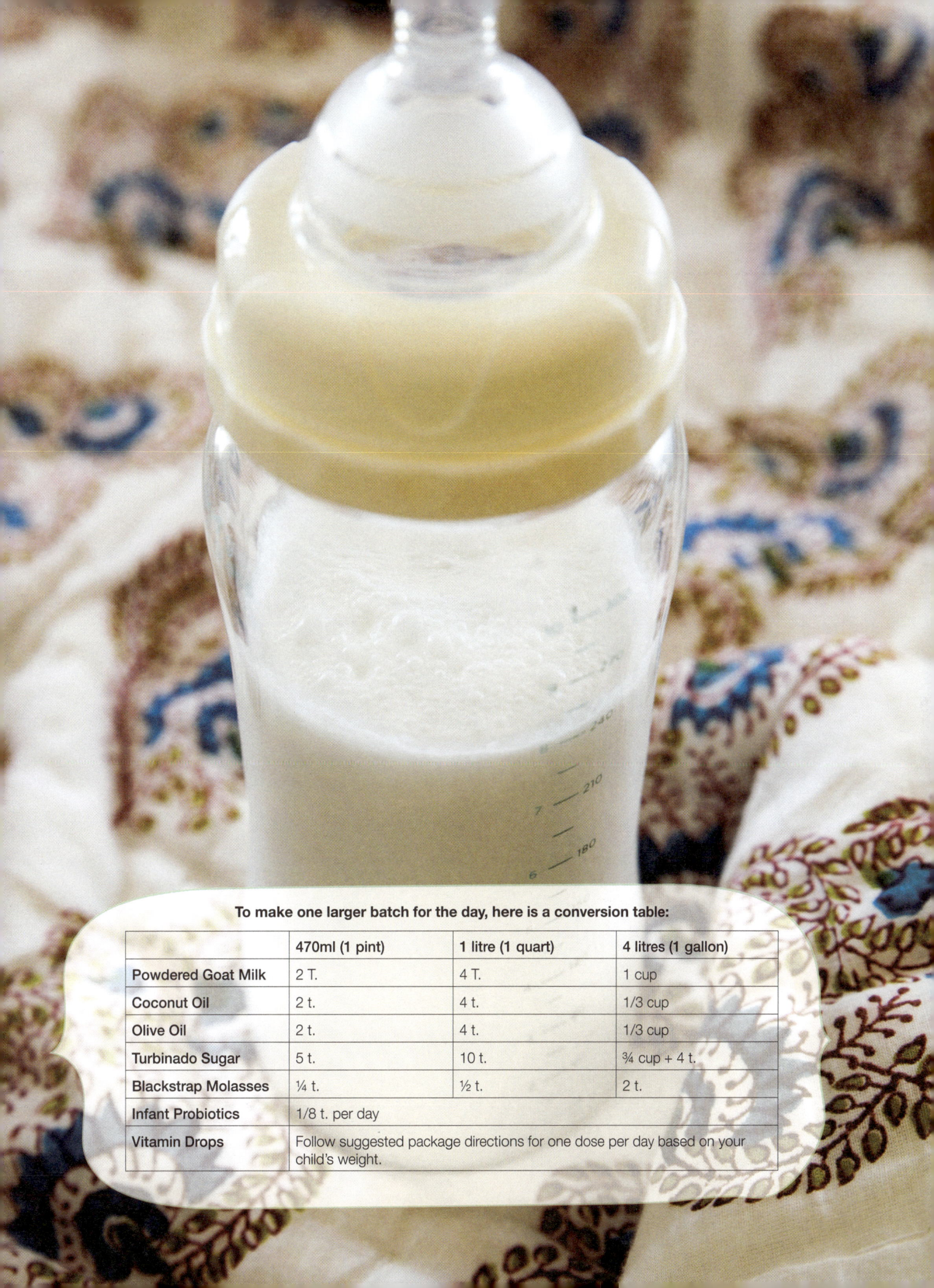

To make one larger batch for the day, here is a conversion table:

	470ml (1 pint)	1 litre (1 quart)	4 litres (1 gallon)
Powdered Goat Milk	2 T.	4 T.	1 cup
Coconut Oil	2 t.	4 t.	1/3 cup
Olive Oil	2 t.	4 t.	1/3 cup
Turbinado Sugar	5 t.	10 t.	¾ cup + 4 t.
Blackstrap Molasses	¼ t.	½ t.	2 t.
Infant Probiotics	1/8 t. per day		
Vitamin Drops	Follow suggested package directions for one dose per day based on your child's weight.		

Recipes: Thirsty

JUICES

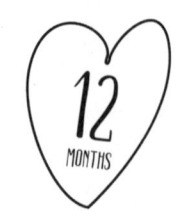

12 MONTHS

raw; vegetarian; vegan; egg-free; grain-free; for adults too; great for lunchboxes
Makes 3 cups

• •

There are so many recipes for fruit and vegetable juices that I highly recommend buying a separate recipe book for this. Books focusing exclusively on juices give great insights into what juices to use when (for an immune boost, concentration, sleep etc.) as well as the nutrient content of each juice. I have included some of our favourite combinations here – although I usually just add whatever I have in the fridge and hope for the best!

When making juices try buy organic fruits and vegetables. If these are unavailable, soak your produce in a hydrogen peroxide solution or in water with ½ cup white vinegar and 2 T. sea salt added. Allow to soak for 10 minutes, then rinse. This should remove most of the pesticides.

Cucumbers are useful to add bulk and reduce costs! They have a high water content so significantly add to the volume of the juice as well as being a great source of vitamins K, C and B5, potassium, magnesium, manganese.

BEGINNER'S JUICE

This one is a little sweeter to entice your little one into the world of juices!

This juice is high in: folate, magnesium, potassium, vitamins A, B6 and C, silica, beta-carotene, phytochemicals chlorophyll, iron, lutein, calcium, bromelain, and bioflavonoids.

2 pineapples, skin removed
6 carrots
1 cucumber

Put all the ingredients through a juicer, pour into a sippy cup or straw bottle and serve.

• •

WATERMELON COOLER

You do not need to spend time deseeding the watermelon – the seeds contain important nutrients like protein, magnesium, manganese, phosphorus, zinc and iron and several amino acids. The skin is edible too!

This juice is high in: the phytonutrient lypocene, folate, magnesium, potassium, manganese, vitamins A, B, C and K.

½ a watermelon
(rind removed unless organic)
1 cucumber
½ lemon *(rind removed unless organic)*

Put all the ingredients through a juicer (watermelon rind and all), pour into a sippy cup or straw bottle and serve.

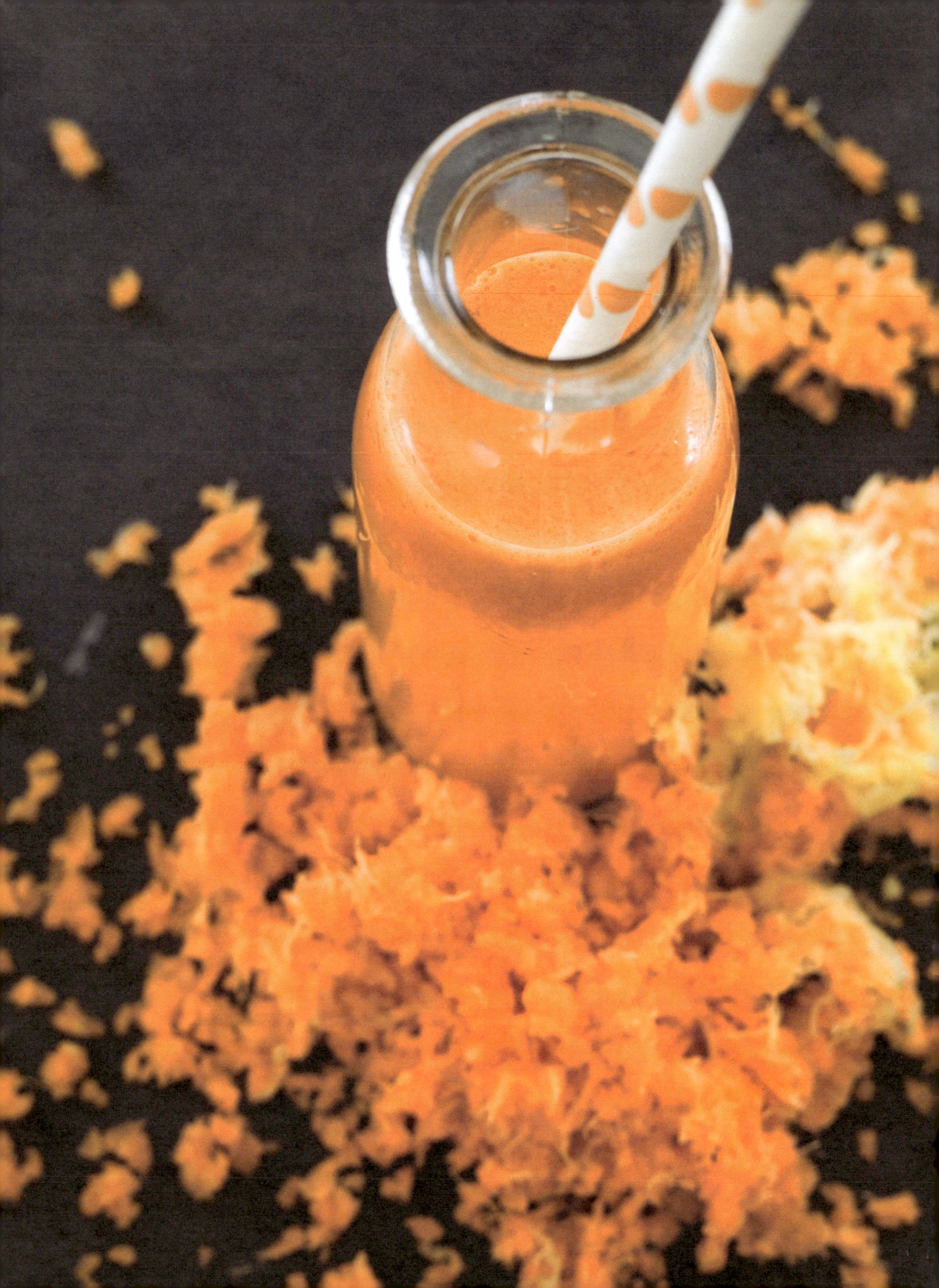

Recipes: Thirsty

EVERYDAY VEGGIE JUICE

This is what I generally make everyday.

Beetroot is a great laxative but it can turn your little one's poop red – do not get a fright! Use beetroot on alternate days as it is high in nitrates.

This juice is high in: folic acid, magnesium, potassium, vitamins A, B6 and C, silica, beta-carotene, phytochemicals chlorophyll, iron, lutein, calcium, bromelain, and bioflavonoids.

5 carrots
1 cucumber
5 leaves spinach or kale
a handful parsley
2 stalks celery *(with leaves)*
1 beetroot *(with stalks and leaves)*
4 apples or 1 pineapple
½ lemon *(rind removed if not organic)*
optional - ½ cup sprouts, such as lentil or chickpea sprouts *(for added enzymes and protein)*

Put all the ingredients through a juicer, pour into a sippy cup or straw bottle and serve.

WEEKEND BREAK

Sometimes on the weekend we are in a rush to get to the beach, or we may have gone away and there was no space in the car for the juicer and all the ingredients, so I quickly make Mila one of these. (It also gives me a break from cleaning the juicer!).

Naartjies are a great source of vitamins A, B and C, calcium, magnesium, phosphorous and potassium.

6 naartjies (tangerines)

Cut the naartjies (tangerines) in half.

Place a sieve over a bowl.

Using a fork to hold the centre of the fruit, squeeze the naartjies with your other hand allowing juice to fall into the sieve. The sieve will catch the pips.

Pour the juice from the bowl into a sippy cup or straw bottle, top up with water and serve.

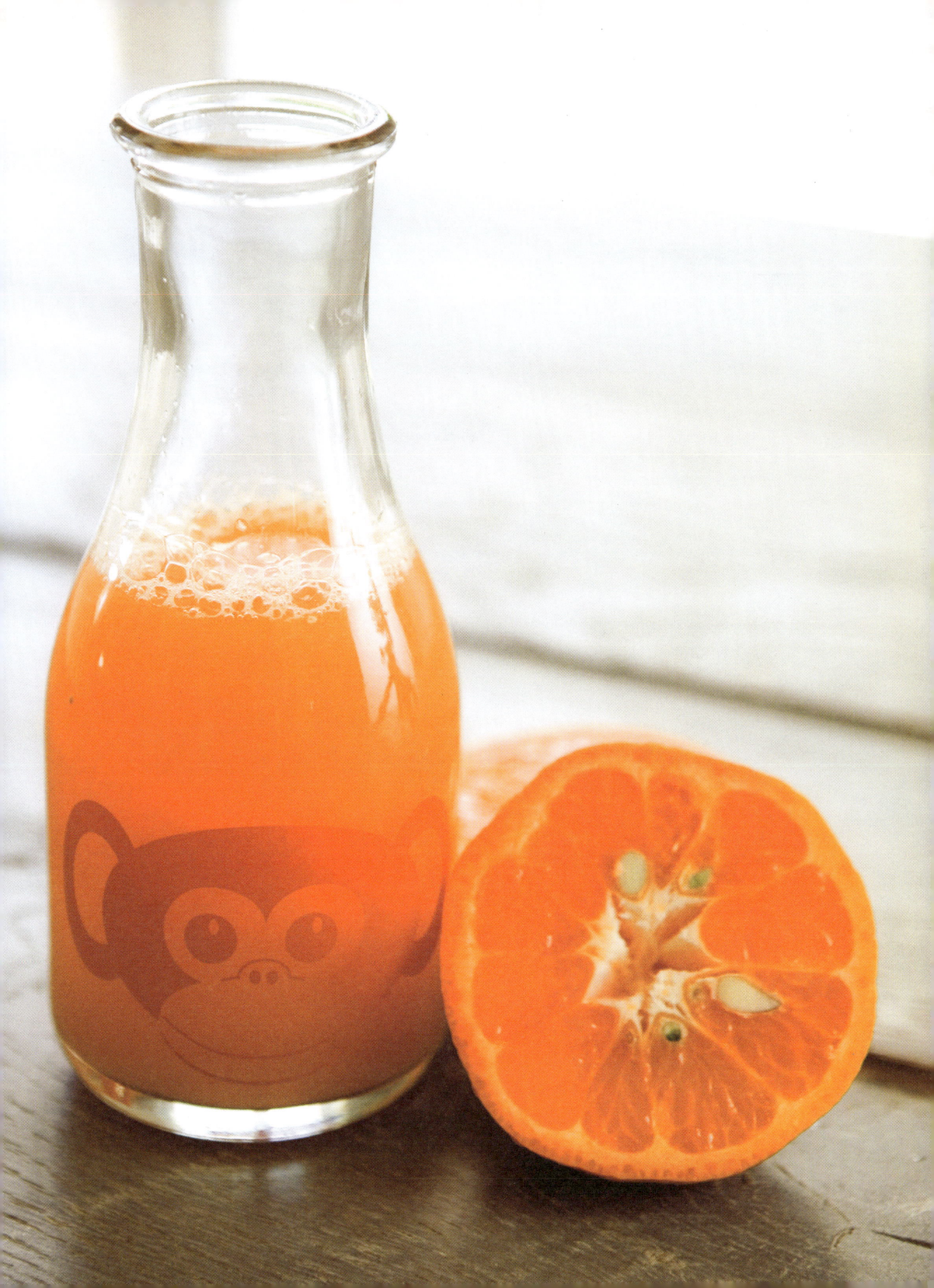

Recipes: Thirsty

SMOOTHIES

You are only limited by available produce and your imagination when it comes to creating smoothies! This is really something you can experiment with by using fruit and vegetables that are in season and those which are your little one's favourites.

Check the glossary to learn about the superfood powders as these add a nutritional boost without affecting the flavour too much.

Other great additions to smoothies are: nuts (almonds, cashews and macadamias); seeds (sunflower seeds, pumpkin seeds, flax seeds, sesame seeds, chia seeds); and oils (avocado oil, flax oil, hemp oil, coconut oil). These all add the protein and omega oils which your little one needs.

To thin the smoothies, add water or cooled herbal teas to the mix. I tend to make warm smoothies with hot tea in winter - the herbal teas have medicinal benefits too, so I use whichever one suits my needs.

If your combination is too 'bitty' for your little one, pass it through a sieve before serving.

*Superfoods are foods that are exceptionally high in vitamins, minerals and overall nutritional value. Often sold as powders, they are sourced from all over the world and include things such as baobab, maca, hemp, moringa, lucuma and camu camu.

SUPER SMOOTH

raw; superfood; vegetarian; egg-free; grain-free; for adults too; great for lunchboxes

Makes 2 cups

When I started Mila on smoothies she did not like any which had 'bits' in them. This recipe works well for those with texture sensitivities. The Superfood* powders add extra nutrition without adding any texture.

If you would like an ice-cold smoothie, cut up and freeze the banana before blending.

This smoothie is a good source of vitamins E, C and B's, calcium, fibre, iron, potassium, magnesium, manganese, phosphorous, iron, antioxidants and protein.

. . . .

1 banana, peeled

½ cup coconut milk *(be sure to find one without preservatives)*

½ cup water

1 t. raw honey, or maple syrup *(only use honey if your little one is older than 12 months)*

¼ t. vanilla powder

¼ t. baobab powder

¼ t. green powder *(optional – this may affect the flavour too much for your little one's liking)*

Place all the ingredients in a blender and blend until smooth.

Pour into a sippy cup or straw bottle and serve.

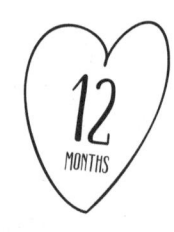

12 MONTHS

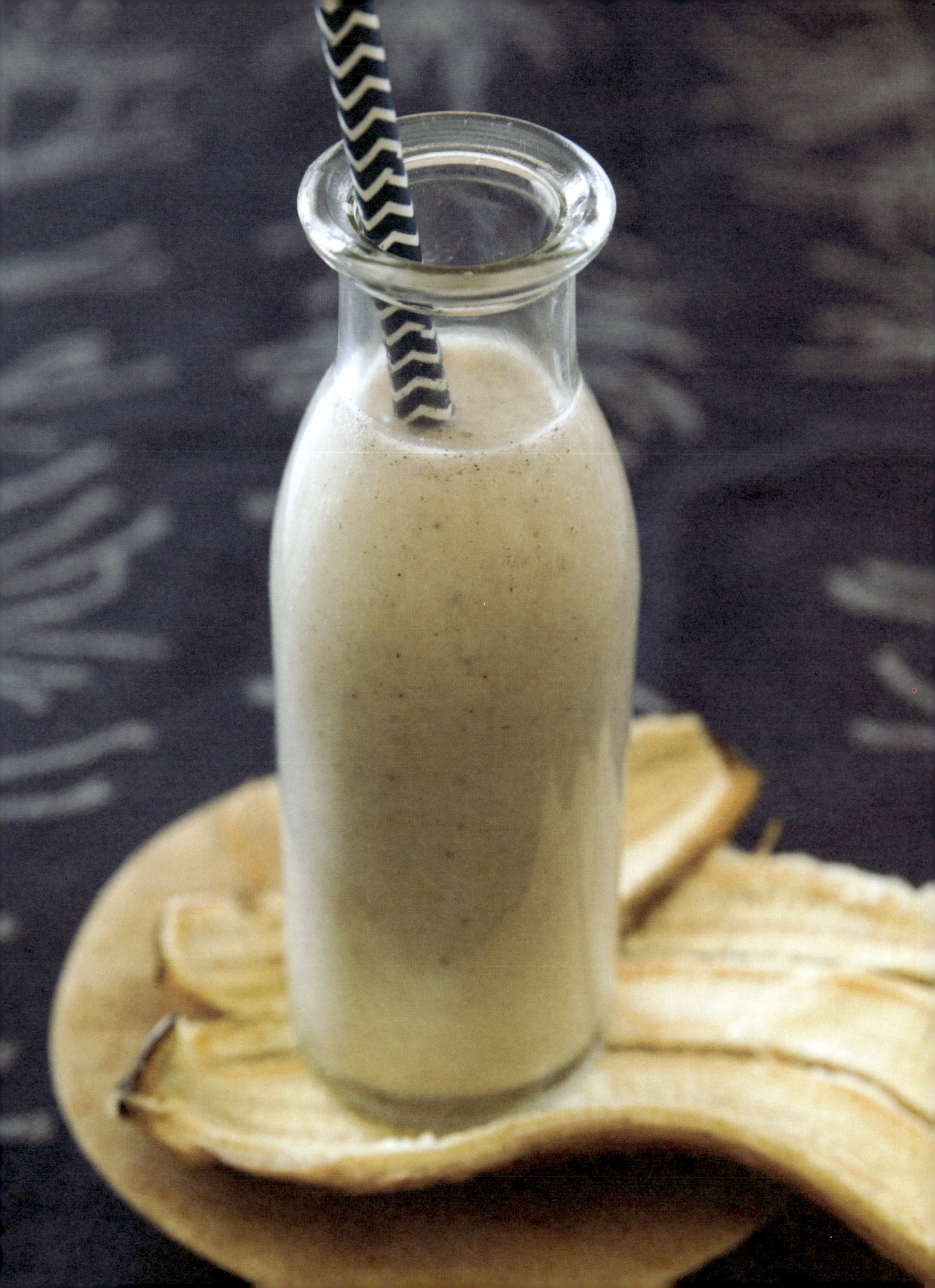

Recipes: Thirsty

BERRY BLAZE

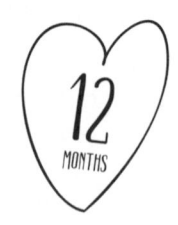

raw; vegetarian; egg-free; grain-free; for adults too; great for lunchboxes

Makes 2 cups

12 MONTHS

This smoothie is a good source of phytonutrients, vitamins C and K, manganese, folate, fibre, iodine, potassium, omega-3 fatty acids and magnesium.

1 cup mixed berries, fresh or frozen *(such as strawberries, blueberries, raspberries)*

1 cup baby leaf spinach *(or 1 t. green powder)*

½ an avocado, peeled

1 cup water, or coconut milk *(be sure to find one without preservatives)*

2 dates, soaked

1 t. honey, or maple syrup *(only use honey if your little one is older than 12 months)*

Place all the ingredients in a blender and blend until smooth.

Pour into a sippy cup or straw bottle and serve.

> REMEMBER YOUR LITTLE ONE MAY 'OBJECT' TO THE SMOOTHIE NOT BECAUSE OF ITS TASTE, BUT RATHER BECAUSE OF THE TEXTURE. IF IT IS BEING REJECTED, TRY PASSING IT THROUGH A SIEVE TO REMOVE ANY 'BITS' AND THEN SERVING AGAIN. ALTERNATIVELY, FREEZE THE SMOOTHIE AND SERVE AS AN ICE LOLLY.

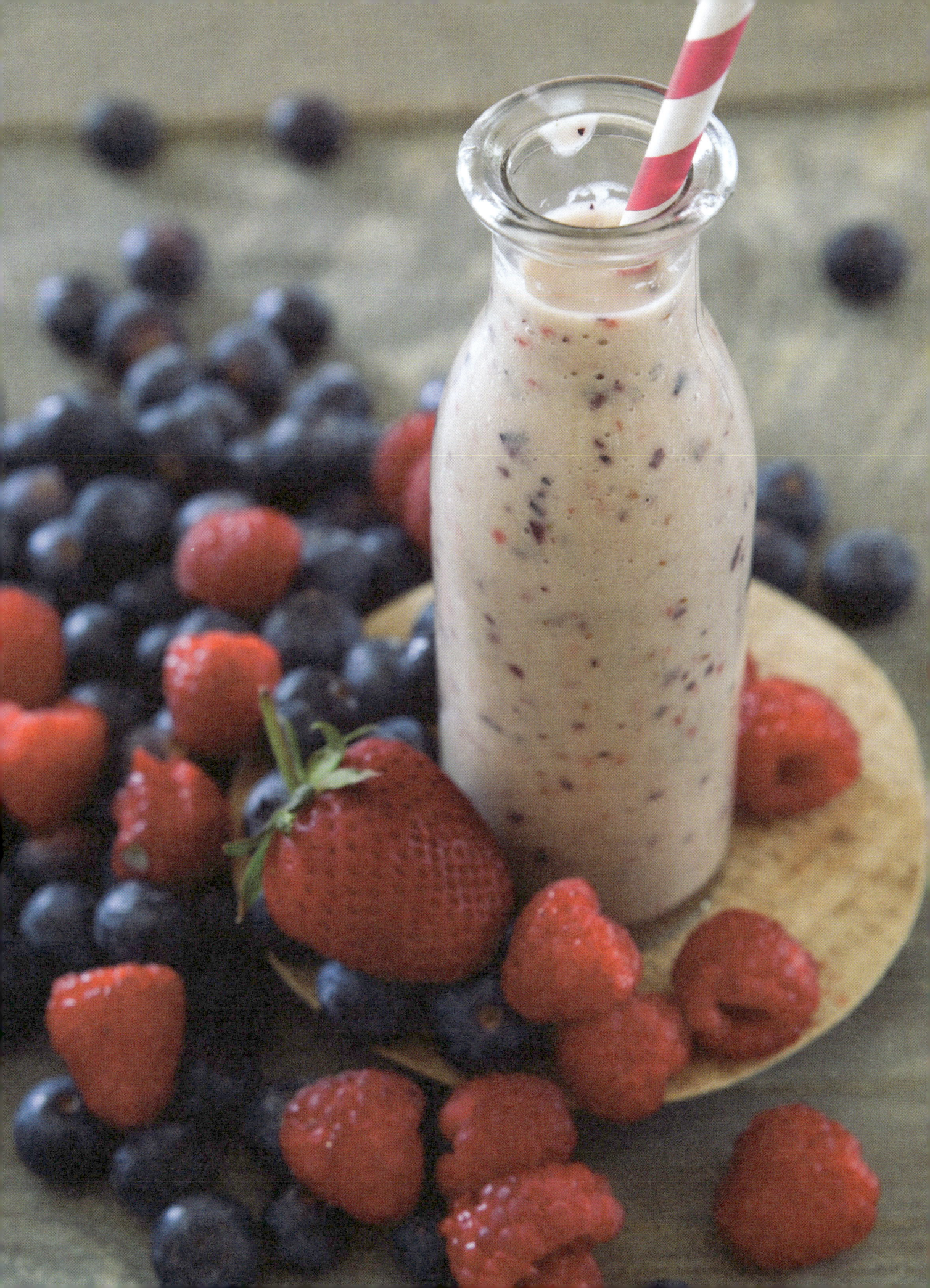

Recipes: Thirsty

GRASS GREEN

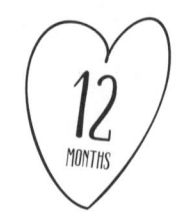

12 MONTHS

raw; vegetarian; vegan; egg-free; grain-free; for adults too; great for lunchboxes

Makes 2 cups

This recipe uses fresh greens, but you can turn any smoothie into a green smoothie by adding a teaspoon of green powder.

This smoothie is a good source of fibre, omega 3's, vitamins A, B's, C, K, and E, manganese, tryptophan, calcium, potassium, iron, magnesium, protein, folate, phosphorous, and phytonutrients.

1 cup shredded kale or spinach
1 banana, peeled
1 apple
2 dates, soaked
¼ cup frozen peas
½ cup preservative-free coconut milk *(or water)*
½ cup water

Place all the ingredients in a blender and blend until smooth.

Pour into a sippy cup or straw bottle and serve.

CREATE-YOUR-OWN SMOOTHIE FORMULA

I encourage you to make your own smoothie recipes!

There are endless possibilities and you should not be limited to the ones in this book, or by my ingredients that may, or may not be, in season. Here is a smoothie 'formula' that will guarantee some success as you experiment to find what works for you and your little one.

½ cup liquid + 1 handful greens + ½ cup fruit + 1 creamy fruit + ½ T. fats + 1 t. extras

Liquid = *Nut milk, coconut milk, coconut water, water.*
Greens = *kale, spinach, Swiss chard, peas, green string beans.*
Fruit = *strawberries, blueberries, raspberries, grapes, mangoes, peaches, nectarines, apricots, pears, apples, pineapples.*
Creamy Fruit = *banana, avocado.*
Fats = *nuts (almonds, cashews and macadamias); seeds (sunflower seeds, pumpkin seeds, flax seeds, sesame seeds, chia seeds); and oils (avocado oil, flax oil, hemp oil, coconut oil).*
Extras = *sweeteners (honey, dates), flavours and spices (vanilla powder, cinnamon, nutmeg, ginger); superfoods (baobab, maca, lucuma, camu camu, green powder, raw cacao).*

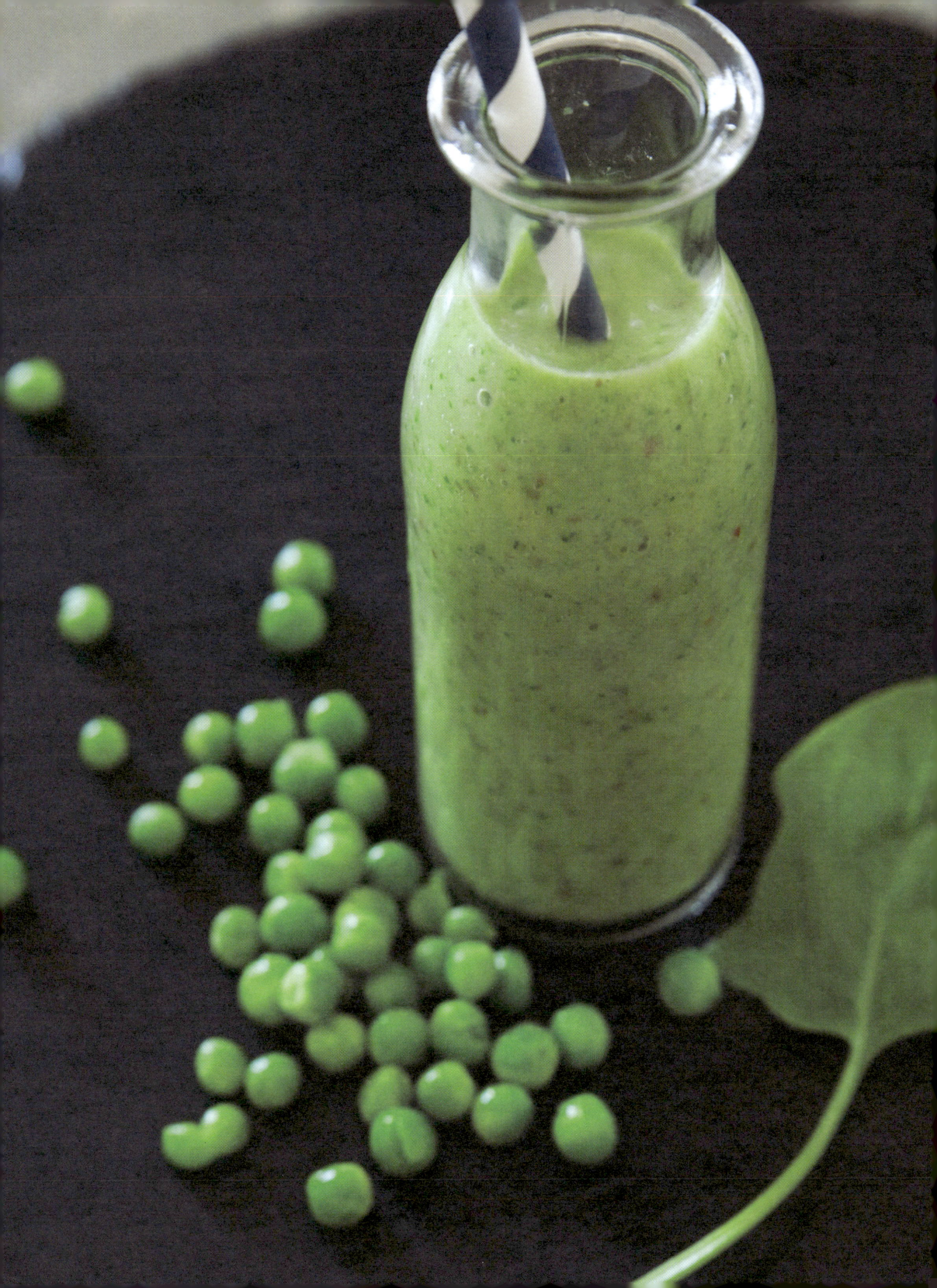

Recipes: Thirsty

ICED TEA

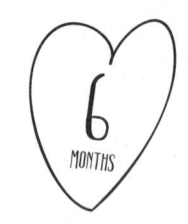

6 MONTHS

vegetarian; egg-free; grain-free; for adults too; great for lunchboxes

Makes 1 l. (1 qt.)

• •

Mila went through a stage where she got bored of plain Rooibos tea. She had also seen her cousin drinking ice tea from a can. In an attempt to entice her back to drinking tea, I turned it into a 'fancy' drink – flavoured iced tea! As soon as it became something special and out of the ordinary, she happily drank it! (It is also delicious and you can keep changing the flavour.)

Rooibos tea is naturally caffeine-free and is full of antioxidants which help protect your body from free radicals. It is a good source of copper, iron, magnesium, calcium, zinc and potassium - making it beneficial for healthy bones and strong teeth.

Rooibos can soothe digestive disorders – such as constipation, diarrhoea, stomach cramps, colic and nausea.

• •

1 l. (1 qt.) boiling water
4 Rooibos tea bags
1 peach, finely chopped
1 apple, finely chopped
2 T. honey, optional
(if your little one is older than 12 months and if you want to use this drink as a sweet treat)
Ice cubes

Place all the ingredients (except the ice cubes) in a glass jug, or teapot.

Stir, cover and allow to brew for 10 minutes. (If you want the tea to be stronger, rather add more tea bags instead of increasing the brewing time).

Add the ice cubes to cool the tea down.

Pour though a sieve into a sippy cup or straw bottle and serve.

You can add some ice cubes and fruit to the straw bottle (if you are using one) – the sound it makes when your little one shakes it adds some excitement to the whole drink!

Keep the rest of the tea in the fridge. The tea should last for 24 hours in the fridge if you have added fruit to it. Plain Rooibos tea will keep in the fridge for up to 2 weeks.

This really is a very basic recipe and you can experiment with different flavours by adding some of the following:

- *Fruit: mango, passion fruit (granadilla), raspberries, blueberries, nectarines, plums, dates, pineapple, orange, naartjies (tangerine), lemon.*
- *Spices: cinnamon, nutmeg, vanilla, ginger, cardamom.*
- *Herbs: mint, lemongrass, peppermint, lavender.*

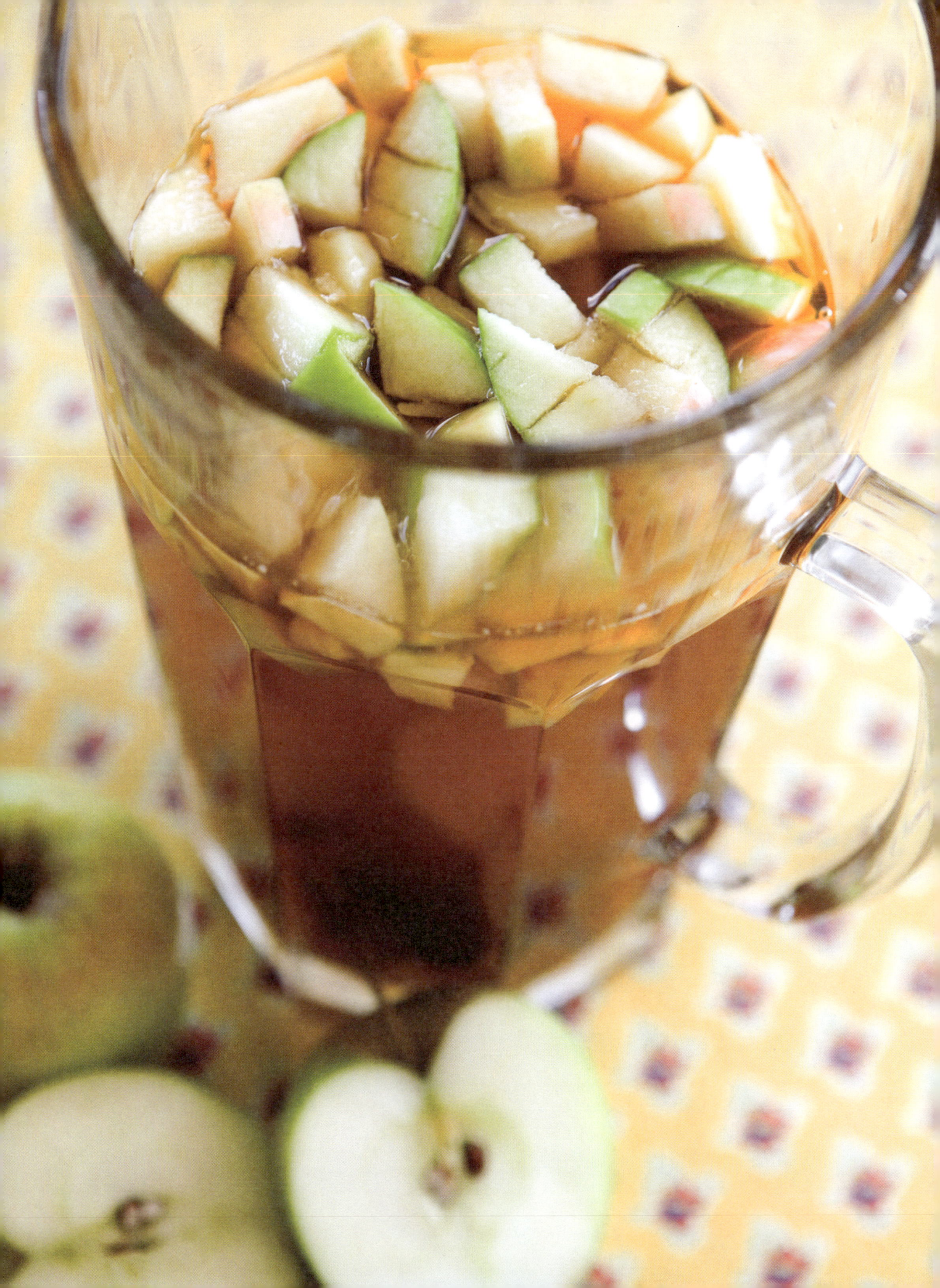

Recipes: Thirsty

NUT MILK

raw; superfood; vegetarian; vegan; egg-free; grain-free; for adults too; great for lunchboxes

Makes 1 l. (1 qt.)

• •

Every now and then I would alternate one of Mila's Goat Milk Formulas with a nut milk – just to add some variation and to get different nutrients into her diet. I prefer to use almonds as they are alkalising on the system and high in antioxidants. Almond milk is a good source of iron, copper, zinc, magnesium, manganese, calcium, phosphorous, potassium and selenium and is low in sodium.

It must be said that almond milk does not have a high enough fat content to be a stand-alone replacement for goat's milk (or breast milk). If you are vegan, you will need to supplement this milk with additional fats from avocados etc. To boost the fat and protein content of the nut milk, I add hemp seeds since they are a good source of Omega oils (3&6), amino acids, protein, calcium, Vitamins A, E, B12 and D as well as folate, potassium, phosphorous, riboflavin, magnesium, iron and zinc.

This milk can be used as a substitute for goat's milk in any of the recipes in this book – provided your little one does not have a nut allergy.

• •

1 cup raw, organic almonds
¼ cup hemp seeds
4 dates
3 cups filtered water
1 t. alcohol-free vanilla extract or powder

Cover the almonds with water and soak overnight. In a separate bowl, cover the dates with water and allow to soak overnight too.

Drain the almonds and rinse well. Place in a high-speed blender.

Drain the dates and add them to the blender along with all the other ingredients.

Blend for a minute or so.

For a smoother consistency, pour the nut milk through a nut milk bag (or cheesecloth).

Serve or store in a sealed glass jar in the fridge for up to 3 days.

Variations:

- *You can try creating different flavours by adding: raw cacao nibs or powder, cinnamon or nutmeg to name but a few.*
- *If your little one does have a nut allergy, try making pure hemp milk instead. Replace the cup of almonds in this recipe with ½ cup hemp seeds (so you will use a total of ¾ cup of seeds altogether).*

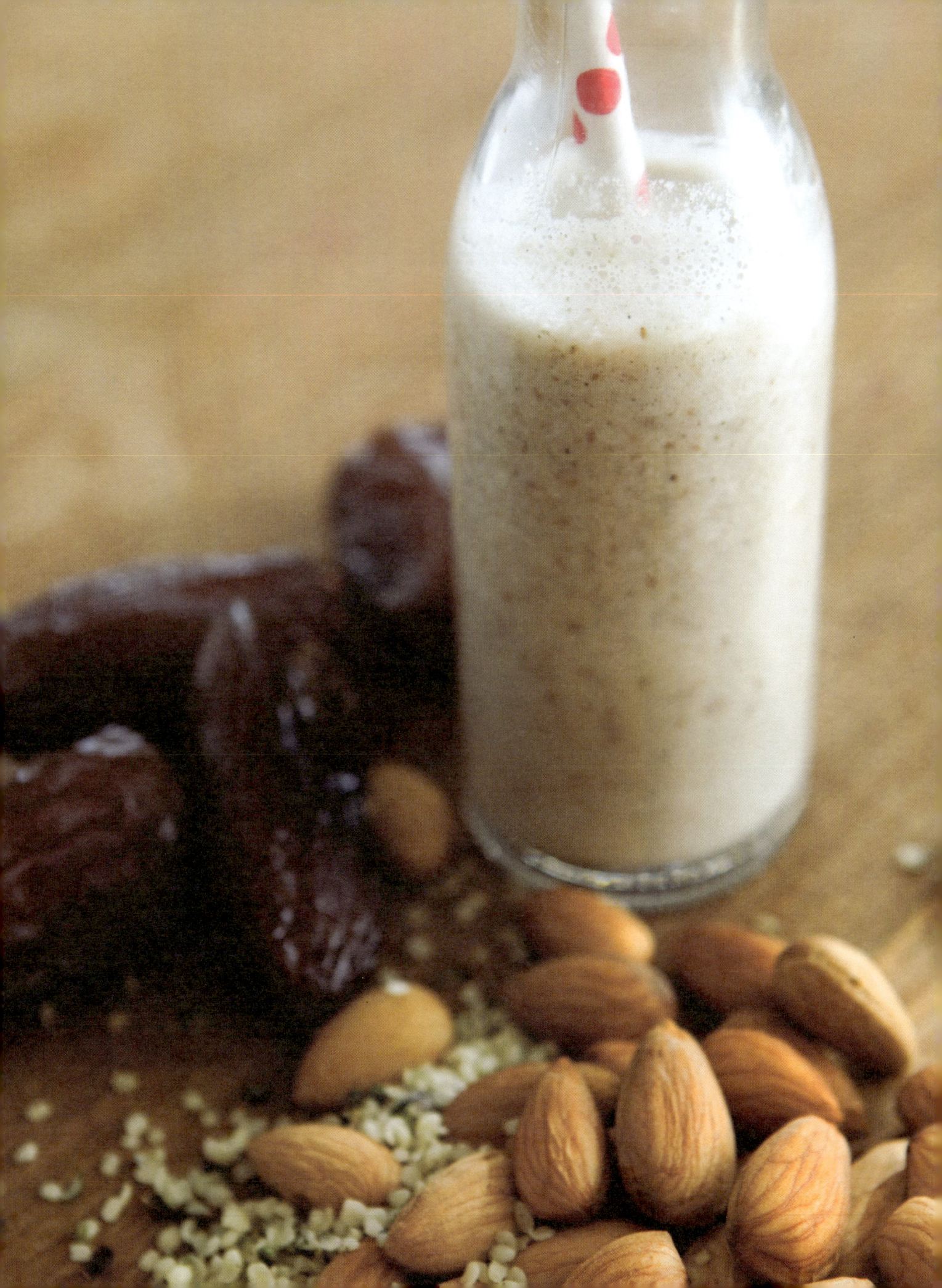

Recipes: Off the Spoon

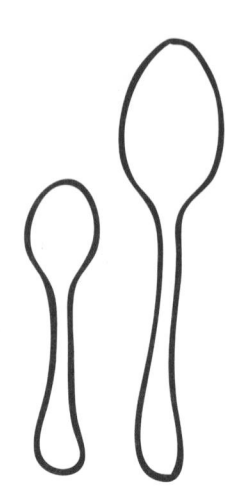

It is an exciting and somewhat daunting time when you prepare to give your little one solids for the first time!

Please refer to the section **"What to Introduce When"** to see which foods you should begin with. Familiarise yourself with this information, purchase the necessary equipment, get the camera ready and take a deep breath!

I first introduced Mila to solids when she was 4 months old under the mistaken impression that it would help her sleep through the night. Her sleeping got worse and after further research I realised that her under developed digestive system now had to work even harder to digest its food, meaning she was not having a very peaceful sleep at all.

I also made the mistake of giving Mila rice porridge as her first food – the poor little thing had cramps and serious constipation as a result. Despite the very successful marketing of Baby Cereals that they are baby's best first food, babies have limited enzyme production - and enzymes are necessary for the digestion of food. The specific enzymes required for the digestion of carbohydrates, and grains in particular, are only available in sufficient quantities when your little one is a year old, and only fully available when the molar teeth are developed. This is usually when your little one is around 28 months old. As such, cereals, pasta, grains and breads should be the last foods to be introduced and, when they are, they must be properly prepared by means of pre-soaking or fermenting.

SO IF NOT CEREALS AND PORRIDGES WHAT FOOD CAN YOU START WITH?

As you begin to wean your little one at 6 months, it is essential that the food that is replacing the breast milk or formula contains fat, iron, zinc and protein. While your little ones will not have the enzymes necessary to digest grains, they do produce the functional enzymes and digestive juices necessary for digesting proteins and fats. It stands to reason, then, that for ease of digestion as well as meeting nutrient requirements, your little ones' first foods should be animal foods (meat, organ meats, and eggs) as opposed to carbohydrates (grains and cereals).

FOLLOW YOUR LITTLE ONE'S LEAD.

When you begin with solids it is important to remember that most of the nutrition is still coming from your breast milk (or formula). Do not get stressed about how much your baby is, or is not eating – follow his/her lead. Food, at this stage, is about learning how to chew and swallow and about textures (as well as a whole lot of other neural development) – it is not so much about getting full or nourished.

Recipes: Off the Spoon

PURÉES → 162-180
THE FIRST EGG → 182
PORRIDGE → 184
MUESLI → 186
GREEN YOGHURT → 188
YOGHURT (DAIRY-FREE VERSION) → 188
RAW TOMATO AND BASIL SOUP → 190
BUTTERNUT SOUP → 192
DHAL → 194

Essential Nutrients

PURÉES

These are not really recipes but more ideas for food combinations and some guidelines on cooking methods and times.

When I began feeding Mila solids I followed the three-day wait rule - which is simply, feed your little one the same food for three days before introducing another one. This allows you to easily identify a food that may be causing an allergic reaction or digestive troubles. I therefore created individual food purées to start with. I made big batches and froze them in ice cube trays (covered and sealed in a zip lock bag).

Once I was confident that Mila did not react badly to a few different foods, I began to combine them in a purée mix. To reduce waste and save time (and my sanity), I kept making individual puréed food ice cubes. I would then take a couple different flavours out at a time and make a combination of those. To these I would add spices or superfoods just before serving. If she did not like that combination, it was easy and quick enough to make another one from scratch.

You will notice that this section is therefore composed of fairly simple purée 'combinations', more than recipes. There are some incredible purée 'meal' recipes available and I encourage you to look for them if you feel you would like to be a bit more adventurous – or more of a chef than a scientist!

PREPARING PURÉES

In terms of cooking various meat, fruits and vegetables for purées, steaming is the best way to preserve the nutrients. As such, you may want to invest in an electric steamer – the fact that you can set the timer, turn it on and walk away is very convenient! Alternatively, you can use a stove-top steaming basket.

You can sauté the food by placing it in a small saucepan with enough boiling water to cover the bottom of the pan. Cover and simmer – allowing the steam to do more of the cooking than the water. You will need to make sure that the saucepan does not cook dry. Use the cooking water to thin the purées so as not to discard valuable nutrients.

You can also bake your meat, fruit and vegetables. Use a relatively low oven heat (140-160°C / 280-320°F) for a longer period of time, instead of using high heat, in order to preserve nutrients. Be sure to never feed your little one any food which has been charred as this blackened food is carcinogenic.

I highly recommend in investing in a small blender to make the purées. I was fortunate enough to get one from my mom – it has worked hard and saved me a lot of time. Alternatively, you can mash the food with a fork and then pass it through a strainer to make sure it is very smooth for the first stage of feeding. If you are using raw fruit or vegetables, you can finely grate them to make the purée.

By the third month of solids you can make the purées a little coarser to introduce your little one to texture. I would continue to purée meats until they are smooth in order to aid their digestion.

> Essential Nutrients

FOOD COMBINATIONS

When creating your purée combinations, it may be worth taking the Body Ecology food combining principle into account. According to Donna Gates of the Body Ecology nutrition protocol, animal protein and starches (including grains) should not be combined in the same meal, as they require different enzymes to digest. These enzymes neutralise each other and inhibit digestion. If your little one is struggling with her digestion, it may be worth trying different food combinations to see if it helps.

NUTRIENTS

Please see the glossary pages for more information on each ingredient. Please also see the Nutrient Enhancer section for all the nutrient boosters you can add to a purée.

FLAVOUR

I strongly believe in introducing your little one to an array of flavours as early as possible. To spice your purées up (as well as adding additional nutrients), you can add a pinch of any of the following spices:

- ♥ **Cinnamon:** works well with savoury and sweet; fruit and vegetables.
- ♥ **Coriander:** works well with meat.
- ♥ **Nutmeg:** works well with savoury and sweet; fruit and vegetables.
- ♥ **Clove:** works well with savoury and sweet; fruit and vegetables.
- ♥ **Vanilla powder:** works well with sweet fruit.
- ♥ **Ginger:** works well with savoury and sweet; fruit, vegetables and meat.
- ♥ **Cardamom:** works well with savoury and sweet; fruit, vegetables and meat.
- ♥ **All Spice:** works well with savoury and sweet; fruit and vegetables.

Fresh herbs add flavour and nutrients. Try some of the following:

- ♥ **Basil:** works well with savoury and sweet; fruits, vegetables and meat.
- ♥ **Oreganum:** works well with vegetables and meat.
- ♥ **Coriander:** works well with vegetables and meat.
- ♥ **Thyme:** works well with vegetables and meat.
- ♥ **Rosemary:** works well with vegetables and meat.

> **NOTES FOR ALL PURÉES:**
> - ☐ REFERS TO AN ICE-CUBE PORTION, YOU CAN INCREASE QUANTITIES BY USING RATIOS.
> - ♡ PREPARATION IS SIMPLE: BLEND, PURÉE OR MASH ALL THE INGREDIENTS TOGETHER.
> - ♡ ADD A SPLASH OF ORGANIC EXTRA VIRGIN OLIVE OIL, FLAXSEED OIL, HEMP OIL OR COCONUT OIL.
> - ♡ MELT IN SOME ORGANIC GRASS FED GHEE OR BUTTER (IF YOU ARE NOT AVOIDING DAIRY).
> - ♡ ADD SOME ORGANIC EGG YOLK.
> - ♡ ADD 1/8 T. KEFIR OR JUICE FROM FERMENTED VEGETABLES.
> - ♡ IF YOUR LITTLE ONE IS UNWELL, ADD SOME NATURAL ANTIBIOTICS LIKE TURMERIC, STEAMED GARLIC OR ONION.
> - ♡ ADD ANY OF THE OTHER NUTRITIONAL ENHANCERS REMEMBERING TO FOLLOW THE 3-DAY RULE FOR THESE TOO.

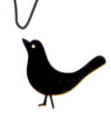

'FIXERS'

If you need to change the consistency of your purée, here are some 'fixers':

- ♥ **To thin the purée:** use breast milk, coconut milk, water (boiled and cooled, or filtered), or bone broth.
- ♥ **To make the purée thicker:** use mashed avocado, puréed lentils, ground chia seeds, arrowroot powder or tapioca flour.

Recipes: Off the Spoon

FRUIT

AVOCADO

ideal first food

What a convenient nutritious first food! Simply peal, pit, scoop out the flesh, mash with a fork and serve!

If you are not using the rest of the avocado for yourself, only cut out a slice for your little one. The rest of the avo (with skin on and pip in) can be store in an airtight container in the fridge for days. Avo tends to discolour when cut - simply cut the discoloured section off.

Avocado can also be stored in the freezer. Peel the whole fruit, pit and cut into baba-size slices. Make a lemon bath by adding freshly squeezed lemon juice to a bowl of water. Dip the slices of avo in the bath, then transfer to a parchment covered baking tray. Place the tray in the freezer. Once frozen, transfer the slices to a zip lock bag and keep in the freezer.

Avocados are high in unsaturated fats, which are important for normal growth and development of the central nervous system and brain. They are a good source of bone supportive vitamin K as well as heart-healthy dietary fibre, vitamin B6, vitamin C, and folate. Avocados are also a good source of energy-producing vitamin B5 and muscle-healthy potassium.

AVO PURÉES:

1☐ avocado + 1☐ banana

1☐ avocado + 1☐ banana + 1☐ pear

1☐ avocado + 1☐ mango + water or breast milk (for desired consistency)

1☐ avocado + 3☐ peach

1☐ avocado + 1☐ butternut / pumpkin + 1☐ peach

1☐ avocado + 1☐ apple + ½☐ chicken

BANANA

ideal first food

Simply peel, mash and serve! You can add some breast milk (or water) to make a slightly thinner consistency in the first few days of weaning.

For a different flavour, try baking bananas. Place the bananas (with their peels on) on a roasting tray and bake at 180°C (350°F) for 20 minutes. Allow the bananas to cool, then peel and mash.

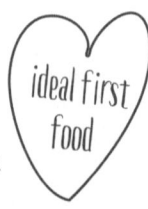

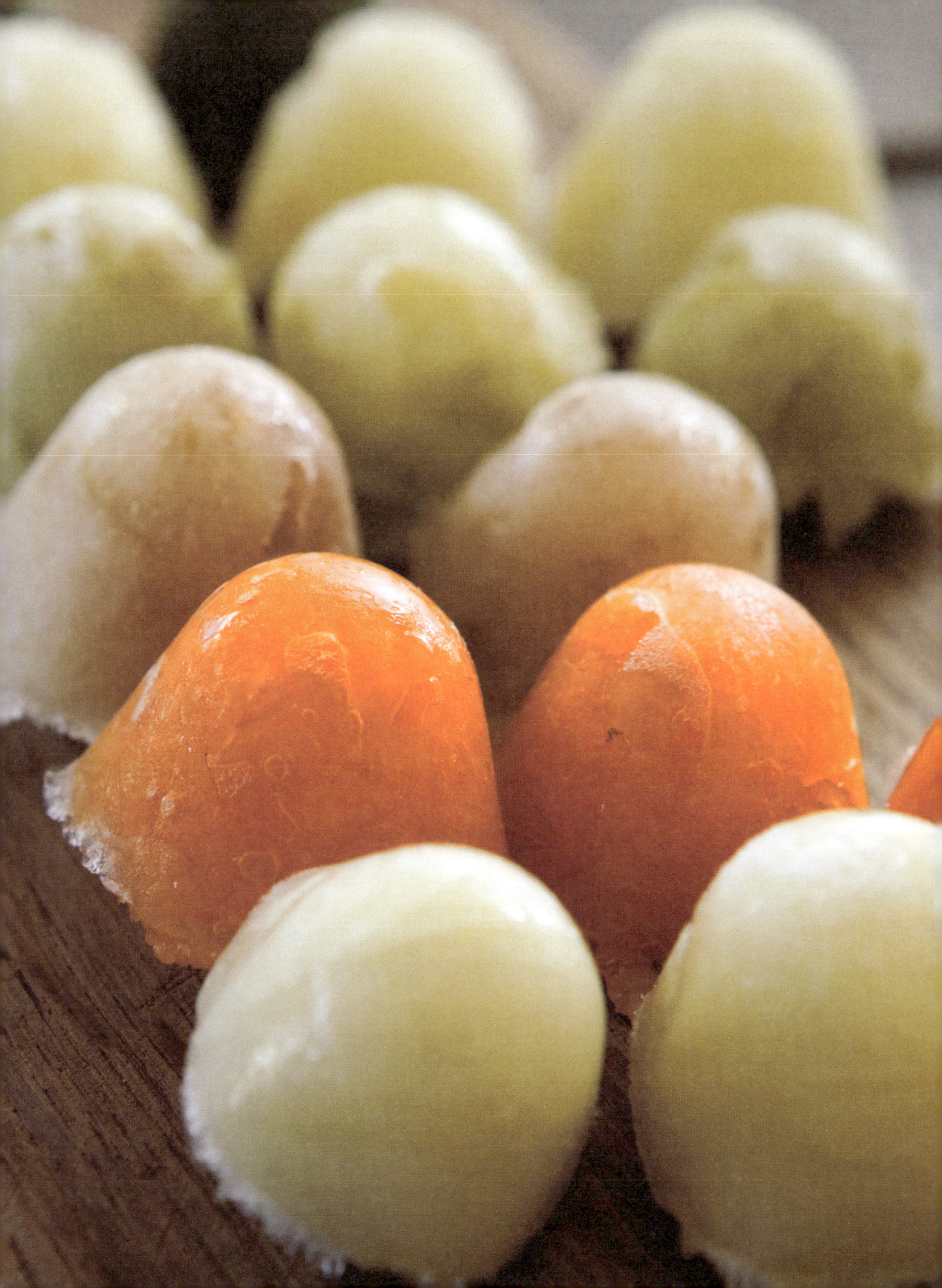

Recipes: Off the Spoon

Left over peeled bananas can be stored in the freezer. Simply cut into baba-size pieces. Make a lemon bath by adding freshly squeezed lemon juice to a bowl of water. Bath the banana chunks and then transfer to a parchment covered baking tray. Place the tray in the freezer. Once frozen, transfer the chunks to a Ziploc bag and keep in the freezer.

Bananas should only be eaten once they are very ripe or have black spots on the skin.

Ripe banana is a great food to add to porridge or grains because it contains amylase enzymes that are needed to digest carbohydrates and which your little one does not produce in sufficient quantities until he/she is over a year old.

BANANA PURÉES:

1☐ banana + 1☐ avocado

1☐ banana + 1☐ pear

1☐ banana + 1☐ apple

1☐ banana + 1☐ sweet potato + a sprinkle of nutmeg

1☐ banana + 1☐ butternut / pumpkin + a sprinkle of cinnamon

1☐ banana + 1☐ amaranth (as porridge or as whole grains if your little one is older)

APPLE

Wash, peel and core the apples. (Apples are one of the Dirty Dozen, they must be peeled.)

ideal first food

Cut into chunks and place in a steamer, or a small pot with 2-4 cm (1-2") of boiling water.

Steam for approximately 8 minutes. The apple is cooked when a fork can easily slide through it. Be careful not to overcook the apple as it will loose valuable nutrients. Under cooking the apple will result in it going brown once it has cooled.

Cool, mash or blend into a purée and serve or freeze.

You can add a pinch of cinnamon, nutmeg or vanilla powder to your apple. If you are storing the rest of the purée, only add the spices right before serving as freezing spices will cause them to lose their flavour.

Apples can also be baked. Core the apples, leaving the peels on. Sprinkle some cinnamon into the apples, then place in a roasting tray with enough water to just cover the bottom. Bake at 160°C (320°F) for 30-40 minutes. Allow the apples to cool, then scoop the flesh out of the skins and purée.

Cooked apple purée is a great remedy for constipation.

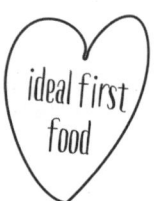

APPLE PURÉES:

1› apple + 1› banana + ½› broccoli

1› apple + 1› sweet potato + ½› liver

1› apple + ½› broccoli + ½ t. coconut oil or butter

1› apple + 1› lentils + pinch of cumin

1› apple (steamed or raw) + 1› avocado + ½ › chicken

PEAR

ideal first food

Pears do not need to be cooked – when they are ripe they are soft and gentle on the digestive system. Simply wash, peel, cur from the core and mash or purée.

Should you wish to steam a pear, cut into chunks and do so very briefly (4 minutes).

Do not forget to add some spices like cinnamon, nutmeg, ginger or vanilla.

Pears can also be baked. Leaving the skin on, core the pears, cut in them half and sprinkle with one of the spices. Place the pears in a roasting tray with enough water to just cover the bottom. Bake at 160°C (320°F) for 25 minutes. Allow the pears to cool, then scoop the flesh out of the skins and purée.

PEAR PURÉES:

1▢ pear + 1▢ apple + pinch of nutmeg, cinnamon, ginger or vanilla

1▢ pear + 1▢ butternut + pinch of cinnamon

1▢ pear + 1▢ sweet potato + 1▢ butternut + pinch of nutmeg

1▢ pear + 1▢ avocado + ½ ▢ liver / chicken / lamb

PEACH

7-8 months

Peaches do not need to be cooked if they are ripe – simply wash, pit and mash or purée. Peeling the peach is optional, although doing so will make it easier to digest.

Should you wish to steam them, cut into chunks and do so very briefly (4 minutes).

Peaches can also be baked. Leaving the skins on, cut the peaches in half and remove the pip. Place them in a roasting tray (skin side up) with enough water to just cover the bottom.

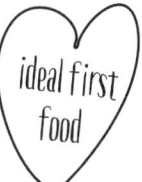

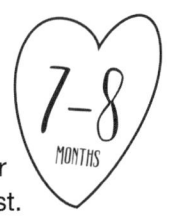

Recipes: Off the Spoon

Bake at 160°C (320°F) for 20 minutes (or until the skin puckers). Allow the peaches to cool, then scoop the flesh out of the skins and purée. You can also purée the peach with the skin on – it will be very soft after baking.

PEACH PURÉES:

1▢ peach + 1▢ banana + pinch of cinnamon or vanilla

1▢ peach + 1▢ butternut + pinch of cinnamon

1▢ peach + 1▢ sweet potato + pinch of nutmeg

1▢ peach + ½▢ chicken

1▢ peach + ½▢ ostrich + pinch of dried ginger

MANGO

7-8 MONTHS

Mangoes have a high fibre content that your little one may struggle with at first so it is best to only introduce these after other foods.

Mangoes are best eaten raw – so simply peel, cut the meat from the pip and mash or blend.

MANGO PURÉES:

1▢ mango + 1t. coconut milk/cream + pinch of vanilla powder

1▢ mango + 1▢ sweet potato + + 1t. coconut milk/cream + pinch of cinnamon

1▢ mango + ½▢ chicken + pinch of turmeric

BERRIES

8-12 MONTHS

These include strawberries, blueberries, raspberries, grapes etc.

I did not make any berry purées for Mila as they are all on the Dirty Dozen list and I wasn't able to source organic ones. I did introduce them as fingers foods at a later stage making sure I had soaked them in a hydrogen peroxide solution first.

They are best served raw.

Please note: Strawberries are a high potential allergen food.

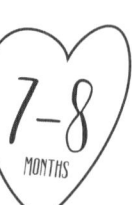

Recipes: Off the Spoon

MELONS

8-12 months

It was quite amusing the first time I tried to make a melon purée – it simply becomes a juice due to the high water content! I therefore delayed introducing melons until Mila was eating finger foods. If you find the melon pieces are too slippery for your little one to pick up, try coating them in almond or coconut flour.

There are a wide variety of melons: Cantaloupe (or Spanspek in South Africa), papaya, paw paw, watermelon etc. Please see the glossary section for more information on each.

VEGETABLES

SWEET POTATO

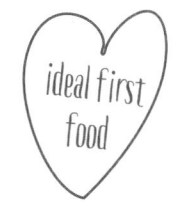

ideal first food

Sweet potatoes can be steamed or baked however baking really brings out their sweetness.

TO BAKE

Wash the sweet potatoes well, then place them in a roasting dish. Drizzle some olive oil or coconut oil over them and bake at 180°C (350°F) for approximately 1 hour. Cooking time will depend on the size of the sweet potato. Your potato will be cooked when a fork easily slides all the way through it. Once done, cut them lengthwise and scoop out the flesh. Cool, mash or blend into a purée and serve or store.

TO STEAM

Wash and peel the sweet potatoes. Cut into small chunks and place in a steamer or a small pot with 2-4 cm (1-2") of boiling water. Steam for approximately 15 minutes, or until soft. Cool, mash or blend into a purée and serve or store.

You can add a pinch of cinnamon or nutmeg to your sweet potato. If you are storing the rest of the purée, only add the spices right before serving as freezing will cause the spices to lose their flavour.

SWEET POTATO PURÉES:

1 sweet potato + 1 apple + ½ > liver / ostrich

1 sweet potato + 1 banana + a sprinkle of nutmeg

1 sweet potato + 1 pear + 1 butternut + pinch of nutmeg

1 sweet potato + 1 peach + pinch of nutmeg

1 sweet potato + 1 mango + 1t. coconut milk/cream + pinch of cinnamon

1 sweet potato + ½ broccoli + ½ chicken

Sweet potato actually combines well with everything!

Recipes: Off the Spoon

BUTTERNUT

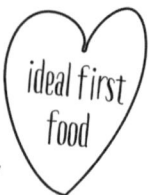

ideal first food

Butternut can be steamed or baked. Baking a butternut really brings out the nutty flavour and buttery texture – and you do not have so peel it (a BIG time saver!)

TO BAKE

Wash the butternut well, cut in half lengthwise and scoop out the seeds. Place skin-side up in a roasting dish with 2-4 cm (1-2") of water. Bake at 180°C (350°F) for approximately 1 hour. Cooking time will depend on the size of the butternut – it will be cooked when the skin is a dark tan colour and a fork slides easily all the way through it. Once done, scoop out the flesh, cool, mash or blend into a purée and serve or store.

TO STEAM

Wash, peel and seed the butternut. Cut the flesh into small chunks and place in a steamer or a small pot with 2-4 cm (1-2") of boiling water. Steam for approximately 15 minutes, or until soft. Cool, mash or blend into a purée and serve or store.

You can add a pinch of cinnamon or nutmeg to your butternut. If you are storing the rest of the purée, only add the spices right before serving as freezing will cause them to lose their flavour.

BUTTERNUT PURÉES:

1 ☐ butternut + 1 ☐ apple + pinch of cinnamon

1 ☐ butternut + 1 ☐ peach + 1 ☐ avocado

1 ☐ butternut + 1 ☐ banana + a sprinkle of cinnamon

1 ☐ butternut + 1 ☐ sweet potato + 1 ☐ pear + pinch of nutmeg

1 ☐ butternut + 1 ☐ apple + ½ ☐ chicken, ostrich, lamb or beef

Do not forget to try the other members of the squash family like pumpkin, gem squash, baby marrow, and patty pans.

BROCCOLI

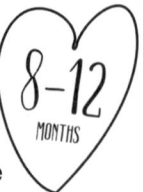

8-12 MONTHS

Break the head of broccoli into smaller florets and wash well by soaking in a hydrogen peroxide or vinegar water solution for 10 minutes. Rinse and cut off all remaining stalks.

Place in a steamer or a small pot with 2-4 cm (1-2") of boiling water.

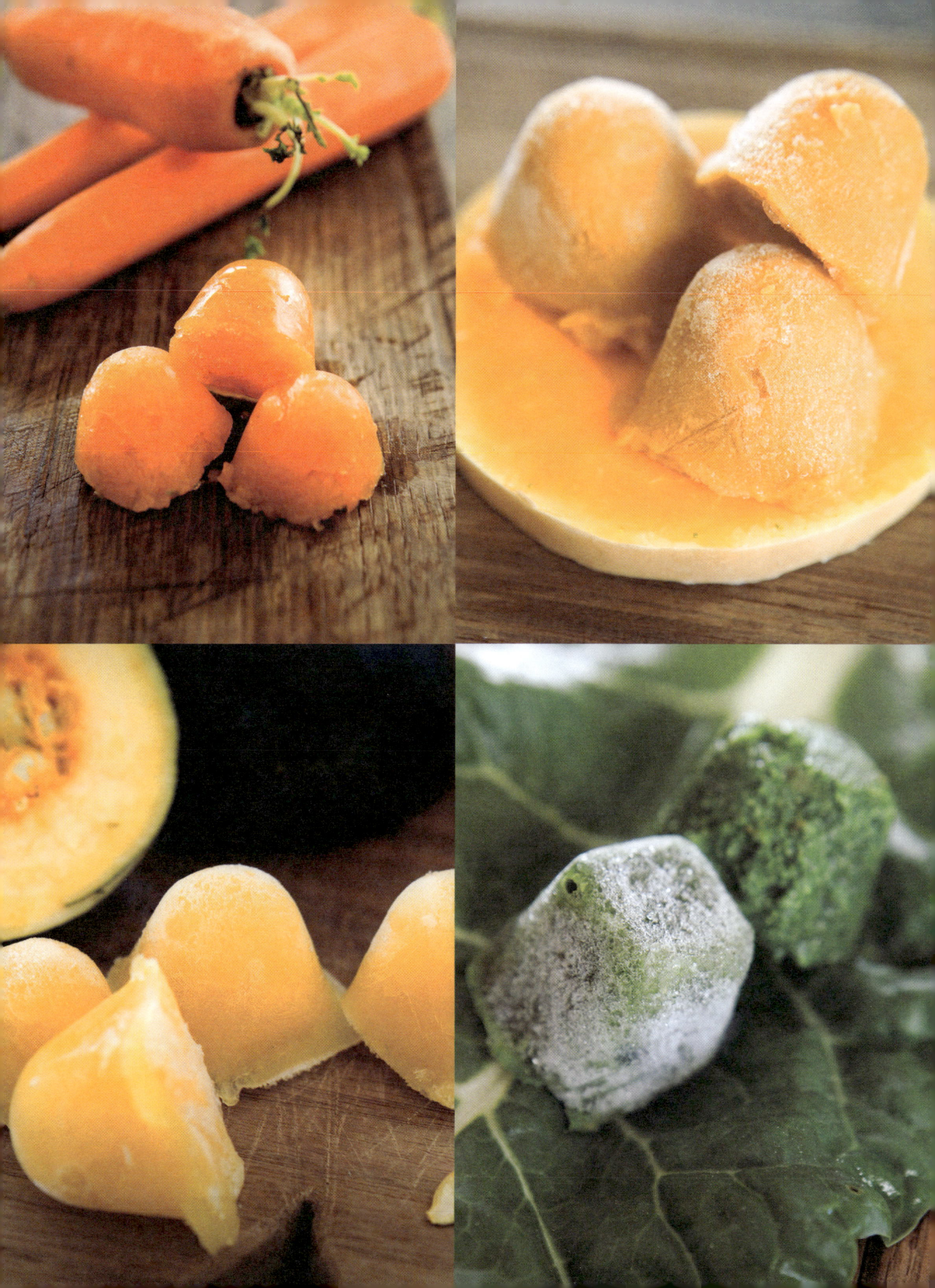

Recipes: Off the Spoon

Steam for approximately 8 minutes or until soft. Be sure not to overcook it as it quickly loses all its colour and nutrients.

Cool, mash or blend into a purée and serve or store.

Broccoli has a very strong flavour and as a member of the Brassica family of vegetables, it can cause gas and be difficult to digest. As such it is best to wait until your little one is 8-10 months old before introducing it, and when you do, add small amount to other purées.

BROCCOLI PURÉES:

½ ☐ broccoli + 1 ☐ apple + ½ t. coconut oil, ghee or butter

½ ☐ broccoli + 1 ☐ apple + 1 ☐ banana

½ ☐ broccoli + 1 ☐ sweet potato + ½ ☐ chicken

CAULIFLOWER

8-12 MONTHS

Break the head of cauliflower into smaller florets and wash well by soaking in a hydrogen peroxide or vinegar water solution for 10 minutes. Rinse and cut off all remaining stalks.

Place in a steamer or a small pot with 2-4 cm (1-2") of boiling water.

Steam for approximately 8 minutes or until soft.

Cool, mash or blend into a purée and serve or store.

You can add a pinch of cinnamon or nutmeg to your cauliflower purée. If you are storing the rest of the purée, only add the spices right before serving as freezing will cause them to lose their flavour.

As a member of the Brassica family of vegetables, cauliflower can cause gas and be difficult to digest. Therefore it is best to wait until your little one is 8-10 months old before introducing it.

CAULIFLOWER PURÉES:

1 ☐ cauliflower + ½ t. coconut oil, ghee or butter

1 ☐ cauliflower + 1 ☐ apple + 1 ☐ butternut

1 ☐ cauliflower + ½ ☐ chicken

Recipes: Off the Spoon

SPINACH

(Including Young Leaf Spinach and Swiss Chard)

8-12 MONTHS

Spinach cooks really quickly so you can simply blanch it.

Wash the spinach leaves well, cut out the stem and place the leaves in a colander in the sink.

Pour a kettle full of boiling water over the leaves ensuring the water flows evenly over all the leaves. Allow the spinach to drain for 2 minutes and then blend. You may need to add a liquid to the spinach to help it move in the blender. You can use water, coconut milk or breast milk.

It is delicious blended with a bit of sautéed garlic and onion.

Spinach contains both oxalates and nitrates and it is therefore best to wait until your little one is 8-10 months old before introducing it. When you do introduce it be sure to follow the 3-day rule and start by adding a little at a time to other purées.

I find it best to mix spinach with another purée or coconut milk before freezing to avoid it becoming too watery.

SPINACH PURÉES:

½ ☐ spinach + 1 ☐ coconut milk + 1 ☐ sweet potato

½ ☐ spinach + 1 ☐ apple + 1 ☐ butternut + pinch of nutmeg

½ ☐ spinach + ½ ☐ any meat + 1 ☐ cauliflower

KALE

8-12 MONTHS

Kale is a better choice of leafy greens than spinach since it is much lower in oxalates - oxalates interfere with the absorption of calcium and iron. Kale has about 2 mg of oxalate per cup, while spinach has about 656 mg per cup.

Wash the kale leaves well in a hydrogen peroxide or vinegar water solution to remove the pesticides if it is not organic. *(Kale is on the Dirty Dozen list.)*

Pull the green leaves from the stems (the stems are not eaten).

Boil or steam the leaves for 2 minutes, then drain.

Blend into a purée. Kale is a thick green leaf and it is not really puréed as it is ground up into fine pieces. You may need to add a liquid to the kale to help it move in the blender. You can use filtered water, coconut milk or breast milk.

Serve or store.

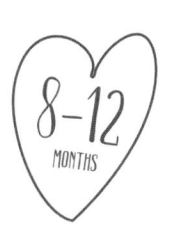

Recipes: Off the Spoon

KALE PURÉES:

1 ☐ kale + 1 ☐ avocado + 1 ☐ banana
1 ☐ kale + 1 ☐ coconut milk + 1 ☐ sweet potato
1 ☐ kale + 1 ☐ apple + 1 ☐ butternut + pinch of nutmeg
1 ☐ kale + ½ ☐ any meat + 1 ☐ cauliflower

There are many other vegetables you can make purées from such as carrots, tomato, beetroot, zucchini, eggplant, parsnips and peas. Please check the introduction chart for some guidelines on when to introduce each one. Be creative and adventurous! The more flavours your little ones taste now; the more varied diet they will eat when they are old enough to choose what they want. Many of these vegetables can also be introduced as finger foods.

PULSES

LENTILS

12 MONTHS

It is best to start with red lentils as these have less fibre; produce less gas; and, cook to a very mushy consistency.

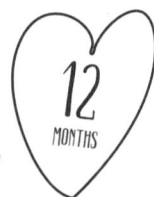

Cover the lentils with warm water and add an acid medium (whey, lemon juice or apple cider vinegar). The ratio of lentils to acid should be 2 tablespoons acid for every 2 cups of lentils. Soak for twelve to twenty-four hours (or overnight), then drain, rinse and cook.

Add one part lentils to two parts boiling water or broth. After the liquid has returned to a boil, turn down the heat, cover and simmer for about 15 - 25 minutes (depending on the variety).

Lentils take on other flavours very well – try adding some ginger, garlic, coriander, cardamom, cinnamon, turmeric and, or nutmeg.

Cool, mash or blend into a purée and serve or store.

LENTIL PURÉES:

1 ☐ lentil + 1 ☐ carrot + ½ ☐ onion + ¼ ☐ garlic + pinch of curry powder
1 ☐ lentil + ½ ☐ spinach + ½ ☐ onion
1 ☐ lentil + 1 ☐ butternut + 1 ☐ pear
1 ☐ lentil + 1 ☐ sweet potato + ½ ☐ chicken
1 ☐ lentil + 1 ☐ apple + ½ ☐ ostrich

CHICKPEA

(Also known as garbanzo beans)

12 MONTHS

Chickpeas can cause gas so be sure to introduce them slowly and follow these preparation guidelines. Since cooked chickpeas freeze well, I prepare a whole bag of dried chickpeas at a time - as the preparation is quite time consuming. Chickpeas not being used for purée can also be made into hummus for the rest of the family.

Cover the chickpeas with hot water and add an acid medium (whey, lemon juice or apple cider vinegar). Soak for twelve to twenty-four hours (or overnight), changing the soaking water at least once during this time. Drain, rinse and cook.

Cover the chickpeas with boiling water or broth (make sure there is twice as much liquid to chickpeas). After the liquid has returned to a boil, turn down the heat, cover and simmer for 1½ hours.

Drain then mash or blend into a purée and serve or store.

CHICKPEA PURÉES:

1☐ chickpea + 1☐ sweet potato + coconut / breast milk to thin

1☐ chickpea + 1☐ butternut/pumpkin + 1☐ mashed banana

1☐ chickpea + 1☐ avo + ½ ☐ chicken + few drops lemon juice

•••

MEAT

CHICKEN

6-7 MONTHS

Only use pasture-raised free-range or organic chicken.

The light meat of chicken, such as the breast, is higher in protein and lower in fat. The dark meat, such as thighs and legs, is higher in iron and higher in fat – making it the preferable choice.

Although grilled, pan-fried, braaied or barbecued chicken is delicious, these methods of cooking are not recommended for your little one. Any blackened food is carcinogenic and cooking over high heat destroys many valuable nutrients.

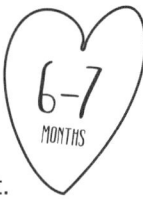

Recipes: Off the Spoon

SLOW COOKER / CROCK-POT

This is a great way of preparing chicken for the whole family.

Chicken meat on the bone (such as thighs and drumsticks) is best cooked slowly.

Place the chicken in a slow cooker with some carrots, celery, onion, garlic, thyme, salt and bay leaves. Cover with chicken broth, vegetable broth or water (or a combination) and cook on high for 4 hours, or on low for 6 hours.

Reserve the cooking liquid (broth) to use for thinning out purées, adding to other meals, drinking or cooking (you can pour it into an ice-cube tray and freeze it for future use).

Remove the chicken meat from the bone and purée with some of the cooking liquid. Add some vegetable purées and serve or store.

SIMMERING

If you would like to cook chicken breasts, poaching them is a great method to use.

Dice the chicken breasts and place the meat in a saucepan with just enough water or chicken broth to cover. You can also add some freshly pressed apple juice – this not only sweetens the chicken but tenderises it too.

Bring the contents of the saucepan to a boil and then turn the heat down to a simmer. Simmer for approximately 10-20 minutes (depending on the size of your chicken pieces). The chicken is cooked when it has turned white and the juices run clear.

Place the chicken pieces in a blender with some of the cooking water and purée. Add some vegetable purées and serve or store.

STEAMING

By far the quickest and easiest way of preparing chicken is to steam it.

To season the chicken in a steamer you can sprinkle the meat with dried herbs or spices. Alternatively cover the chicken pieces with a layer of lemon or orange slices (citrus tenderises the chicken thanks to its acidity). For a earthier taste you can cover the chicken with a layer of nori sheets.

Simply place the chicken in a steamer for 10 minutes or until the chicken is cooked through (the meat should be opaque and the juices should run clear).

Remove the chicken meat from the bone and purée with some broth, reserved steaming water and nori (if used). Add some vegetable purées and serve or store.

ROASTING

This is a great way of preparing chicken for the whole family.

Preheat your oven to 160°C (320°F).

Take a whole chicken and rub it all over with olive oil. Season with herbs such as dried basil, oreganum, rosemary or thyme, and/or spices such as paprika. Sprinkle with some sea salt

Recipes: Off the Spoon

and a squeeze of lemon juice.

Place the chicken in a roasting dish just big enough to hold it (using a roasting dish that is too big causes the cooking juices to evaporate and then the chicken tends to dry out).

Place in the oven for 2 hours, basting every now and then with the cooking juices.

Remove the chicken meat from the bone and purée with some broth or water – do not use the cooking juices from the roasting tray as the fat content would be too high for your little one.

Add some vegetable purées and serve or store.

You can also roast individual chicken pieces. Using the same method as above a general rule is that you should cook the meat for 20 minutes per 450g/pound.

CHICKEN PURÉES:

½ ☐ chicken + 1☐ lentils + 1☐ sweet potato

½ ☐ chicken + 1☐ avocado + 1☐ apple

½ ☐ chicken + 1☐ pear + 1☐ avocado

½ ☐ chicken + 1☐ peach

½ ☐ chicken + 1☐ mango + pinch of turmeric

½ ☐ chicken + 1☐ sweet potato + ½ ☐ broccoli

½ ☐ chicken + 1☐ butternut + 1☐ apple

½ ☐ chicken + 1☐ lentils + 1☐ sweet potato

LAMB

Only use free-range grass-fed lamb.

Lamb cooked on the bone is far more tender than other cuts of lamb. You will need to slow cook it though.

6-7 MONTHS

Although grilled, pan-fried, braaied or barbecued lamb is delicious, these methods of cooking are not recommended for your little one. Any blackened food is carcinogenic and cooking over high heat destroys many valuable nutrients.

SLOW COOKER / CROCK-POT

This is a great way of preparing lamb for the whole family.

Good cuts to use include lamb knuckles, lamb neck, lamb chops and lamb shanks.

Heat some ghee, butter or coconut oil in a large frying pan and brown the lamb on all sides. Place the lamb in a slow cooker with some carrots, celery, onion, garlic, rosemary, bay leaves

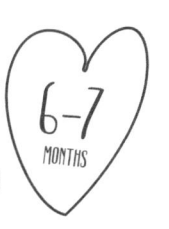

Recipes: Off the Spoon

and sea salt. Cover with lamb broth, vegetable broth or water (or a combination) and cook on low for 6 hours.

Reserve the cooking liquid (broth) to use for thinning out purées, adding to other meals, drinking or cooking (you can pour it into an ice-cube tray and freeze for future use).

Remove the lamb meat from the bone and purée with some of the cooking liquid. Add some vegetable purées and serve or store.

STEAMING

A good cut to use for steaming is the lamb loin.

Cut the lamb into medallions and season with spices such as coriander or herbs such rosemary or oreganum.

Place the lamb in a steamer for 10 minutes or until the lamb is cooked though.

Purée the lamb with some broth or reserved steaming water. Add some vegetable purées and serve or store.

ROASTING

This is a great way of preparing lamb for the whole family.

Good cuts to use include lamb shoulder and leg of lamb.

To slow roast a shoulder or leg of lamb, heat your oven to its maximum temperature.

Rub both sides of the lamb with olive oil or macadamia nut oil. Line the bottom of a roasting pan with fresh rosemary and garlic cloves (skin on). Place the lamb on top of the herbs and cover with more rosemary and garlic. Cover the roasting pan with tin foil and place in the oven. Turn the oven down to 170°C (325°F). Roast the lamb for 4 hours, or until it falls off the bone.

Remove the lamb meat from the bone and purée it with some broth or water. Add some vegetable purées and serve or store.

The roasted garlic with have a nutty flavour and is a delicious addition to the meat purée.

LAMB PURÉES:

½ ☐ lamb + 1☐ sweet potato + ½ ☐ carrot

½ ☐ lamb + 1☐ avocado + 1☐ apple

½ ☐ lamb + 1☐ butternut + 1☐ apple

Recipes: Off the Spoon

BEEF

6-7 MONTHS

Only use free-range or organic grass-fed beef.

Beef cooked on the bone is far more tender than other cuts of beef and therefore easier to purée smoothly. You will need to slow cook it though.

Although grilled, pan-fried, braaied or barbecued beef is delicious, these methods of cooking are not recommended for your little one. Any blackened food is carcinogenic and cooking over high heat destroys many valuable nutrients.

SLOW COOKER / CROCK-POT

This is a great way of preparing beef for the whole family.

Good cuts to use include beef shin, chuck steak, oxtail and brisket. (These also happen to be the cheaper cuts of meat).

Heat some ghee, butter or coconut oil in a large frying pan and brown the beef on all sides. Place the beef in a slow cooker with some carrots, celery, onion, garlic, rosemary, bay leaves and salt. Cover with beef broth, vegetable broth or water (or a combination) and cook on low for 6 hours.

Reserve the cooking liquid (broth) to use for thinning out purées, adding to other meals, drinking or cooking (you can pour it into an ice-cube tray and freeze for future use).

Remove the beef from the bone and purée with some of the cooking liquid. Add some vegetable purées and serve or store.

STEAMING

A good cut of beef to use for steaming is the beef loin.

Cut the beef loin into medallions and season with spices such as coriander or herbs such as oreganum.

Place the medallions in a steamer for 10 minutes or until the beef is cooked though.

Purée the beef with some broth or reserved steaming water. Add some vegetable purées and serve or store.

ROASTING

This is a great way of preparing lamb for the whole family.

Good cuts to use include silverside, blade, topside, standing rib, centre rump and rump eye.

Preheat your oven to 160°C (320°F).

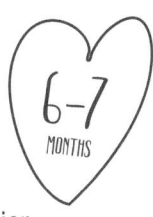

Rub all sides of the beef with olive oil or macadamia nut oil. Line the bottom of a roasting pan with fresh oreganum, carrots and garlic cloves still in their skin – the garlic helps to tenderise the meat. Place the beef on top of the herbs and vegetables. Place the roasting pan in the oven and roast the beef for 25 minutes per 500 grams (1 pound). The beef will be cooked to medium.

Allow the beef to rest for 5 minutes then carve and slice into pieces. Purée the beef with some broth or water. Add some vegetable purées and serve or store.

The roasted garlic with have a nutty flavour and will be a delicious addition to the meat purée.

BEEF PURÉES:

½ ☐ beef + 1☐ sweet potato + ½ ☐ apple

½ ☐ beef + 1☐ carrot + 1☐ pear

½ ☐ beef + 1☐ gem squash + 1☐ butternut + roasted garlic to taste

LIVER

6-7 MONTHS

Please read the section Unlearn: Liver is Dangerous to see what an important, nutrient-dense, great first food liver is.

Please choose pasture raised organic or free-range chicken, or grass fed calf or lamb liver. Livers are highly perishable – either cook or freeze them on the day of purchase. They can be frozen for 1 month.

Besides freezing and grating the raw liver into any purée, you can also cook and purée the liver in the following way.

Clean the liver thoroughly before cooking by rinsing and cutting away any connective tissue. Roughly chop the liver and place in a saucepan with enough broth to cover the livers. Bring to the boil. Turn the heat down, cover and simmer for 5 - 8 minutes. Transfer the livers to a blender and add some of the cooking broth. Blend, adding more broth to achieve the desired consistency.

Add some vegetable purées and serve or store.

LIVER PURÉES:

½ ☐ liver + 1☐ sweet potato

½ ☐ liver + 1☐ avocado

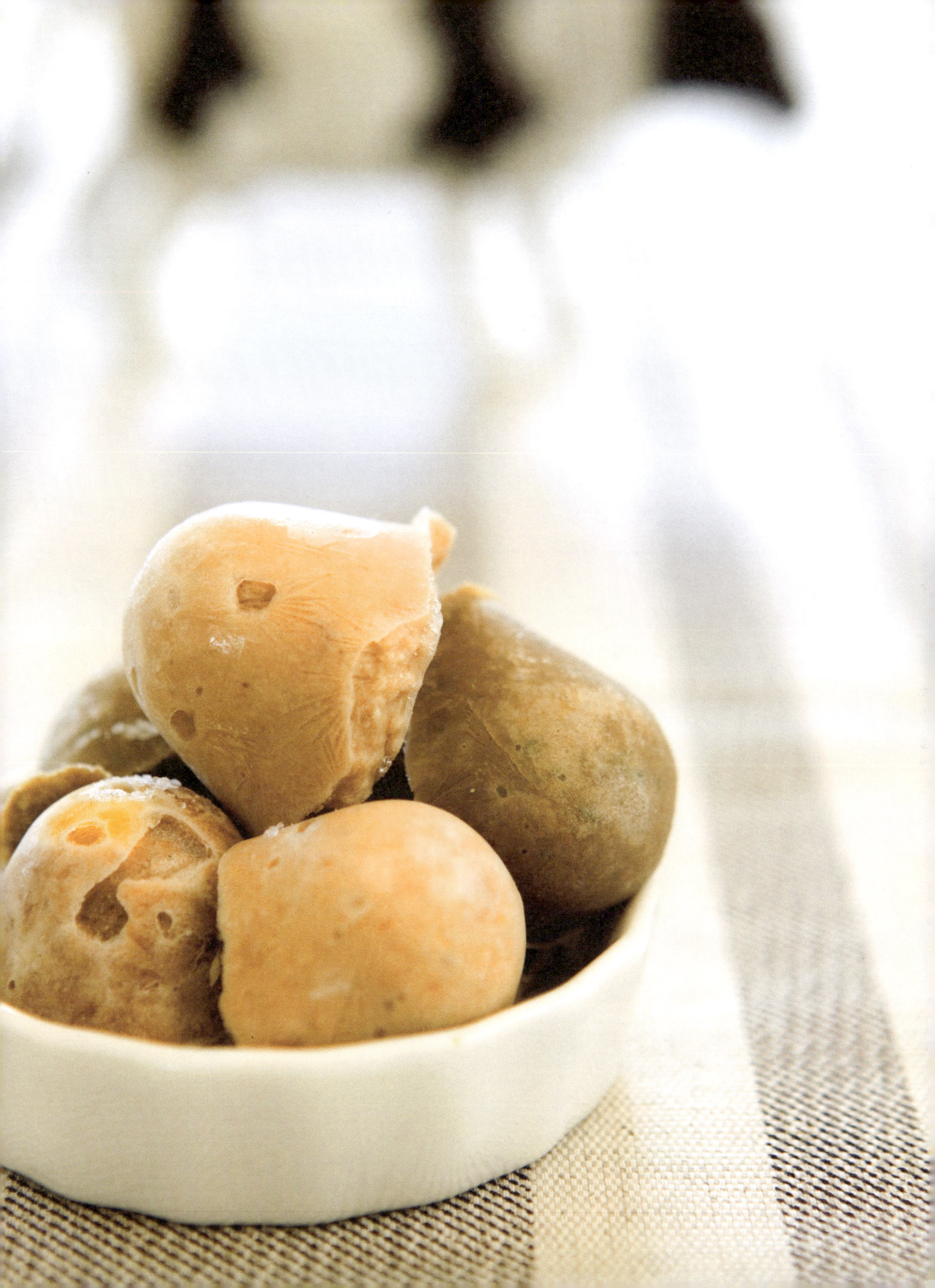

Recipes: Off the Spoon

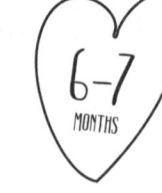

THE FIRST EGG

6-7 MONTHS

vegetarian; grain-free; for adults too; great for lunchboxes

••

Eggs have had a bad reputation as a high allergen food, and it has in the past been recommended that they should only be introduced after the age of 1. This is unfortunate since egg yolks are one of the most nutrient dense foods. They are easily digested with nutrients that are easily absorbed. The Weston A. Price Foundation (and others) are now recommending that pasture-raised organic egg yolks should be one of your little one's first foods. The egg whites should only be introduced after your little one is a year old – it is the egg whites which are allergenic, not the yolks.

The First Egg can be eaten on its own or added to any of your purée combinations as a nutritional enhancer.

According to Sally Fallon Morell, The First Egg can be introduced to your little one as early as 4 months. If your little one does not tolerate it well, try again a month later.

*The liver should only be added when your little one is 6 months old. It must be frozen for 2 weeks prior to using it as this will ensure the elimination of pathogens and parasites.

••

1 organic egg
(from a pasture-raised hen)

½ t. grated raw organic liver, (frozen for 14 days*) - *optional*

Boil the egg for approximately 3½ minutes (longer at higher altitudes).

Place in a bowl and peel off the shell.

Remove egg white.

The yolk should be soft and warm, not hot and not runny.

If you wish to add liver, grate it on the small holes of a grater while frozen. Allow it to warm up and stir it into egg yolk.

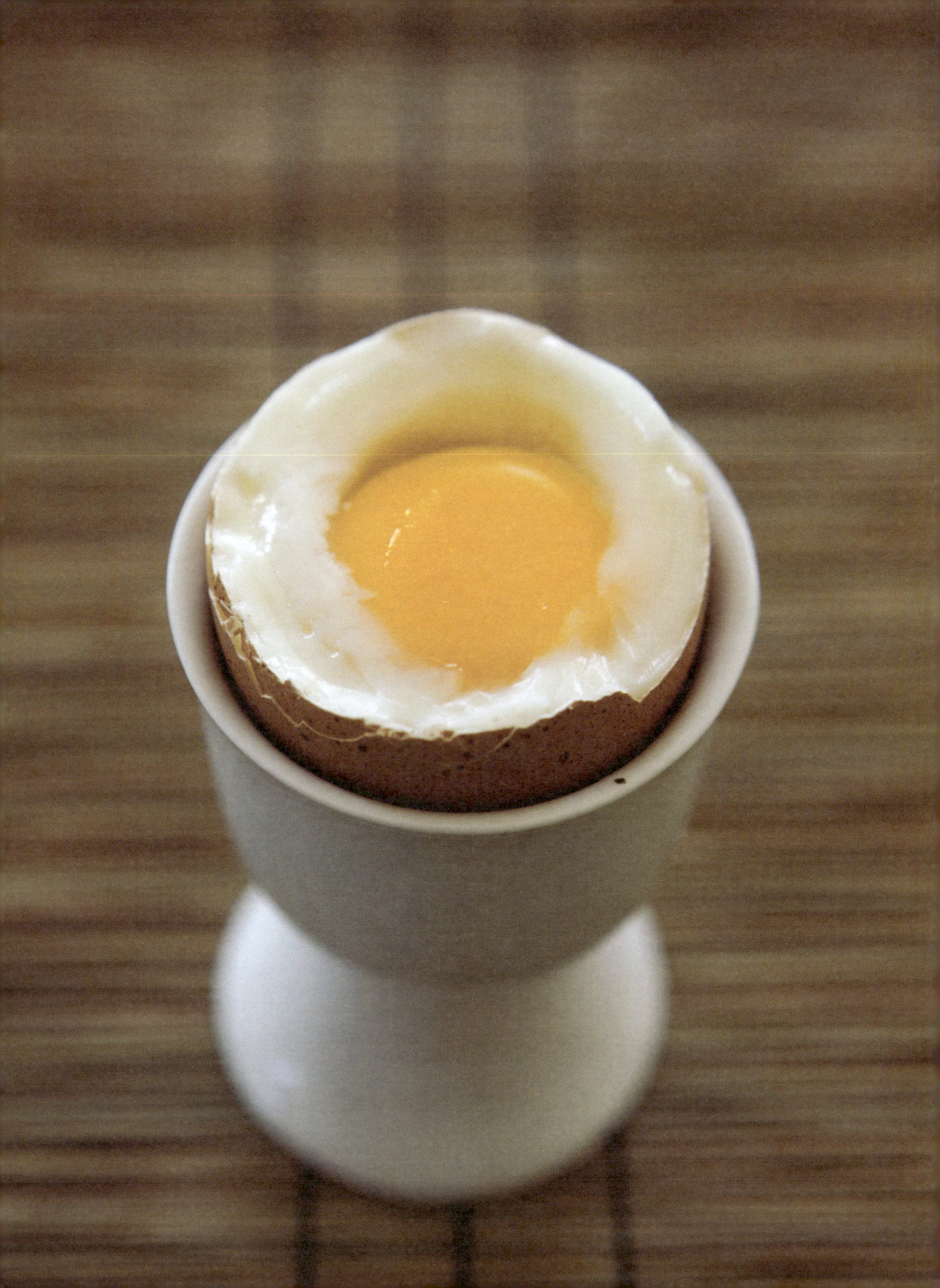

Recipes: Off the Spoon

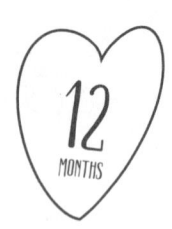

PORRIDGE

vegetarian; egg-free; for adults too

Makes enough for baby, mom and dad.

....

Remember, grains are very difficult for your little one to digest and they should ideally not be introduced until they are at least a year old, and if possible it should be delayed until they are 2 years old.

When I started feeding Mila solids I was unaware of the need to pre-soak grains, or that they should not be introduced in the first year. Already colicky and constipated, the grains seriously aggravated her digestion. But I carried on – thinking it was simply her body's way of getting used to solid food. Now that she is 3 years old, I have taken her off all grains in an attempt to heal her gut which I believe was injured, in part, due to the early introduction of grains.

If you do want to feed your little one grains, use one of the four traditional grains (millet, quinoa, amaranth, and buckwheat) or short-grain brown rice.

....

1 cup grains *(millet, short grain brown rice, amaranth or quinoa) – soaked and dehydrated*

1 cup water, or coconut milk

1 T. organic maple syrup

1 t. cinnamon

2 t. grass fed ghee or butter*

¼ cup finely chopped fruit (such as apple, peach, raisins) – *optional, and only if your little one is comfortable with chewing and lumpy bits!*

Grind the grains with a pestle and mortar or coffee grinder. The younger your little one the finer you will want this to be.

Place the grains in a saucepan and add the water (or coconut milk), maple syrup, cinnamon and fruit.

Gently simmer for a 10 minutes.

Pour into bowls, allow to cool and serve.

Left over porridge can be kept in the fridge for 2 – 3 days.

---

*The fat soluble vitamins in the ghee or butter assist in the absorption of the nutrients from the grains. They also slow down the release of glucose (from the grains) into the bloodstream, keeping your little one's blood sugar more stable.

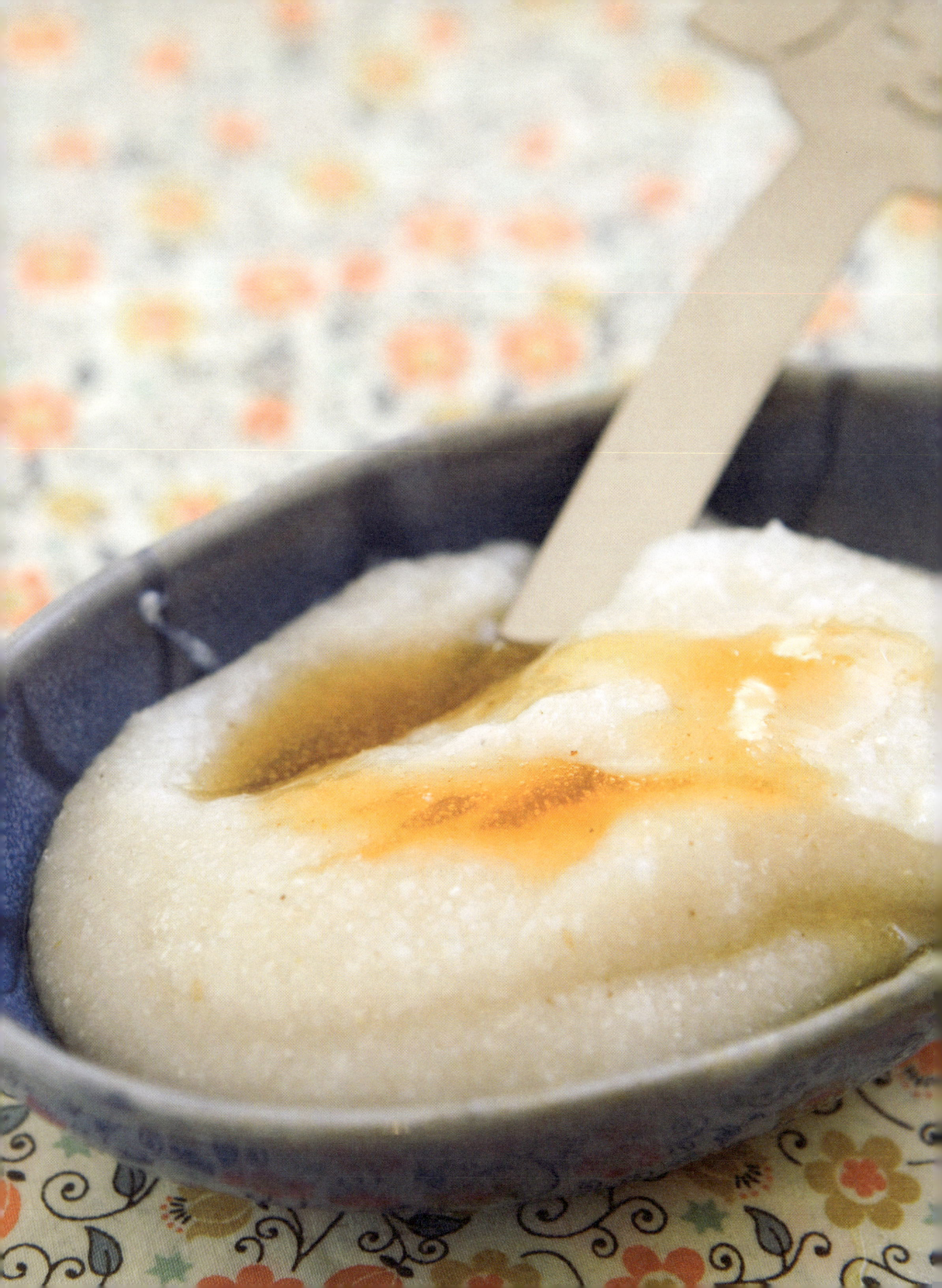

Recipes: Off the Spoon

MUESLI

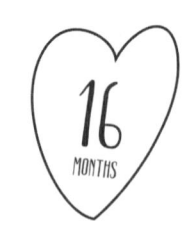

16 months

raw; superfood; vegetarian; egg-free; for adults too

Makes a one week supply for baby, mom and dad. (Or a 1 month supply for baby.)

Now that your little one is happily chewing solids you may want to add a breakfast cereal into the mix. Before you grab a box with brightly coloured cartoon characters, or even a healthy looking bag of muesli, be warned... many breakfast cereals available in the supermarkets are loaded with sugar, artificial colours and chemical flavourings. They have been produced at high temperature and pressure which destroys most of the original ingredients' natural nutrients and changes the chemical structure of the grains making them toxic.

These cereals (and baby porridges) have had to be fortified with synthetic vitamins in order to replace the lost nutrients. The synthetic replacements are not recognised by your little one's body, are difficult-to-digest and are not a suitable substitute for the real thing - in fact the body tries to eliminate them as quickly as possible.

Standard breakfast cereals cause a spike in blood sugar leaving your little one hungry soon after the meal; more inclined to 'naughty' behaviour; and, craving more sugar or carbohydrates. Also, because these gains have not been soaked, fermented or sprouted they contain phytic acid - an anti-nutrient. Which means, they actually draw good nutrients out of your little one's body.

Bottom line... breakfast cereals are so popular because of clever marketing and because they are convenient – not because they are a good start to the day!

This raw muesli recipe may be time consuming to make, but it can be made in bulk and has a long shelf-life. It is also suitable for the whole family – there is no need to chop it into smaller pieces for older children or yourself.

The buckwheat and seeds in this recipe are an excellent source of protein and healthy fats making it a great way to start the day.

Mila (and I) have been enjoying this since she was 16 months old.

---

2 cups raw buckwheat groats
¼ cup raw almonds
¼ cup raw sunflower seeds
¼ cup raw pumpkin seeds
2 apples
2 T. cinnamon
4 T. raw honey
½ cup raisins
¼ cup hemp seeds
¼ cup chia seeds
¼ cup shredded coconut

Optional superfood extras: baobab, moringa, lucuma

Day 1: Morning

Place the buckwheat in a bowl and cover with filtered water. Allow to soak for 12 hours.

Evening

Pour the soaked buckwheat into a sieve and rinse VERY well. The buckwheat produces a slimy substance that must be rinsed off. Place the sieve over the soaking bowl and leave the buckwheat to sprout. Alternatively use a glass sprouting jar.

Day 2: Morning

Rinse the buckwheat very well and then continue sprouting.

Evening

Rinse the buckwheat very well and continue sprouting.

Now place your almonds, sunflower seeds and pumpkin seeds in separate bowl, cover with filtered water and soak.

Day 3: Morning

Rinse the almonds, sunflower seeds and pumpkin seeds and spread out on dehydrator sheets.

Rinse the buckwheat very well and place in a mixing bowl.

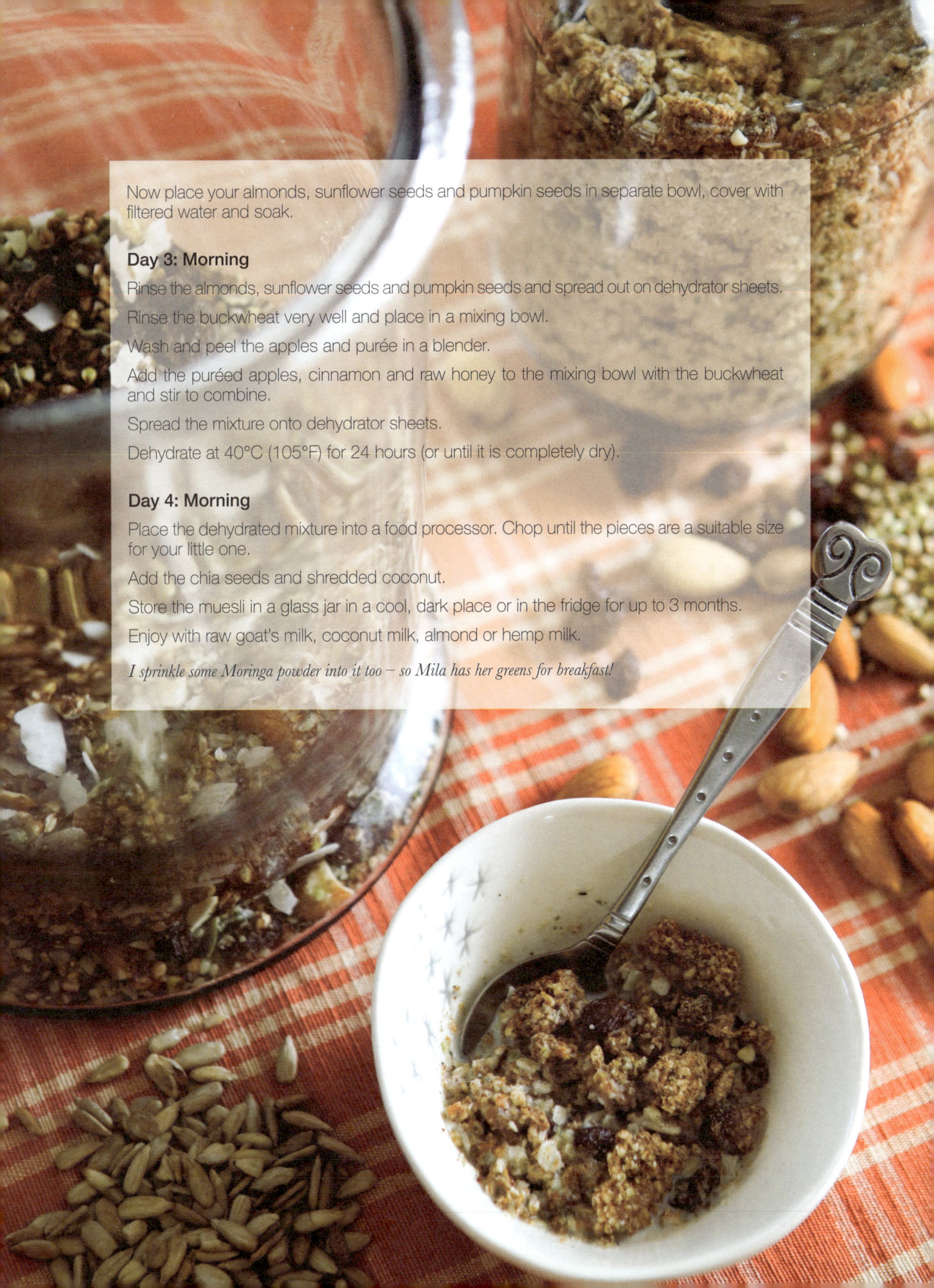

Wash and peel the apples and purée in a blender.

Add the puréed apples, cinnamon and raw honey to the mixing bowl with the buckwheat and stir to combine.

Spread the mixture onto dehydrator sheets.

Dehydrate at 40°C (105°F) for 24 hours (or until it is completely dry).

Day 4: Morning

Place the dehydrated mixture into a food processor. Chop until the pieces are a suitable size for your little one.

Add the chia seeds and shredded coconut.

Store the muesli in a glass jar in a cool, dark place or in the fridge for up to 3 months.

Enjoy with raw goat's milk, coconut milk, almond or hemp milk.

I sprinkle some Moringa powder into it too – so Mila has her greens for breakfast!

Recipes: Off the Spoon

GREEN YOGHURT (DAIRY VERSION)

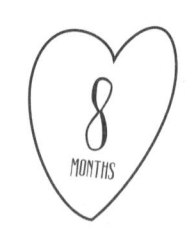

8 MONTHS

superfood; vegetarian; egg-free; for adults too; great for lunchboxes

Makes one serving.

3 T. yoghurt or kefir

½ t. green powder *(a blend of blend of organic wheat, barley and alfalfa grasses, sea vegetables and chlorella)*

1 t. raw honey *(or organic maple syrup if your little one is younger than a year old)*

Mix all the ingredients together and serve!

• •

YOGHURT (DAIRY-FREE VERSION)

vegetarian; vegan; egg-free; for adults too; great for lunchboxes

Makes 1 l. (1 qt.)

2 cans preservative-free coconut milk

1 t. agar agar powder

1 t. infant probiotic powder or contents from capsules

1-2 T. raw honey or maple syrup *(only use honey if your little one is older than a year)*

Sterilise the glass jars you will be using as storage containers by running them through the dishwasher, or filling with boiling water.

If you are do not have a yoghurt maker or dehydrator, heat your oven to 40°C (100°F).

Place the coconut milk in a saucepan and sprinkle the agar agar powder on top.

Heat the milk over medium heat until it begins to simmer, then lower the heat and whisk continuously for 7 minutes.

Turn the heat off and allow the milk mixture to cool until it is just warm to the touch.

Add the sweetener of choice and the contents of the probiotic capsules – whisk to combine.

Pour the mixture into the sterilised jars and seal tightly.

If you are using an oven, turn the heat off (but leave the light on as a source of heat). Place the glass jars in the oven and leave for 12 – 24 hours.

Alternatively, use a yogurt maker or place into a dehydrator at 45°C (100°F). Set the timer for 12 to 24 hours.

After the 'culturing' time, put your yoghurt into the fridge and cool for 6 hours before serving.

Keep the yoghurt refrigerated and use within 2 weeks.

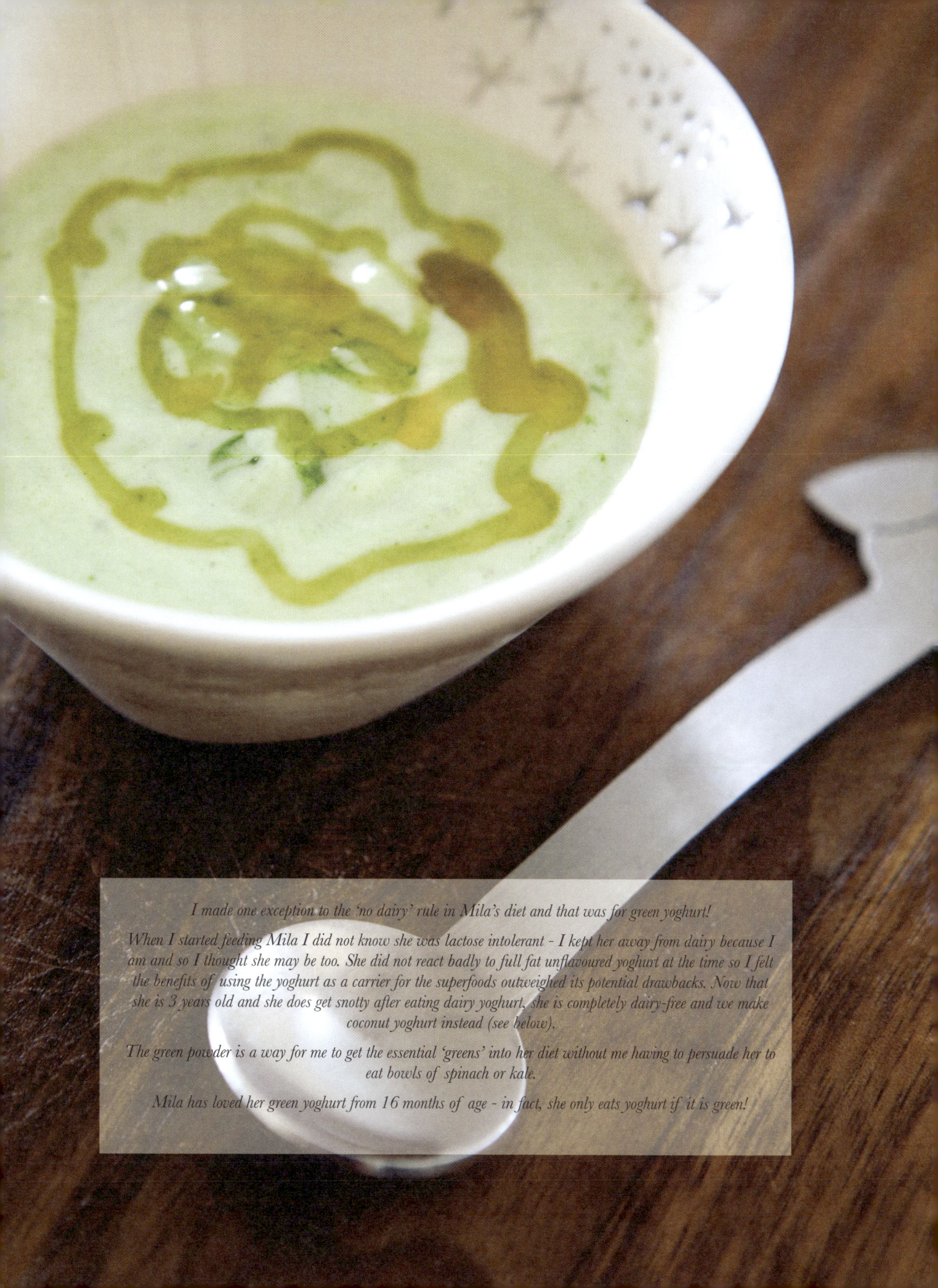

I made one exception to the 'no dairy' rule in Mila's diet and that was for green yoghurt!

When I started feeding Mila I did not know she was lactose intolerant - I kept her away from dairy because I am and so I thought she may be too. She did not react badly to full fat unflavoured yoghurt at the time so I felt the benefits of using the yoghurt as a carrier for the superfoods outweighed its potential drawbacks. Now that she is 3 years old and she does get snotty after eating dairy yoghurt, she is completely dairy-free and we make coconut yoghurt instead (see below).

The green powder is a way for me to get the essential 'greens' into her diet without me having to persuade her to eat bowls of spinach or kale.

Mila has loved her green yoghurt from 16 months of age - in fact, she only eats yoghurt if it is green!

Recipes: Off the Spoon

RAW TOMATO AND BASIL SOUP

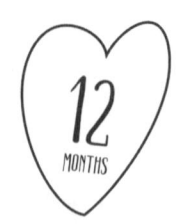

12 MONTHS

raw; vegetarian; vegan; egg-free; grain-free; for adults too; great for lunchboxes

Makes 1 cup (8 oz.)

This is a nutritious and really quick soup to make recipe.

Mila was eating this soup from 16 months – but it can be introduced to your little one earlier.

Tomatoes may be a bit acidic so watch for any reaction such as nappy rash.

This soup is a great source of anti-inflammatory essential fatty acids, protein, magnesium and vitamins A, B1, C, and K.

1 vine-ripened tomato
pinch Himalayan or sea salt
¼ cup macadamia or cashew nuts, activated
¼ cup basil leaves

Place all the ingredients in a blender and blend until smooth. Add water to thin if necessary.

Leftover soup can be stored in a fridge for 2 days or frozen.

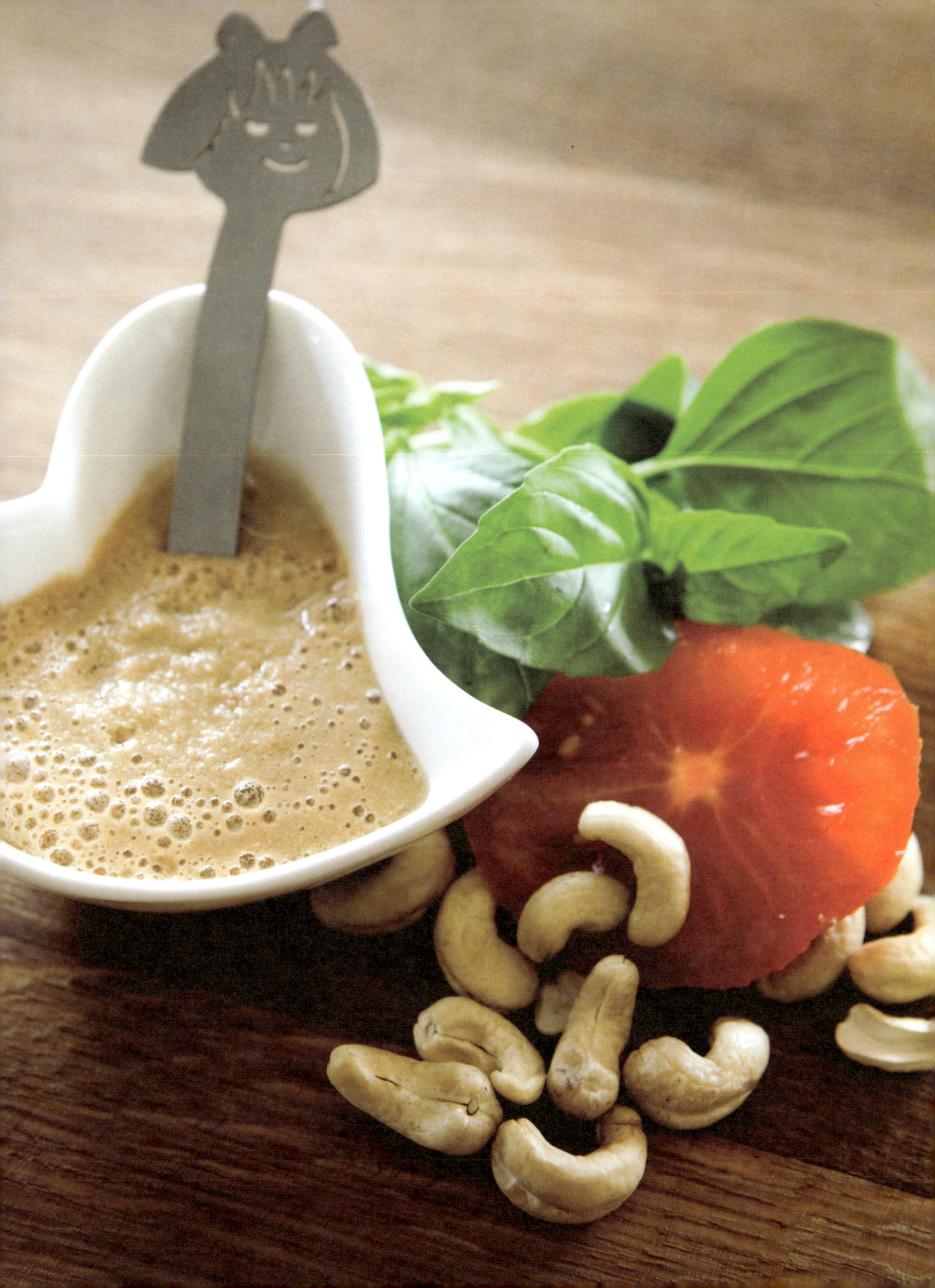

Recipes: Off the Spoon

BUTTERNUT SOUP

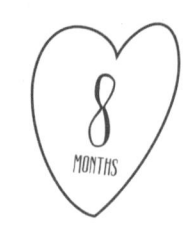

8 MONTHS

egg-free; grain-free; for adults too; great for lunchboxes

Makes 1 l. (1 qt.)

Mila has never been a big soup eater, but I keep on trying as it is a nutrient-dense food largely due to the homemade broth. It is an ideal food if your little one is unwell as it is easy to digest and the ingredients have antioxidant and anti-inflammatory benefits.

The homemade chicken broth used is this soup has immune boosting and digestion enhancing benefits. It is a rich source of easily absorbed calcium, magnesium, phosphorous and other trace minerals that support the adrenal glands and the growth of strong bones and teeth. Its gelatine content is a good source of protein that supports the body's connective tissues, promotes healthy hair, skin, teeth and nails.

The tahini adds additional healthy fats as well as calcium, protein, magnesium and iron.

Once made, it is a quick and convenient meal as you can quickly reheat frozen portions.

1 T. coconut oil, ghee or butter *(if you are not avoiding dairy)*
3 T. onion, chopped
1 cup butternut, peeled and chopped
¼ t. cinnamon
¼ t. nutmeg
salt to taste
1 apple, peeled and chopped
2 cups Mila's Meals chicken broth
¼ cup tahini *(if your little one is older than 1 years old)*

In a saucepan sauté the onion in the coconut oil (ghee or butter) until soft.

Add the butternut, cinnamon, nutmeg and salt and sauté for a few minutes.

Add the apple and chicken broth. Bring to the boil, then reduce heat and simmer for 10 – 20 minutes (or until the butternut is soft).

Pour the mixture into a blender. Add the tahini and blend until smooth.

Allow to cool slightly and serve.

Leftover soup can be kept in the fridge for a couple of days, or frozen.

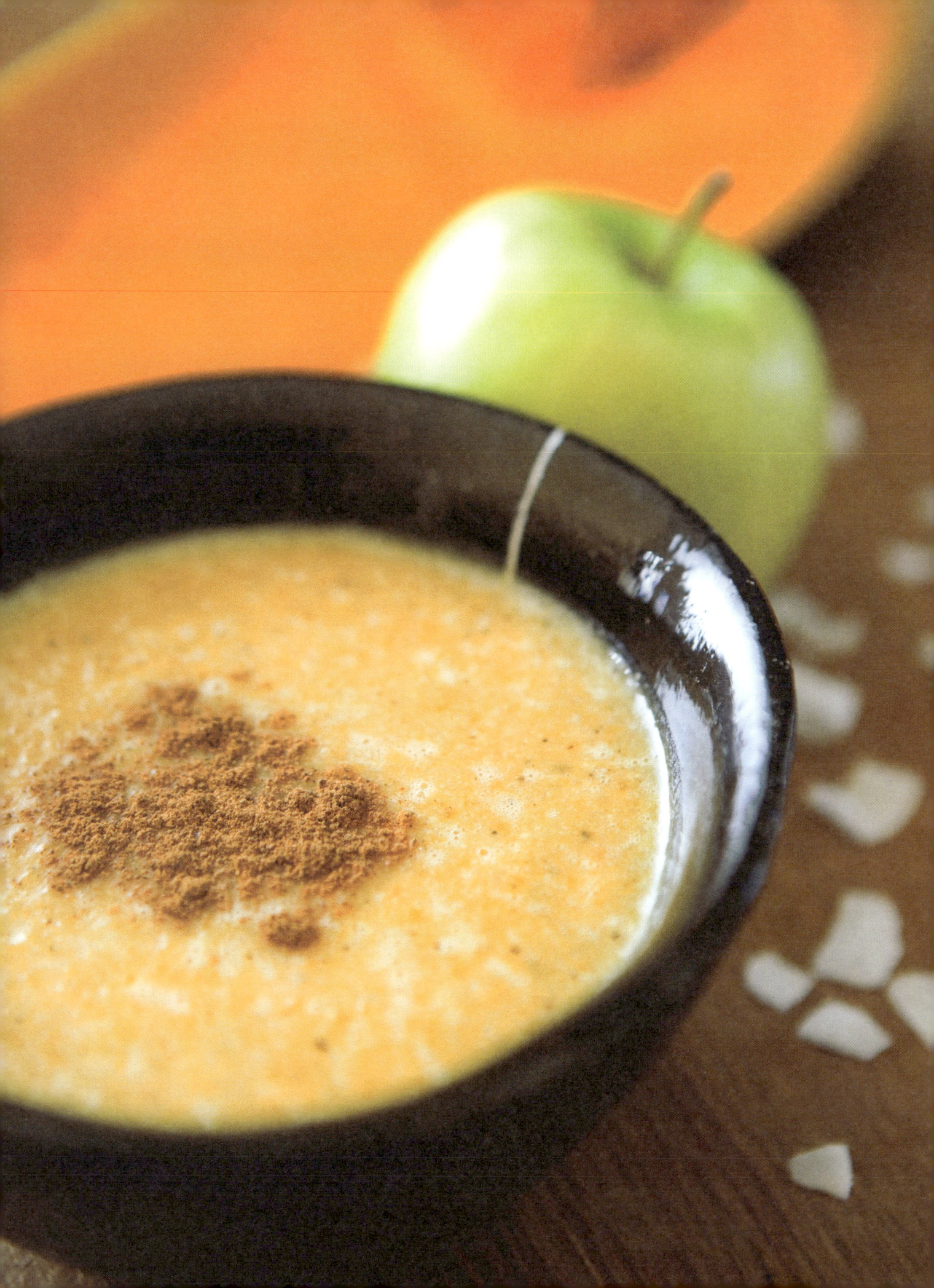

Recipes: Off the Spoon

DHAL

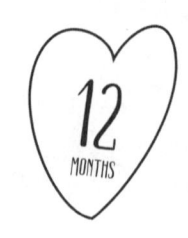

12 MONTHS

vegetarian; vegan; egg-free; grain-free; for adults too

Makes 4 cups / 750g (26 oz.)

• •

Lentils are an affordable, nutrient dense food and make a great substitute for meat thanks to their protein content.

They must, however, be properly prepared. While they do have less phytic acid (an anti-nutrient) than other legumes, lentils should be soaked before cooking. Soaking the lentils helps to break down the phytates and releases beneficial nutrients which can then be easily absorbed by your little one.

Lentils are considered to be one of the most nutritious of all legumes as they are loaded with folate, potassium, calcium, zinc, iron, and B vitamins. Pairing them with bone broth, another excellent source of minerals, provides even more nutritional support.

• •

1½ cups dry lentils (red lentils are the easiest to digest)

2 T. apple cider vinegar, lemon juice, kefir, or whey

2 ½ cups Mila's Meals chicken broth

1 t. fresh ginger, grated

2 bay leaves

1 cinnamon stick

1 T. coconut oil (butter or ghee, if you are not avoiding dairy)

1 small onion, finely chopped

1 clove garlic, crushed

1 t. turmeric

1 t. cumin

½ t. Himalayan or sea salt

Place the lentils in a mixing bowl, cover with filtered water and stir through the apple cider vinegar, lemon juice, kefir, or whey.

Allow to soak for 7 hours (or up to 18 hours).

Rinse the lentils well then place them in a saucepan.

Add the chicken broth, ginger, bay leaves and cinnamon stick and simmer (covered) for 15 - 25 minutes.

Just before the lentils are finished cooking, sauté the onion, garlic, turmeric, cumin and salt in a frying pan until the onions are soft.

Remove the bay leaves and cinnamon stick from the lentils.

Whisk the onion mixture into the lentils.

Allow to cool and serve.

Left over dhal can be refrigerated for 3 days or frozen for up to 6 months.

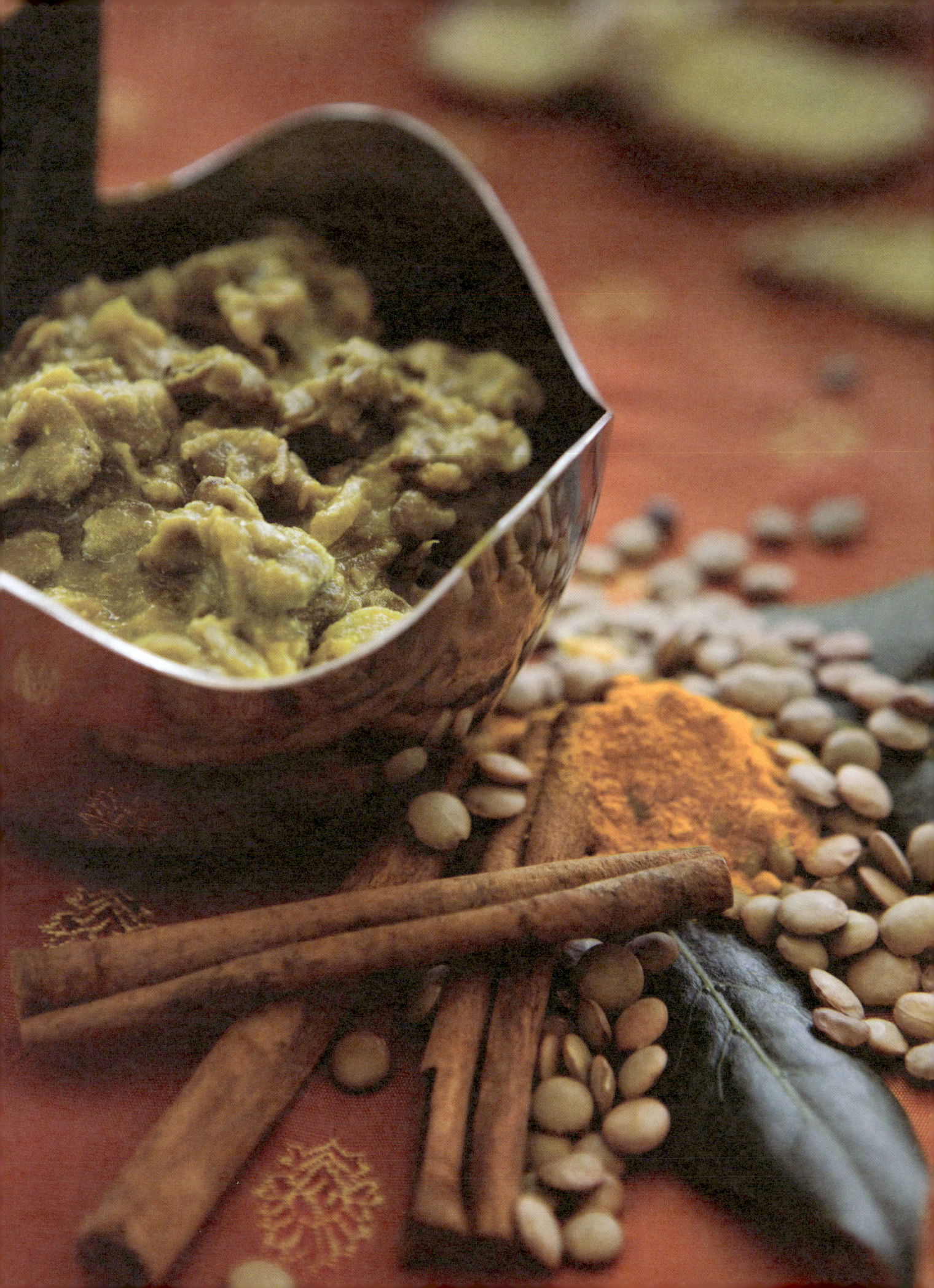

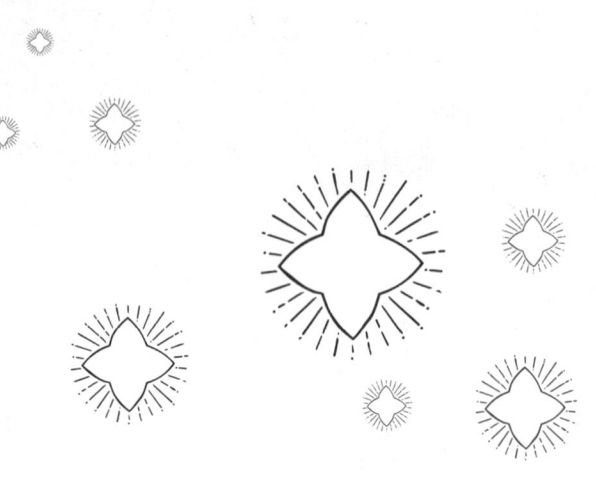

Recipes: Out & About Finger Foods

Recipes: Out & About Finger Foods

PLAIN & SIMPLE FRUIT & VEGGIES → 198
DRIED FRUITS → 200
FRUIT LEATHER → 202
KALE CHIPS → 206
ZUCCHINI CRISPS → 210
MAPLE SYRUP TEETHING BISCUITS → 212
RUSKS → 214
SWEET POTATO MUFFINS → 216
MORNING GLORY MUFFINS → 218
BUTTERNUT & APPLE MUFFINS → 220
NANA CAKES → 222
SIMPLE SEED CRACKERS → 224
VEGGIE CRACKERS → 226
CHEESY CRACKERS → 228
OAT BARS → 230

Recipes: Out & About Finger Foods

PLAIN & SIMPLE – FRUIT & VEGGIES

raw; vegetarian; vegan; egg-free; grain-free; for adults too; great for lunchboxes

Fruit and veggies are a perfect first finger food – easy to prepare, colourful and highly nutritious! By using his/her thumb and forefinger to pick up the food, your little one is developing their fine motor skills, taking the first steps towards independence and probably having a lot of (messy) fun too!

In the very beginning start with those fruit and vegetables that are soft when raw, or lightly steam the harder ones. The food should be easy to handle but should not present a choking hazard. A whole grape, for example, is too big and impossible to bite into smaller pieces without teeth (the gums cannot get a grip on the slippery skin). You can cut those type of food into 'fingers' or dice them. To make slippery diced foods easier to pick up with tiny fingers, coat them with almond flour, coconut flour or psyllium husks.

Remember to wash fruit and veggies thoroughly and, if they are not organic, it is best to peel them. In the early stages of eating solids, Mila preferred all her fruit peeled, as the skins were harder to chew and tended to get stuck in her throat.

Offer a variety of different fruit and veggies to vary the nutrient intake but also allow your baby to learn about different tastes, textures, colours and smells. Some of Mila's favourites are listed below.

EARLY STAGES OF CHEWING SOLIDS

+9 MONTHS

(Foods that are easy to gum, or dissolve easily in the mouth.)

- **Watermelon:** Seeds removed, cut into fingers.
  Oh my goodness Mila eats a lot of this! This is, in my mind, the perfect finger food! No need to cook it, it does not go brown, it is easy to hold, it has a high water content... and it is DELICIOUS!

- **Litchis:** Peeled and pip removed.
  Another great one! Absolutely no preparation needs to be done at home – just throw them in your bag as you run out the door. The skin protects the fruit while you are travelling, and you can peel them as you need them. Mila eats a lot of litchis on the beach!

- **Banana:** diced.
- **Pear:** steamed and diced (you can add a little nutmeg when steaming).
- **Apple:** steamed and diced (you can add a little cinnamon when steaming).
- **Peach:** peeled, steamed and diced.
- **Avocado:** diced.
- **Pumpkin / Butternut:** steamed and diced.
- **Sweet Potato:** steamed and diced.
- **Broccoli:** cut into florets and steamed.

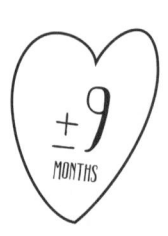

WHEN THERE ARE MORE TEETH

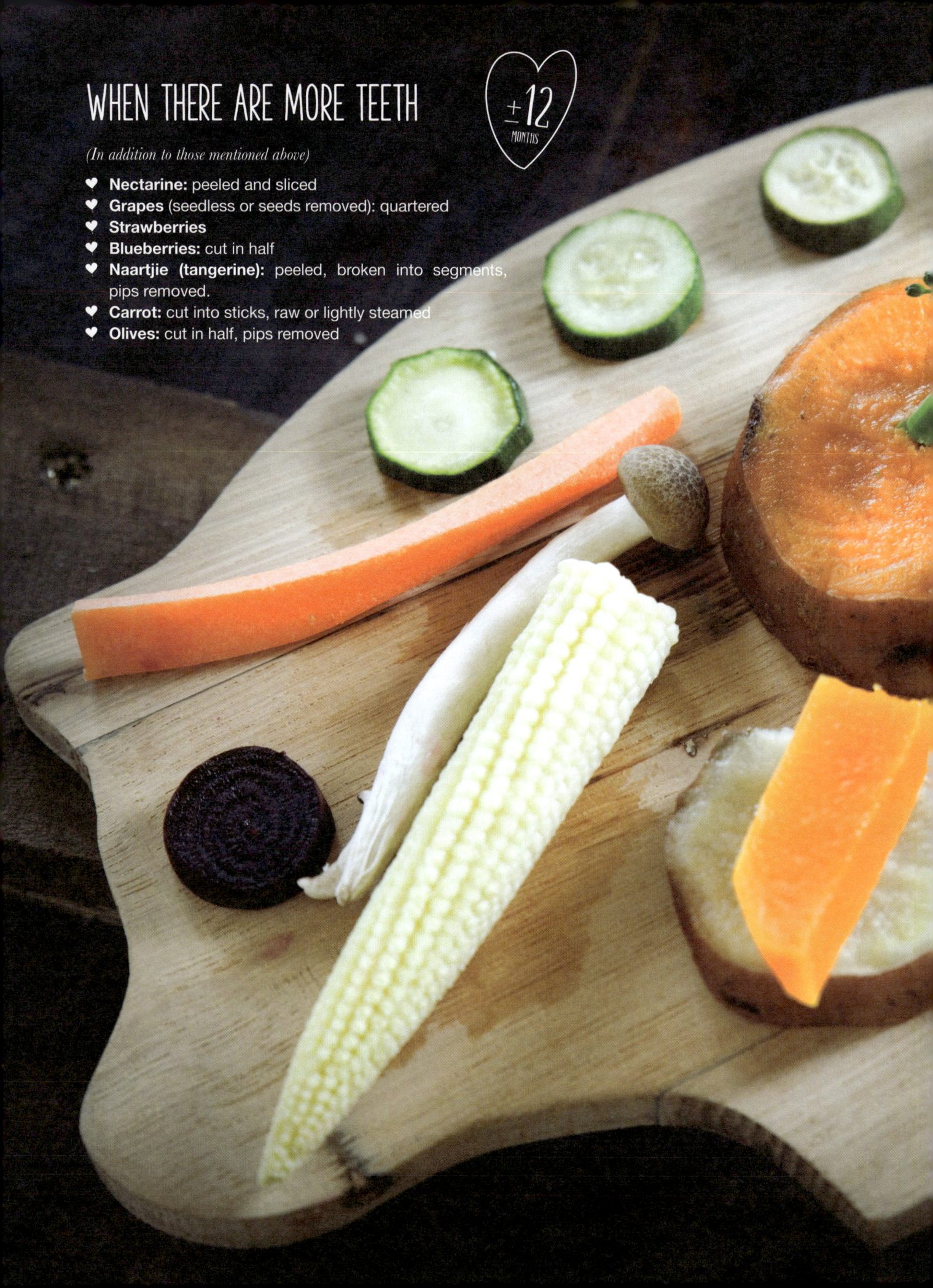

± 12 MONTHS

(In addition to those mentioned above)

- ♥ **Nectarine:** peeled and sliced
- ♥ **Grapes** (seedless or seeds removed): quartered
- ♥ **Strawberries**
- ♥ **Blueberries:** cut in half
- ♥ **Naartjie (tangerine):** peeled, broken into segments, pips removed.
- ♥ **Carrot:** cut into sticks, raw or lightly steamed
- ♥ **Olives:** cut in half, pips removed

Recipes: Out & About Finger Foods

DRIED FRUITS

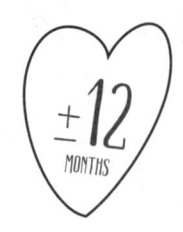

±12 MONTHS

raw; vegetarian; vegan; egg-free; grain-free; for adults too; great for lunchboxes

• •

What a convenient no-mess, no-fuss snack food that can live in the nappy bag in case of those emergency hunger situations! They make a great addition to school lunchboxes too.

Most dried fruit available in the supermarkets are covered in preservatives, GM vegetable oils, colorants and artificial flavourings. Just being able to make these alone made me pleased that I had invested a dehydrator.

This is a great way to eat seasonal fruits even when they are out of season! Towards the end of summer, I stock up on mangoes and dehydrate big batches of them to see use through the winter months.

• •

Fruit of your choice, sliced
(Mila loves apple, mango, pineapple, plum, peach, nectarine, strawberry)
Lemon juice, freshly squeezed
Water
Spices of you choice for example: cinnamon, vanilla powder, dried ginger. *(Vanilla powder on dried apple rings is delicious!)*

The amount of lemon juice and water obviously depends on how much fruit you are preparing. I use a ratio of 1:4.

Wash your fruit thoroughly.

Place the lemon juice and water in a bowl.

If you are using non-organic fruit, remember to peel it.

(Mila will only eat the dried apples if they do not have the skin on, as it tends to get a bit tough when dried.)

Place the peeled fruit in the lemon water as soon as you have peeled it to avoid discolouration.

Slice some of your fruit into thin even slices. Using a mandolin really helps.

Place the sliced fruit in the lemon water and allow it to soak while you carry on peeling or slicing the rest of the fruit.

Remove the sliced fruit from the lemon water, drain it briefly on some kitchen towel then place it on the dehydrator trays or baking sheets.

Continue with this process (peeling, slicing, soaking) until all your fruit is prepared.

Dehydrate in a dehydrator or oven at 45-55°C (110-130°F) for approximately 8 hours. You will know your fruit is ready when you cannot squeeze out any moisture when you pinch the fruit. Alternatively put the fruit into a plastic bag or glass jar while warm, and if condensation forms on the inside, you need to dry them out a bit more.

Store in a sealed container in a cool, dark place.

For longer storage periods, store the dried fruit in a vacuum-sealed bag in a cool, dark place or in the freezer.

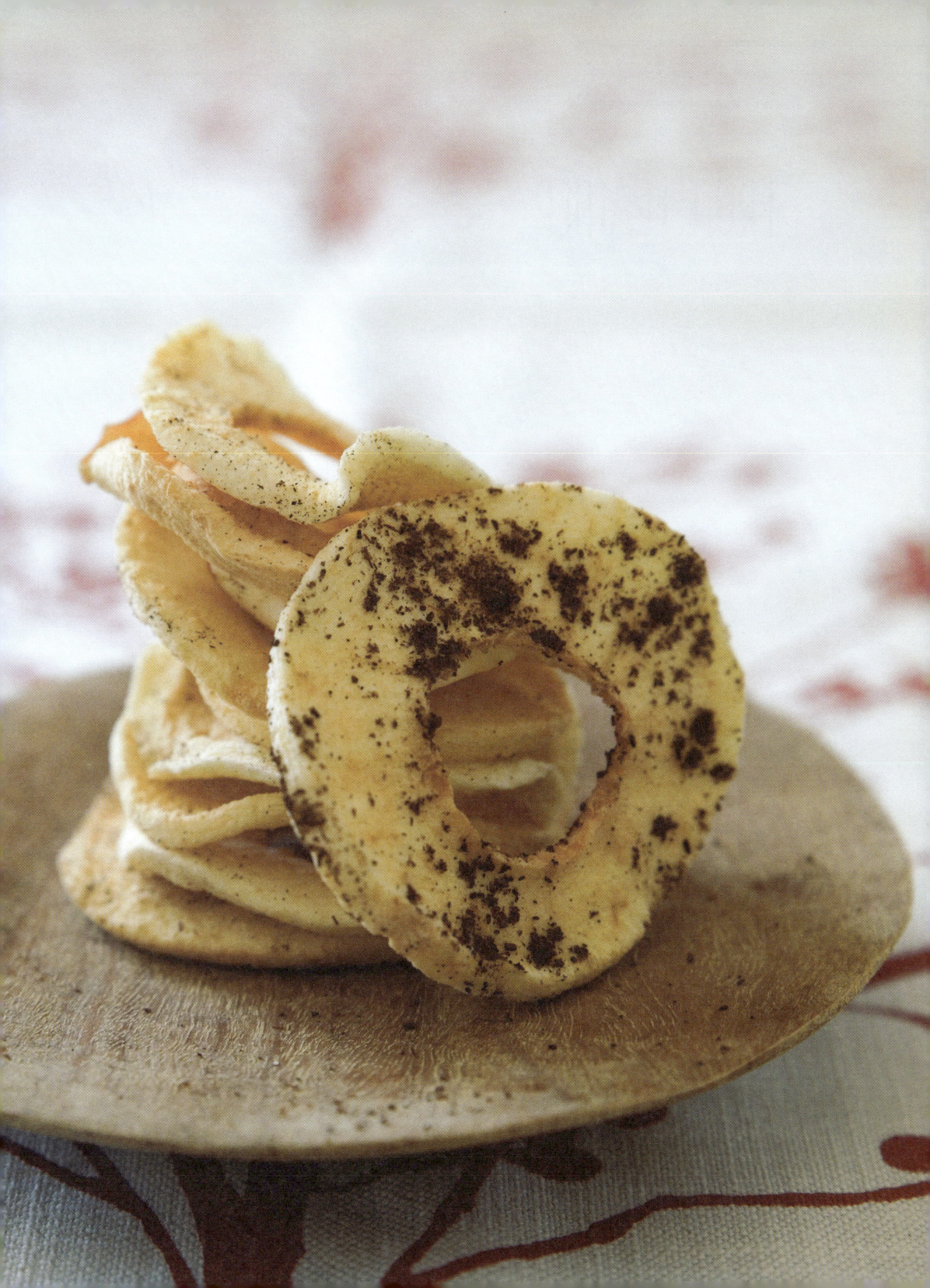

Recipes: Out & About Finger Foods

FRUIT LEATHER

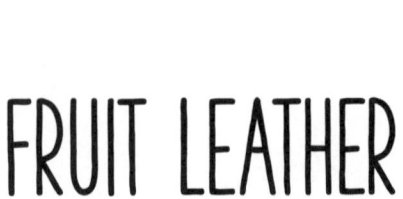

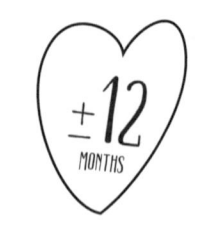

± 12 MONTHS

superfood; vegetarian; vegan; egg-free; grain-free; for adults too; great for lunchboxes

Makes 2 trays / 20 fruit leather rolls

· ·

Another great no-mess, no-fuss snack food that can live in the nappy bag and a very, very sneaky way to get the vegetables in! Now that Mila is 3years old and totally against eating anything that looks like a vegetable, I permanently have a batch of 'fruit' leather drying in the dehydrator.

Our go to combination is blueberry leather – I simply use left over roast vegetables from the night before, a bag of frozen blueberries and the superfoods. It could be simpler! And Mila eats it for breakfast, lunch and dinner – so she is actually eating vegetables three times a day… without even knowing it!

Most fruit leathers (rolls) available in the supermarkets have added sugars or high fructose corn syrup, GM vegetable oils and transfats as ingredients, as well as being covered in preservatives – please read the labels.

Mila started eating these when she was 12 months old.

· ·

In an oven:
If you do not have a dehydrator, you can dry the fruit leather in the oven. Turn the oven on at its lowest setting and use the shelf furthest away from the heating element. Line a baking sheet with greased parchment paper and spread the mixture as above. When drying the leather, leave the oven door open slightly to allow for airflow. Drying times will vary according to your oven and the ambient humidity, but with an oven set at 50°C (120°F) it will take approximately 6 hours.

Tips and variations:
- *Applesauce is added to make the leather smoother and more pliable. It is also a great extender (thus reducing the overall cost) and can balance the tartness of other fruits.*
- ***Fruit leather can be a great remedy for constipation – use beetroot as the cooked vegetable, and liquorice tea as the liquid.***
- *If you are using the fermented apple sauce be sure to dehydrate at 45°C (110°F) to ensure the viability of the probiotics.*
- *Be adventurous by adding some spices like vanilla, cinnamon, ginger, nutmeg or cloves.*
- *Add extra texture by sprinkling shredded coconut, chia seeds or chopped sesame or sunflower seeds on top of the mixture before drying.*
- *Additional fibre can be added by including psyllium husks to the mixture before drying.*

Recipes: Out & About Finger Foods

- **2 cups raw fruit, or fruit combination of your choice** *(for example, berries, bananas, mango, peaches, nectarines, pears, pineapple)*
- **1 cup cooked apple or pear** *(or Mila's Meals fermented apple sauce)*
- **1 cup cooked sweet potato, butternut or beetroot** *(or a combination of these veggies)*
- **1 T. moringa** *(optional)*
- **1 T. baobab powder, or maca** *(optional)*
- **1 t. green powder** *(blend of chlorella, spirulina, wheatgrass and barley grass) (optional)*
- **1 cup water or herbal tea**
- **2 T. ground chia seeds** *(optional)*
- **honey, maple syrup or stevia to taste** *(optional)*
- **1 T. lemon juice**
- **2 T. coconut oil**

Wash the chosen fruit thoroughly. De-stem, pit, peel etc. as necessary.

Place the raw fruit, cooked apple/pear, cooked vegetables and superfoods in a blender and blend.

Check the consistency. If it is too thick to pour, add a little water or herbal tea until a pouring consistency is reached. If it is too thin, add fruit that has a lower water content such as banana, or add ground chia seeds (one tablespoon at a time).

Check the taste. If it is too tart, add your sweetener of choice until the desired sweetness is reached. Keep in mind that the flavours will intensify as they dehydrate.

If you are using fruit that discolours (such as apples and bananas) add a little lemon juice to the mixture. Be sure not to add too much as this will affect the flavour. Approximately 2 teaspoons per 2 cups of mixture should be sufficient.

Spread the mixture evenly onto greased, solid dehydrator trays to a thickness of approximately ½ cm (⅛"). If you do not have solid sheets you can line mesh sheets with parchment paper. Do not use wax paper or tin foil.

Dehydrate at 45-55°C (110-130°F) for 10 hours then flip the mixture onto a mesh sheet and continue drying for another hour. Check on the leather to make sure it is not getting too dry (crunchy). If it peels away from the sheet easily it is dry. Remember that under-dried fruit will not keep.

Allow the leather to cool; remove from the sheets, cut into long strips and roll up.

Sore in a glass jar in a cool, dark place for up to one month, or in the freezer for up to a year.

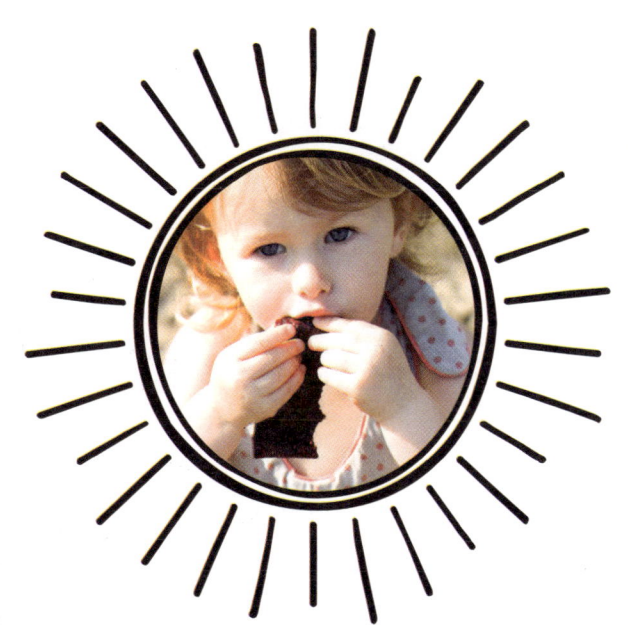

IMAGE ON NEXT PAGE →

203

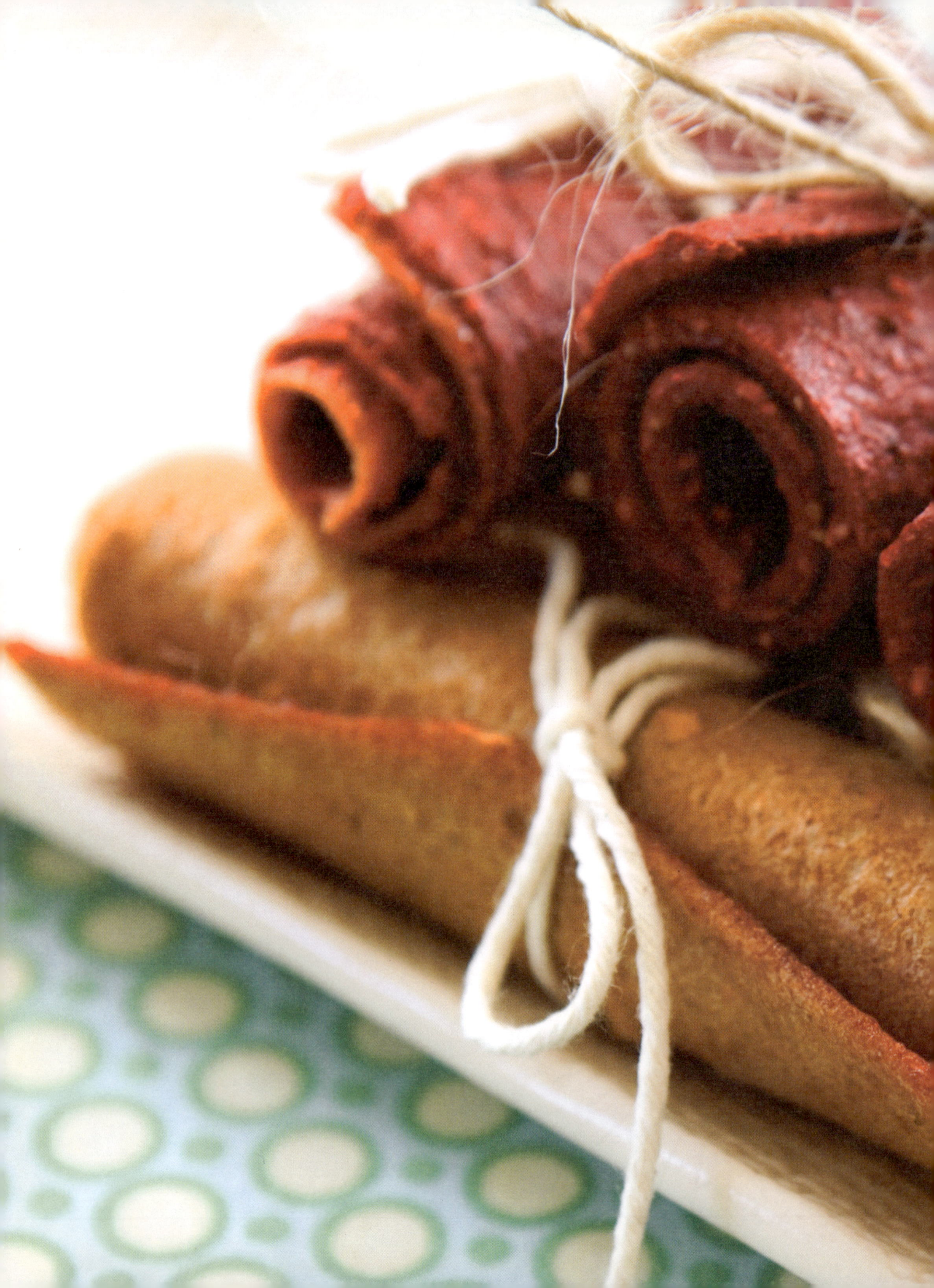

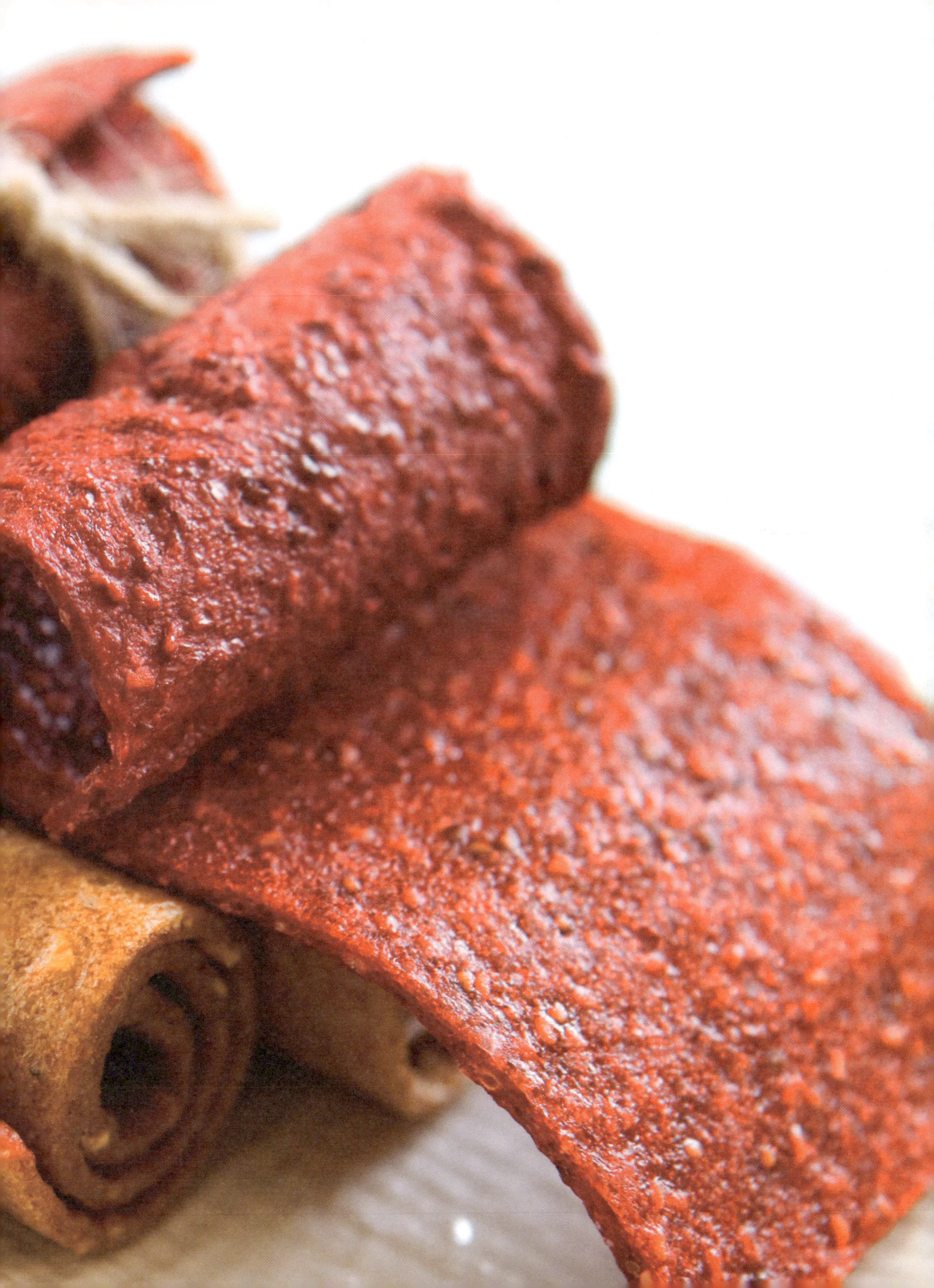

Recipes: Out & About Finger Foods

KALE CHIPS

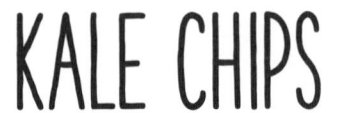

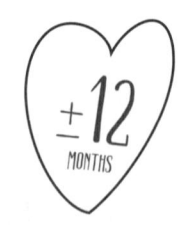

±12 MONTHS

All 3 flavours below use 1 bunch of washed and spun dry kale (±20 kale leaves). Remove the spine. No need to tear into smaller pieces as they shrink when they are dried.

Be careful not to over dry your chips as they will become tough and loose their flavour.

Store your kale chips in an airtight container. They can also be stored in the freezer for lasting freshness. They do not need to be defrosted before eating – simply remove from the freezer, let rest for a minute then enjoy!

PLAIN SALTED KALE CHIPS

raw; vegetarian; vegan; egg-free; grain-free; for adults too; great for lunchboxes

3 T. olive oil
1 t. Himalayan or sea salt *(finely ground)*

Combine the oil and salt in a large bowl. Add in the kale and massage the oil into the leaves until they are well coated. Place the leaves on mesh dehydrator sheets and dry at 45°C (110°F) for 4 – 6 hours or until crisp.

. . . .

HERBY KALE CHIPS

raw; vegetarian; vegan; egg-free; grain-free; for adults too; great for lunchboxes

3 T. olive oil
2 t. fresh thyme or oreganum, finely chopped
1 clove garlic, minced

Place the kale in a large mixing bowl. Grind the oil, herbs and garlic with a pestle and mortar. Pour over the kale and massage into the leaves until they are well coated. Place the leaves on mesh dehydrator sheets and dry at 45°C (110°F) for 4 – 6 hours or until crisp.

. . . .

In an oven:
- *This recipe uses a dehydrator. If you do not have one, you can dehydrate the kale chips in the oven.*
- *Turn the oven on at the lowest setting and leave the door slightly open to allow for airflow - my oven was set to 60°C (135°F). Line a baking sheet with parchment paper. Place the seasoned kale on the paper and dry in the warm oven for approximately 6 hours. Turn the oven off after 6 hours leaving the kale chips in the warm oven (with the door closed) for another hour. The chips should be completely dry and crispy. If not, turn on the oven again for another half an hour and then leave them in the turned off warm oven for an additional half an hour.*
- *These chips wont technically be raw, as anything over 45°C (115°F) is no longer raw, but they are a whole lot healthier than the store-bought crisps and cheaper than the ready-made kale chips from health food shops.*

Recipes: Out & About Finger Foods

CHEESY KALE CHIPS

raw; vegetarian; egg-free; grain-free; for adults too; great for lunchboxes

1 cup cashew nuts, soaked overnight

¼ cup warm water

1 T. nutritional yeast

½ t. Himalayan or sea salt

2 T. lemon juice

1 T. onion, finely chopped

2 T. raw honey (or organic maple syrup if your little one is younger than a year old)

2 T. olive oil

Blend the cashew nuts, water, nutritional yeast, salt, lemon juice, onion, honey (or maple syrup) and olive oil until smooth. Pour over the prepared kale and massage in until all the leaves are well coated. Place on mesh dehydrator sheets and dry at 45°C (110°F) for 4 - 6 hours or until crisp.

This is a great way to feed your little one vegetables – and a highly nutritious (green) one at that.

Kale is one of the most nutrient-dense vegetables on the planet. 1 cup of kale has 684% of the RDA (recommended daily amount) of vitamin K, 206% of the RDA of vitamin A, and 134% of vitamin C. It has more calcium by weight than milk, and that calcium is 25% more bioavailable than that in milk!

A special mention must also be made of kale's protein content – like meat, it has all the essential amino acids and 9 non-essential ones (amino acids are the building clocks of protein within the body). With this exceptionally high amount of protein (especially for a vegetable) it has recently been nick-named the "new beef" and is a useful addition to any, but especially, a vegetarian, diet. The protein is more bioavailable than meat protein and the body has to expend less energy to make use of it. Mila has never been a big meat-eater but by eating these chips and by having kale in her veggie juice every morning, I am assured she is getting a healthy dose of protein.

Kale is also a great source of omega 3 fatty acids, iron, magnesium, folate and vitamins A, B, C, E and K.

RECIPE ON PREVIOUS PAGE

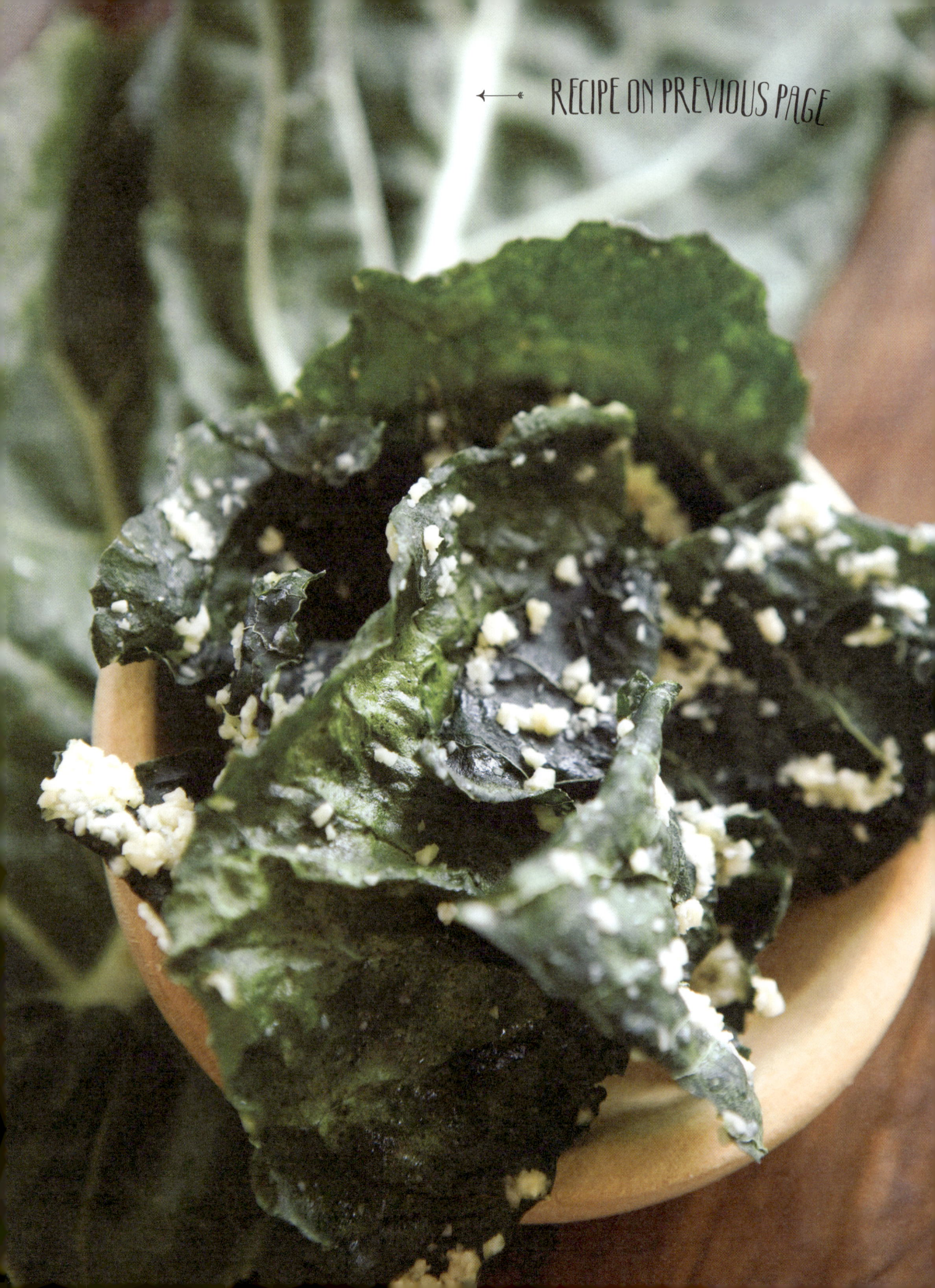

RECIPE ON NEXT PAGE →

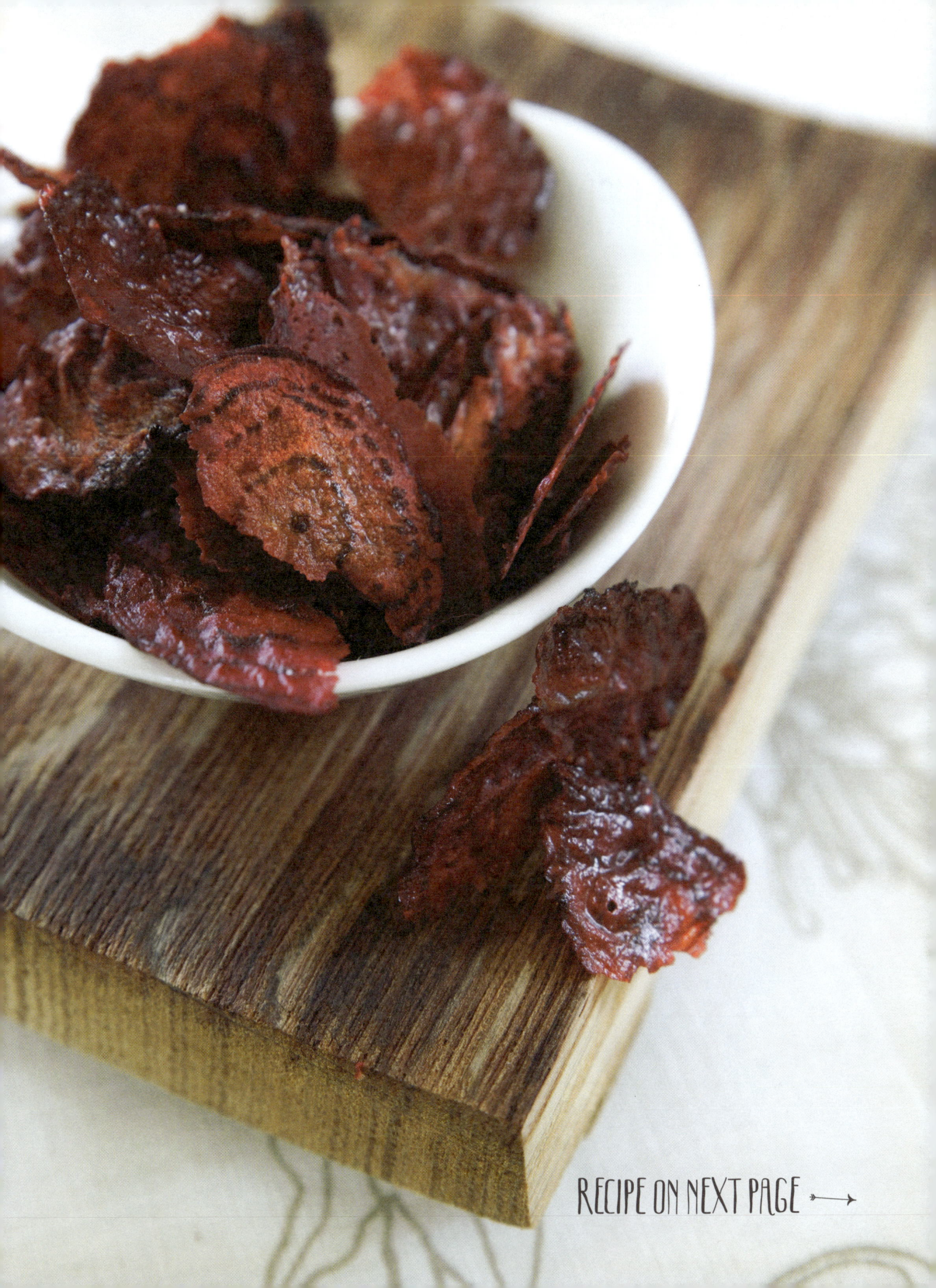

Recipes: Out & About Finger Foods

ZUCCHINI CRISPS

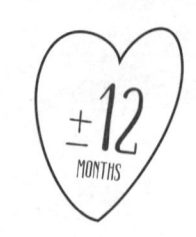

± 12 MONTHS

vegetarian; vegan; egg-free; grain-free; for adults too; great for lunchboxes

Makes 1 small bowl

Oh wow – these are delicious!

They make a great finger food once your little one is chewing well, and they are a nutritious alternative to deep fried, MSG enhanced commercial crisps which are often available at social events.

Now that Mila is three, and still refusing to eat anything that resembles a normal cooked vegetable, these are an excellent (and easy) way for me to feed her vegetables. Who would have thought your little one could have crisps for dinner!

1 large zucchini or 4 baby marrows
2 T. olive oil
Himalayan or sea salt

Preheat your oven to 100°C (220°F).

Line two large baking sheets with parchment paper. Using a pastry brush (or painting brush), brush the parchment paper with olive oil.

Thinly slice the zucchini or baby marrows (a mandolin is great for this).

Place the slices on the parchment paper and brush with olive oil.

Sprinkle the salt over all the slices (less is more!).

Bake in the oven for approximately 2 hours – they should be crispy, not soggy or brown.

Cool and serve.

These can be stored in an airtight container for 3 days. If they get a little soggy, simply 'refresh' in the oven until crispy again.

Variations:
- I have used this method to make crisps with sweet potato, butternut, beetroot and parsnips – I have to say parsnips were my favourite!
- If you do not have 2 hours to spend in the house while your crisps are cooking, you can turn the oven temperature up to 170°C (340°F) and cook the crisps for 20 – 35 minutes, depending on which vegetable you are using.

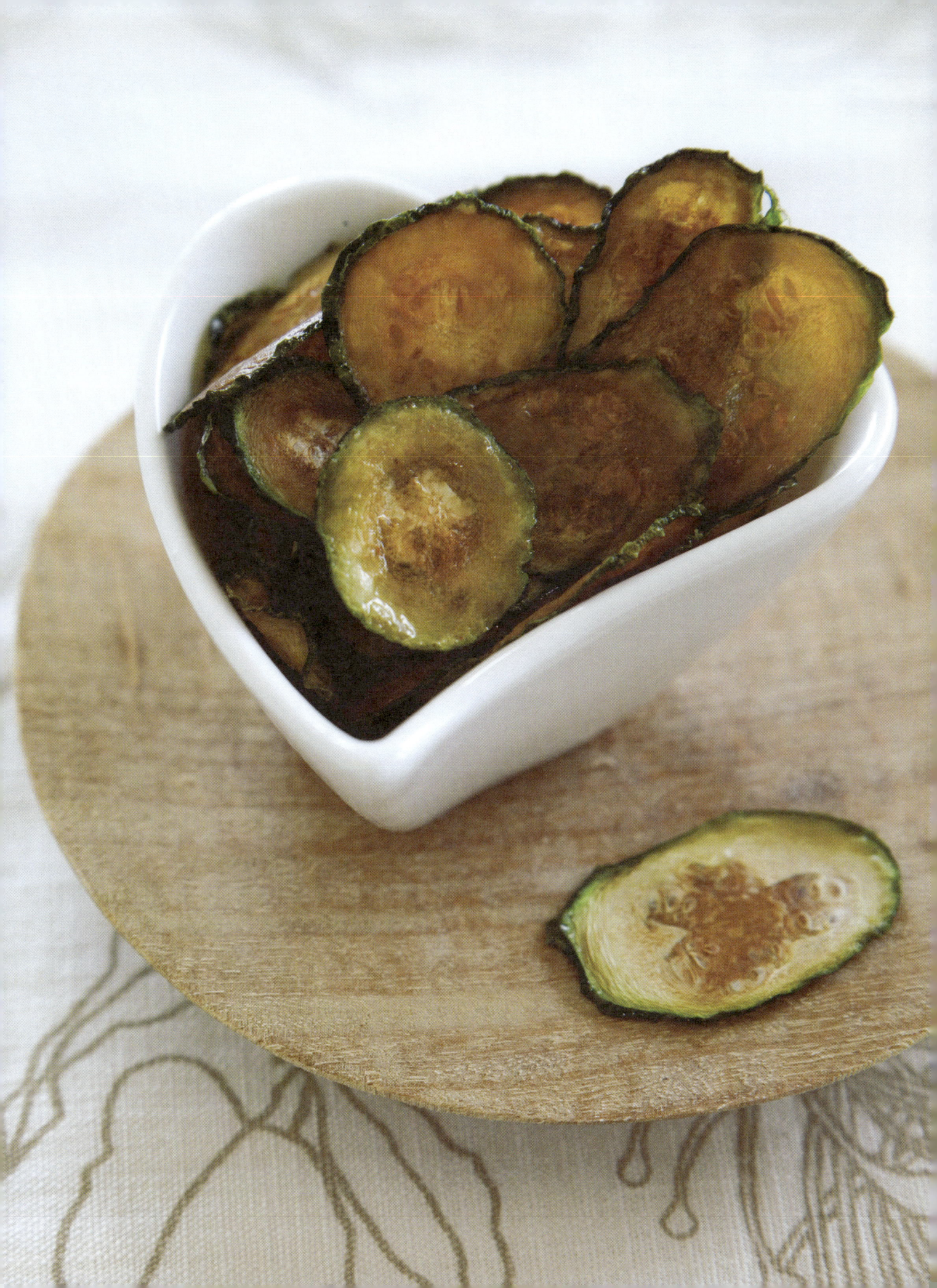

Recipes: Out & About Finger Foods

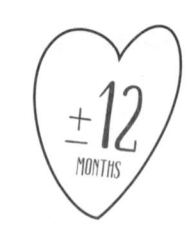

± 12 MONTHS

MAPLE SYRUP TEETHING BISCUITS

vegetarian; vegan; egg-free; for adults too; great for lunchboxes

Makes ±10 biscuits (depending on the size of your cookie cutters)

One of these biscuits would keep Mila busy for at least 20 minutes - which was very handy when we were out and about and she had to sit in the stroller while I was preoccupied with what I was doing.

They are also great as an afternoon snack when your little one wakes up from his/her sleep.

These biscuits are a complete protein, high in fibre and omega oils. They are very hard and do not crumble so there is no choking hazard.

Mila was eating these when she was 10 months old – but they do contain grains, so you may want to wait until your little one is 12 months old.

- 1 cup amaranth, ground to flour
- ¾ cup rice flour
- ½ cup tapioca starch
- 2 t. aluminium-free baking powder
- 1 t. cinnamon
- ½ cup ground flaxseed
- ¼ cup organic maple syrup
- ¼ cup coconut oil
- ½ cup applesauce
- 1 t. vanilla extract *(organic, sugar-, flavouring- and colourant-free)*

Preheat the oven to 180°C (350°F).

Melt the coconut oil (by placing it in a bowl resting in hot water).

Combine all the dry ingredients in a bowl.

Combine the liquid ingredients in a separate bowl.

Mix the dry and liquid ingredients together, stirring thoroughly until it forms a ball.

Place the mixture between 2 sheets of parchment paper and roll out to approximately 1 cm (½") thickness.

Cut out the biscuits using cookie cutters.

Gather remaining mixture together, roll and cut again. Repeat until all the mixture has been used.

Place biscuits on a baking tray lined with baking paper.

Bake for approximately 20 minutes.

Allow to cool on the baking trays then serve.

Biscuits can be stored in a sealed container in a cool, dark place for up to 1 month. For longer storage, keep them in the freezer.

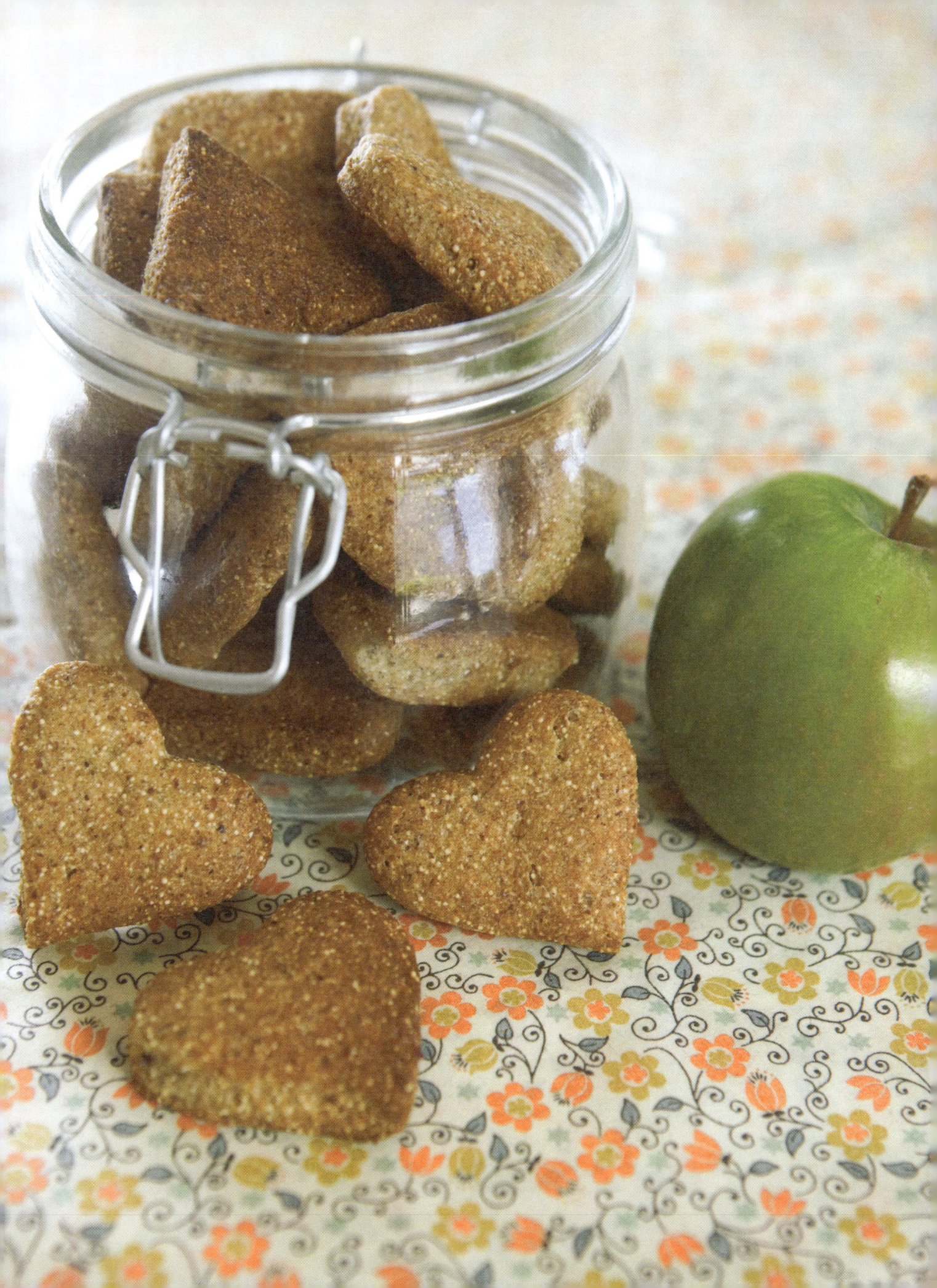

Recipes: Out & About Finger Foods

RUSKS

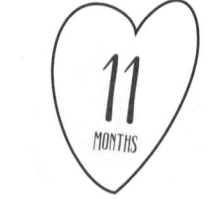

11 MONTHS

vegetarian; vegan; grain-free; for adults too; great for lunchboxes

Makes 30 rusks

A rusk is a hard, dry biscuit also known as twice-baked bread. They are a traditional South African early morning or tea time snack and are typically dunked in tea before being eaten.

Rusks make a great finger food for teething little ones – although they can crumble, so your little one may need to be supervised while eating them until he/she is chewing well enough. Even now that Mila is a little older, she enjoys dipping rusks into her Rooibos tea as a pre-breakfast snack.

- 2 cups almond flour
- 2 T. coconut flour
- 5 eggs
- 2 bananas, mashed
- ¼ cup Mila's Meals date jam
- 1 T. coconut oil, melted
- 2 T. honey *(or maple syrup if you are a vegan or if your little one is younger than a year)*
- ¼ cup flaxseeds, ground
- ¼ cup sunflower seeds, ground
- ¼ t. Himalayan or sea salt
- 1 t. nutmeg
- ½ T. vanilla powder
- ½ T. cinnamon
- ½ t. baking soda *(bicarbonate of soda)*
- ½ t. aluminium-free baking powder

Preheat the oven to 180°C (350°F).

Grease two 14.5 cm x 8 cm (5.57" x 3") bread loaf tins. You can also line the bottom of the pans with parchment paper to ensure the loaves fall out easily once cooked.

Place the almond flour, coconut flour, eggs, banana, date jam, coconut oil and honey in a mixing bowl. Beat with an electric beater for 2 minutes. This softens the rather dry flours as they have the opportunity to absorb moisture before being cooked.

Add the flaxseeds, sunflower seeds, salt, nutmeg, vanilla powder, cinnamon, baking soda and baking powder and beat to combine.

Pour the batter into the tins. They should be three quarters full.

Bake for 30 minutes.

Remove the loaves from the pans and allow them to cool on a wire rack.

When completely cool, slice into 3 cm (1") thick slices. Then slice those slices in three.

Turn your oven on to its lowest setting.

Place the rusks on a baking tray and dehydrate in the oven with the door slightly ajar. This can take up to 10 hours so you may want to do this overnight.

Alternatively, if you have a dehydrator, place the rusks on the silicone trays and dehydrate at 45°C (113°F) for 10 hours.

The finished rusks should be very dry and hard.

Store the rusks in a glass jar or other airtight container.

The rusks will last for up to 2 months.

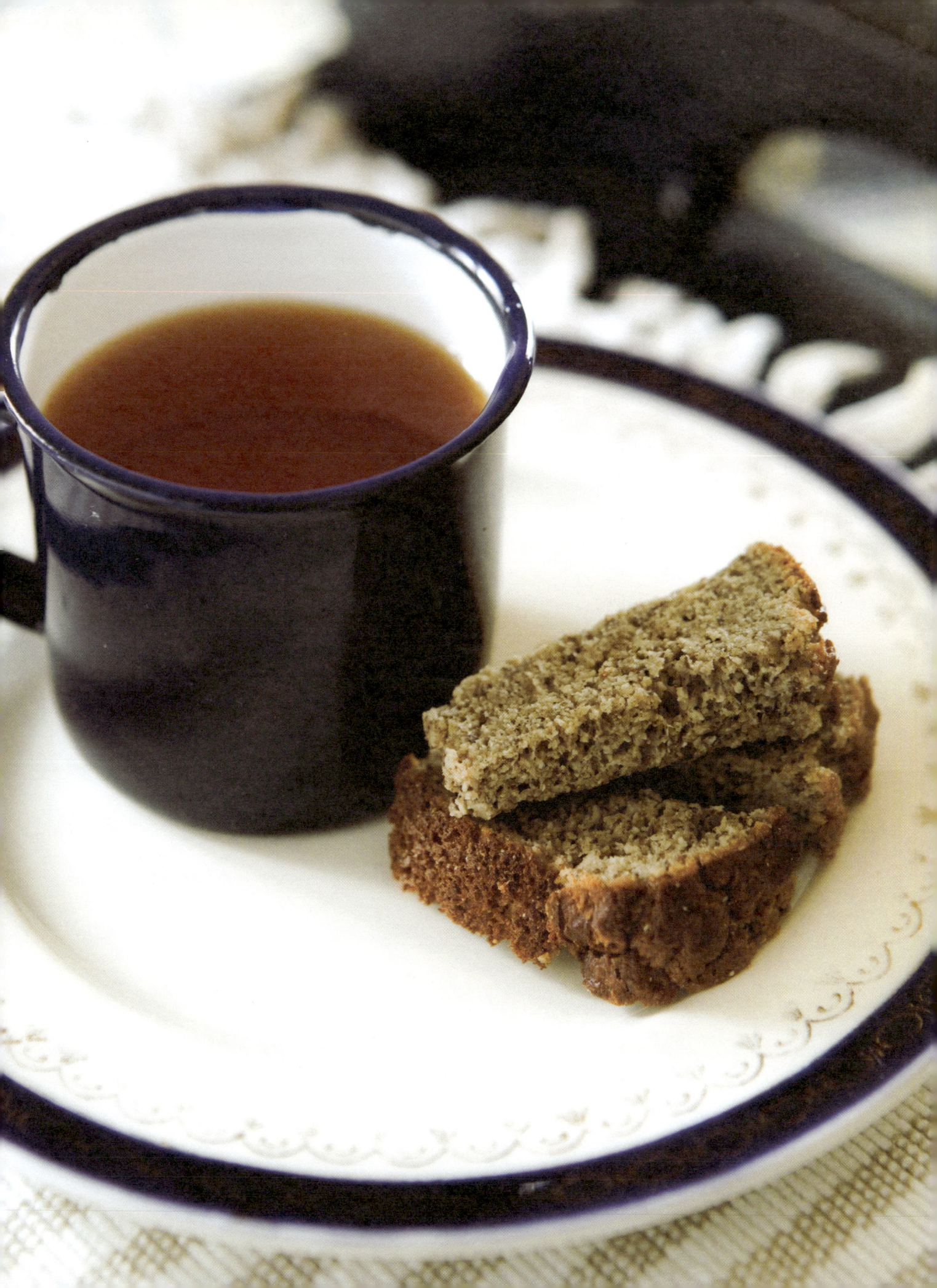

Recipes: Out & About Finger Foods

SWEET POTATO MUFFINS

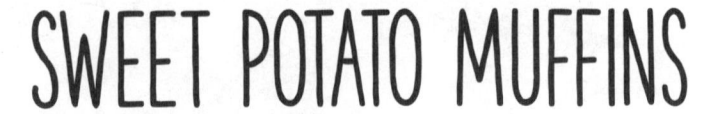

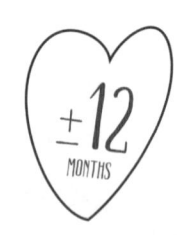

±12 MONTHS

vegetarian; for adults too; great for lunchboxes

Makes 12 baby muffins plus 6 adult ones

Mila has been eating these since she was 12 months old.

The muffins freeze well for up to a month. Simply take one out to defrost in the morning and you'll have an out-and-about snack ready by mid-morning.

Alternatively reheat briefly in the oven making sure the fruit is not too hot for your little one.

1 cup rolled oats*

1 cup sorghum flour*

½ t. baking soda

1 t. aluminium-free baking powder

¾ t. nutmeg

¾ t. cinnamon

1 cup sweet potato, steamed and mashed

2 T. raw honey *(or organic maple syrup if you are vegan or your little one is younger than a year old)*

3 T. coconut oil *(or ghee or butter)*, melted

2 T. dried cranberries

¼ cup coconut milk

1 egg

Preheat the oven to 180°C (350°F).

Sieve the oats, sorghum flour, baking soda, baking powder and spices together in a bowl.

In a separate bowl, mix together the mashed sweet potato, honey (or maple syrup), coconut oil, cranberries, milk and egg.

Add this mixture to the dry ingredients and mix together until the ingredients are all completely moistened - but do not over-mix.

Grease your baby muffin pans with coconut oil and spoon in the mixture making sure it reaches the brim of the pan. (Remember to make some bigger ones for dad!)

Cook for 20 minutes until risen and golden.

Allow the muffins to cool slightly in the pan before removing and eating, or leave to cool completely on a wire rack.

Place in a container, seal and freeze as soon as they have cooled.

---

*If you would like to soak the grains first (and I recommend that you do), simply place the oats and sorghum flour in a bowl and stir in the milk. Cover with a dish towel and allow to soak overnight. In the morning, mix the soaked mixture, baking soda, baking powder and spices together in a bowl and the proceed with the recipe as above.

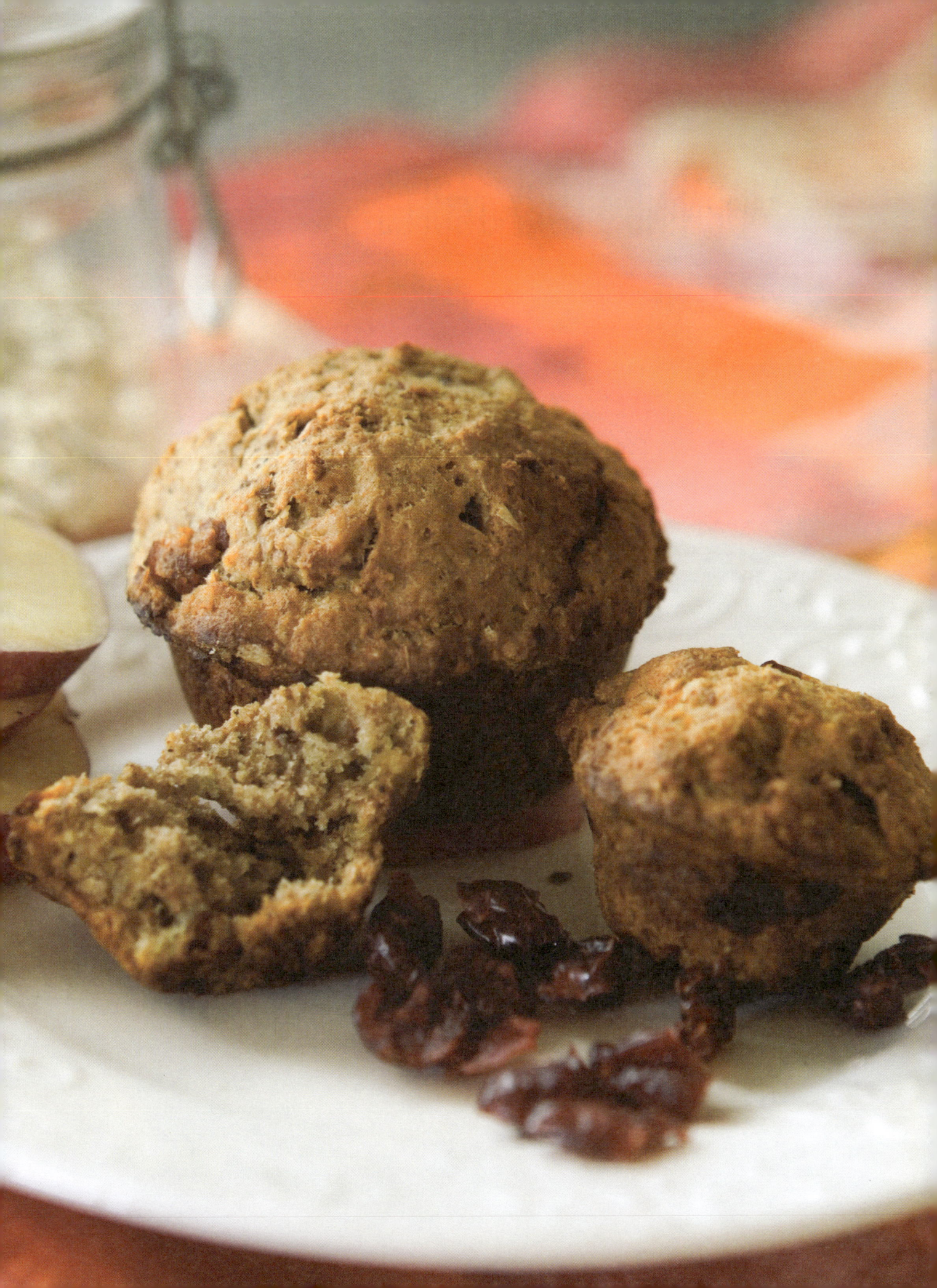

Recipes: Out & About Finger Foods

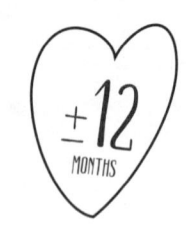

MORNING GLORY MUFFINS

±12 MONTHS

vegetarian; for adults too; great for lunchboxes

Makes 12 baby muffins plus 6 adult ones

• •

These are a great way to sneak in some veggies!

The muffins freeze well for a month. Simply take one out to defrost in the morning and you will have an out-and-about snack ready by mid-morning.

Alternatively reheat briefly in an oven making sure the fruit is not too hot for your little one.

• •

2 egg yolks*

⅔ cup coconut oil, melted

2 T. coconut sugar (or honey if your little one is older than a year)

1 teaspoon vanilla powder

1 cup carrots, finely grated or chopped (±2 carrots)

1 cup zucchini, finely grated or chopped (±3 baby marrows)

½ cup seedless raisins, finely chopped

½ cup coconut flakes, finely chopped

1 pear/apple, peeled, cored, and finely chopped

½ cup goat's milk (or any dairy-free alternative)

½ cup quinoa flour**

¼ cup sorghum flour**

¼ cup brown rice flour**

½ cup potato starch

½ cup tapioca flour

1 t. baking soda

1 t. aluminium-free baking powder

2 t. ground cinnamon

2 t. guar gum

½ t. Himalayan or sea salt

Preheat oven to 180°C (350°F).

Place the eggs, coconut oil, coconut sugar and vanilla powder into a bowl and whisk.

Add the carrots, zucchini, raisins, coconut flakes, apple and milk and stir well to combine.

In a separate bowl sieve together the flours (quinoa, sorghum, brown rice, potato and tapioca), baking soda, baking powder, cinnamon, guar gum and salt.

Add the dry ingredients to the wet and stir well to form a batter.

Spoon the batter into greased muffin tins and bake until cooked through, approximately 15 – 20 minutes.

Allow the muffins to cool slightly in the pan before removing and eating, or leave to cool completely on a wire rack.

Place in a container, seal and freeze as soon as they have cooled.

Variations:
- *If you would prefer not to use eggs then use this replacement:
  ¼ cup applesauce and ¼ cup warm water mixed with 2 T. ground flax (allow this to sit for 10 minutes before using, it will get 'slimy')
- **If you would like to soak the grains first (and I recommend that you do) place the quinoa, sorghum and brown rice flours in a bowl with the milk. (There is no need to soak the tapioca flour or potato starch as they are not grains.) Stir to combine, cover with a dish towel and leave to soak overnight. In the morning, add the eggs, coconut oil, coconut sugar and vanilla powder to the soaked grains and whisk. Then continue with the recipe as above.

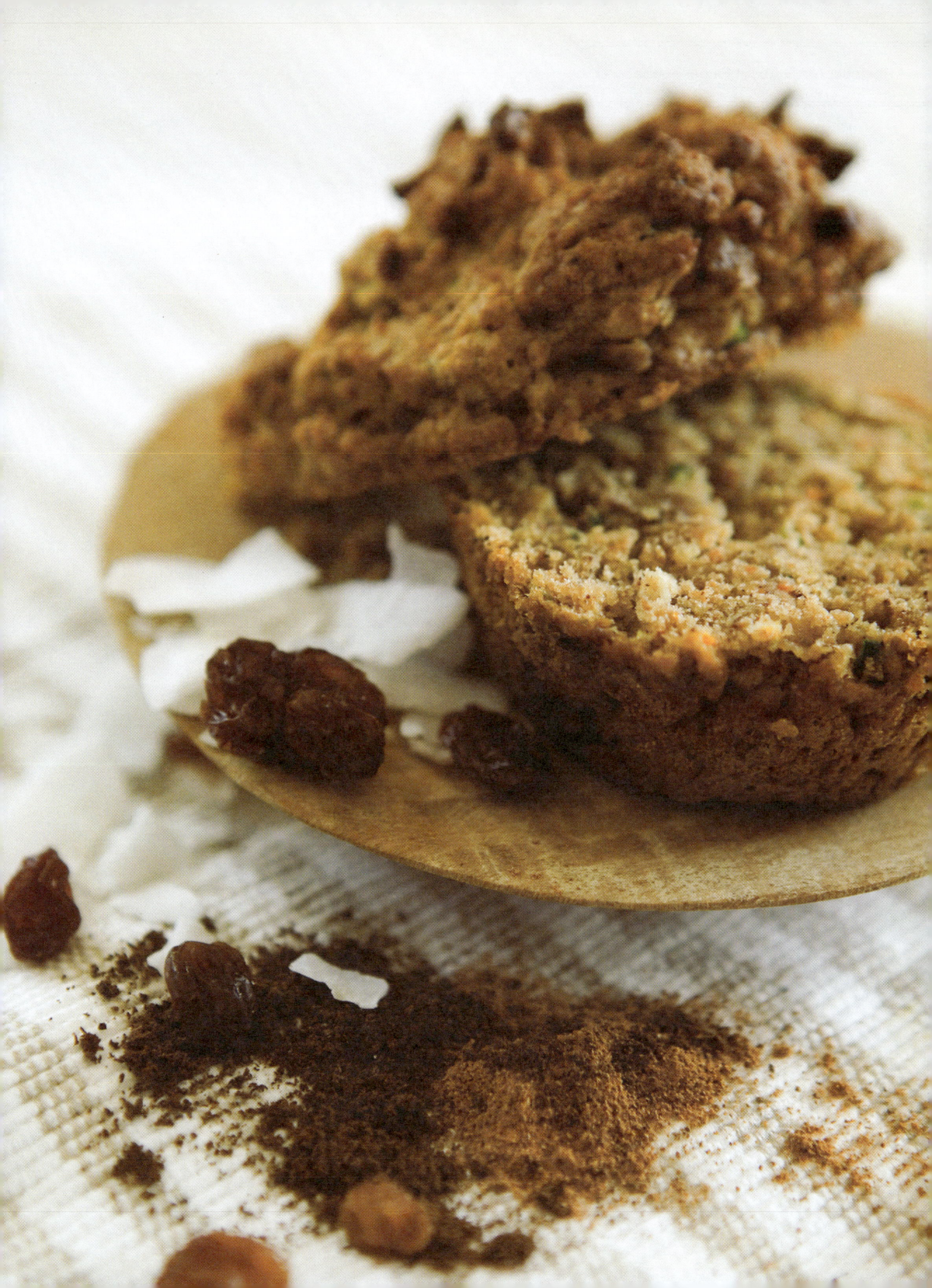

Recipes: Out & About Finger Foods

BUTTERNUT & APPLE MUFFINS

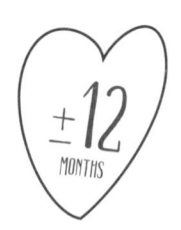

±12 MONTHS

vegetarian; for adults too; great for lunchboxes

Makes 12 baby muffins plus 6 adult ones

These muffins are great way to sneak the vegetables in! They are highly nutritious: rich in omega oils from the flaxseeds; vitamins and minerals from the fruits and vegetables; and, a complete protein thanks to the flours, egg and milk.

½ cup ground oats*
¾ cup ground flaxseeds
1 cup sorghum flour*
½ cup tapioca flour
1 t. aluminium-free baking powder
1 t. baking soda
1 t. Himalayan or sea salt
1½ t. ground nutmeg
1½ t. ground cinnamon
2 T. coconut sugar *(or honey, maple syrup or stevia – you will only need ½ t. stevia)*
4 T. dried cranberries or raisins
1½ cups goat's milk, coconut milk or any other dairy-free alternative
1 t. vanilla extract
2 medium eggs, beaten
3 apples, grated
2 cups butternut, grated

Preheat the oven to 170°C (340°F).

Combine dry ingredients in a large bowl and mix well.

Combine the wet ingredients in a separate bowl.

Mix the dry and wet ingredients together, stirring thoroughly.

Spoon the mixture making into greased baby muffin tins, ensuring it reaches the brim of the pan. (Remember to make some bigger ones for dad!)

Cook for 20 minutes until risen and golden.

Allow the muffins to cool slightly in the pan before removing and eating, or leave to cool completely on a wire rack.

Place in a container, seal and freeze as soon as they have cooled. Frozen, they keep well for up to 1 month.

*If you would like to soak the grains first (and I recommend that you do) place the oats and sorghum flour in a bowl with the milk. (There is no need to soak the tapioca flour as it is not a grain.) Stir to combine, cover with a dish towel and leave to soak overnight. In the morning, add the rest of the ingredients to the soaked grains and mix well. Then continue with the recipe as above.

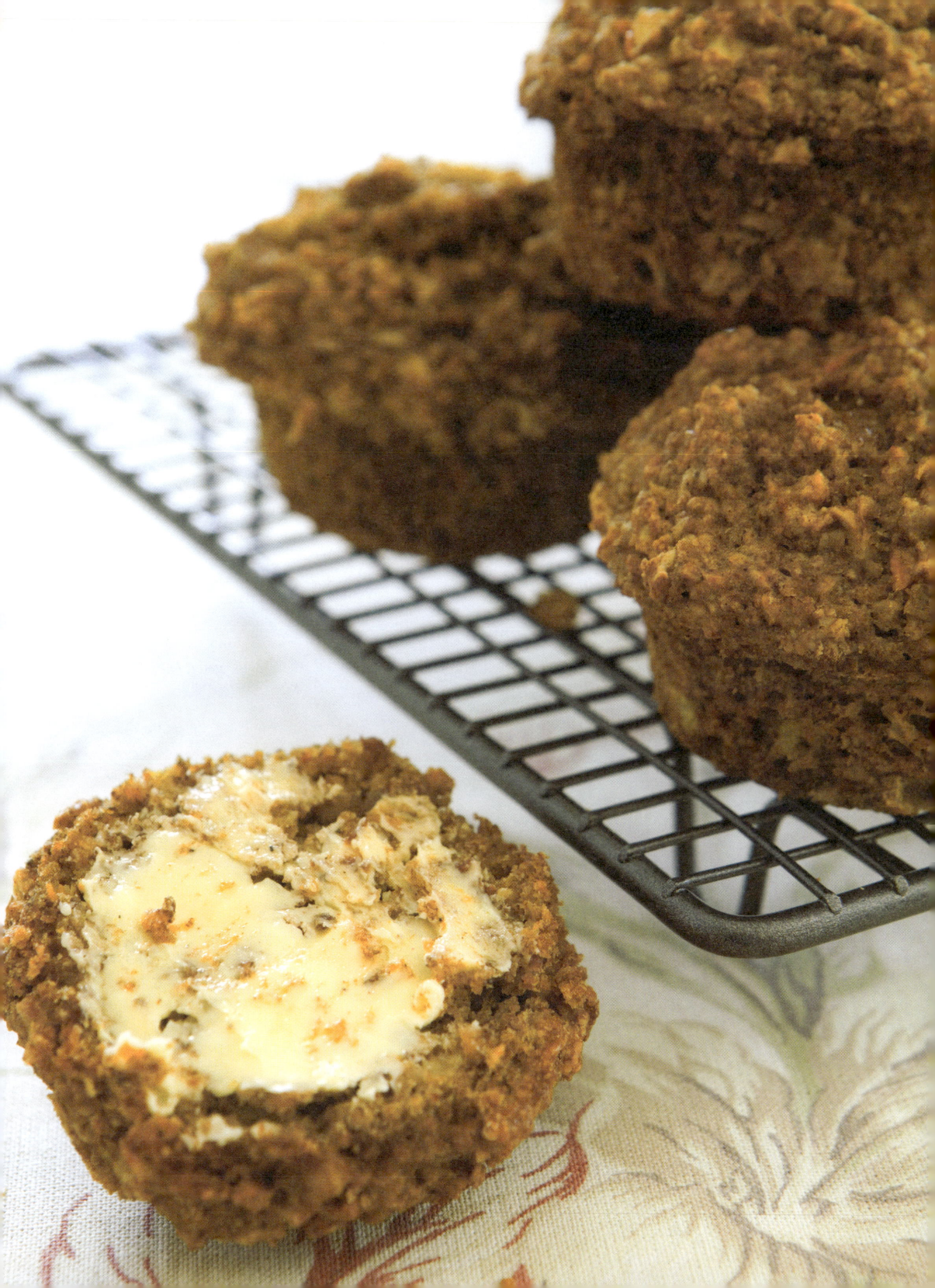

Recipes: Out & About Finger Foods

NANA CAKES

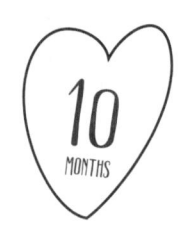

10 MONTHS

raw; superfood; vegetarian; vegan; egg-free; grain-free; for adults too; great for lunchboxes
Makes approximately 40 little 'cakes'

- 4 bananas
- 1 cup dates, pitted and soaked
- 1½ cups almond flour
- 1 T. lemon juice, freshly squeezed
- 1 T. baobab powder (optional)
- coconut oil for greasing

Place all the ingredients in a food processor and blend until smooth.

Grease solid dehydrator sheets with coconut oil.

Scoop spoonful's of mixture onto the dehydrator sheets and spread out into flat round shapes.

Dehydrate at 45°C (115°F) for 8 hours. Transfer the 'cakes' and to mesh dehydrator sheets. Dehydrate for a further 2 hours.

Allow the nana cakes to cool then place in an airtight container in the freezer for storage.

Leave nana cakes out overnight to defrost or toast in the toaster. *(I turn my toaster up-side-down to get the nana cakes out again!)* Alternatively, gently heat in a dry frying pan on the stove.

In the oven:
Turn the oven on to the lowest setting and leave the door slightly open to allow for airflow. Line a baking tray with baking paper and grease with coconut oil. Scoop a spoonful of mixture onto the tray and spread out into flat round shapes. "Bake" for approximately 2 hours.

These nana cakes wont technically be raw, as anything over 45°C (115°F) is no longer raw, but they are still really delicious!

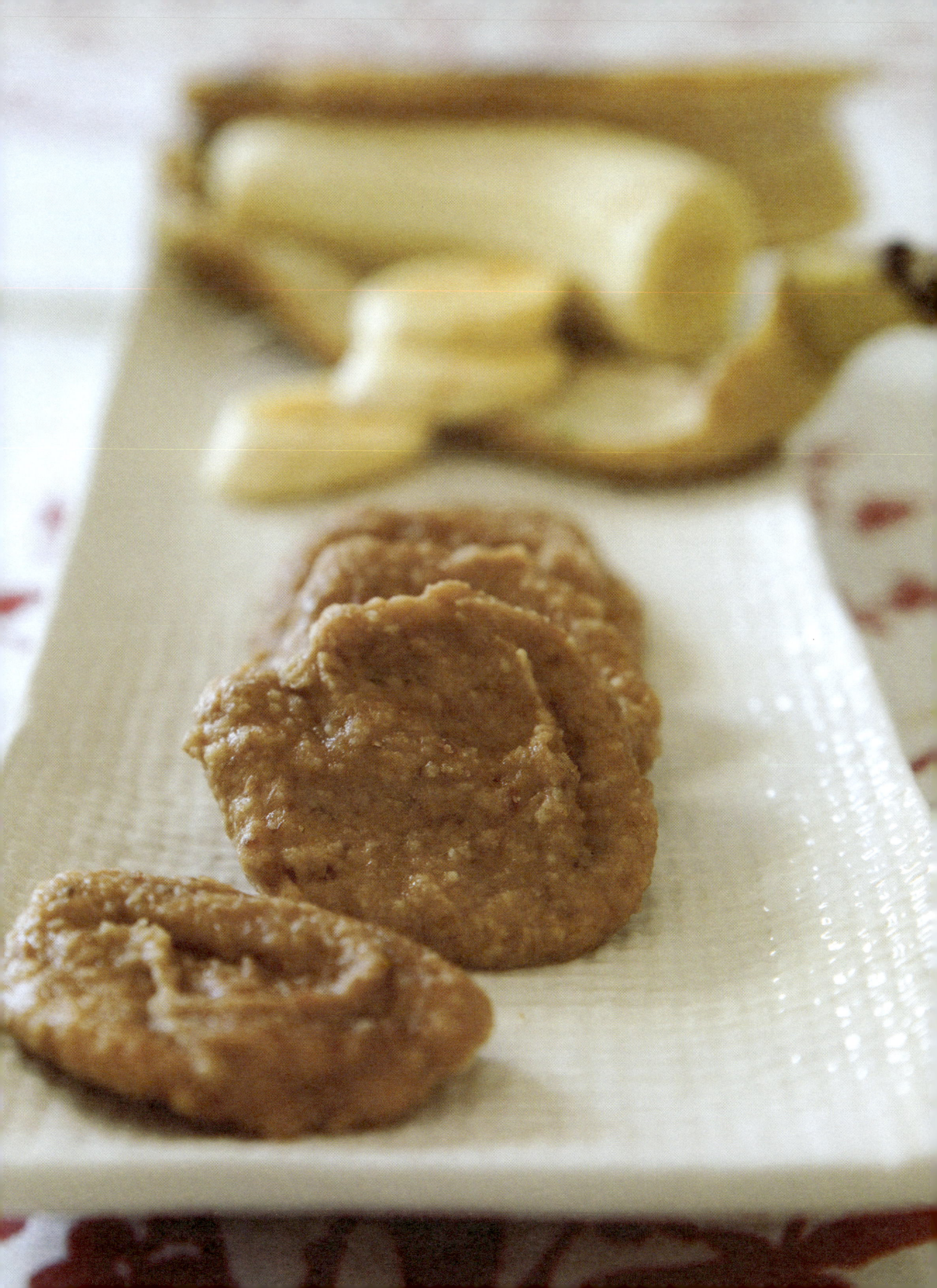

Recipes: Out & About Finger Foods

SIMPLE SEED CRACKERS

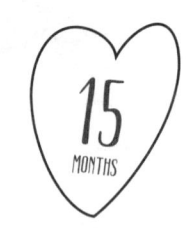

15 MONTHS

raw; vegetarian; vegan; egg-free; grain-free; for adults too; great for lunchboxes

These crackers are a whole lot more nutritious than the store-bought ones which are exposed to incredibly high, damaging heat. They are a great source of omega fatty acids, fibre, protein vitamins B and E and magnesium.

- **1 cup flaxseeds, ground** *(I find a coffee grinder works the best)*
- **½ cup sunflower seeds, soaked* and ground**
- **½ cup pumpkin seeds, soaked* and ground**
- **¾ cup water**
- **¼ cup olive oil**
- **1 t. Himalayan or sea salt**

Place all the ingredients in a mixing bowl and mix well.

Add a little water (if necessary) to create a pliable consistency. If the mixture is too dry it will be difficult to spread onto the dehydrator trays or baking sheets.

Transfer the mixture to solid dehydrator trays or lined baking sheets, pressing it out with wet hands until it is about ½ cm (¼") thick.

Dehydrate in a dehydrator set to 45°C (115°F) for 12 hours, or the oven (set to its lowest temperature) for approximately 4 hours.

Remove the crackers and cut into desired shapes.

Return the crackers to the dehydrator for another 12 hours, or the oven for an additional hour.

Allow to cool, then store in an airtight container in the fridge or freezer for lasting crispness.

Eat as is or with your little one's favourite topping. *(See "Dips Dips & Spreads" for some ideas.)*

---

*If you have not pre-soaked and dehydrated the sunflower and pumpkin seeds, place them in a bowl, cover with warm filtered water and add 1 t. salt. Cover with a dish towel and allow to soak overnight or for 12 hours. Strain and rinse.

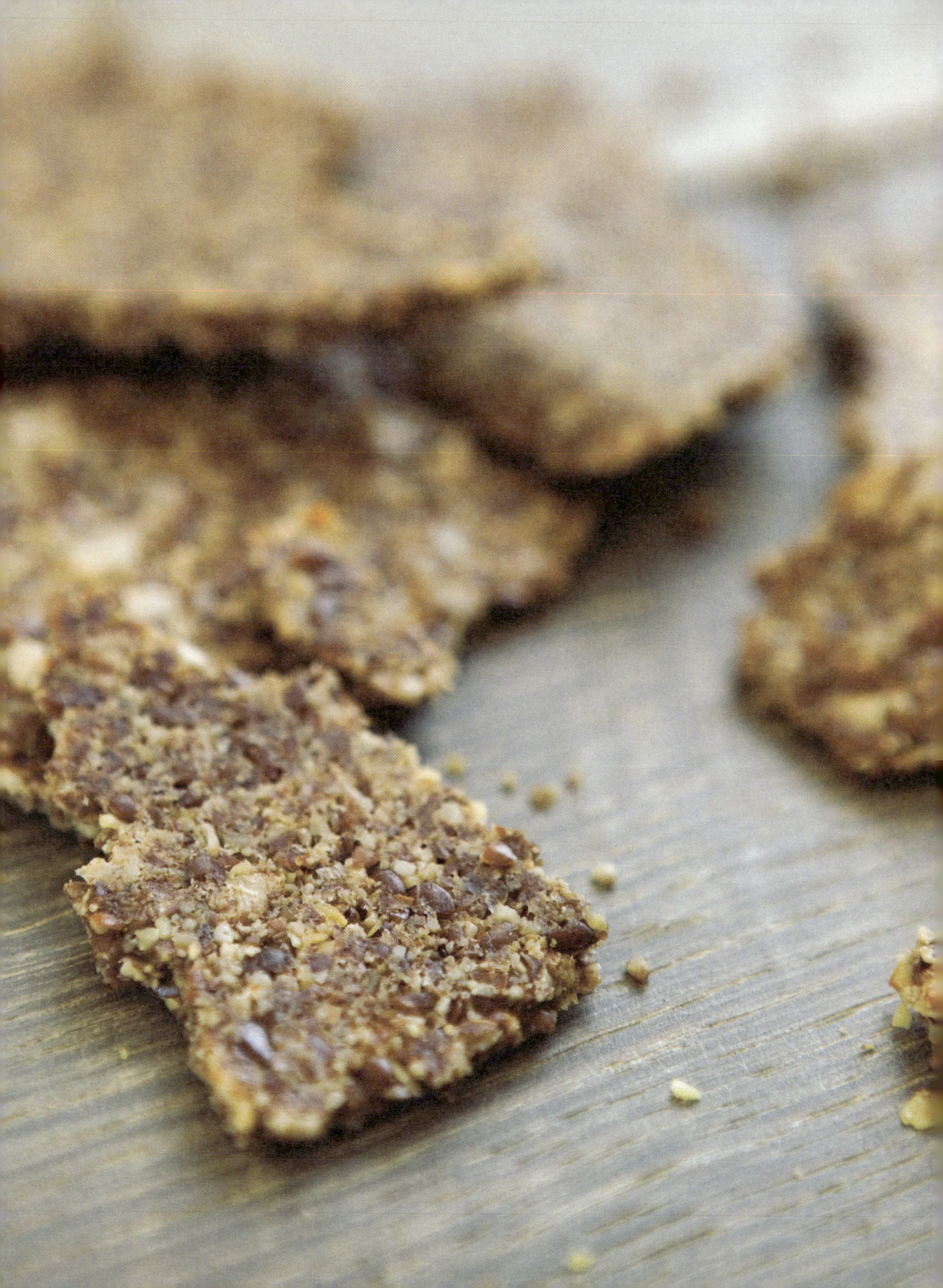

Recipes: Out & About Finger Foods

VEGGIE CRACKERS

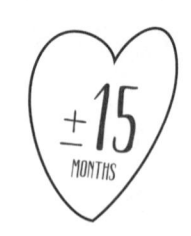

±15 MONTHS

raw; vegetarian; vegan; egg-free; grain-free; for adults too; great for lunchboxes

This is a great way to use the pulp left over after you have made a veggie juice and an excellent way to get the veggies in, as well as the omega oils and fibre.

4 cups vegetables, finely grated or chopped (*For example, carrots, sweet potato, parsley, spinach and apple.*)
2 cups flaxseeds, ground
1 cup sunflower seeds*, ground
¼ cup olive oil
1 T. tamari
1 T. lemon juice
1 t. Himalayan or sea salt
¼ t. cayenne pepper (*optional*)
(water)

Place all the ingredients in a mixing bowl and mix well.

Add a little water (if necessary) to create a pliable consistency. If the mixture is too dry it will be difficult to spread onto the dehydrator trays or baking sheets.

Transfer the mixture to solid dehydrator trays or lined baking sheets, pressing it out with wet hands until it is about ½ cm (¼") thick.

Dehydrate in a dehydrator set to 45°C (115°F) for 12 hours, or the oven (set to its lowest temperature) for approximately 4 hours.

Remove the crackers and cut into desired shapes.

Return the crackers to the dehydrator for another 12 hours, or the oven for an additional hour.

Allow to cool, then store in an airtight container in the fridge or freezer for lasting crispness.

Eat as is or with your little one's favourite topping. *(See Dips Dips & Spreads for some ideas.)*

---

*If you have not pre-soaked and dehydrated the sunflower seeds, place them in a bowl, cover with warm filtered water and add 1 t. salt. Cover with a dish towel and allow to soak overnight or for 12 hours. Strain and rinse.

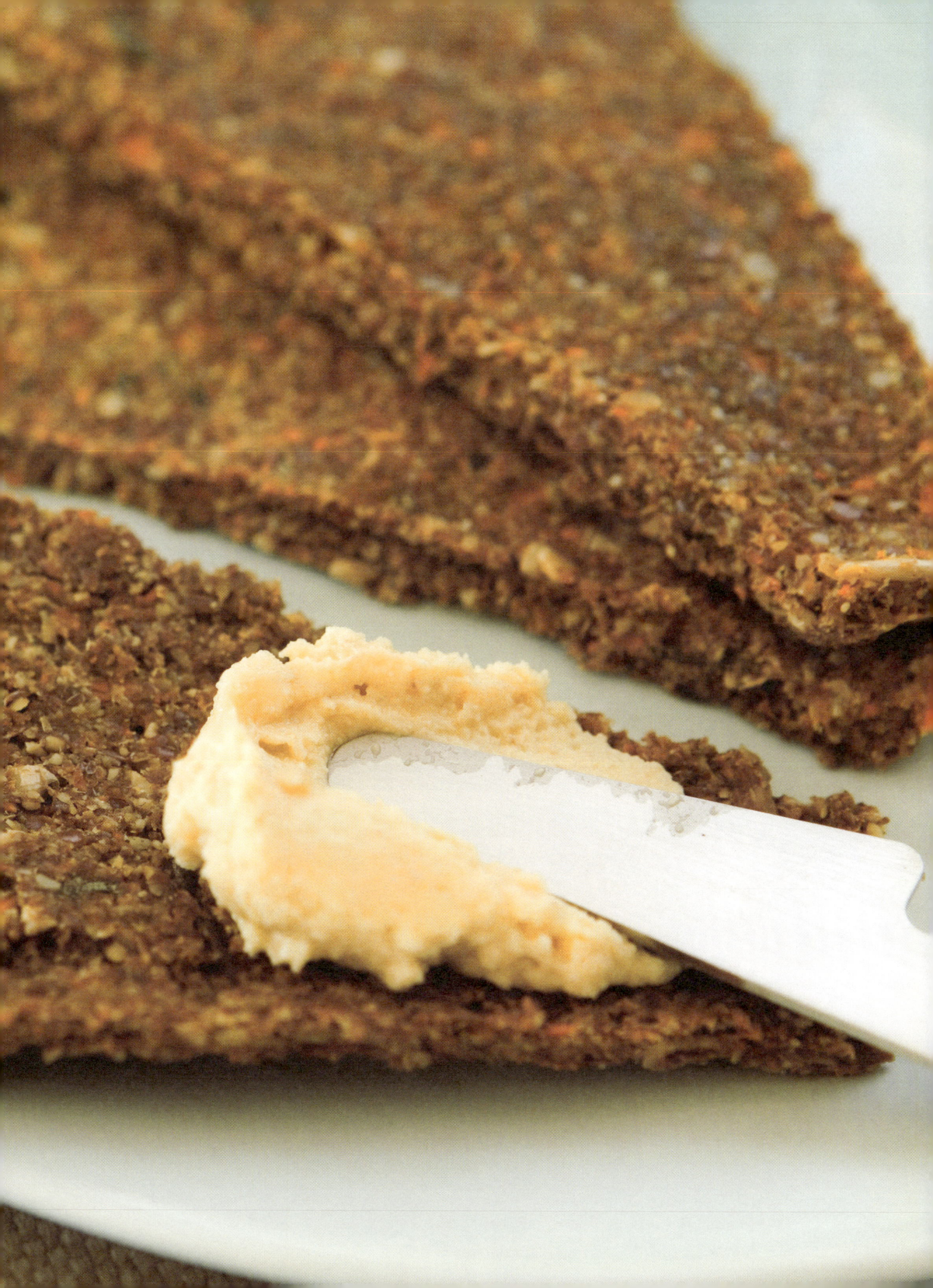

Recipes: Out & About Finger Foods

CHEESY CRACKERS

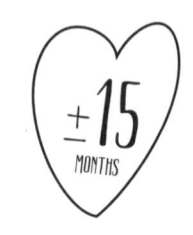

±15 MONTHS

raw; vegetarian; vegan; egg-free; grain-free; for adults too; great for lunchboxes

- 1 cup flaxseeds, ground
- 1 cup water
- 2 cups almonds, soaked over night, drained and rinsed
- ½ cup coconut flour
- 3 T. nutritional yeast
- 1 t. paprika
- 1 T. olive oil
- ½ cup spinach or kale, finely chopped
- Himalayan or sea salt and pepper to taste

Mix together ground flax and water. Set aside.

Place almonds in food processor and process until finely chopped. Place in a large bowl.

Add the nutritional yeast, coconut flour, paprika, olive oil and spinach or kale. Mix well.

Add the flax/water mixture. Mix together well using your hands.

Transfer the mixture to dehydrator trays or baking sheets lined with parchment paper, pressing it out with wet hands until it is about ½ cm (¼") thick.

Dehydrate in a dehydrator set to 45°C (115°F) for 8 hours, or the oven (set to its lowest temperature) for approximately 3 hours turning over and cutting into desired shape half way through.

Allow to cool, then store in an airtight container in the fridge or freezer for lasting crispness.

Eat as is or with your little one's favourite topping. (See Dips Dips & Spreads for some ideas.)

Variation:
- *Substitute the spinach/kale with chopped red bell pepper.*

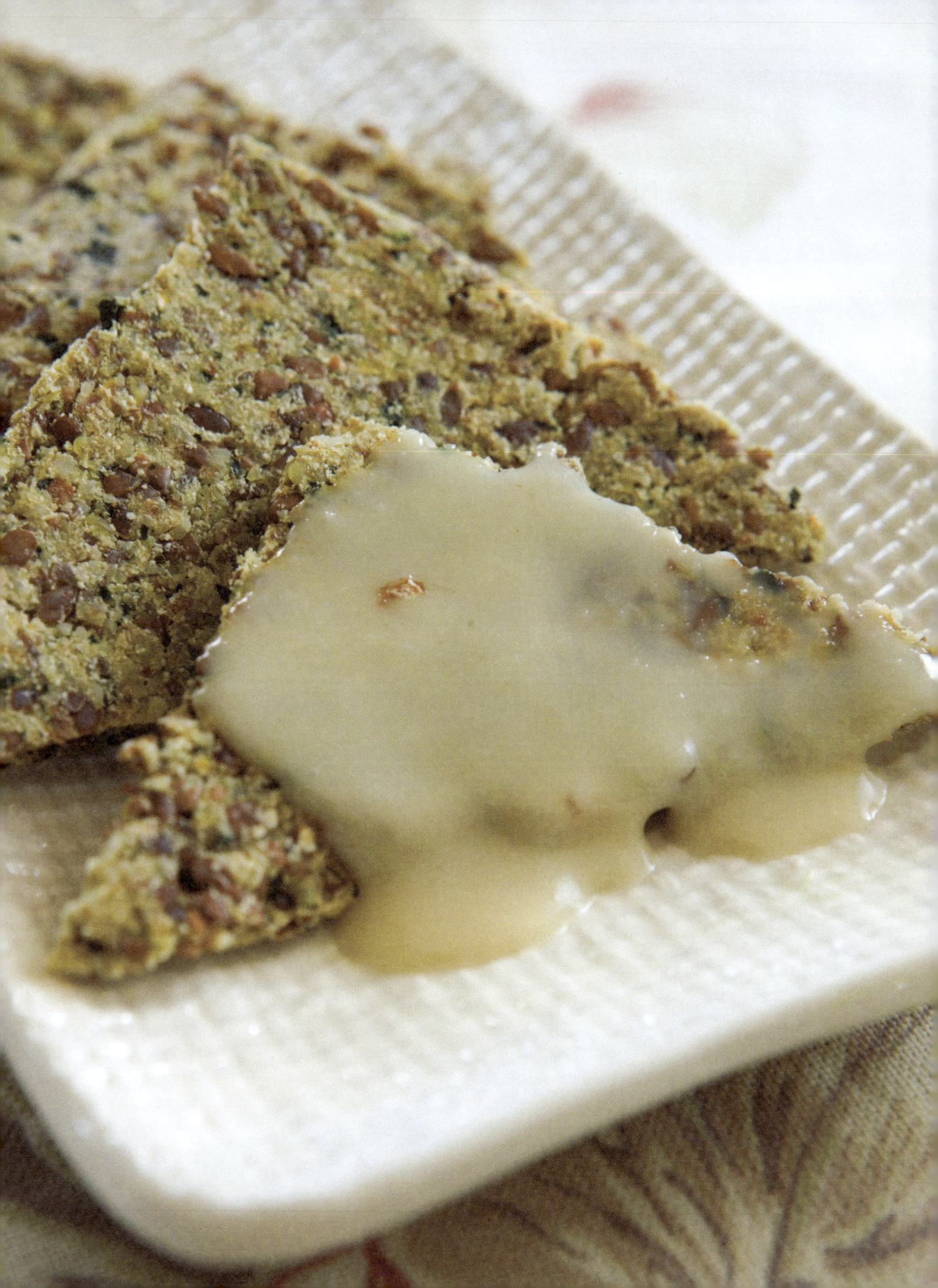

Recipes: Out & About Finger Foods

OAT BARS

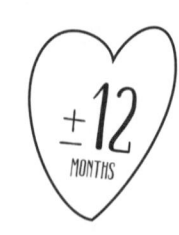

+12 MONTHS

raw; superfood; vegetarian; vegan; egg-free; for adults too; great for lunchboxes

Makes 15

• •

Mila started eating these when she was 15 months old, however I think they can be introduced earlier.

You can play around with this recipe adding more fruit (such as bananas and apples) or different superfoods.

Oats do not contain gluten however, most oats that you buy in the supermarket have been processed in an environment that also processes grains such as wheat, rye and barley. Since these grains contain gluten, there will be cross-contamination. As a result, most oat brands available are not suitable for celiacs and those following a strict gluten-free diet. You can find certified gluten-free oats which have been processed in a gluten-free facility.

• •

- 5 dates, soaked for 2 hours and pitted
- 1 cup certified gluten-free oats, soaked overnight
- ¼ cup preservative-free raisins, finely chopped
- ½ cup apple juice, freshly pressed
- ¼ cup water
- ½ t. vanilla powder
- 1 T. raw cacao powder or cinnamon
- ½ t. green powder
- ½ cup cashew nuts, soaked overnight (optional)
- 2 T. raw honey or maple syrup (optional)

Place all the ingredients in a food processor and blend until smooth.

Spread the mixture onto solid dehydrator sheets.

Dehydrate in a dehydrator set to 45°C (115°F) for 6 hours then remove and cut into desired shapes.

Return the oat bars to the dehydrator for an additional 12 hours. Check on the oat bars to make sure they are not getting too dry. *I left them in for too long once, and they were more like dog biscuits which Mila refused to eat!*

In the oven:
Spread the mixture onto baking sheets lined with greased parchment paper. Set your oven to its lowest temperature. Leave the door slightly ajar for airflow and cook for 4 hours.

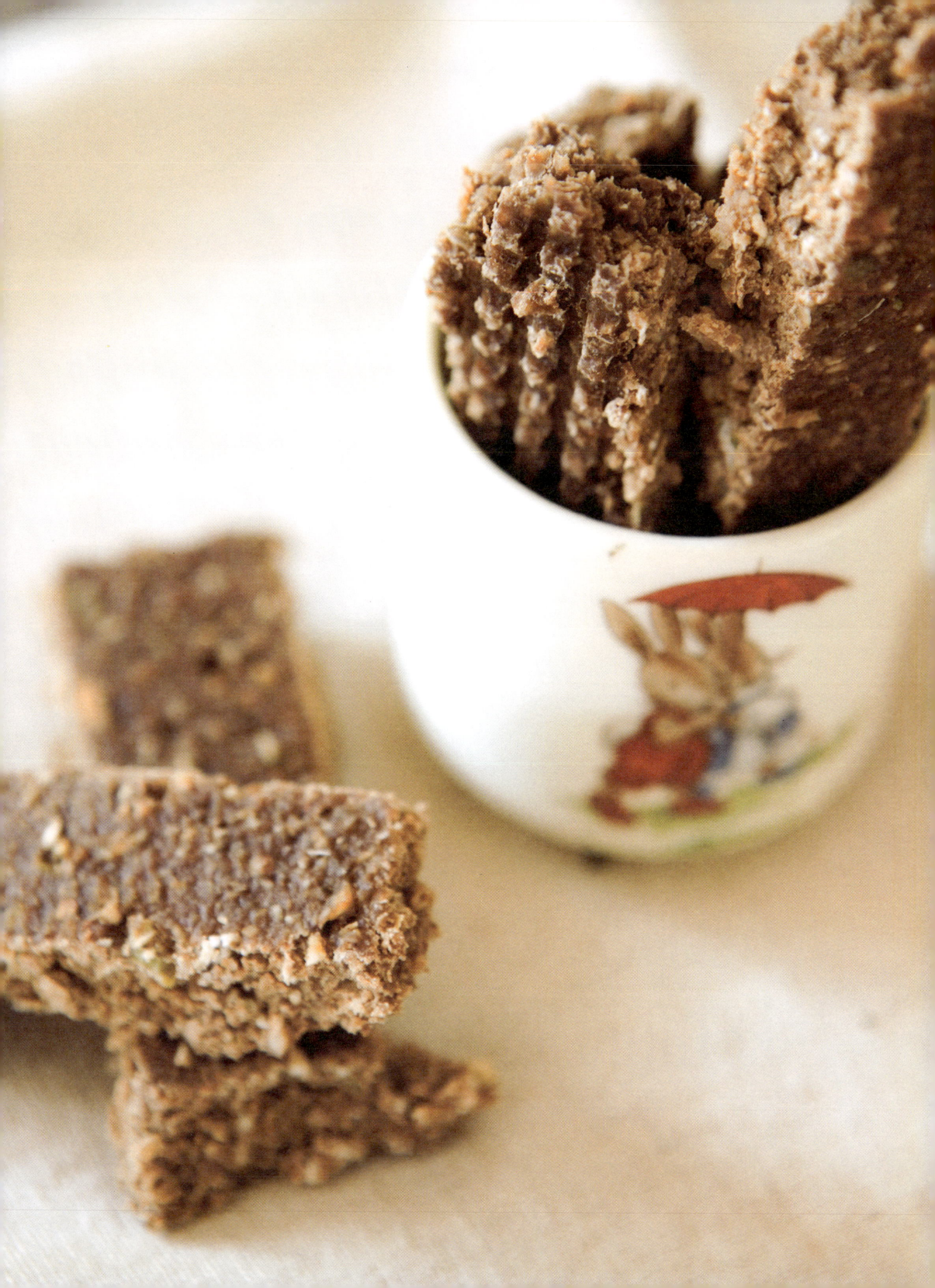

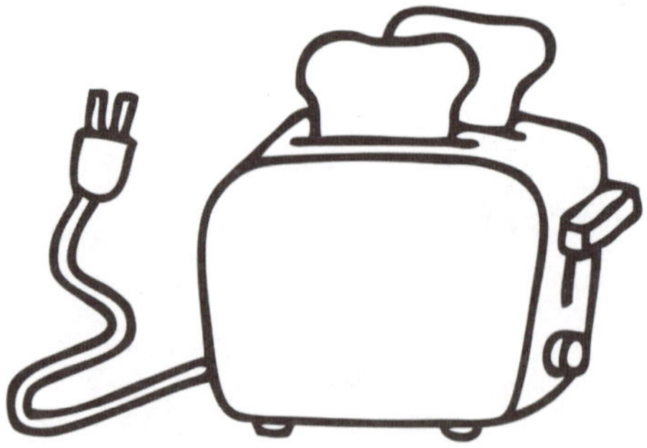

Recipes:
Eating In Finger Foods

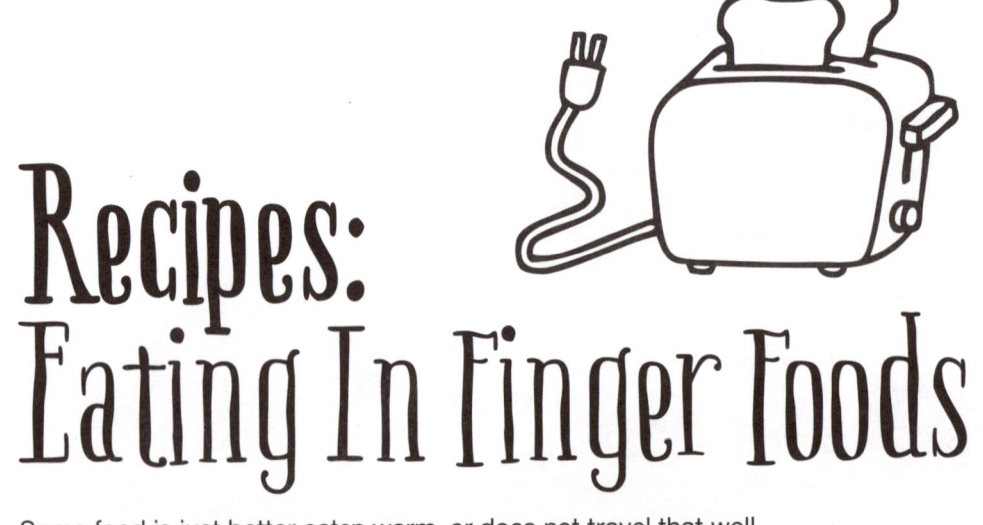

Some food is just better eaten warm, or does not travel that well.

Recipes: Eating In Finger Foods

SWEET POTATO BREAD → 234
CHICKPEA FLATBREAD → 236
RÖSTI → 238
'ONTBIJTKOEK' – SPICED BREAKFAST CAKE → 240
RAISIN AND BANANA FLAPJACKS → 242
BUTTERNUT & CRANBERRY FRITTERS → 244
CHICKPEA BITES → 246
QUINOA BITES → 248
VEGGIE BITES → 250
CHICKEN BALLS → 252
SWEET POTATO GNOCCHI → 254
MOCK FISH FINGERS → 256
REAL FISH FINGERS → 258
FISHCAKES → 260
CHICKEN NUGGETS → 262
BUFFALO WINGS → 264
SWEET POTATO CHIPS → 266
PIZZA → 268
PESTO 'PANCAKE' (CRÊPE) → 270
REAL PANCAKES (CRÊPES) → 272

Recipes: Eating In Finger Foods

SWEET POTATO BREAD

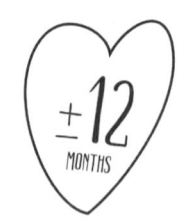

±12 MONTHS

vegetarian; vegan; egg-free; for adults too; great for lunchboxes

Makes: 1 big loaf or 2 small loaves.

••

It took me a LONG time to perfect gluten-free, yeast-free bread! Many loaves were inedible, and much money was spent at the health food store as Mila went through her 'toastie' stage. I am very proud of this recipe, and it is the only one of my breads that Mila has not only eaten, but also thoroughly enjoyed!

Mila's "toastie stage" (when she would only eat toast for breakfast) lasted for 4 months. As toast became such a big part of her diet, I really wanted it to be more than just a filler of processed flours. Which is why I have added the sweet potato and the flax seeds.

Instead of just being a base for nutritious toppings, this bread is highly nutritious itself. Sweet potatoes are an excellent source of vitamins A, B and C and the flax seeds add omega-3 essential fatty acids and fibre. Both these ingredients have both anti-oxidant and anti-inflammatory benefits and can both prevent and relieve constipation.

••

- 1 cup white rice flour*
- ¾ cup potato starch
- ¼ cup tapioca flour
- ¼ cup flaxseeds, ground
- 2 T. coconut sugar
- 1 t. aluminium-free baking powder
- ½ t. baking soda
- ¼ t. Himalayan or sea salt
- 1 t. guar gum
- ⅓ cup coconut oil, melted
- 1¼ cup coconut milk, or goat's milk *(you may need more)*
- 1 T. raw, unfiltered apple cider vinegar
- 1¼ cup sweet potato, cooked and mashed

Variations:
- *You can replace the sweet potato with butternut and add a pinch of cinnamon to the mix.*
- *Play around with flavours by adding spices (cinnamon, nutmeg), herbs (dried oreganum, basil, rosemary) and ground seeds (sunflower seeds, pumpkins seeds).*

Preheat your oven to 160°C (325°F) and grease your loaf tin/tins. I use two 14.5 x 7.5 cm (5.75 x 3") tins.

Mash your sweet potatoes (which should be at room temperature).

In a small mixing bowl add the apple cider vinegar to the coconut milk.

In a separate bowl, sieve all the dry ingredients together.

Add the coconut oil and the sweet potato to the coconut milk mixture.

Add the dry ingredients to the wet mixture and stir until well combined. The mixture should be like a thick cake batter. If it is too dry, add more milk slowly until you reach the desired consistency.

Scoop the batter into the greased loaf tin and quickly place in the preheated oven.

Bake the bread for approximately 60 minutes. The bread is done when you insert a knife / toothpick into the centre and it comes out clean.

Remove the loaf from the pan and place on a wire rack to cool.

This bread is delicious eaten as is with butter or almond butter. It makes a great slice of toast too.

For freshness, it is best to slice the entire loaf, place in a freezer bag and freeze. Simply toast individual slices to thaw them as you need them.

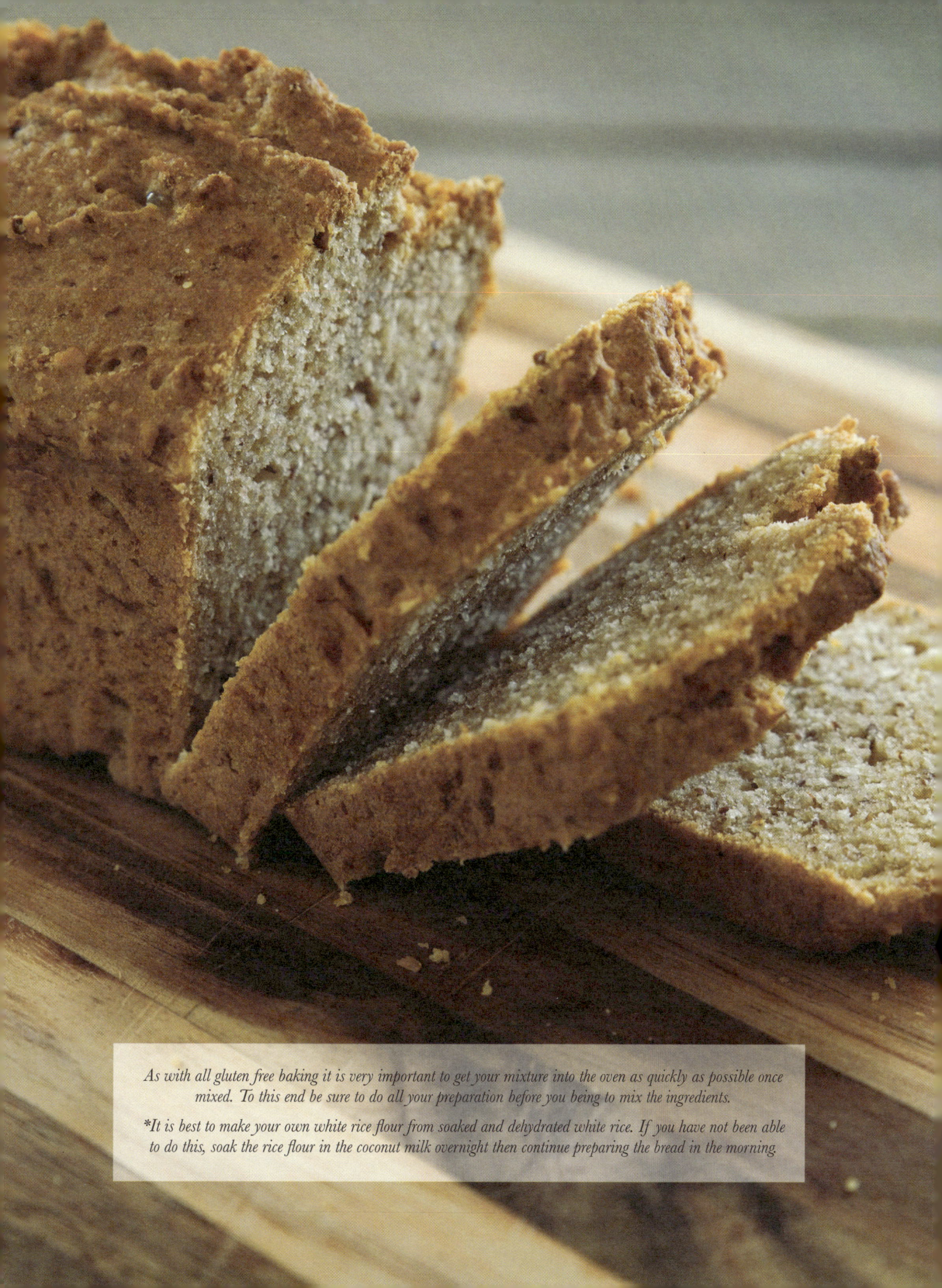

As with all gluten free baking it is very important to get your mixture into the oven as quickly as possible once mixed. To this end be sure to do all your preparation before you being to mix the ingredients.

*It is best to make your own white rice flour from soaked and dehydrated white rice. If you have not been able to do this, soak the rice flour in the coconut milk overnight then continue preparing the bread in the morning.

Recipes: Eating In Finger Foods

CHICKPEA FLATBREAD

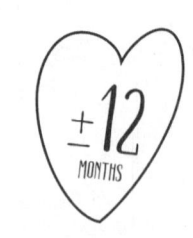

+12 MONTHS

vegetarian; vegan; egg-free; grain-free; for adults too; great for lunchboxes

Makes: 15 squares - 10 cm x 10 cm (4" x 4")

• •

I feel people rely on bread too much. Yes, it is convenient, but there are many other foods which can be used as a 'base' for sandwiches or other toppings. A big black mushrooms works well as a hamburger bun, nut butter is just as delicious between two slices of apple, perhaps even more so. Other bread/sandwich substitutes include rice paper, cucumber, potato rösti, and this flatbread – which is so easy to make, and so delicious.

• •

- 3 cups chickpea (garbanzo) flour
- 3 cups water
- 1 T. Himalayan or sea salt
- ½ T. lemon juice or apple cider vinegar
- 2 t. dried oreganum
- ½ cup sundried tomatoes, chopped and soaked in warm water
- ½ cup olives, chopped
- ¼ cup cold-pressed olive oil

Place your chickpea flour and water in a mixing bowl. Stir with a whisk to remove any lumps.

Add in the salt, apple cider vinegar and oreganum.

Cover and allow to soak for 3 hours or overnight.

Preheat your oven to 200°C (400°F).

Pour the olive oil into a large baking tray.

Sprinkle the sundried tomatoes and olives onto the bottom of the tray.

Gently, pour the chickpea flour mixture into the tray.

Place in the oven and cook for 20 minutes, or until golden brown on top.

Allow to cool, cut and serve.

Leftover flatbread can be stored in the freezer. When you or your little one wants a slice, simply pop it into the toaster.

Variations:
- *For a plain flatbread simply leave out the herbs, tomatoes and olives.*
- *For a cheesy one, add some grated goat cheese.*

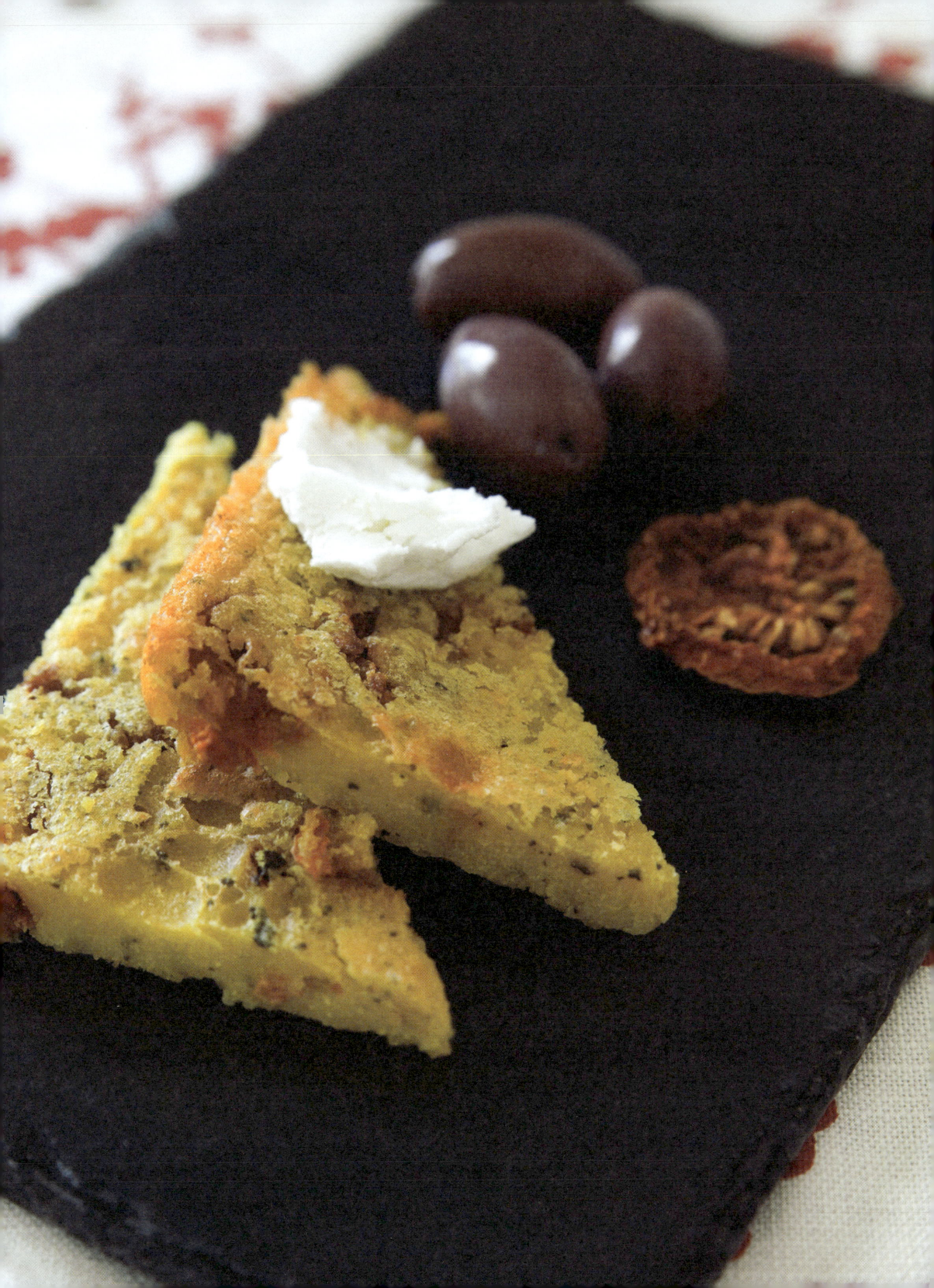

Recipes: Eating In Finger Foods

RÖSTI

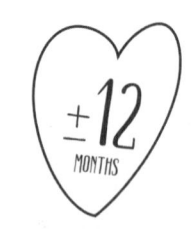

± 12 MONTHS

vegetarian; grain-free; for adults too; great for lunchboxes

Makes: 20 toddler-sized rösti

• •

*You can make rösti with just about any root vegetable or combination thereof.
They are a great breakfast bread replacement and make an excellent base for poached eggs. They are also, of course, a great finger food for your little one.*

Please see the glossary pages for more information on each ingredient.

• •

4 medium white potatoes, or 2 sweet potatoes
1 organic egg
¼ cup tapioca flour
pinch salt and pepper
pinch turmeric
pinch dried oreganum
coconut oil for frying

Wash, peel and grate the potatoes. Squeeze out and discard the excess liquid and place into a bowl.

Stir in the egg, flour, and seasoning.

Mix well.

Heat the oil in a frying pan over medium to high heat.

Drop in tablespoons of mixture, press down with the back of the spoon and gently cook for 15 minutes turning halfway through cooking.

The rösti should be golden brown and crispy on the outside and the potato cooked all the way through.

Variations:
- *Try adding some beetroot for pink rösti!*
- *Adding a cup of parsnips and carrots works well too.*

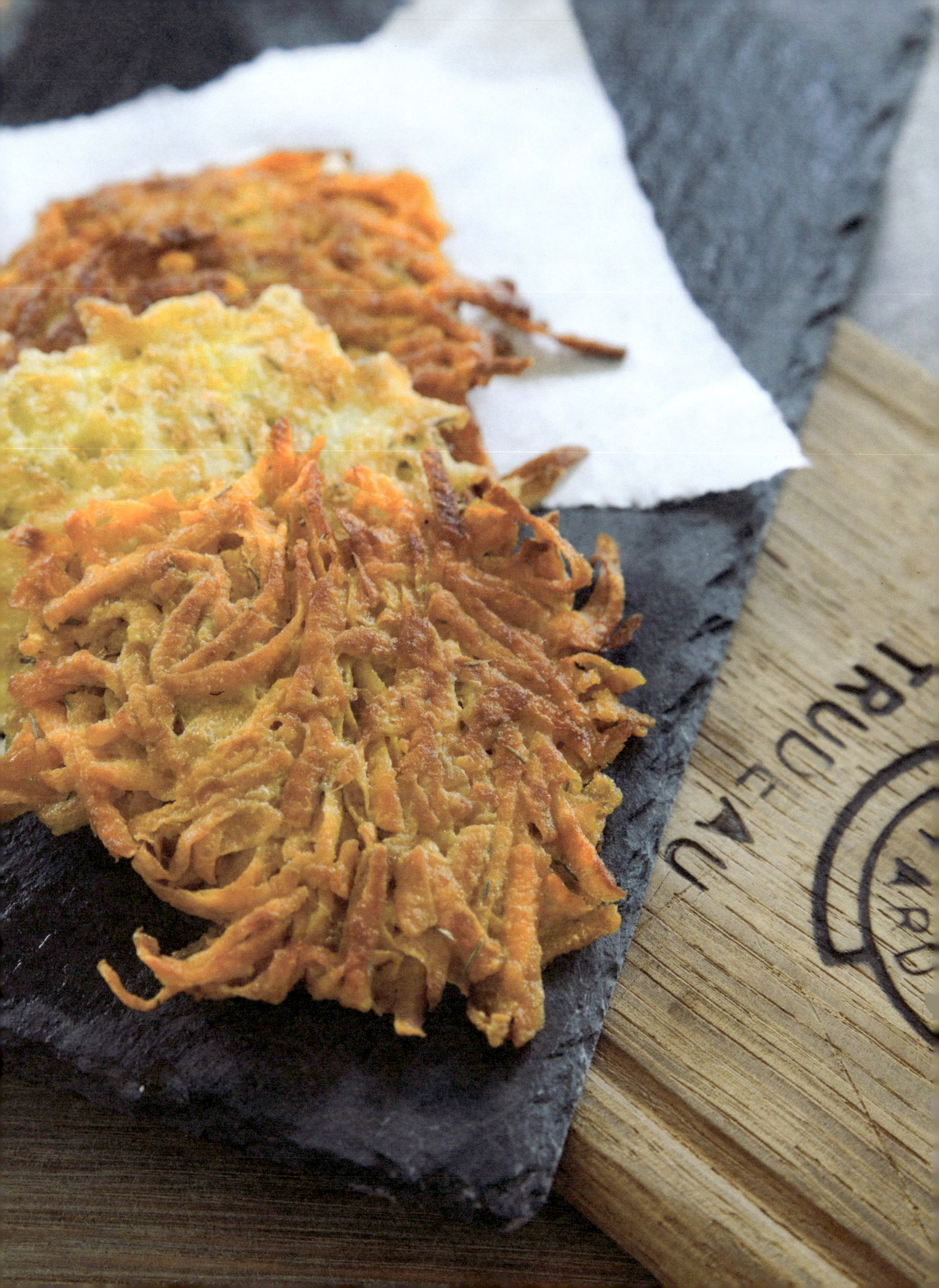

Recipes: Eating In Finger Foods

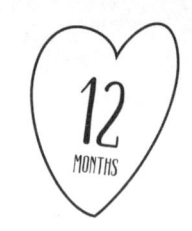

12 MONTHS

'ONTBIJTKOEK' – SPICED BREAKFAST CAKE

vegetarian; grain-free; for adults too; great for lunchboxes

Makes 2 mini loaves - 14½ x 8 cm (5½ x 3")

•••

The original ontbijtkoek is made with wheat or rye flour, sugar and milk – this recipe is my gluten, dairy and sugar-free adaptation!

Ontbijtkoek (Dutch for Breakfast Cake) is another food I remember fondly from my childhood. My dad is Dutch and we would often have this 'cake' at my Ouma's house with our afternoon tea. Traditionally, it is eaten for breakfast.

It is more of a spiced bread than a cake and with my addition of butternut, it makes for a wholesome and nutritious breakfast or afternoon snack. Traditionally served with a thick layer of butter spread over it, I use almond butter instead – it is delicious!

•••

- 1¼ cups almond flour*
- 3 organic eggs
- ¼ t. Himalayan or sea salt
- 1 T. cinnamon
- 1 t. nutmeg
- 1 t. ground ginger
- ½ t. cloves
- ½ cup butternut, roasted, cooled and mashed (it is important to not steam the butternut as it will have too much moisture for the bread)
- 3 T. raw honey
- 2 T. unsulphured blackstrap molasses
- 1 T. coconut oil, melted
- ½ t. baking soda
- ½ t. aluminium-free baking powder

Preheat the oven to 180°C (350°F).

Grease two 14½ x 8 cm (5½ x 3") loaf pans. Line the bottom of the pans with parchment paper to ensure the loaves fall out easily once cooked.

Place the almond flour and eggs in a large mixing bowl and beat with an electric beater for 2 minutes. This allows the rather dry almond flour to absorb some moisture before being cooked.

Add the salt, cinnamon, nutmeg, ginger, and cloves and beat to mix.

In another mixing bowl beat together the butternut, eggs, honey, molasses and coconut oil. Add this mixture to the almond flour mixture.

Add the baking soda and baking powder and beat until combined.

Scoop the batter into your prepared loaf pans and bake for 40 minutes, until a knife inserted into the middle comes out clean.

Place the cake on a wire rack to cool, then wrap in tin foil for 24 hours before eating – this creates the delicious sticky crust!

Cut and serve as is, or pop in the toaster and spread with butter.

The remaining cake can be stored in a sealed container for up to 3 days. For longer storage, freeze slices for up to 1 month.

*I recommend making your own almond flour by grinding soaked and dehydrated almonds.

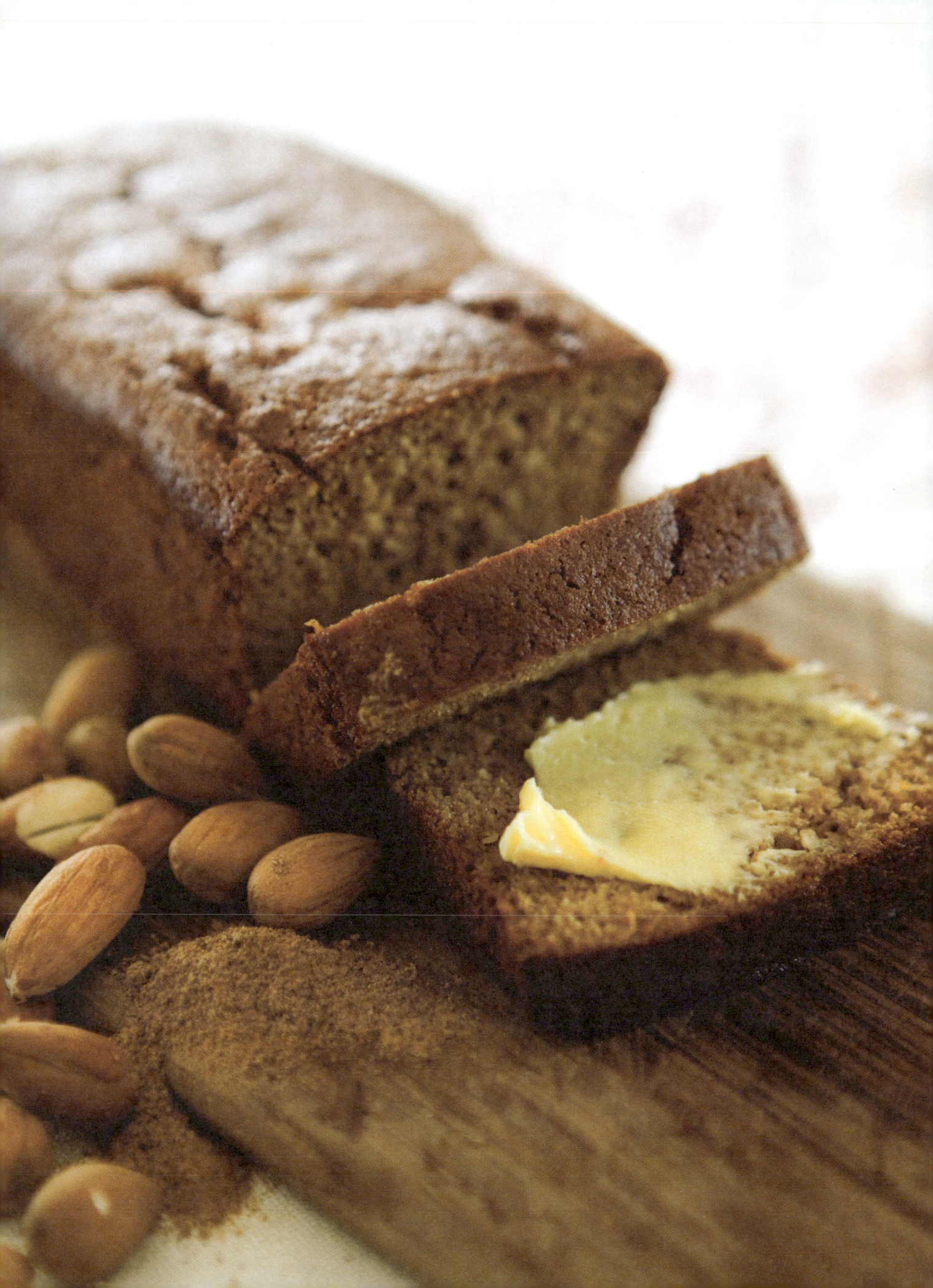

Recipes: Eating In Finger Foods

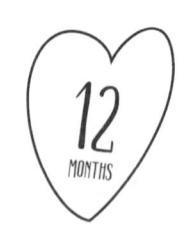

RAISIN AND BANANA FLAPJACKS

12 MONTHS

vegetarian; egg-free; for adults too; great for lunchboxes

Makes 30 toddler sized flapjacks

• •

This is a really quick and easy recipe that makes a great breakfast or mid morning snack.

These flapjacks are a high fibre, nutritionally dense meal filled with anti-inflammatory omega-3 essential fatty acids, energy-producing vitamin B1, manganese, selenium, magnesium, phosphorus, zinc and copper.

Pure oatmeal does not contain gluten. However, most oats that you buy in the supermarket have been processed in an environment that also processes grains such as wheat, rye and barley. Since these grains contain gluten, there will be cross-contamination. As a result, most oat brands available may not be suitable for celiacs and those following a strict gluten-free diet.

• •

¾ cup goat's milk*
½ cup chickpea flour, or sorghum flour
¾ cup rolled oats
1 t. raw, unfiltered apple cider vinegar
3 T. flaxseeds, ground
2 T. raisins, chopped
1 banana, mashed
½ t. aluminium free baking powder
½ t. baking soda
Coconut oil for frying

Place the milk, flour, oats and apple cider vinegar in a mixing bowl. Whisk together, cover and leave to soak overnight.

In the morning, put your soaked mixture in a blender or food processor with all the other ingredients and process until smooth.

Heat a little coconut oil in a frying pan over medium-high heat (just enough to lightly coat the bottom of the pan). Spoon the batter in, forming individual flapjacks in your size of choice (approximately ½ cm / ¼" thick).

Flip the flapjacks over once little bubbles start to form on the top side and the batter has set.

Cook for a few more minutes on the second side until golden.

Serve as they are! For a special treat spread them with some maple syrup, honey or Mila's Meals chocolate sauce.

Cooked flapjacks can be stored in the freezer for up to 1 month. Simply pop in the toaster to defrost and reheat.

Variations:
- *You can also use almond milk, rice milk or coconut milk. Use an additional ¼ cup if using a coconut milk which has guar gum as an ingredient as it tends to be thicker.
- Make blueberry flapjacks by omitting the banana and raisins and adding 1 cup of blueberries and 4 dates instead.

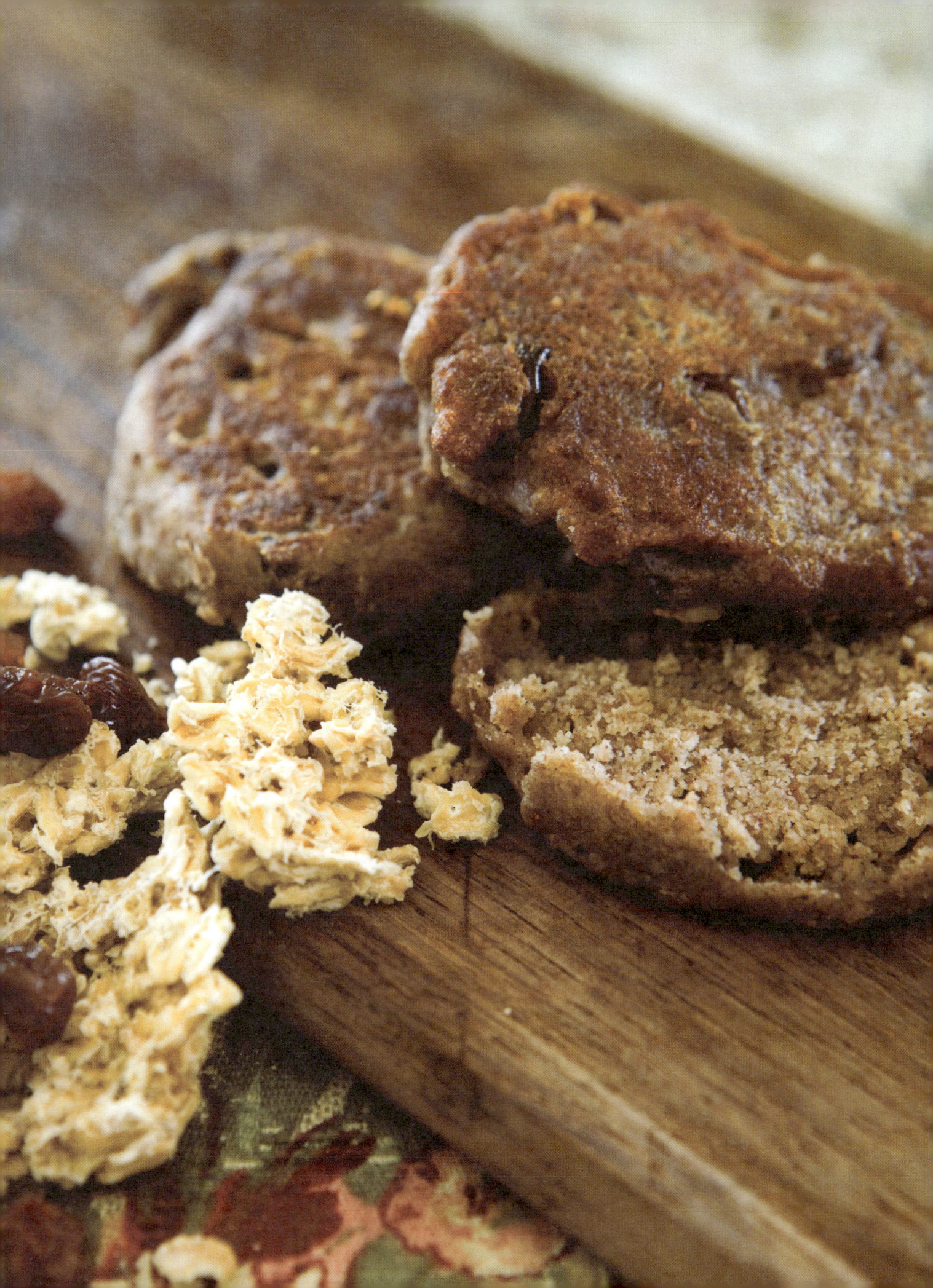

Recipes: Eating In Finger Foods

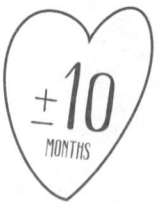

±10 MONTHS

BUTTERNUT & CRANBERRY FRITTERS

vegetarian; grain-free; for adults too; great for lunchboxes

Makes 30 toddler sized flapjacks

• •

Fritters are a South African classic! *My sister-in-law, Ady, is well known for hers and she makes them for every big family meal. I simply had to come up with a gluten- and sugar-free alternative to avoid the food envy at these occasions!*

Fritters are a wonderful way to use up left over veggies and purées. You are only limited by your imagination when it comes to what flavour you would like your fritters to be.

This particular recipe is one of Mila's favourites and she has been eating them since she moved on from purées at 9 months old – but I did not know to delay introducing grains, legumes and nuts! Since the chickpea flour is made from a legume it may be difficult to digest and it may be best to wait until your little one is closer to a year before introducing it. Watch for any signs of discomfort after feeding it to him/her.

Butternut is an excellent source of vitamins A, B's, C and K and fibre. Mixed with the cranberries you get a meal with an astonishing array of phytonutrients which offer antioxidant, anti-inflammatory, and anti-cancer health benefits. The addition of chickpea flour makes this meal a source of protein too – perfect for the little one's who are not too keen on meat.

• •

1/3 cup chickpea flour

½ T. freshly squeezed lemon juice

½ cup coconut milk (or other dairy-free alternative)

1 cup butternut, cooked and puréed

2 eggs, beaten

4 T. cranberries, chopped

⅓ cup potato flour

⅓ cup tapioca flour

1 t. aluminium-free baking powder

½ t. baking soda

1 t. cinnamon

½ Himalayan or sea salt

Coconut oil for frying

Variations:
- *Replace the butternut with sweet potato.*
- *Replace the butternut with finely grated baby marrow, the cranberries with goats cheese, and the cinnamon with black pepper.*

Place the chickpea flour, lemon juice and milk in a mixing bowl and whisk to combine. Cover with a dish towel and leave to soak for 8 hours or overnight.

Once the soaking is complete, add the butternut purée, beaten eggs and cranberries. Mix well.

In a separate bowl, mix the dry ingredients with a whisk (the potato flour, tapioca flour, baking powder, baking soda, cinnamon and salt).

Add the dry ingredients to the butternut mixture and mix well to form a thick batter (while being careful not to over mix).

Heat just enough coconut oil in a frying pan to coat it.

Scoop tablespoons of the batter into the pan.

Fry them until they are firm and golden on the underside then flip over for another couple of minutes. Test to see if the fritters are done by pressing lightly on them. If they are done, they will spring back. Transfer to some kitchen towel to drain and cool.

Serve as is - or with some raw honey drizzled on top!

Left over fritters can be frozen and placed in the toaster to defrost and reheat as and when you need them.

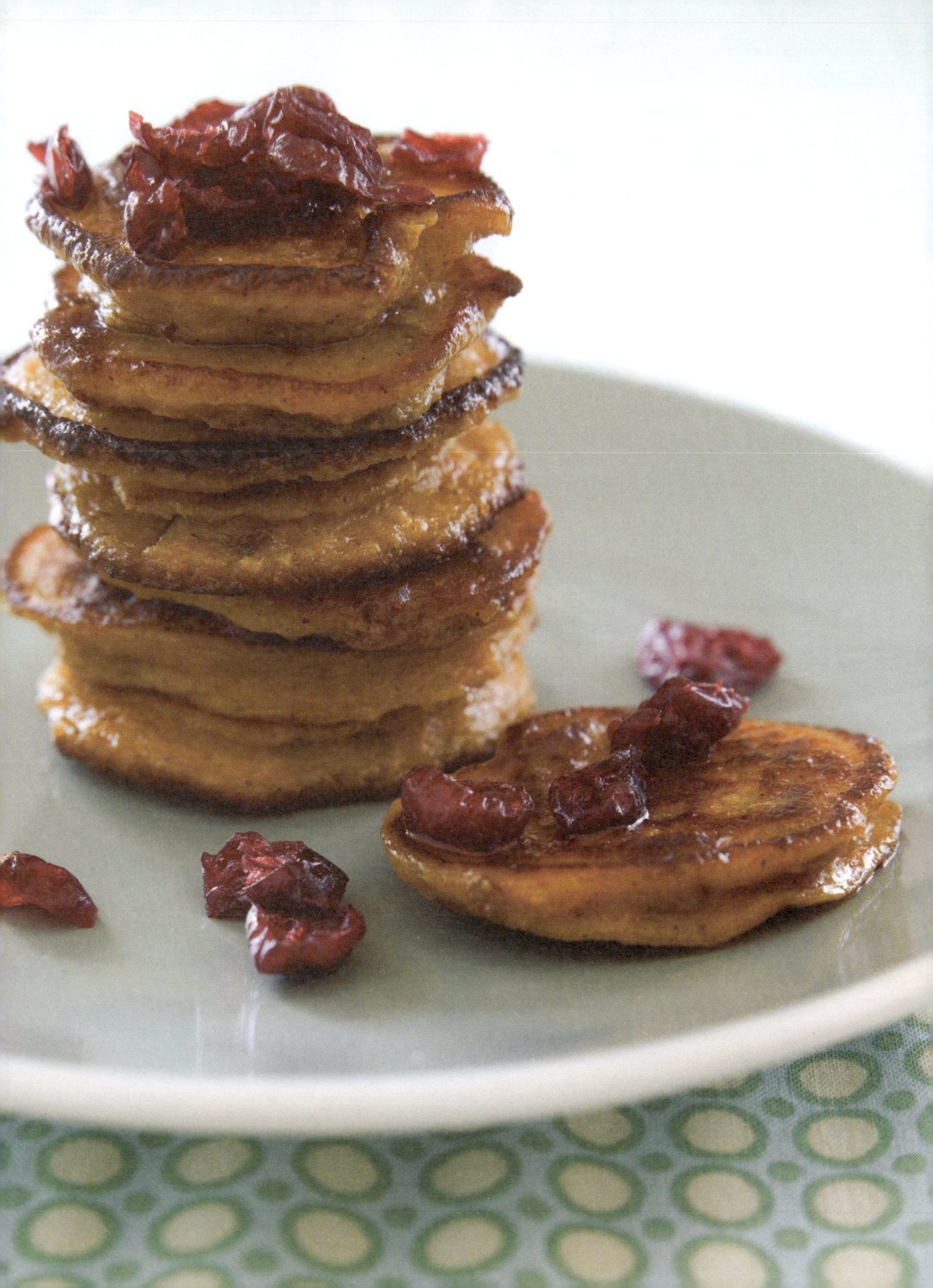

Recipes: Eating In Finger Foods

CHICKPEA BITES

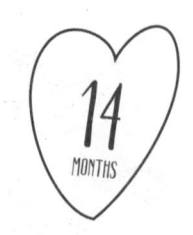

14 MONTHS

vegetarian; grain-free; for adults too; great for lunchboxes

Makes 24

As the preparation of dried chickpeas takes a long time, I usually cook the whole bag, use what I need and then freeze the rest for the next recipe that requires them. That way, I am not tempted to use the canned ones! Cooked chickpeas can be frozen for up to a month.

These chickpea bites are a really useful all-in-one meal which Mila was eating from 14 months old. They are a great source of protein, fibre, magnesium, phosphorus, zinc and iron. The chickpeas and flaxseeds both have anti-inflammatory and anti-oxidant properties.

To cook your chickpeas:

Place the dried chickpeas in a big bowl. Cover with hot water and add an acid medium (whey, lemon juice or apple cider vinegar). The amount of acid will depend on the quantity of chickpeas you are preparing – for a full bag of chickpeas, I use 2 T. of apple cider vinegar. The chickpeas will swell and absorb a lot of water so make sure your bowl is big enough and you have covered them with enough soak water. Soak for twelve to twenty-four hours (or overnight), changing the soaking water at least once during this time. Drain and rinse.

Place the chickpeas in a large pot on the stove and cover with boiling water or broth (make sure there is twice as much liquid to chickpeas). Return the liquid to a boil, then turn down the heat, cover and simmer for 1½ hours.

---

4 T. oats, ground and soaked overnight in lemon water

½ small onion, chopped

1 clove garlic, crushed

2 cups chickpeas, soaked and cooked

2 organic egg yolks

1 T. flaxseed, ground

½ t. cumin powder

½ t. coriander powder

½ t. Himalayan or sea salt

2 T. coconut oil

1 T. lemon juice, freshly squeezed

coconut oil for cooking

Drain the soaked oats from any excess water.

In a medium pan, heat 1 T. of the oil over a medium-high heat. Cook the onion and garlic for about 4 minutes, until the onion is soft and translucent. Let the it cool.

Add all the ingredients to a food processor or blender. Process until combined and as smooth as you would like it. It should have a moist, dough-like consistency. If it is too moist, add some extra ground flax seeds.

Spoon out 1-2 T. and use wet hands to form a round chickpea bite, and flatten to approximately ½ cm (¼") thickness.

Heat a little oil in a frying pan over medium-high heat. Add the chickpea bites and cook for approximately 5 minutes on each side, until lightly browned.

Cool to handling temperature and serve, on their own, or with some hummus or plain yoghurt.

The chickpea bites can be stored in the freezer for up to one month.

To reheat, place them in a warm oven until heated through.

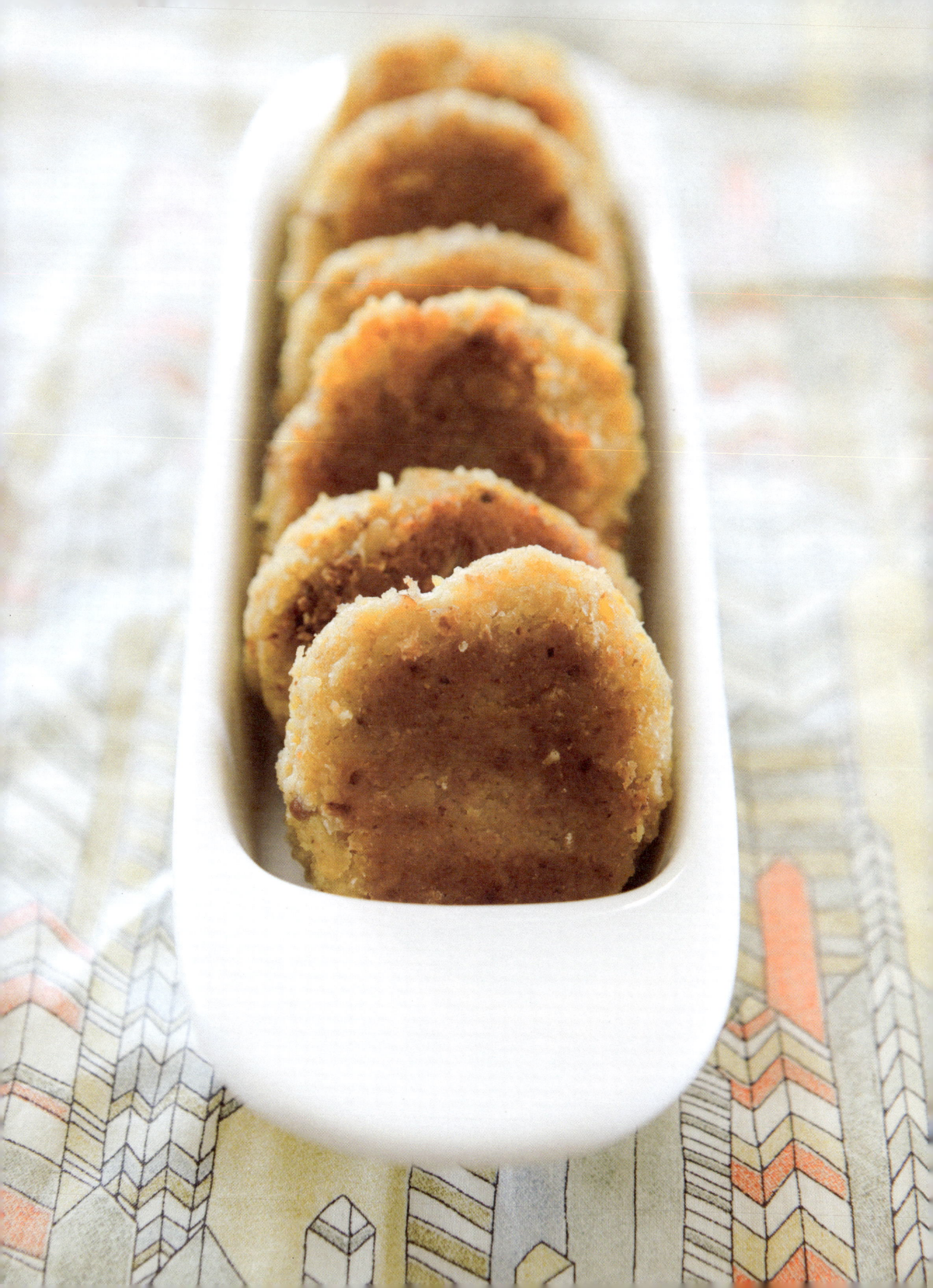

Recipes: Eating In Finger Foods

QUINOA BITES

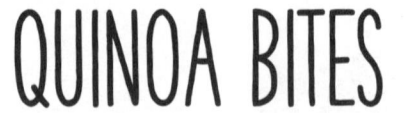

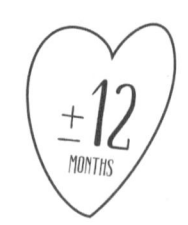

±12 MONTHS

vegetarian; for adults too; great for lunchboxes

Makes 12 (using a small muffin pan)

This is a great way to use up left over quinoa, and simple enough to cook from scratch.

Quinoa is a nutrient dense food - a complete protein and a valuable source of healthy fats, calcium, phosphorus, magnesium, vitamins E and B, fibre and iron.

Mila loves these and has been eating them since she was 12 months old.

To cook your quinoa:

Place ¾ cup quinoa in a bowl and cover with plenty warm filtered water. Add 1 T. apple cider vinegar. Cover with a dish towel and allow to soak overnight or for up to 24 hours. Strain the quinoa and rinse well. Place the quinoa in a pot with 1 cup water. Bring to the boil. Cover and simmer for 15 minutes or until all the liquid is absorbed. The quinoa grains get little 'tails' when cooked.

1 cup fresh spinach
2 cups soaked and cooked quinoa
2 organic eggs, beaten
¼ cup fresh parsley, finely chopped
½ cup hard goat's cheese, finely grated
1 t. paprika
pinch Himalayan or sea salt
pinch freshly ground black pepper

Preheat the oven to 180°C (350°F).

Grease a muffin pan with some coconut oil, ghee or butter.

Wilt the spinach leaves by placing them in a sieve and pouring boiling water over them. Chop finely.

Add all the ingredients to a large bowl and mix well.

Spoon the mixture into the prepared muffin pan and push down with the back of a spoon. These will not rise so fill the muffin pan to the height you would like your quinoa bite to be.

Place in the oven and bake for approximately 20 minutes until golden.

Allow to cool slightly, then place all the quinoa bites on a wire rack until cool enough to eat.

Serve as is or with your little one's favourite dip.

Leftover quinoa bites can be frozen for up to one month.

To reheat, place them in a warm oven until heated through.

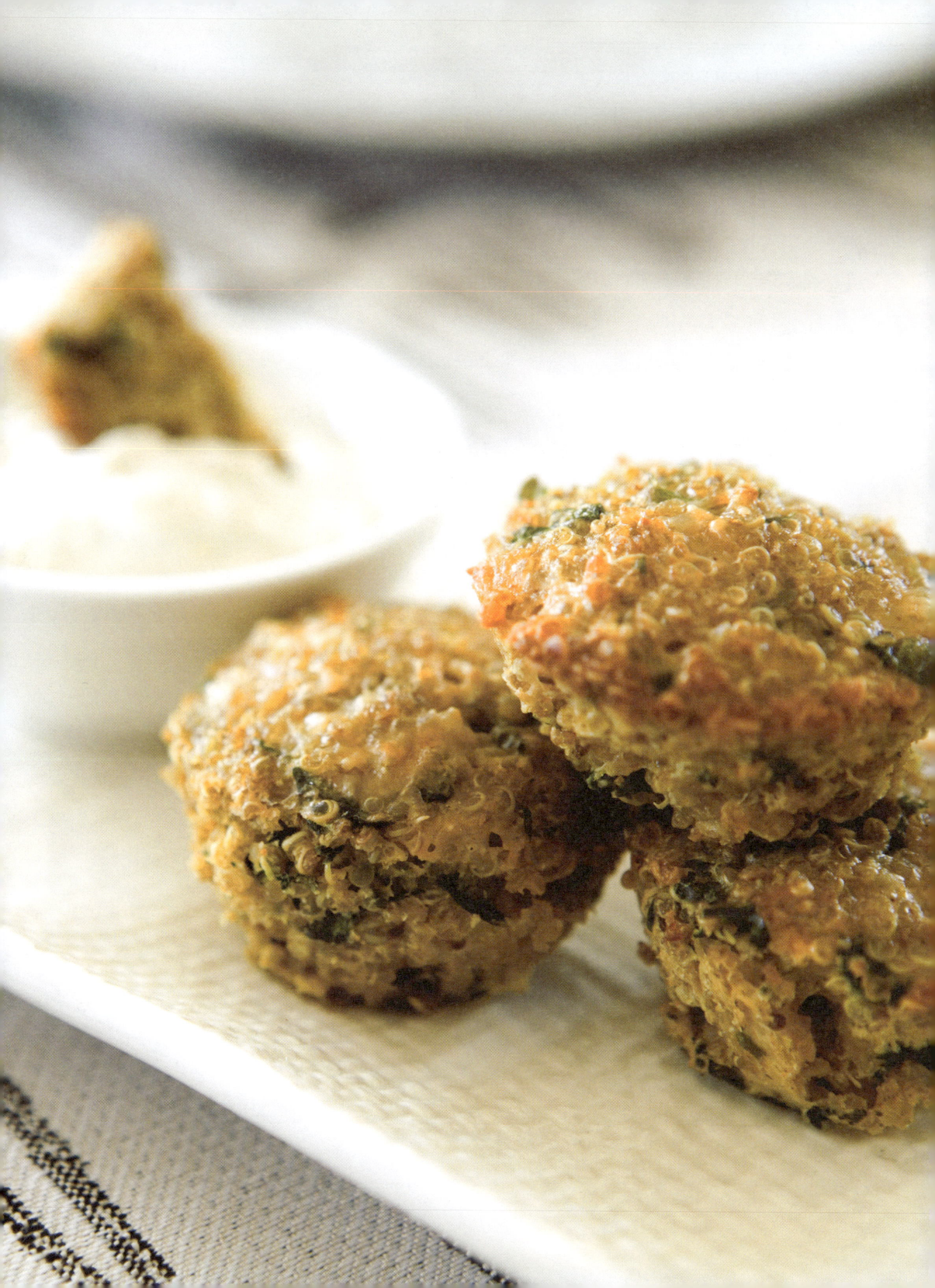

Recipes: Eating In Finger Foods

VEGGIE BITES

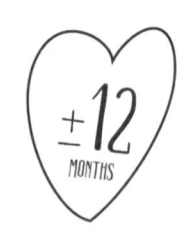

±12 MONTHS

vegetarian; for adults too; great for lunchboxes

• •

These veggie bites are rich in fibre, iron and protein.

To soak your lentils:

Cover the lentils with warm water and add an acid medium (whey, lemon juice or apple cider vinegar). The ratio of lentils to acid should be 2 tablespoon acid for every 2 cups of lentils. Soak for twelve to twenty-four hours (or overnight), then drain, rinse and cook.

• •

1 cup red lentils, soaked overnight
2 cups water or bone broth
pinch of curry powder
1 T. onion, chopped
¼ cup sweet potato, peeled and finely grated
¼ cup butternut, peeled and finely grated
1 T. celery, chopped
1 clove garlic, crushed
2 T. coconut oil
2 sundried tomatoes, soaked and puréed – or 2 T. Mila's Meals All Good Tomato Sauce
small pinch cayenne pepper
pinch Himalayan or sea salt
1 egg, beaten
4 T. tapioca flour
2 T. goat cheese *(optional)*

Preheat your oven to 190°C (375°F).

Rinse the lentils and place in a small saucepan.

Add the water or broth and curry powder and bring to the boil.

Reduce the heat and simmer for approximately 20 minutes (until the lentils are soft and mushy). Drain.

While the lentils are cooking add the onion, sweet potato, butternut, celery and garlic to a food processor and process until finely chopped.

Heat the coconut oil in a frying pan, add the processed ingredients and sauté until tender.

Add the puréed sundried tomatoes, cayenne pepper and salt and cook for another couple of minutes.

Add this mixture to the lentils and stir to combine. Allow to cool.

Once the lentil mixture is cool, add the beaten egg, tapioca flour and cheese (if using) and stir well.

Spoon the mixture into a greased baking tray and push down.

Place in the oven and bake for approximately 30 minutes (or until firm and cooked through).

Cut into squares and allow to cool to a safe eating temperature.

Serve as is or with your little one's favourite dip.

Leftover veggie bites can be frozen for up to one month.

To reheat, place them in a warm oven until heated through.

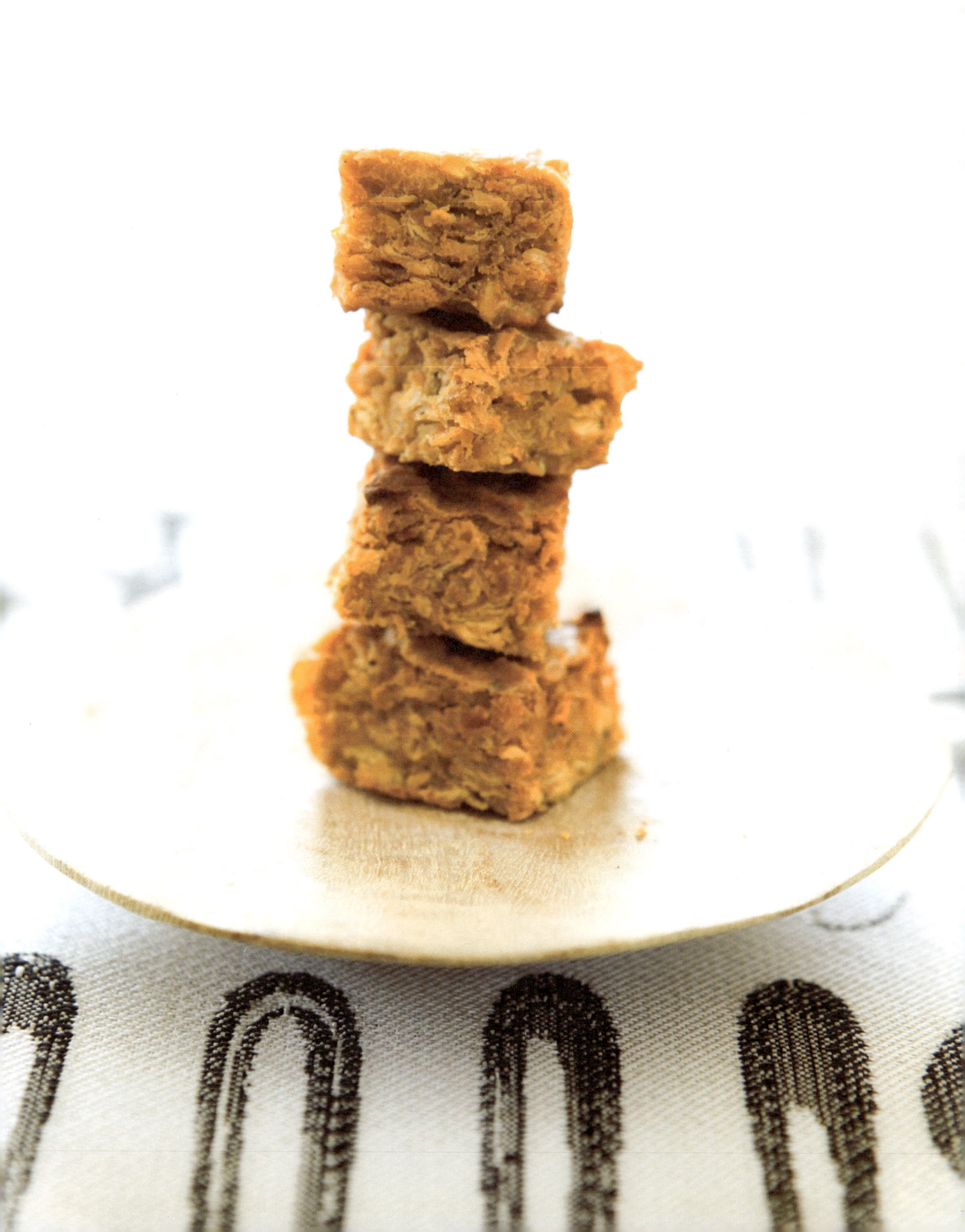

Recipes: Eating In Finger Foods

CHICKEN BALLS

10 MONTHS

egg-free; for adults too; great for lunchboxes

Makes 20 balls

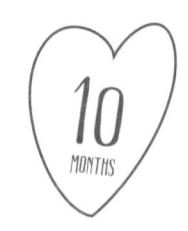

Mila has never been a very big meat eater but these have always gone down very well. This was, in fact, her very first introduction to meat. By the time I introduced meat to Mila she had entered her "I-will-not-eat-anything-off-a-spoon phase" – so these worked very well!

Chicken is an excellent first food for your little one - little did I know when I started feeing Mila! It is an excellent source of protein, vitamin B's, choline, selenium and iron.

1 T. onion, chopped
½ t. garlic, crushed
1 T. coconut oil, butter or ghee
110 g free-range or organic chicken breast or thigh meat, cut into chunks *(±2 chicken thighs)*
½ apple, peeled and grated
2 T. coconut flour
1 T. fresh parsley, chopped
2 T. goats cheese *(optional)*
pinch black pepper, freshly ground
pinch Himalayan or sea salt
3 cups Mila's Meals chicken stock

Sauté the onion and garlic in the coconut oil, butter or ghee.

Place the chicken, apple, breadcrumbs, parsley, onion, garlic, salt, pepper and cheese (if using) in a food processor and blend until smooth.

Place the chicken stock in a saucepan and bring to the boil.

While the stock is coming to a boil, take spoonful's of the chicken mixture and roll into bite-sized balls.

Using a slotted spoon, place a few chicken balls at a time into the boiling stock. Reduce to a simmer and poach for 5 minutes.

Remove the cooked balls and place them in a sieve to drain, then continue poaching the rest.

Allow to cool to a safe eating temperature, and serve. These are great as is, or with a tomato sauce dip.

The chicken balls can be frozen for up to 1 month. Take them out of the freezer in the morning and allow to defrost in the fridge for an easy addition to a lunch or dinner time meal.

They can be eaten cold, or reheated by placing in kettle boiled water for a couple of minutes.

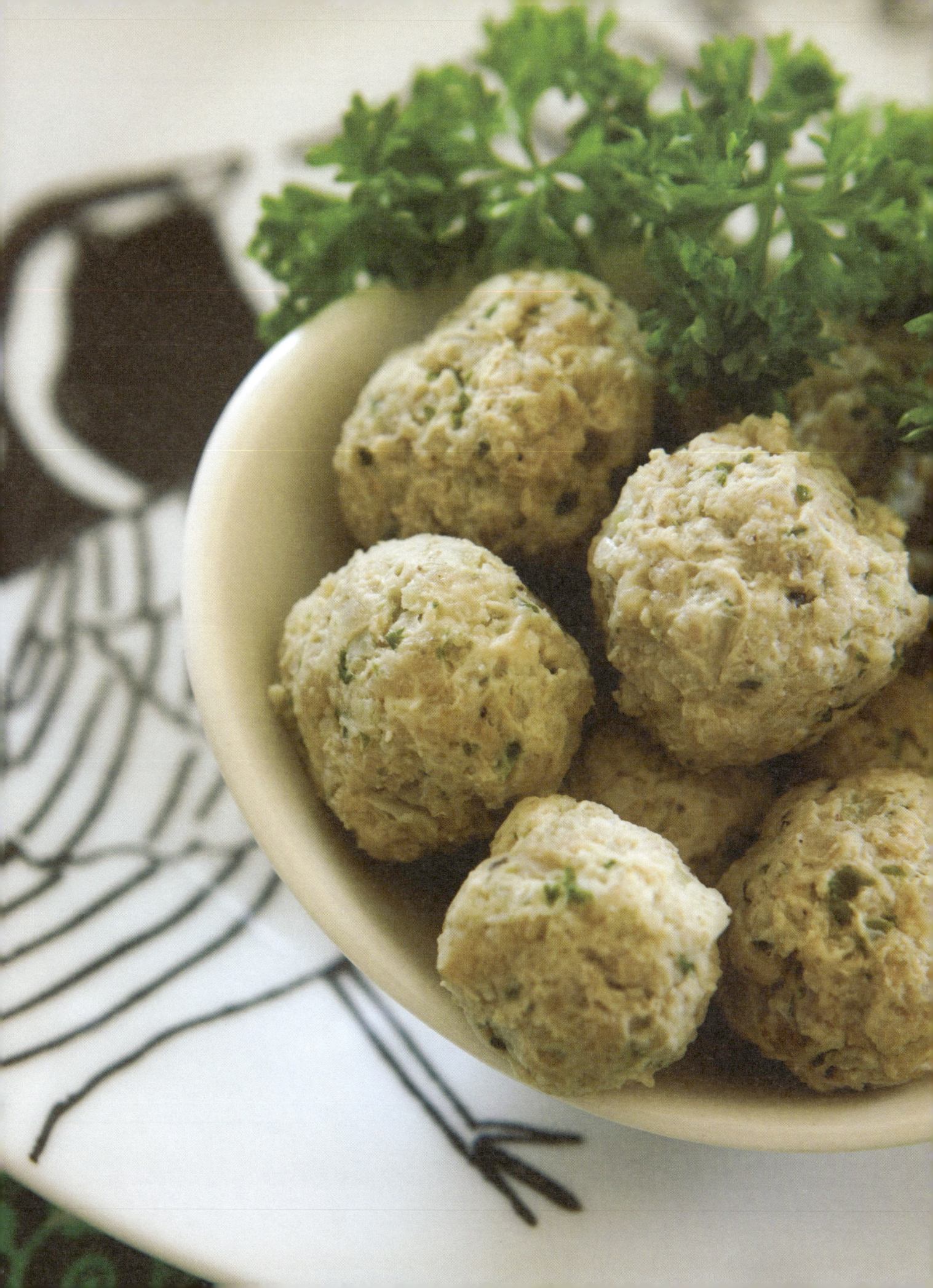

Recipes: Eating In Finger Foods

SWEET POTATO GNOCCHI

♡ 11 MONTHS

vegetarian; egg-free; for adults too; great for lunchboxes

Makes... a lot!

In the beginning of her food journey, Mila never really took to pasta. I tried the gluten free store-bought varieties a number of times but she refused to eat them (she obviously knew what I did not!). When she did eventually eat pasta, it made her constipated - so it immediately got taken off the menu. I found this frustrating as pasta can be such a quick and easy meal to prepare – and a great way to sneak the veggies in when you cover it with a homemade vegetable or tomato sauce. I then thought of gnocchi! Traditionally made from potatoes and wheat flour, I decided to create a sweet potato, gluten-free option instead.

Sweet potatoes are considered one of the healthiest vegetables. They are an excellent source of vitamin A (in the form of beta-carotene), which is essential for cell growth and good vision. Sweet potatoes are also a very good source of vitamin C, manganese, copper, fibre, niacin, and potassium.

• •

200 g sweet potato, peeled, cooked and cooled

1 egg

2 t. fresh sage, finely chopped

1 t. Himalayan or sea salt

½ t. ground black pepper

2 T. goat cheese, finely grated *(optional)*

¾ cup white rice flour

½ cup tapioca flour

¼ cup potato starch

Allow the sweet potato to come to room temperature *(either cool it down if it has just been cooked, or warm it up in the oven if you have kept it in the fridge).*

Peel the sweet potatoes, place in a large mixing bowl and mash.

Add the egg and stir to combine. Then add the sage, salt, pepper and goat cheese and stir again.

In a separate bowl mix your flours well. *(I find shaking them in a plastic bag works well too!)*

Add 1 cup of the mixed flour to the sweet potato mixture. Mash with a fork until it comes together and then knead with your hands. The dough should be slightly sticky – if it is too sticky add more flour until the correct consistency is reached.

Divide the dough into 4 equal balls. Roll each ball into a rope approximately 1cm (½") thick and cover with a slightly damp dish towel once rolled. Cut each rope into the gnocchi size of your choice and place on a baking tray lined with greaseproof paper. Cover the tray with a damp dish towel while you are preparing the rest of the gnocchi (to prevent the dough from drying out).

Bring a large saucepan of water or broth to the boil.

Add the gnocchi in small batches with a slotted spoon. It will sink to the bottom. After about 2 minutes you will see the gnocchi floating to the top. Wait another minute and then remove it with the slotted spoon. Continue adding gnocchi to the water until you have cooked as much as you need for this meal.

Serve warm with your little one's favourite sauce. Alternatively, quick-fry the gnocchi in some coconut oil, ghee or butter with additional sage.

The rest of the uncooked gnocchi can be frozen. Simply place the baking tray with the prepared gnocchi in the freezer. Once the gnocchi is frozen you can move it from the baking tray to a plastic freezer bag. There is no need to defrost the gnocchi before cooking – a perfect quick meal!

You can plan ahead for this meal to make the preparation quicker. The sweet potatoes need to be cooked and cooled – so roast them (and more) for dinner the night before you plan on making the gnocchi. Simply wash, pat dry, rub with coconut oil and roast at 180°C (350°F) for 1 hour. Keep them in the fridge until you need them.

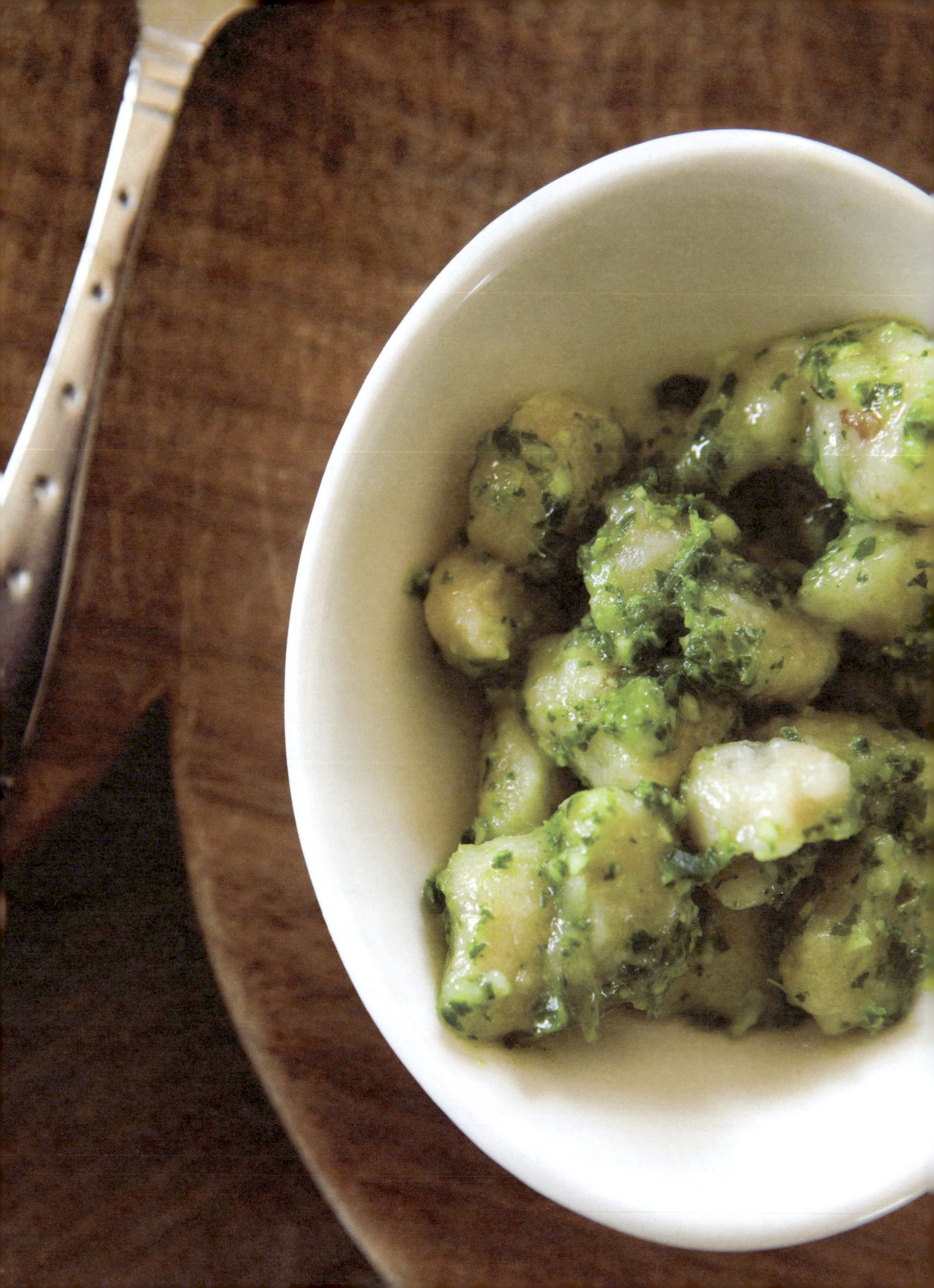

Recipes: Eating In Finger Foods

MOCK FISH FINGERS

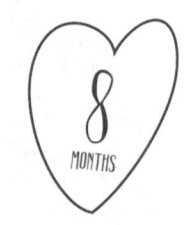

egg-free; grain-free; for adults too

Makes 6 toddler portions

8 months

These are not fish fingers in the conventional sense! I discovered, while cooking sole for myself, that the fish meat retains is shape really well when removed from the bone – making it an ideal finger food, and eliminating the need for a batter (which many other fish varieties require in order to hold their shape)! Another great benefit of using sole is that there is one easy-to-remove bone!

As well as being a complete protein, sole is a source of omega-3 fatty acids and useful amounts of vitamin B12 and potassium.

Fish is considered safe to introduce from 6 months old. Sole (and other white flesh fish) are considered some of the safest to introduce. They are the most easily digestible and lowest on the allergen list.

---

1 sole, cleaned
1 T. lemon juice, freshly squeezed
pinch of Himalayan or sea salt
pinch of black pepper, freshly ground
pinch of paprika
1 T. coconut oil, for frying

Heat the coconut oil in a frying pan over medium heat.

Place the sole in the frying pan and season with half the lemon juice, salt, pepper and paprika.

Flip over after 5 minutes and season with the rest of the seasoning.

After 5 minutes, check the fish is completely cooked by pulling some flesh away from the bone. It should be opaque all the way through and fall off the bone easily.

Pull the meat off the bone with a fork, being careful to retain its shape. Cut into finger size strips and serve.

Sole is, however, on the SASSI* orange list so it is best saved for a special occasion. You can use angelfish as an alternative as it has similar flat, thin fillets.

*The Southern African Sustainable Seafood Initiative (SASSI) was established to drive change in the local seafood industry by working with suppliers and sellers of seafood, as well as informing and inspiring consumers to make sustainable seafood choices. SASSI provides a few easy-to-use tools with seafood species categorised by a red, orange, green 'traffic light' system. For more information, visit: www.wwfsassi.co.za

The SASSI Consumer Guide

GREEN – BEST CHOICE
These are the most sustainable seafood choices, from the healthiest and most well-managed fish populations. These species can handle current fishing pressure or are farmed in a way that does not harm the ocean.

ORANGE – THINK TWICE
There are reasons for concern either because the species is depleted as a result of overfishing and cannot sustain current fishing pressure or because the fishing or farming method poses harm to the environment and/or the biology of the species makes it vulnerable to high fishing pressure.

RED – DON'T BUY
Red list species are either from unsustainable populations, have extreme environmental concerns, lack appropriate management or are illegal to buy or sell in SA. 'No sale' species are illegal to sell and are reserved for recreational fishers who require a valid fishing permit and must adhere to specific regulations.

GREEN
- Anchovy
- Angelfish
- Calamari/Squid (various species)
- Dorado (SA line caught)
- Gurnard (SA offshore trawl)
- Hake (SA trawl)
- Hottentot
- Kob (farmed in SA)
- King mackerel
- Queen mackerel
- Monk
- Mussels
- Oysters
- Rainbow trout (farmed in SA)
- Sardines (SA)
- Snoek (SA)
- Yellowfin tuna (SA pole caught)
- Yellowtail (SA)

ORANGE
- Cape dory
- Carpenter (SA line caught)
- Dorado (SA pelagic longline)
- East Coast spiny lobster
- Englishman
- Geelbek/Cape salmon (SA line caught)
- Hake (SA demersal longline)
- Kingklip
- Octopus
- Panga (SA line caught)
- Pangasius/Basa (farmed in Vietnam)
- Prawns (various species)
- Catface rockcod
- White-edge rockcod
- Yellowbelly rockcod
- Red roman
- Atlantic salmon (farmed in Norway)
- Santer
- Sole (East Coast)
- Swordfish (SA pelagic longline)
- Bigeye tuna (SA pelagic longline)
- West Coast rock lobster

RED
- Black musselcracker/Poenskop
- Dageraad
- Jacopever
- Kob (SA inshore trawl)
- Red stumpnose/Miss Lucy
- Scotsman
- Shortfin Mako shark (SA pelagic longline)
- Biscuit skate
- White stumpnose
- Bluefin tuna

ILLEGAL TO SELL IN SA (BELOW)
- **Baardman/Belman**
- **Blacktail/Dassie**
- **Brindle bass**
- **Bronze bream**
- **Cape stumpnose**
- **Galjoen**
- **Garrick**
- **King fish**
- **Natal knife jaw**
- **Natal stumpnose**
- **Natal wrasse**
- **Potato bass**
- **Red steenbras**
- **River snapper**
- **Seventy-four**
- **Spotted grunter**
- **West Coast steenbras**
- **White musselcracker**
- **White steenbras**

Recipes: Eating In Finger Foods

REAL FISH FINGERS

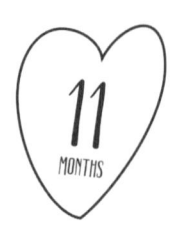

grain-free; for adults too

Makes 15

11 months

I created these especially for one of Mila's friends – CJ – who went through a 'Fish Finger Phase'. He had been used to the store bought variety, so it was important to me that these looked the same as those while tasting good (hence the turmeric in the coating)!

1 hake fillet (*approximately 350 g*)
1 organic egg
2 T. potato or tapioca flour
½ t. onion powder
pinch of Himalayan or sea salt
pinch of black pepper, freshly ground
pinch of paprika

For the coating
2 organic eggs, beaten
2 cups coconut flour or almond flour
1 t. turmeric (*to add a yellow colour*)
coconut oil, for frying

Place the fish, egg, flour, and seasoning in a food processor. Process until fairly smooth.

Line a baking tray with parchment paper.

Scoop the fish mixture into the baking tray and flatten with a spatula. Really squash it all together well.

Place the baking tray in the freezer for ½ hour for the mixture to set.

Cut the slightly frozen fish mixture into fish finger shapes.

Beat the 2 eggs and pour onto a plate.

Mix the turmeric into the coconut or almond flour. Pour the flour onto another plate.

Coat the fish fingers by first dipping them in the beaten egg, followed by the flour.

Heat the coconut oil in a frying pan over medium heat.

Place the fish fingers in the frying pan and cook for 5 minutes on each side.

Allow to cool and serve with Mila's Meals All Good Tomato Sauce

Left over fish fingers can be stored in the freezer for up to 1 month.

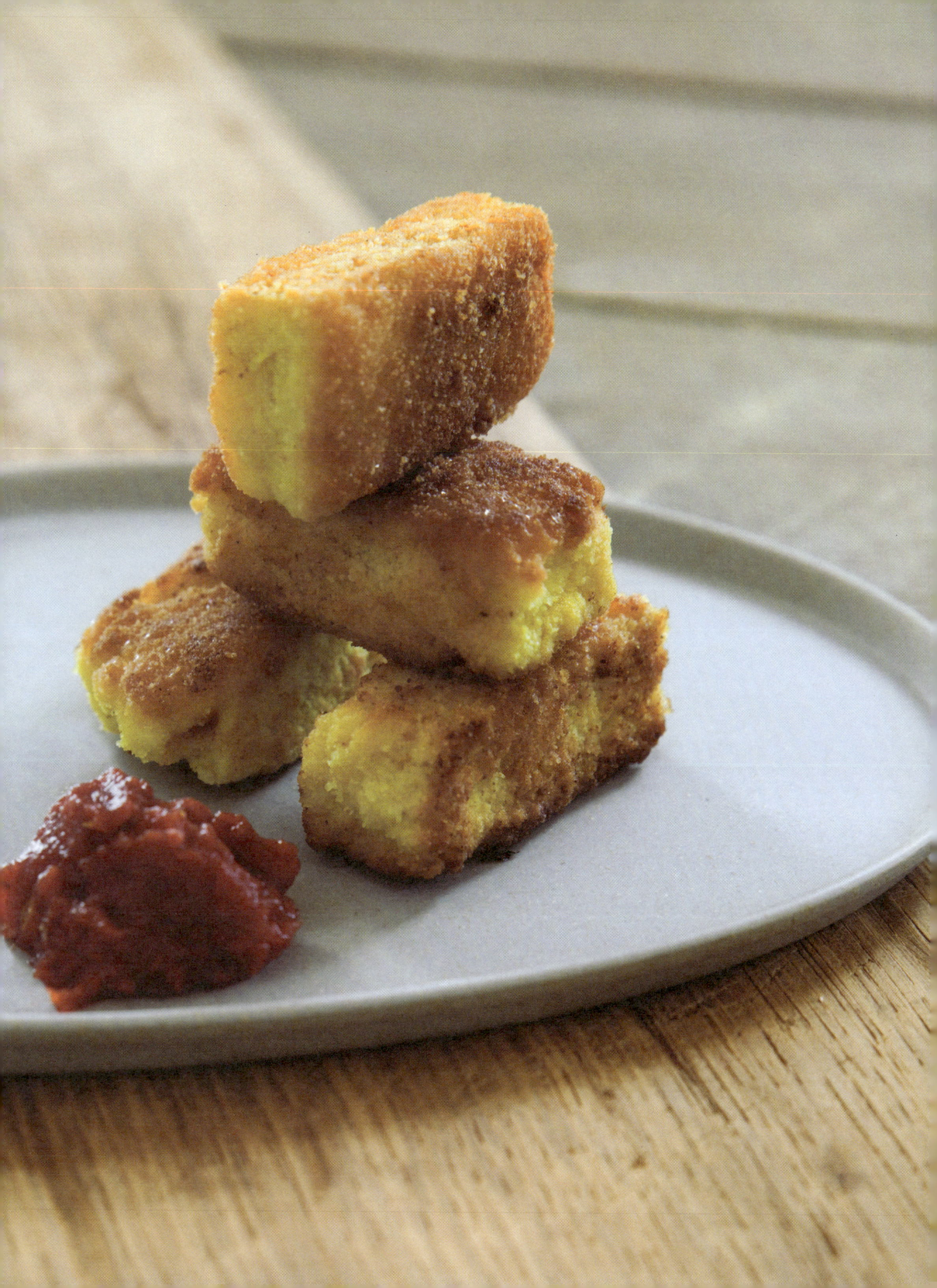

Recipes: Eating In Finger Foods

FISHCAKES

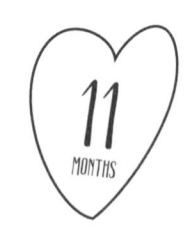

♡ 11 MONTHS

grain-free; for adults too

Makes 12 toddler sized fishcakes plus 2 adult sized ones.

• •

This is a great way to use leftover fish and sweet potatoes from your own dinner. Alternatively, pre-bake the fish and sweet potatoes to use in this recipe.

With all the added vegetables, this is a great all-in-one meal.

Hake is a lean fish of the same family as cod and haddock. It is an excellent source of high-quality protein, is rich in vitamin B and provides a generous amount of phosphorus, magnesium, zinc, selenium, iodine and iron.

Hake is an easy fish to prepare as it has few bones. It is on the SASSI* green list and one of the more affordable fish options.

* The Southern African Sustainable Seafood Initiative (SASSI) was established to drive change in the local seafood industry by working with suppliers and sellers of seafood, as well as informing and inspiring consumers to make sustainable seafood choices. SASSI provides a few easy-to-use tools with seafood species categorised by a red, orange, green 'traffic light' system. For more information, visit: www.wwfsassi.co.za

• •

2 spring onions, chopped or ¼ brown onion, chopped

half a garlic clove, crushed

1 T. coconut oil

1 carrot (50 g), peeled and finely grated

1 zucchini (50g), peeled and finely grated

2 T. parsley, chopped

1 T. lemon juice, freshly squeezed

250g firm fish (like hake), cooked and flaked or mashed

2 sweet potatoes (200 g), cooked, peeled and mashed

2 organic eggs, beaten

¼ t. paprika

¼ t. turmeric

salt and pepper

coconut oil for frying

Sauté the onion and garlic in coconut oil over medium heat for 5 minutes. Then transfer them to a large mixing bowl.

Add the rest of the ingredients and stir to combine.

Using a teaspoon, scoop some of the mixture into your hand. Roll into little balls and then flatten slightly to form the fish cake patty.

Heat some coconut oil in a frying pan over medium-high heat (just enough to lightly coat the bottom of the pan).

Cook the fish cakes for 3-4 minutes on each side, until golden.

Cool to a safe eating temperature and serve with your little one's favourite dip.

Left over fish cakes can be frozen for up to one month. Defrost in the fridge overnight. To reheat, simply place in a dry frying pan for a minute on each side.

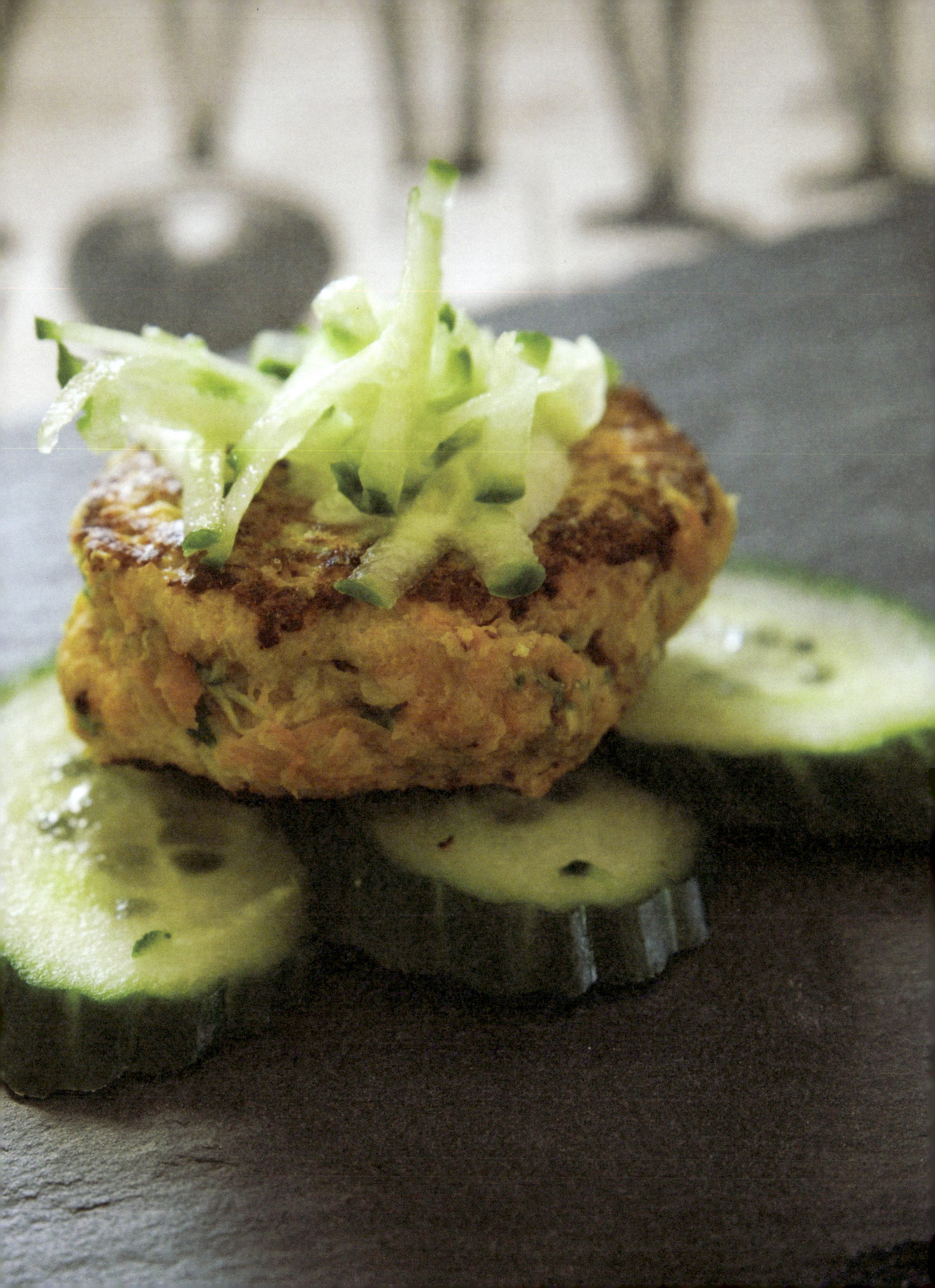

Recipes: Eating In Finger Foods

CHICKEN NUGGETS

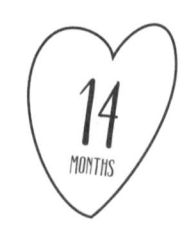

14 MONTHS

grain-free; for adults too; great for lunchboxes

Makes 10

• •

This is a far cry from the conventional store-bought or takeaway chicken nuggets! They are super easy to make and a much healthier alternative.

I usually make double this recipe and use the extra uncoated chicken in a chicken salad for myself.

Chicken is an excellent source of protein, vitamin B, folate, biotin, choline, selenium and iron.

• •

1 organic chicken breast
1 t. paprika
1 t. fresh ginger, finely grated
pinch of Himalayan or sea salt
pinch of black pepper, freshly ground
3 T. lemon juice, freshly squeezed
1 t. sesame oil

For the coating
2 organic eggs, beaten
2 cups coconut flour, desiccated coconut or almond flour
1 t. turmeric *(to add a yellow colour)*
coconut oil, for frying

Rinse the chicken breast and pat dry. Cut into slivers.

In a bowl, combine the spices and ginger with the lemon juice and sesame oil.

Place the chicken pieces in the bowl and massage the marinade into each piece.

Leave the chicken to marinate in the fridge for ½ hour (or overnight).

Beat the 2 eggs and pour onto a plate.

Mix the turmeric into the desiccated coconut or flour. Pour the flour onto another plate.

Coat the chicken pieces by first dipping them in the beaten egg, followed by the flour.

Heat the coconut oil in a frying pan over medium-high heat.

Fry the chicken for approximately 3-4 minutes on each side. Be careful not to over cook it as it will get tough. Cut through a piece to make sure the meat is not pink (undercooked).

Allow to cool to safe eating temperature then serve as is, or with a favourite dip. Kale chips or some steamed veggies make a great accompaniment.

Left over chicken nuggets can be kept in the fridge for 2 days. Alternatively, freeze them for up to a month and defrost as needed.

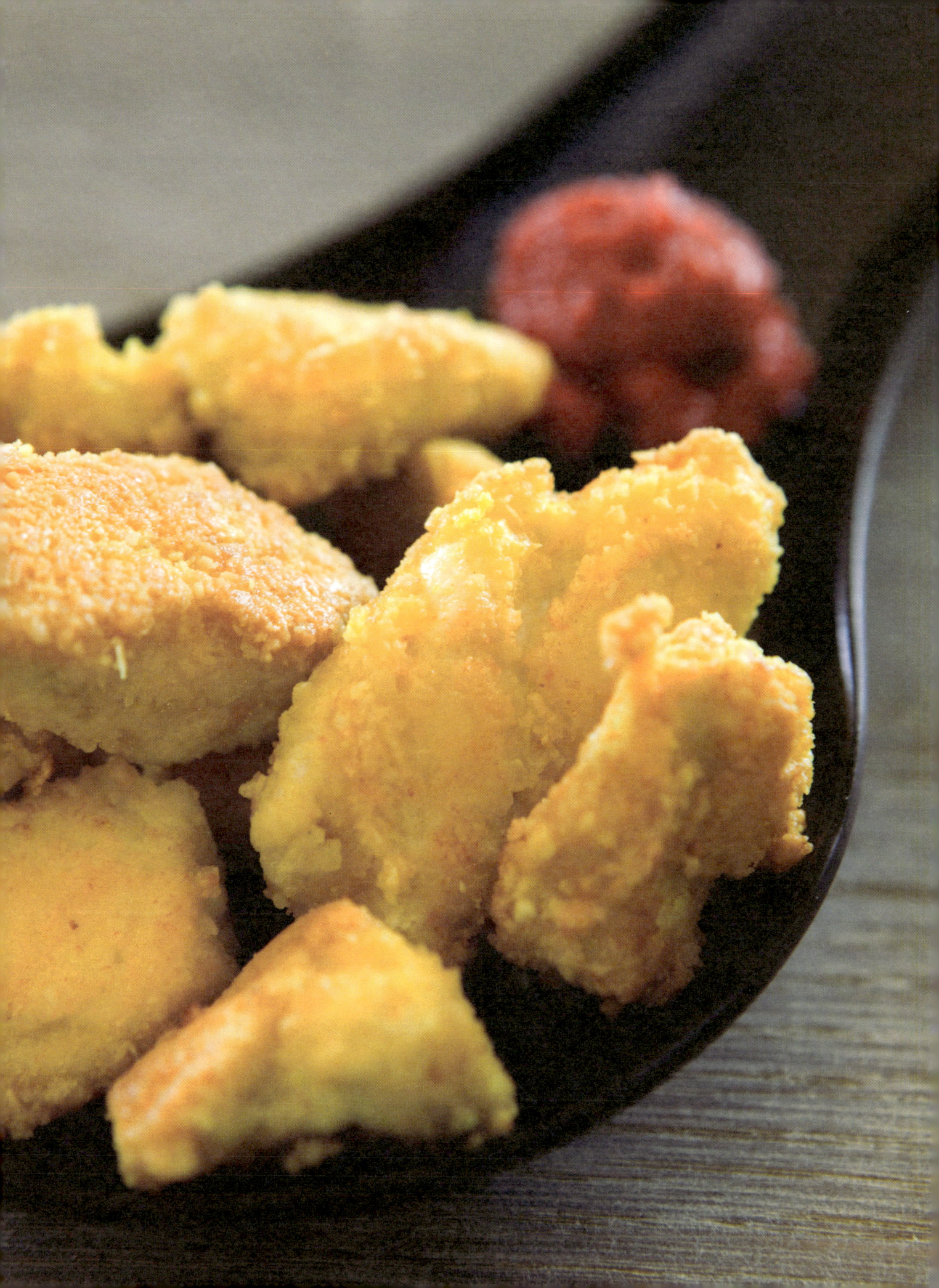

Recipes: Eating In Finger Foods

BUFFALO WINGS

16 MONTHS

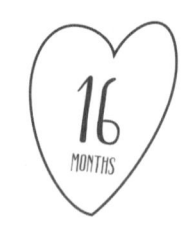

egg-free; grain-free; for adults too; great for lunchboxes
Makes 16

• •

Hot and spicy chicken wings are said to have originated in Buffalo, New York – hence the name Buffalo Wings. In Mila language they are simply called "bones" – but I did not think that would make a very tempting title for this recipe!

Obviously hot and spicy is generally not an option for our little ones – so this is a tame version.

These are a great little finger food – although I only give Mila the piece o the wing with the single thicker bone in it. The other half is for me!

Mila has been eating these since she was 16 months old.

• •

6 - 8 chicken wings
3 T. lemon, squeezed
1 t. paprika
1 T. raw honey
1 T. Mila's Meals All Good Tomato Sauce *(optional)*
pinch Himalayan or sea salt
pinch black pepper, ground

Preheat your oven to 180°C (350°F).

Prepare your chicken wings by separating into 3 parts (the drumstick, the flapper and the wing tip). I use a sharp pair of kitchen scissors for this.

The wing tip can be saved and used to make chicken stock.

Place the rest of the chicken wing parts into an oven dish that is large enough to hold all the chicken wings in a single layer.

In a mixing bowl, whisk together the lemon juice, paprika, honey, tomato sauce, salt and pepper.

Pour the marinade over the chicken pieces.

You can allow this to marinate in the fridge for a couple of hours or overnight, or go straight to cooking.

Place in the oven and bake for 20 minutes.

After 20 minutes, transfer the chicken wings to a plate, pour off the juices from the oven dish and then return the chicken wings - making sure you have flipped them over from the original side facing up. (It is important to pour out the cooking juices if you want the chicken wings to crisp up).

Cook for another 10 minutes until cooked through and lightly crispy.

Allow to cool to a safe eating temperature and serve.

Leftover wings can be stored in the fridge for 2 days, or frozen for 1 month.

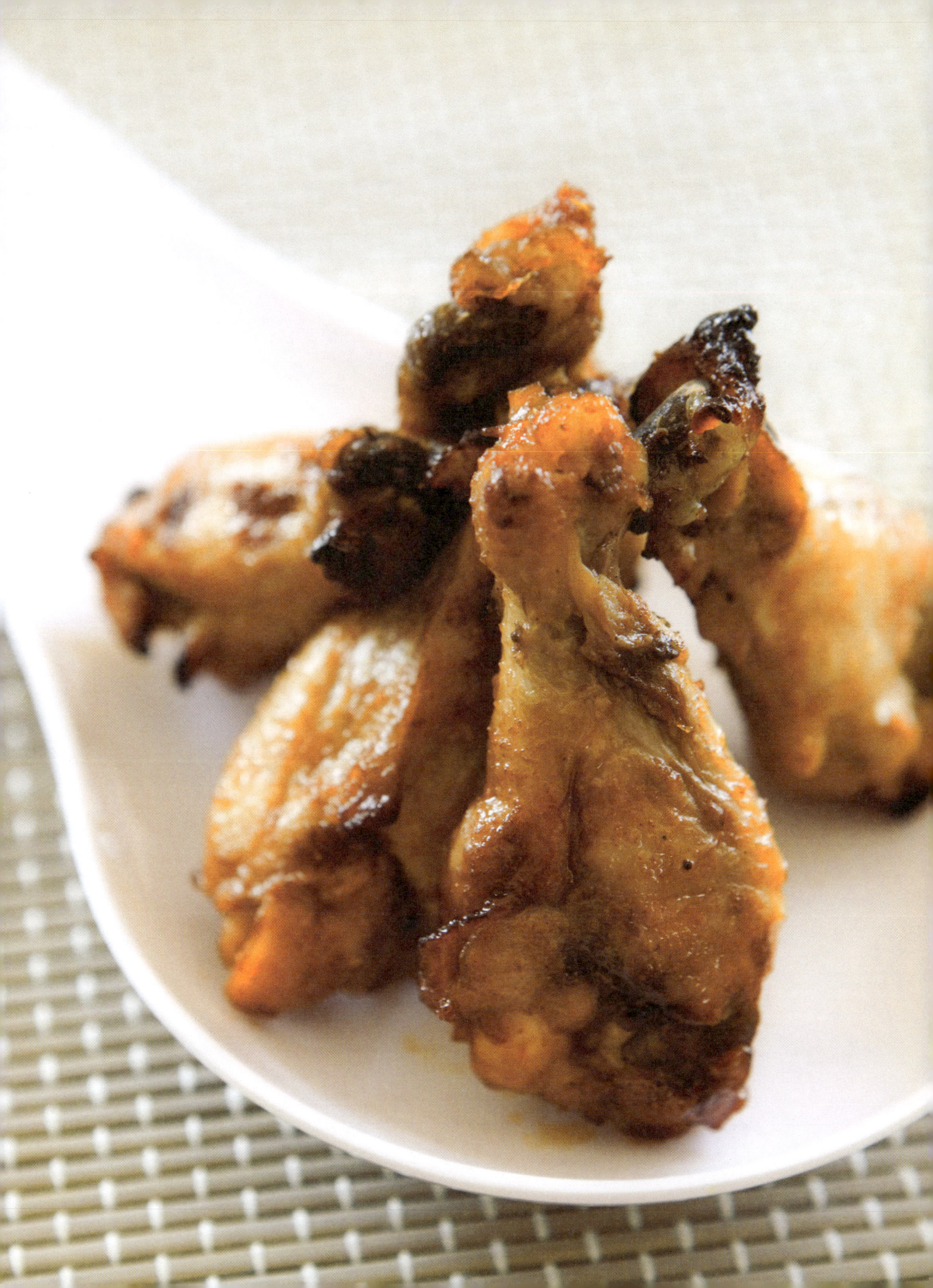

Recipes: Eating In Finger Foods

SWEET POTATO CHIPS

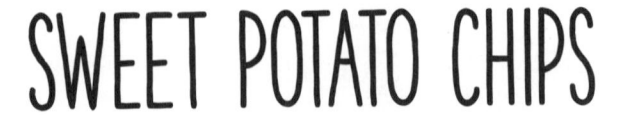

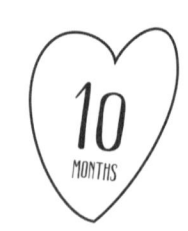

10 MONTHS

vegetarian; vegan; egg-free; grain-free; for adults too

Makes 3 toddler sized servings

I steam, then fry the sweet potatoes so as to minimise the time they spend soaking up the oil. Even though coconut oil is a healthy fat, is stable at high temperatures and helps the bio-availability of the beta carotene, I prefer most of the cooking to be done by steaming.

Sweet potatoes are considered one of the healthiest vegetables. They are an excellent source of vitamin A in the form of beta-carotene, which is essential for cell growth and good vision. They are also a very good source of vitamin C, manganese, copper, fibre, niacin, vitamin B5, and potassium.

1 sweet potato, peeled
coconut oil for frying

Left over steamed sweet potato can be kept in the fridge for 2 days and used for more chips when you need them. Alternatively, you can cut it into sticks and freeze until you want to make more chips. Place the sticks on a baking tray until frozen, then transfer them to a freezer bag (this way they will not stick together as they freeze). Thaw before frying.

Cooked chips can be stored in the fridge for 2 days and reheated as needed.

Variations:
- *Carrots and parsnips make delicious chips too!*

Fried:

Cut the sweet potato into discs approximately 1 cm (½") thick.

Steam for 10 minutes.

Allow to cool to safe handling temperature.

Heat ½ T. coconut oil in a frying pan.

Cut the sweet potato discs into sticks (traditional chip shapes).

Fry the sweet potato for a couple of minutes on each side until lightly brown.

Cool to a safe eating temperature and serve.

These are great as is, or served with any of your little one's dips.

Roasted:

(This is my preferred way to cook them – hands-free, quick and easy!)

Preheat the oven to 200°C (400°F).

Cut the sweet potato into 'fingers' or discs.

Play them in a roasting tray and rub with approximately 2 T. of coconut oil.

Place in the oven and cook for 20 minutes, turning half way through

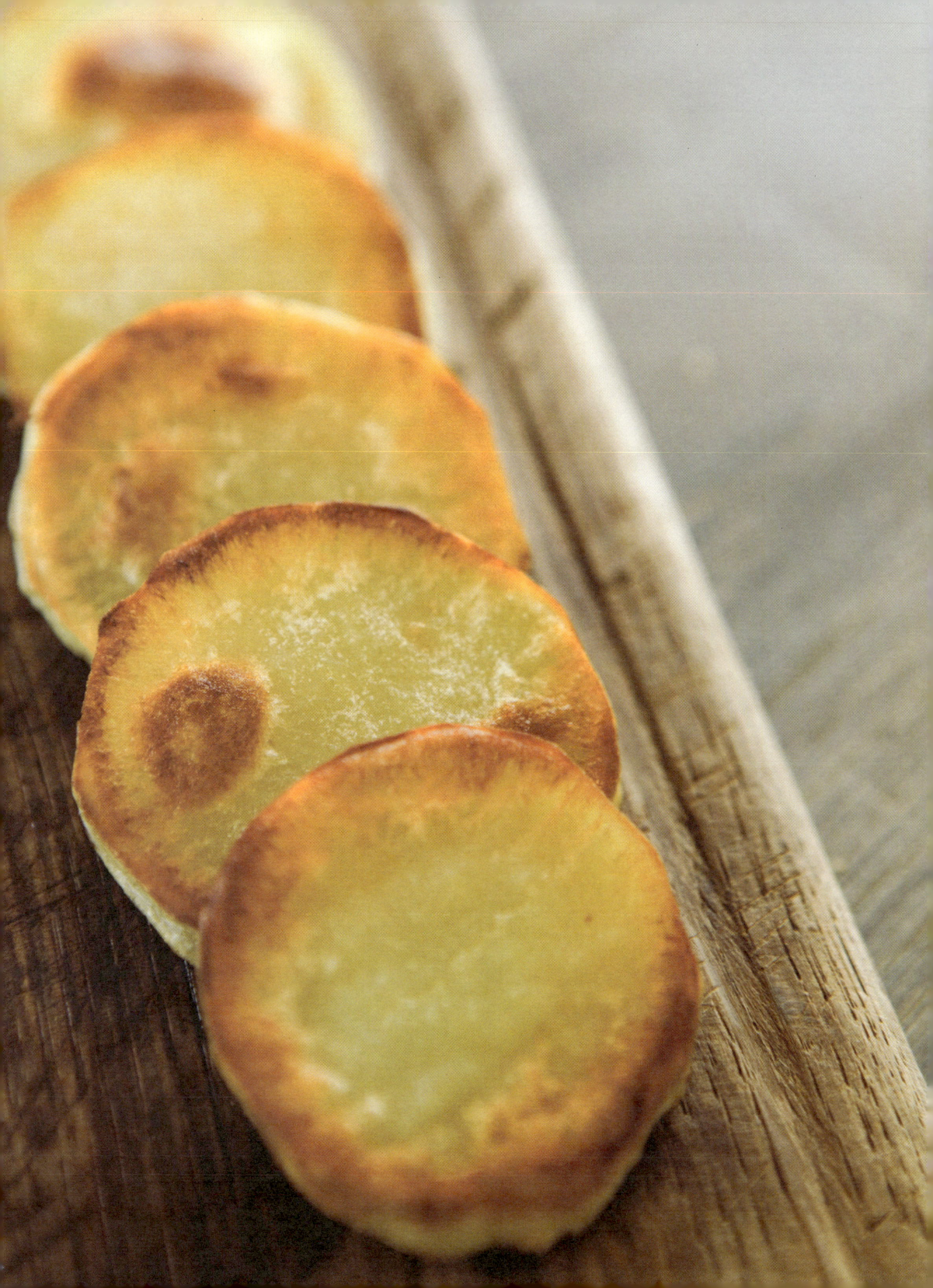

Recipes: Eating In Finger Foods

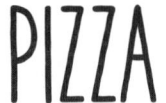

PIZZA

16 MONTHS

vegetarian; egg-free; for adults too

Makes 3 little pizza bases plus 2 adult sized ones

I would suggest saving this meal for special occasions, as I believe melted cheese on top of refined flours is not good for a little one's digestive system. Having said that, Mila did eat pizza every night for a couple of months! Yes, she went through a 'pizza phase'. I soothed my conscience with the fact that her toppings of choice were baby marrows, spinach and olives – so even though she was eating refined flours and cheese, she was eating a large amount of vegetables (that still looked like vegetables)!

Since you can freeze the par-cooked bases, they really do make for a quick and easy meal. You do not even have to defrost them before adding toppings and baking again. It is very handy to have some in the freezer for days that run away with you or, when you are invited to friends for a pizza evening.

Although I usually prefer to make my own flour mix, I use a gluten-free flour premix here (since this is meant to be a quick and easy dinner).

- 2½ cups gluten-free flour mix
- 2 t. aluminium-free baking powder
- 1 t. baking soda
- 1 T. extra virgin olive oil
- 1 cup warm water
- coconut oil for greasing

Pizza topping suggestions:
Mila's Meals All Good Tomato Sauce, goat cheese, pineapple, artichokes, spinach, baby marrow, olives, oreganum, basil.

Preheat your oven to 200°C (400°F).

Lightly grease a baking tray with coconut oil.

Place all the dry ingredients in a mixing bowl and mix well.

Add the oil and the water and stir with a spoon until the dough comes together. It should not be sticky, but it should not be too dry (flaky or crumbly) either.

Knead the dough on a floured work surface for a couple of minutes.

Break the dough into the number of bases you want to make and roll into balls.

Roll the dough into round pizza bases with a rolling pin.

Place the bases on a baking tray, prick them several times with a fork and bake for ±8 minutes. Keep an eye on them – especially the little ones. They can go hard very quickly! You want a lightly pre-cooked pizza base – not a completely cooked one!

Take the bases out of the oven. Either cool and freeze them until you need to use them, or add the toppings of your choice and bake for another 10 minutes.

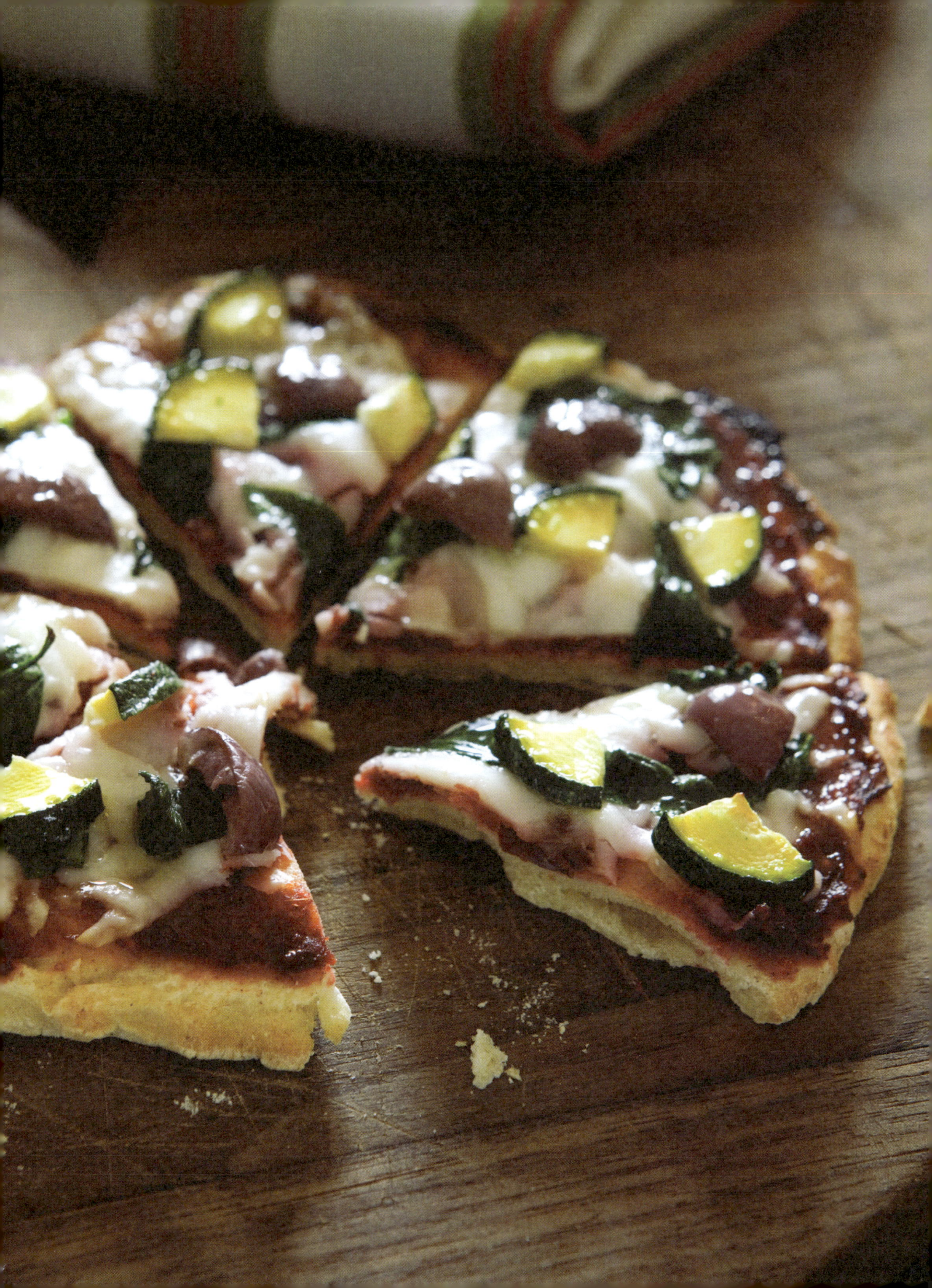

Recipes: Eating In Finger Foods

PESTO 'PANCAKE' (CRÊPE)

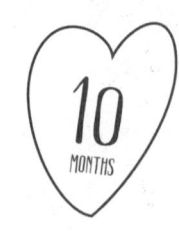

10 MONTHS

vegetarian; grain-free; for adults too

Makes 1 portion

• •

The name might be a little misleading on this one - only part of this that has anything to do with a pancake/crêpe is the final presentation! This is quite simply an egg cooked like you would a pancake and spread with some homemade pesto.

Mila ate these for dinner a few times a week for a couple of months! She is a 'phase-eater'- by that I mean she likes to eat the same thing everyday for a few months. Then, one day, she refuses it – and I have to scramble to find the next meal of choice! But with these being so very quick and easy to make, a great source of high quality protein and with some greens included, I was okay with giving them to her so often.

Eggs are a great source of protein, vitamins A, B's, D and E, choline, folate, selenium, iodine, omega-3 oils, Vitamin A, D and E.

The basil in the pesto is an excellent source of vitamin K and a very good source of iron, calcium, vitamins A and C, fibre, manganese, magnesium, and potassium.

The raw garlic in the pesto is a potent anti-inflammatory, anti-viral and anti-oxidant.

• •

1 free range or organic egg
pinch of turmeric
salt and pepper to taste
coconut oil for frying
1 t. Mila's Meals pesto

Crack the egg into a small bowl and beat it as if you were making scrambled eggs.

Add the turmeric, salt and pepper and beat again.

Melt some coconut oil in a medium sized frying pan (just enough to lightly coat the bottom of the pan).

Pour in the egg mixture and swirl over the bottom of the pan so than it spreads all over (like you would pancake/crêpe mixture).

Cook for a couple of minutes until the top of the egg pancake looks almost cooked.

Flip the egg over and cook for a minute on the second side.

Place the cooked egg on a plate and spread with the pesto.

Roll the egg pancake up and cut into bite size pieces.

Variations:
- *You can spread these 'pancakes' with a variety of different mixtures. We have tried hummus, guacamole, and veggie spread – but pesto is still Mila's favourite!*

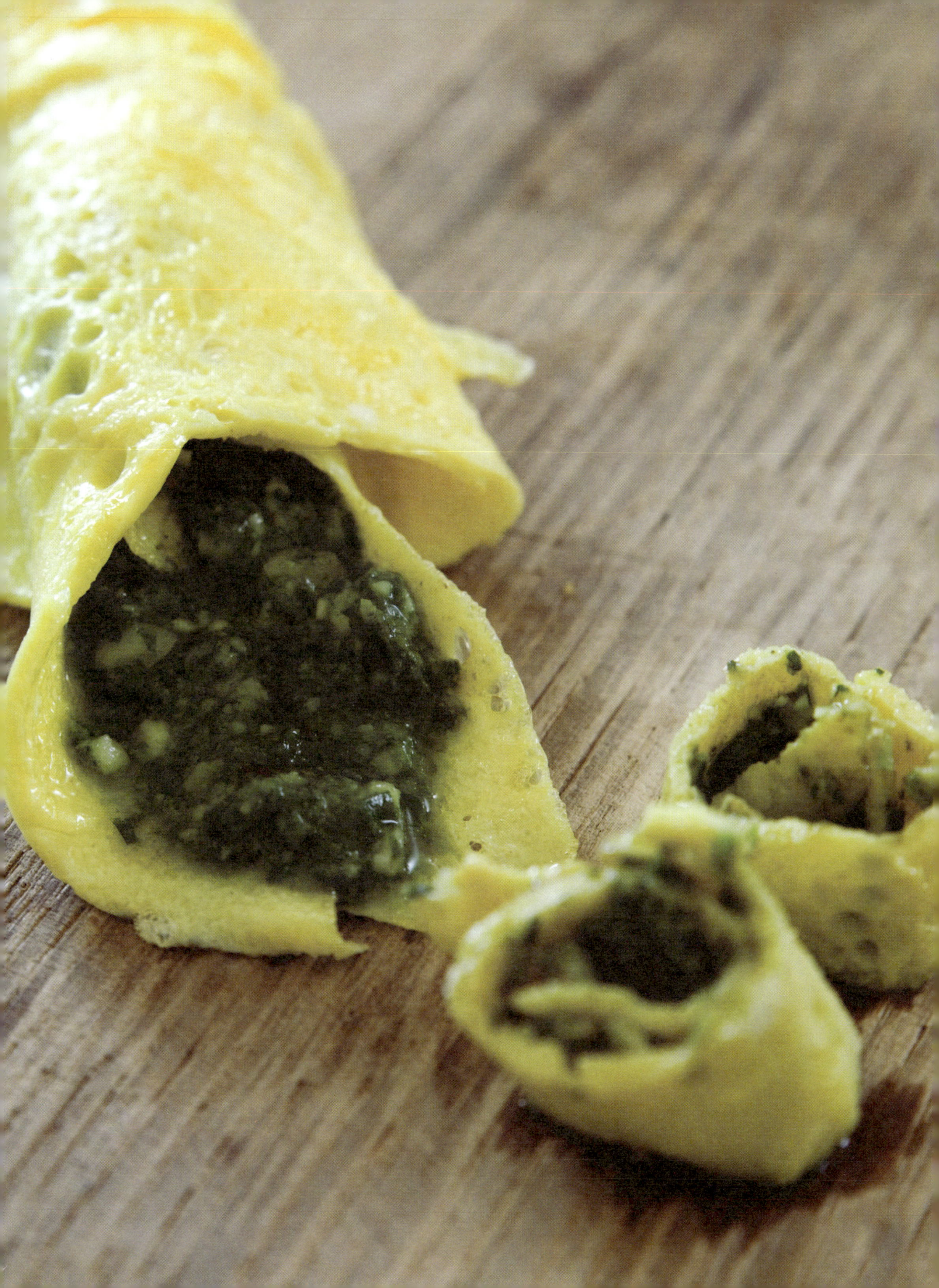

Recipes: Eating In Finger Foods

REAL PANCAKES (CRÊPES)

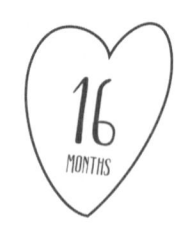

16 MONTHS

vegetarian; for adults too

Makes 25 toddler sized pancakes

These can be a great way to sneak in some vegetables! Fill them with any of the vegetable purées for a quick and easy dinner.

Alternatively turn them into a sweet treat by filling them with steamed apples sprinkled with cinnamon or spread them with honey, maple syrup, jam or Mila's Meals chocolate spread for a really decadent treat!

- 1 cup white rice flour
- ½ cup potato starch
- ¼ cup tapioca flour
- ¼ teaspoon Himalayan or sea salt
- 3 organic eggs, at room temperature, beaten
- 1½ cups goat's milk, or coconut milk
- 2 T. coconut oil, melted
- extra coconut oil for frying

Place the dry ingredients in a large mixing bowl and whisk to combine well.

In a separate small bowl, beat together the eggs, coconut oil and milk.

Create a well in the centre of the dry ingredients and pour in the egg mixture.

Stir slowly from the centre of the bowl - letting the flour mixture fall into the egg mixture and stir until it is all well mixed in.

Cover the bowl and place in the fridge for a couple of hours (or overnight). Before using the batter, allow it to come to room temperature and whisk well.

Heat a non-stick frying pan over medium-high heat. Add just enough coconut oil to lightly coat the bottom of the pan.

Spoon about a ¼ cup of the batter into the centre of the pan. Swirl the pan to spread the mixture evenly across the bottom.

Cook until the bottom of the pancake is lightly golden brown (you will see the top side has set too). Flip the pancake and cook the second slide for another minute. Slide the pancake onto a warm plate and continue to cook the rest of the batter.

Leftover cooked pancakes can be frozen between sheets of parchment paper. Simply thaw and then reheat in a non-stick pan for a minute on each side.

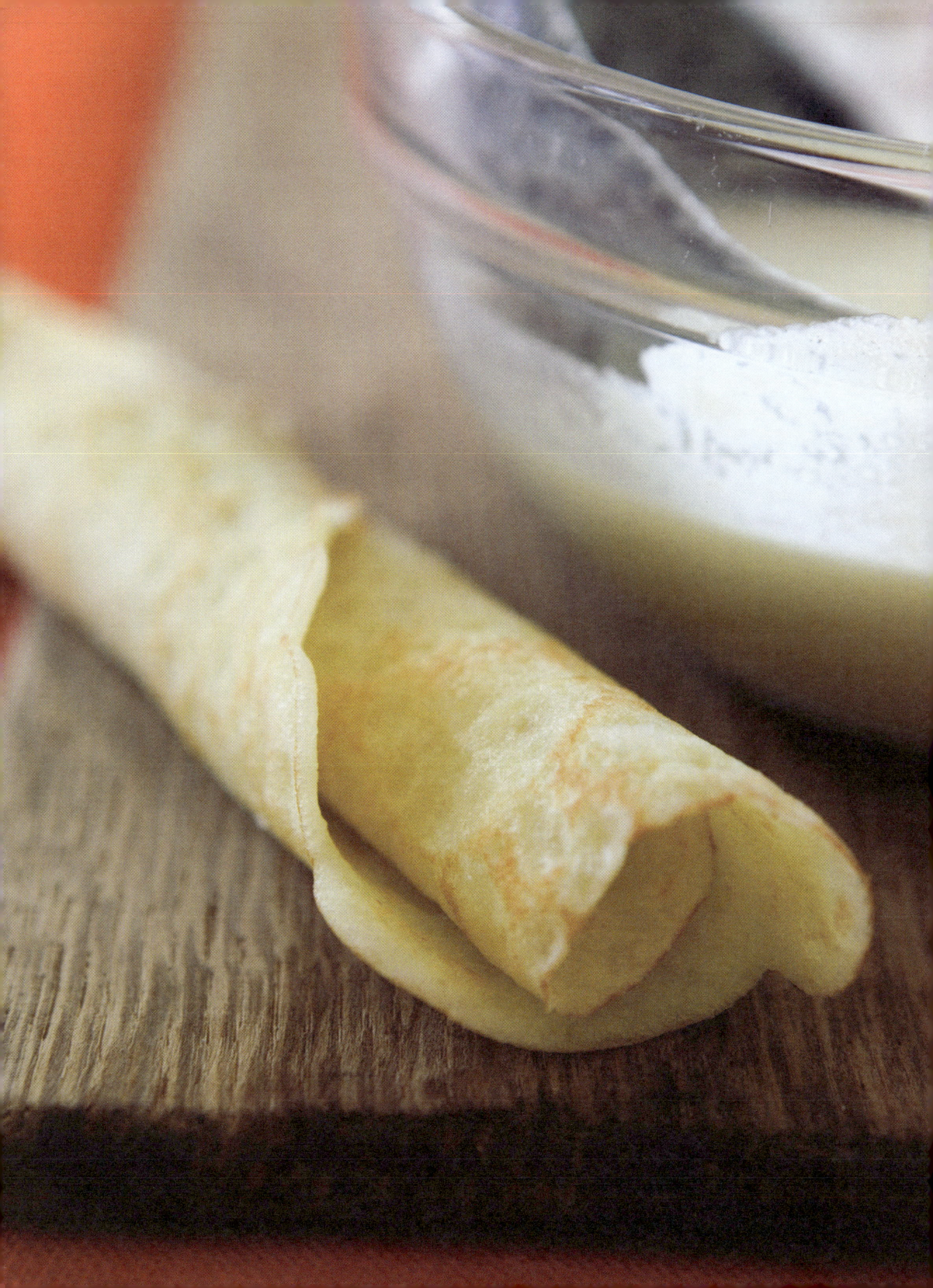

Recipes: Dip Dips & Spreads

Dip Dips are a great way to liven up steamed vegetables, as well as incorporating a variety of additional ingredients and nutrients. They also present an opportunity for a great amount of fun for your little one. Serve them in a little dish on a dinner plate; show him/her how to 'dip dip'; and, watch as they start experimenting with their food.

Mila is usually with me in the kitchen when I am cooking and more often than not she will eat the dips and spreads by the spoonful straight out of the food processor! I encourage this interaction – it is quality time for us, and it is the only way she willingly tries new foods.

The spreads have been a really useful way for me to include vegetables in Mila's diet as she is not too keen on eating hers straight off a plate. Blend them, spread them onto a 'toastie' or cracker – and ta da, she loves them!

All the dips and spreads can be frozen, so you can make a big batch, freeze in ice cube trays and defrost as needed.

Recipes: Dip Dips & Spreads

PESTO → 276
NO-DAIRY CHEESE SAUCE → 278
EGG-FREE MAYONNAISE → 280
ALL GOOD TOMATO SAUCE → 282
HUMMUS → 284
NUT BUTTER → 286
VEGGIE SPREAD → 288
CHICKEN LIVER PÂTÉ → 290
SNOEK PÂTÉ → 292
GUACAMOLE → 294
CHOCOLATE SPREAD → 296
CHOC-NUT SPREAD → 296
DATE JAM → 298
STRAWBERRY JAM → 300

Recipes: Dip Dips & Spreads

PESTO

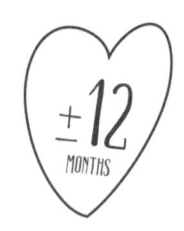

±12 MONTHS

raw; vegetarian, vegan, egg-free, grain-free, for adults too, great for lunchboxes

Makes ½ cup

• •

Mila only started eating pesto after she was 12 months old - I simply had not thought of giving it to her sooner!

Mila went through a 'pesto crazy phase'! She ate it on everything or just by the spoonful! This made for a very happy mama since it is an excellent source of vitamins A, C and K, iron, calcium, magnesium, and potassium. It is also an anti-bacterial and anti-inflammatory.

• •

3 cups fresh basil
1 cup parsley (optional)
½ clove garlic
½ cup almonds, activated or soaked overnight
1 T. lemon juice, freshly squeezed
½ cup extra virgin olive oil
½ t. Himalayan or sea salt

Place all the ingredients in a food processor and blend until well chopped and combined. You may need to add more olive oil.

Spoon into a glass jar, pour a thin layer of olive oil over the top to seal it and keep in the fridge.

Pesto also freezes really well so be sure to make a big batch before basil goes out of season! Freeze in ice cube trays so you can defrost a little cube as needed.

Pesto can be kept in the fridge for 1 week and in the freezer for up to 4 months.

Variations:
- If you would like to feed your little one pesto but would prefer not to use nuts, you can replace these with pumpkin or sunflower seeds.
- I would, ideally, like to use pine nuts in my pesto – but I just cannot justify the cost! You can replace the almonds with pine nuts.
- Pesto is traditionally made with parmesan. You could add ¼ nutritional yeast to this recipe for the cheesy-factor.

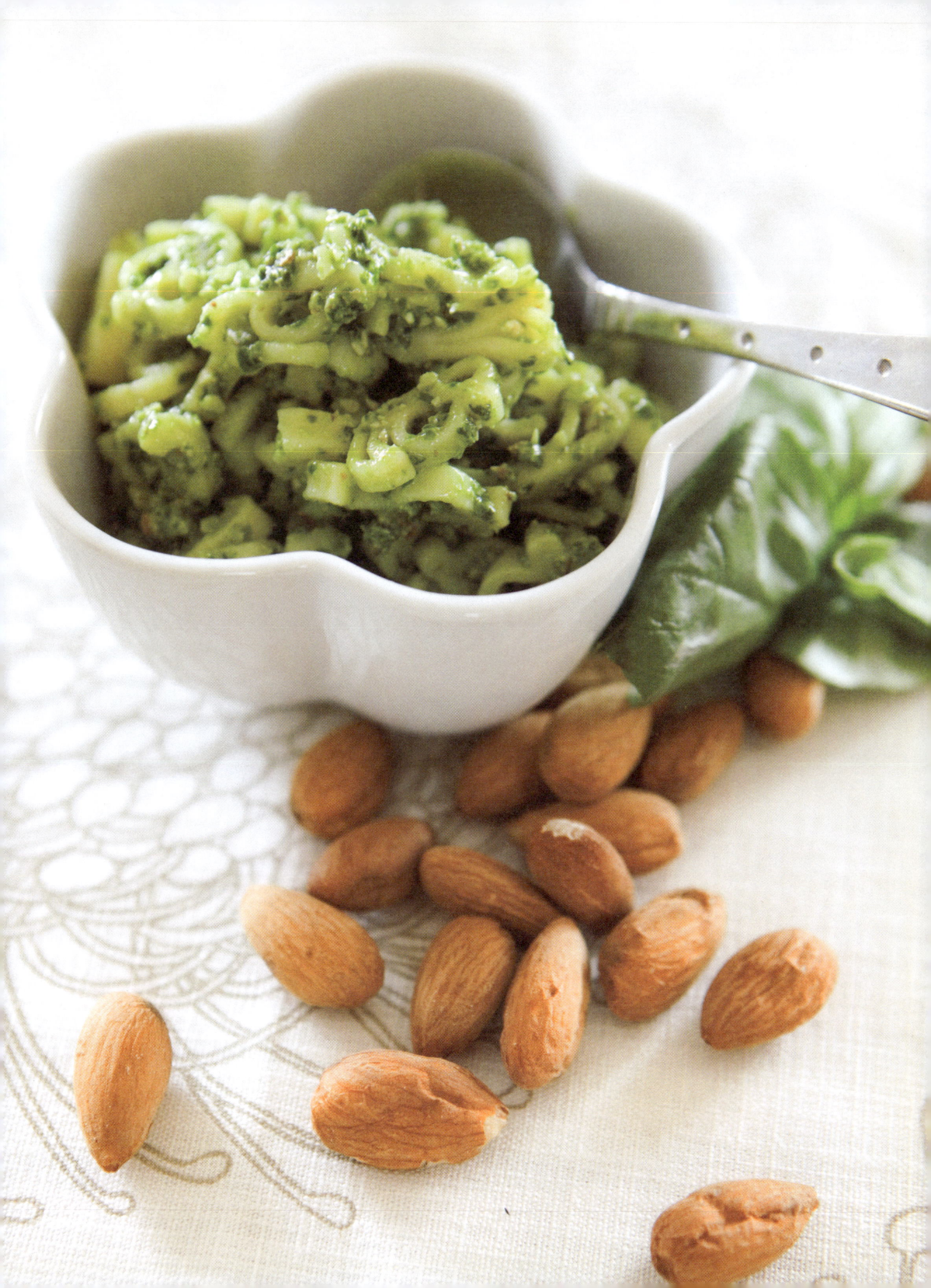

Recipes: Dip Dips & Spreads

NO-DAIRY CHEESE SAUCE

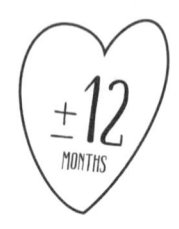

±12 MONTHS

raw; vegetarian; vegan; egg-free; grain-free; for adults too; great for lunchboxes

What would a child's life be without broccoli and cauliflower smothered in cheese sauce? This sauce will fool even the biggest dairy fan!

Nutritional yeast is a nutrient-dense food. It is a very good source of B-vitamins, folate, selenium, zinc, and it is a complete protein. It is gluten-, sugar- and preservative-free.

- **1 cup cashew nuts, soaked**
- **¾ cup warm water**
- **2 T. nutritional yeast**
- **1 T. lemon juice, freshly squeezed**
- **¼ t. Himalayan or sea salt**

Blend all the ingredients in a food processor until the sauce is smooth and warm.

Serve immediately drizzled over broccoli and cauliflower.

This can be stored in the fridge for a couple of days. It will thicken slightly. To thin, simply add some warm water and blend. Alternatively, spread it on some toast like you would cream cheese.

Left over cheese sauce can also be dehydrated until crispy – a great replacement for Parmesan cheese! It can be stored in a glass jar in your pantry.

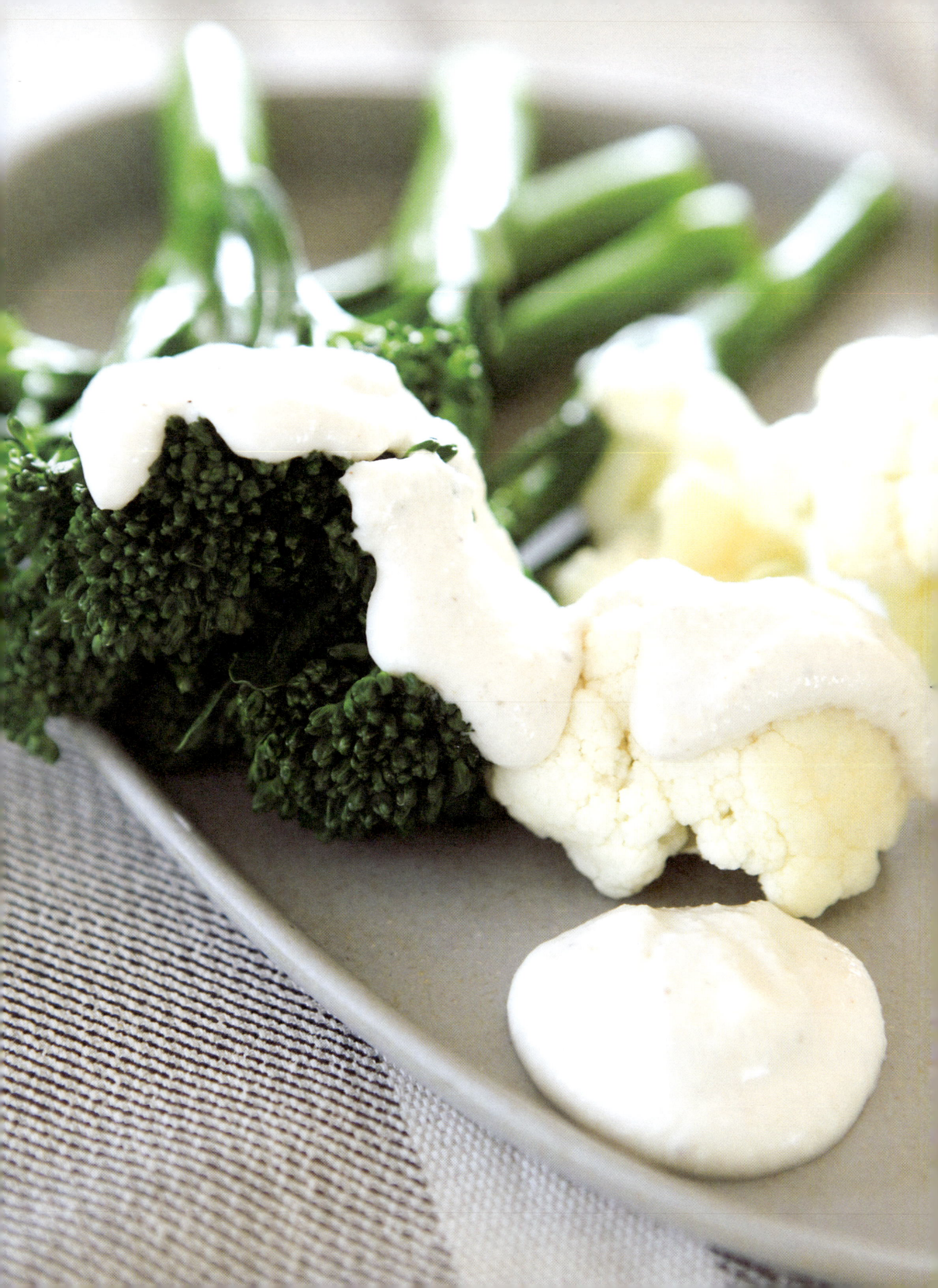

Recipes: Dip Dips & Spreads

EGG-FREE MAYONNAISE

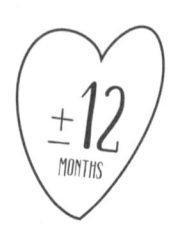

±12 MONTHS

raw; vegetarian; vegan; egg-free; grain-free; for adults too; great for lunchboxes

Makes 3 cups

• •

Conventional, store bought mayonnaise should be avoided at all costs - it is essentially a jar of rancid polyunsaturated fats blended with GMO's, sugar, preservatives and flavourants!

Homemade mayonnaise is not something I wanted to feed to Mila in her first year because of the raw eggs. Even if the chance of salmonella poisoning from fresh eggs is be small, it was still not a chance I was prepared to take. This egg-free mayo made a fantastic substitute.

It is also highly nutritious – a meal in its own right. Unlike conventional mayonnaise, which is simply used to flavour food. Egg-free mayo is a great source of protein and healthy fats.

• •

1 cup cashew nuts, soaked
¼ cup water
¼ cup apple cider vinegar
2 T. coconut oil, melted
1 T. raw honey
¼ t. mustard powder
¼ t. salt

Blend all the ingredients together in a food processor or blender until smooth.

Serve or store in the fridge in a glass jar for 4 days. It will thicken slightly. To thin, simply add some water and blend.

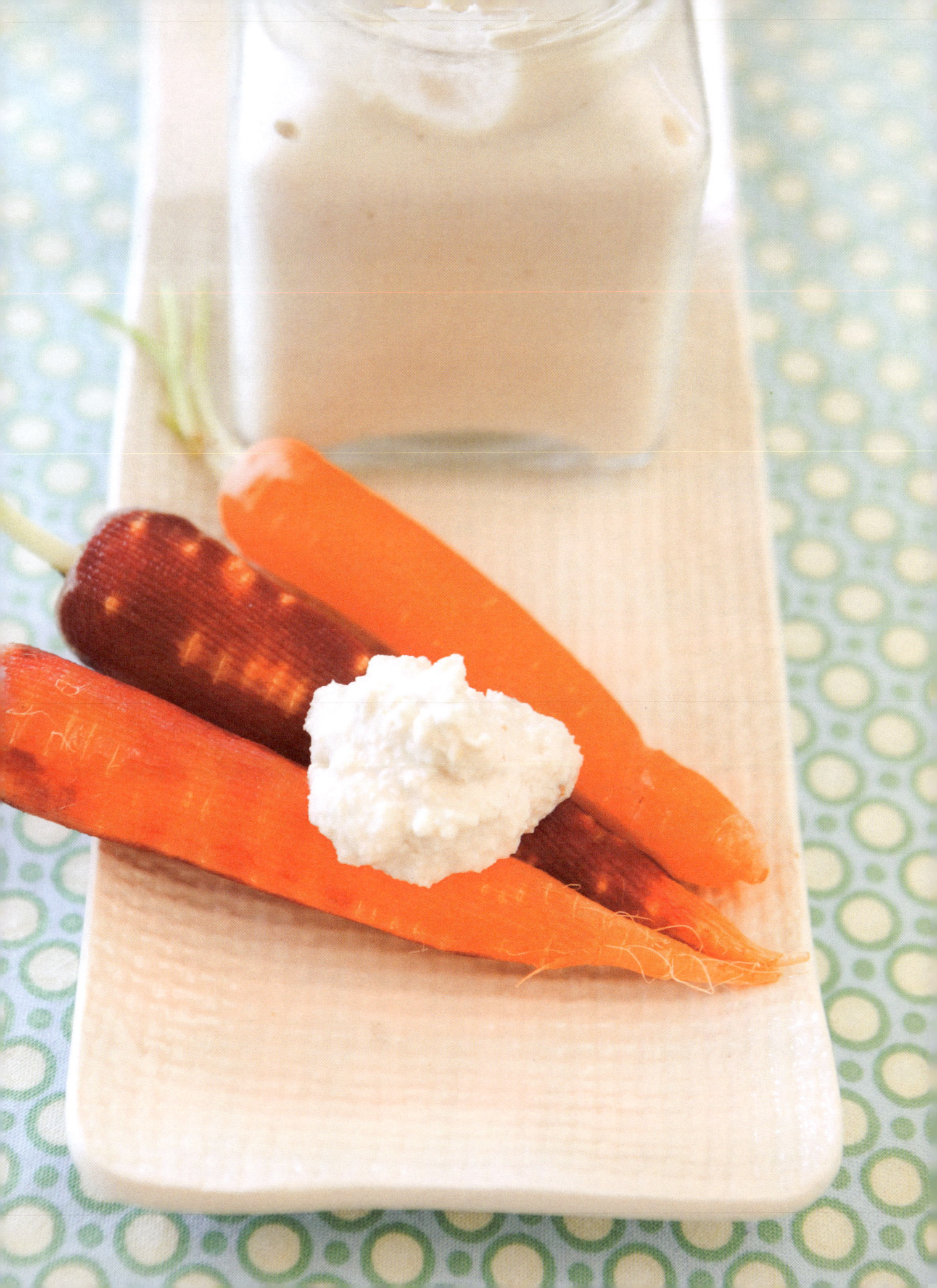

Recipes: Dip Dips & Spreads

ALL GOOD TOMATO SAUCE

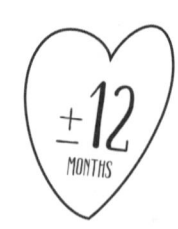

±12 MONTHS

vegetarian; vegan; egg-free; grain-free; for adults too; great for lunchboxes

Makes 250 ml (1 cup)

• •

"Tomato sauce is a good way to get some vegetables into your child's diet" is something I have heard quite often. Unfortunately, store-bought tomato sauces are extremely high in both salt and sugar (usually in the form of high fructose corn syrup from genetically modified corn). This recipe makes a delicious and nutritious alternative.

This tomato sauce makes a great dip, pasta or gnocchi sauce and an excellent tomato base for pizzas.

There is no hard and fast rule on when to introduce tomatoes to your little one. They are not allergenic per se but they can cause nappy rash and eczema flare-ups due to their high acidity. Mila ate her first tomato when she was 10 months old and she loved it – but she did get a nasty nappy rash – her first one ever! Mila has been enjoying this tomato sauce since she was 14 months old.

• •

1 cup sundried tomatoes, chopped and soaked hot water for 1 – 2 hours

2 dates, pitted and soaked

1 T. apple cider vinegar

¼ t. Himalayan or sea salt

3 T. carrot, finely grated (raw or lightly steamed)

2 T. beetroot, finely grated (raw or lightly steamed)

1 t. finely chopped basil OR oregano

½ clove garlic (optional)

¼ t. onion powder

Drain the sundried tomatoes reserving 1 tablespoon of the soak water.

Blend all the ingredients (including the reserved water) until smooth. Add more water if you need a thinner or smoother consistency.

Serve or store in a glass jar in the fridge. It will keep for a couple of weeks in the fridge.

You can also freeze it in ice cubes trays and defrost as and when you need it.

Alternatives:
- For a quick alternative, simply blend 1 cup soaked sundried tomatoes with 2 soaked dates and 1 T. apple cider vinegar.
- You can be more adventurous and hide even more veggies into this sauce! Try butternut, baby marrow and cauliflower.

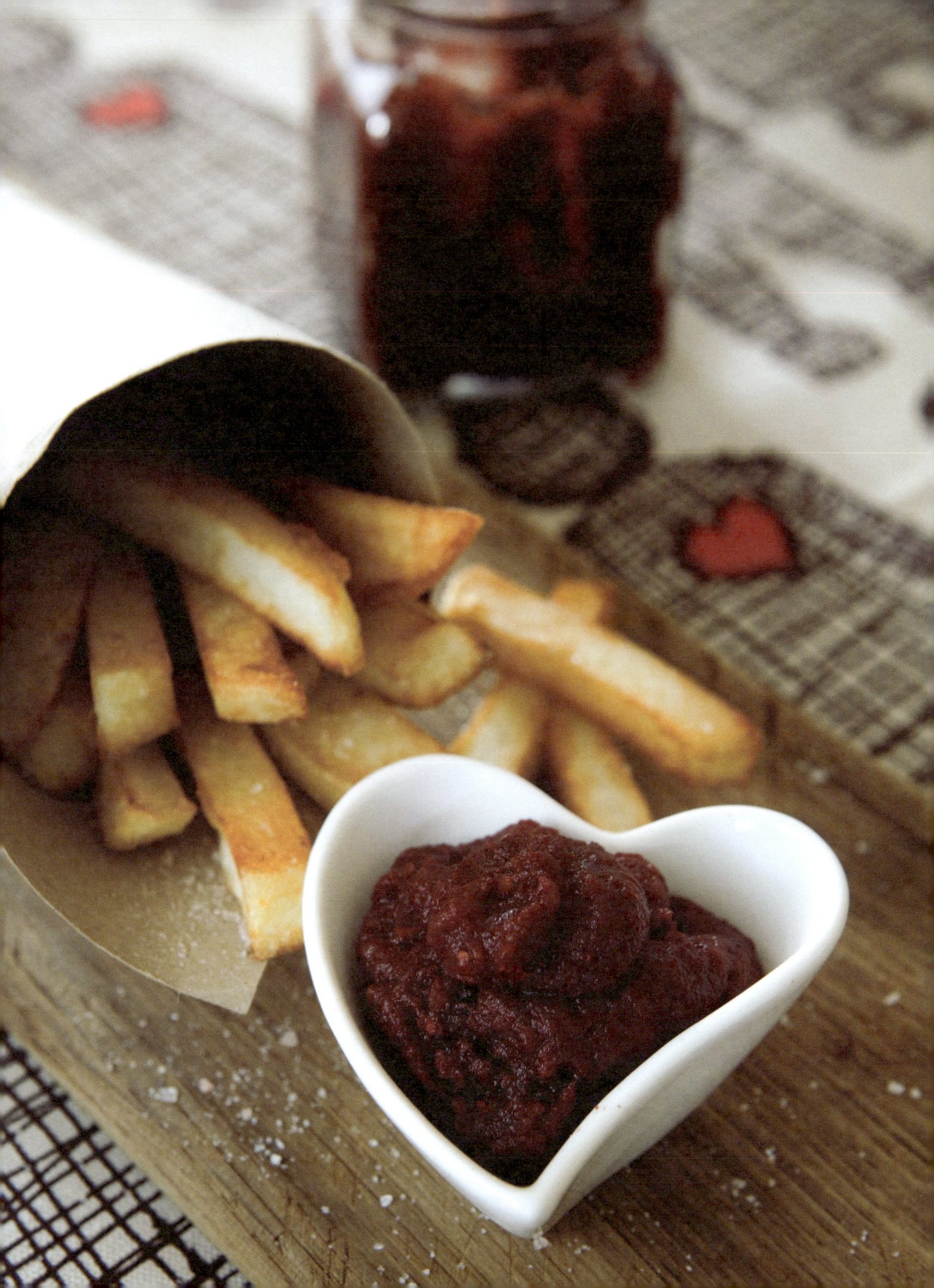

Recipes: Dip Dips & Spreads

HUMMUS

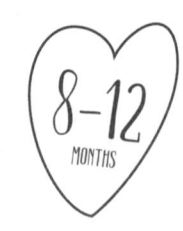

8–12 MONTHS

vegetarian; vegan; egg-free; for adults too; great for lunchboxes

Oh my goodness Mila eats a lot of hummus! She absolutely loves it, and I love the fact that she is eating a high protein food.

The rest of the ingredients have health benefits too. The tahini is also a good source of protein and is high in calcium. The garlic and lemon juice are antioxidants that improve immune function and ward off bacteria and viruses. With plenty of omega 3 fatty acids (necessary for your little one's brain development), iron, vitamin B6, manganese, copper, folate and amino acids, this is one dip you should regularly include on the menu.

Sesame (in the tahini) can cause a very strong allergic reaction in some people. I only introduced it to Mila after she was a year old. If you are nervous about sesame, omit the tahini from this recipe.

- 3 cups chickpeas, soaked and cooked
- 3 T. tahini *(omit if your baby is younger than a year)*
- juice of 2 lemons
- 4 T. extra virgin olive oil
- 1 clove garlic, crushed
- 2 T. cumin, ground
- 1 t. Himalayan or sea salt
- ¼ cup water

To prepare the dry chickpeas, cover 1 cup of chickpeas with warm water, add 1T. apple cider vinegar and allow to soak for 24 hours.

The beans will swell substantially so ensure you use a big enough bowl and that there is plenty of water covering them.

After soaking, rinse the chickpeas (do not use the soak water for cooking).

Place the chickpeas in a pot, cover with water, bring to the boil then simmer for 1½ hours.

Allow the chickpeas to cool, or run under cold water.

Place all the ingredients in a food processor and blend until smooth. You may need to slowly drizzle in more water as the processor is running to obtain the correct smooth consistency.

Hummus can be stored in a sealed container in the fridge for 3 days, or in the freezer for up to 6 months. It may be slightly dry after being frozen. Simply blend with extra water after defrosting.

Variations:
- I often add steamed butternut or sweet potato to Mila's hummus.
- Mila went through a phase where she would only eat green hummus! Simply add a couple of handfuls of fresh basil to the rest of the ingredients in the processor and blend until smooth.
- Beetroot is another great addition - for pink hummus!
- You can turn this into a raw recipe by using sprouted chickpeas instead of cooked.

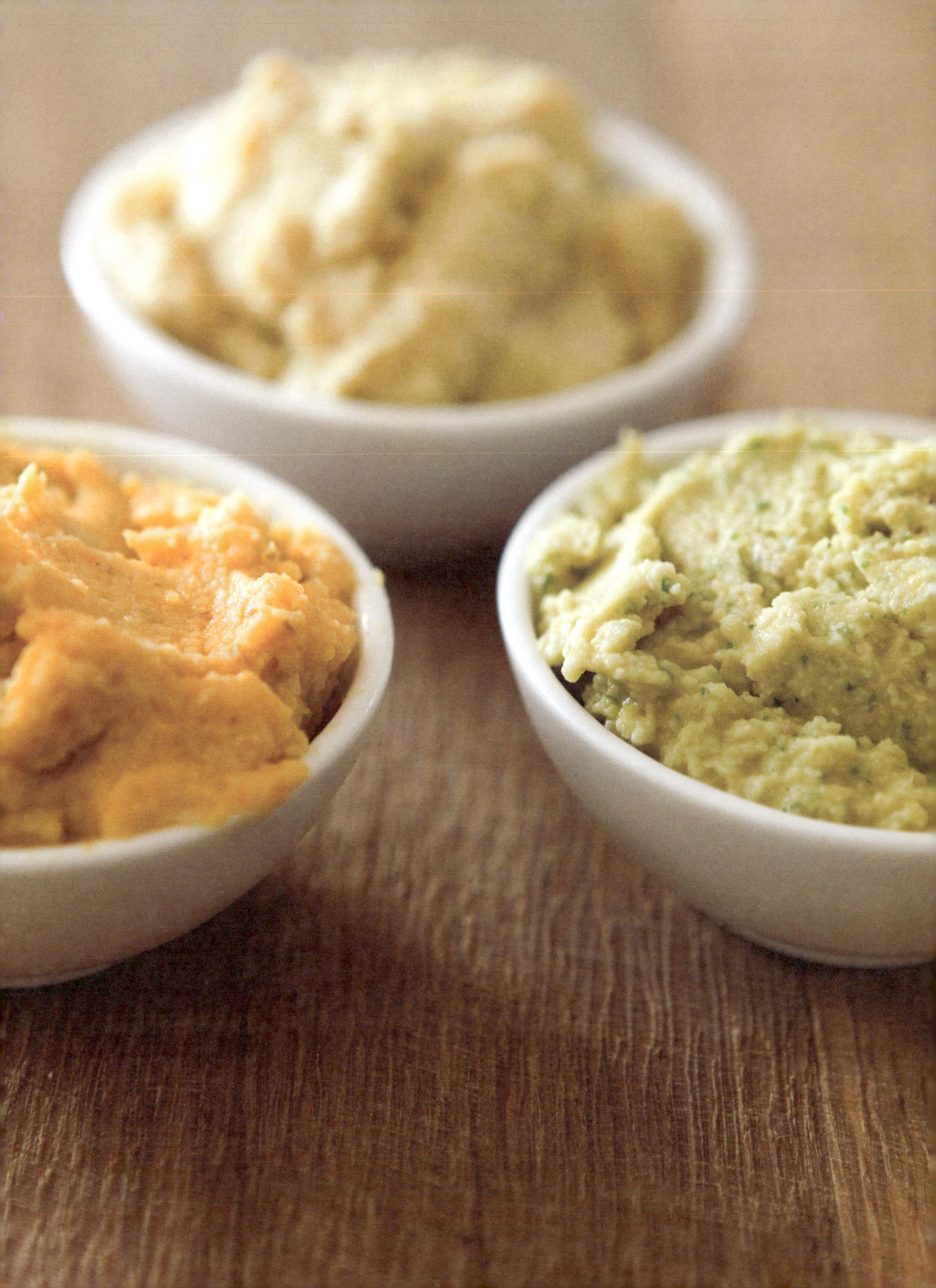

Recipes: Dip Dips & Spreads

NUT BUTTER

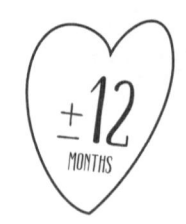

± 12 MONTHS

raw; vegetarian; vegan; egg-free; grain-free; for adults too; great for lunchboxes

Makes 1½ cups

···

You can use any nut to make this nut butter. I use almonds because they are the only nut, and one of the few proteins, that are alkaline forming. I also find they are the most cost effective.

I am happy that Mila loves this nut butter as almonds are a nutrient-dense food – high in protein, healthy fats, fibre, calcium, magnesium, potassium, vitamin E, manganese, copper, riboflavin (vitamin B2), and other antioxidants.

Please see the glossary pages for more information on almonds and how and why to activate them.

···

3 cups almonds (*or any other nut of your choice*)**, activated and dried**
A whole lot of patience!

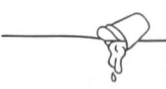

Alternatives:
- *You could also roast your nuts instead of dehydrating them to add a smokier flavour to your nut butter. Roast at 160°C (325°F) degrees for 15 minutes.*
- *Try adding some maple syrup, cinnamon, or vanilla.*
- *If your little one has a nut allergy, you can make a seed butter with sunflower or pumpkin seeds following this same method.*
- *Add some raw cacao powder and honey for a chocolate nut butter.*

Place the almonds in an oven preheated to 120°C (250°F) for 15 minutes, until they are warm to the touch.

Transfer them to a food processor fitted with an "S" blade.

Start the processor and let it run until the almond 'crumble' starts sticking to the sides of the bowl. Stop and scrape down the sides with a plastic spatula every time this happens, and continue processing.

Please do not be tempted to add any liquids to the almond butter as it is processing – this will greatly reduce the shelf life. It may look incredibly dry and crumbly now, but it will turn into smooth creamy butter eventually!

Depending on your processor you will notice a change in the consistency approximately 10 – 15 minutes after you started processing. The almond 'crumble' will start sticking together and move around the bowl in a large clump as the oils are being released. Your processor motor may also start getting a bit warm. If you are worried about burning out your machine, let it rest until cool and then continue.

After approximately 20 – 30 minutes of processing you will have grainy looking nut butter. Continue for a few minutes more until the butter is smooth and creamy.

Place the nut butter in a glass jar and store in the fridge for up to 2 weeks.

This is delicious served on warm toast or as a dip for apples and other fruits.

Photo Credit: Canstock Photo

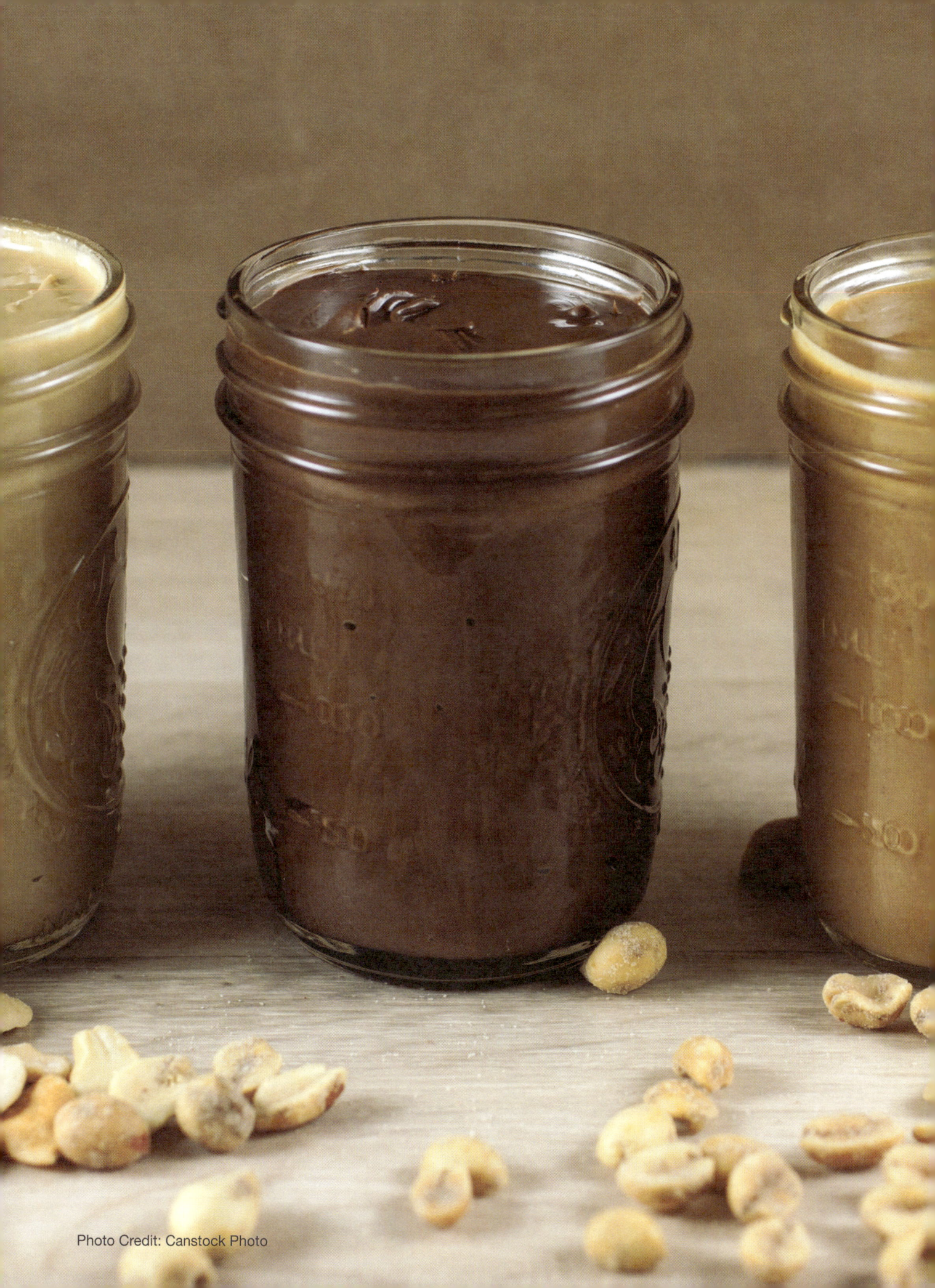

Recipes: Dip Dips & Spreads

VEGGIE SPREAD

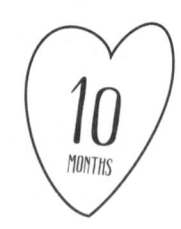

10 MONTHS

vegetarian; vegan; egg-free; grain-free; for adults too; great for lunchboxes

This will make enough roast veggies for dinner and for a spread

• •

Mila refuses to eat vegetables if they still look like vegetables! In an attempt to get her to eat more vegetables, I blended my left over roast veggies one morning and spread them on toast. Ta Da... she loved it!

This meal is so convenient - I make a large portion for myself to eat for dinner and the rest is puréed and frozen in individual portions for Mila.

• •

2 zucchinis
1 small butternut, peeled
1 medium sweet potato
1 medium eggplant
½ onion, peeled
2 cloves garlic, peeled and crushed
3 T. olive oil
½ t. black pepper, ground
1 t. Himalayan or sea salt
2 T. lemon juice, freshly squeezed
Hot water or broth *(for blending if necessary)*

Preheat the oven to 180ºC (350ºF).

Dice the zucchinis, butternut, sweet potato, eggplant and onion into small chunks (the butternut and sweet potato should be in smaller pieces as they will take longer to cook). Place them in a large bowl and add the garlic, olive oil, black pepper, salt and lemon juice and toss them.

Place the vegetables in a roasting dish and roast for approximately 45 minutes (until all the vegetables are soft but not browning).

Allow the vegetables too cool.

Place in a food processor and blend until smooth. If the mixture is too thick, drizzle hot water or broth into the processor while it is running until the mixture is the right consistency.

Serve on toast or crackers.

Can be frozen, or stored in the fridge for 2 days.

Variations:
- *Eggplant, red pepper, and onion.*
- *Sweet potato, eggplant, red pepper, tomato, and onion.*
- *You can add in additional flavours with herbs and spices such as oreganum, thyme, rosemary, cumin and, or dried coriander.*

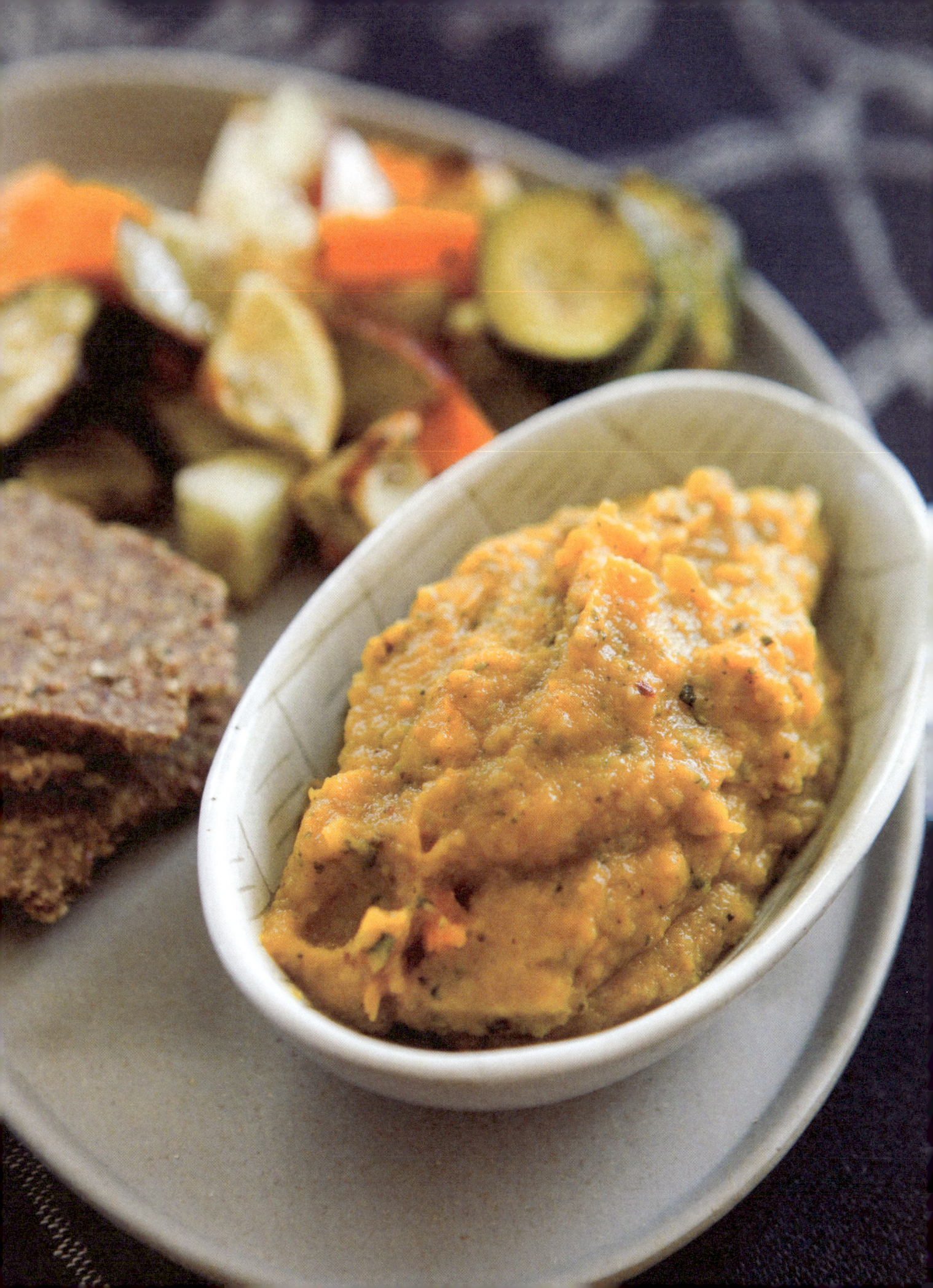

Recipes: Dip Dips & Spreads

CHICKEN LIVER PÂTÉ

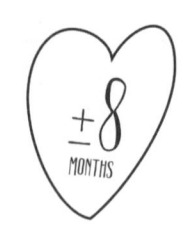

egg-free; grain-free; for adults too; great for lunchboxes

±8 MONTHS

Mila has never been a big meat eater, and worried that she was not getting enough iron and B12, I decided to give liver pâté a try. She loved it and has been eating it since she was 10 months old.
Liver is a highly nutritious food full of preformed vitamin A, B vitamins, vitamin C, copper, folate, zinc, protein, phosphorus, iron, and selenium.

Liver is a highly perishable food. Cook it within 24 hours of purchase or freeze it for up to one month.

---

1 T. coconut oil / butter / ghee
½ cup sweet potato, peeled and grated
¼ onion, finely chopped
½ garlic clove, crushed
250 g organic chicken livers
½ cup Mila's Meals chicken stock
4 T. fresh parsley, chopped
pinch Himalayan or sea salt

Wash the chicken livers and pat dry with kitchen towel.

Add the oil to a saucepan and over medium heat, sauté the sweet potatoes, onions and garlic until soft.

Add the chicken livers and chicken stock. Bring to the boil then lower the heat and simmer for 5 minutes (or until the liver is just cooked through).

Using a slotted spoon, transfer the mixture to a blender, add the fresh parsley and purée until smooth.

Add as much of the cooking liquid as necessary to obtain your desired consistency.

As you will only be using a little bit of this at a time, fill ice cubes trays with the mixture and freeze until needed. I take one cube out in the morning and allow it to defrost in the fridge in time for lunch or supper.

This is great served on toast or crackers, or as a dip for carrot and cucumber sticks.

The cooked pâté can be stored in the freezer for up to one month (remember to label the freezer bag with the date you made it on!).

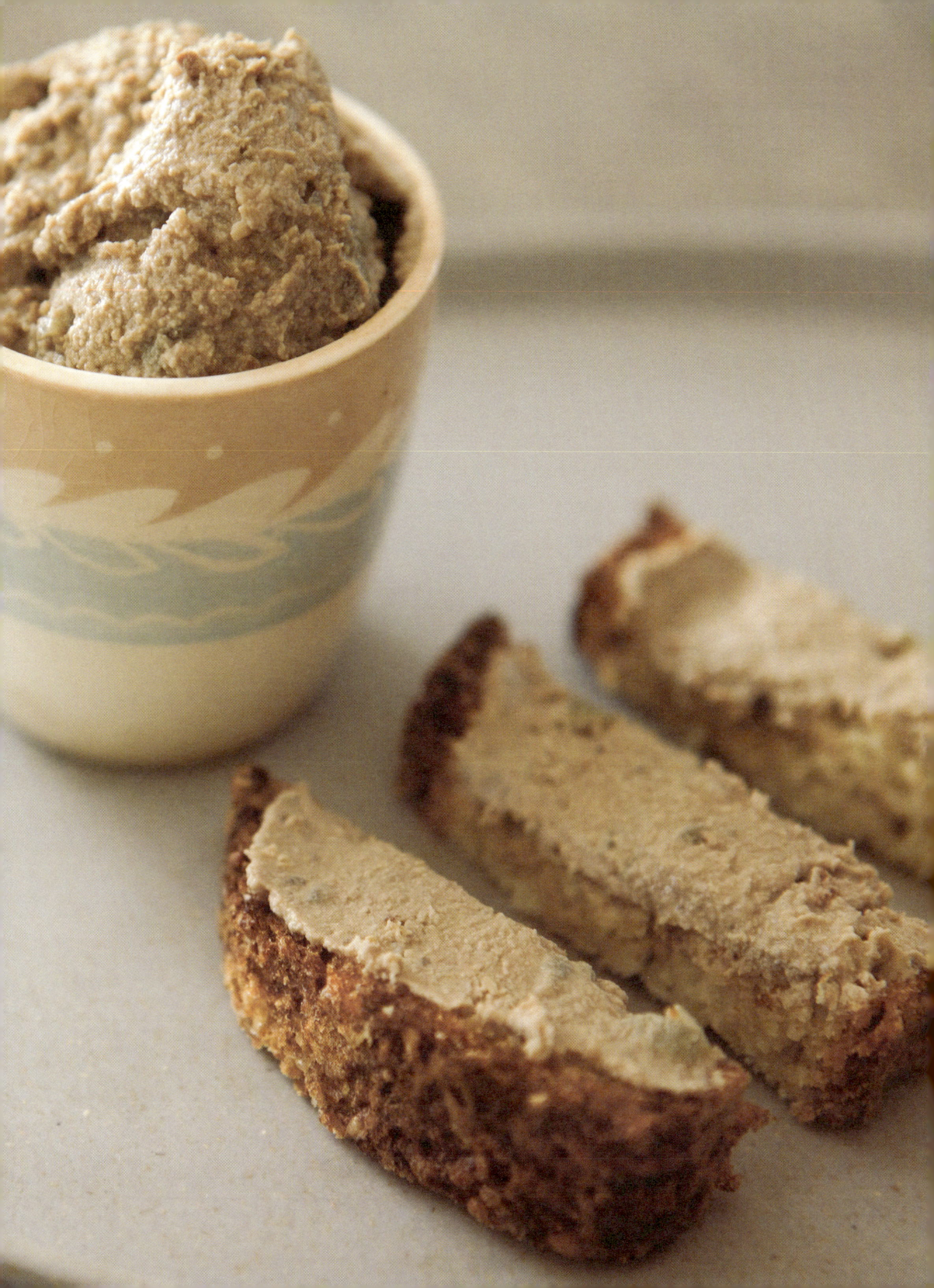

Recipes: Dip Dips & Spreads

SNOEK PÂTÉ

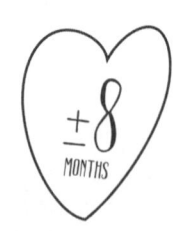

± 8 MONTHS

egg-free; grain-free; for adults too; great for lunchboxes

Snoek pâté is a South African classic! *Traditionally served with crackers or bread, it makes a great lunch or dinner time meal for your little one – and a delicious way to sneak fish into those that otherwise would refuse to eat it!*

To obtain the traditional pink colour, store bought varieties use red food colouring – beetroot juice is a much healthier option. Also beware of the sugars, GM oils and other nasties hiding in the ready-made versions.

½ brown onion, finely chopped
½ clove garlic
1 T. coconut oil
2 T. lemon juice, freshly squeezed
200 g smoked snoek
150 g sweet potato, cooked
2 T. ghee, or melted coconut oil
black pepper
1 t. beetroot juice *(freshly pressed)*

Sauté the onions and garlic in the coconut oil over medium heat until the onions are translucent.

While the onions are cooking, remove the fish from the bone and place in a blender or food processor.

Add the onions, garlic, lemon juice, sweet potato, ghee or coconut oil and pepper.

Process until you reach your desired texture.

With the processor or blender running, add a drop of beetroot juice at a time until you achieve your desired lightly pink colour.

Serve, or refrigerate in a sealed container where it will last for 5 days. Alternatively store in the freezer for up to a month.

Variations:
- If you are using the orange variety of sweet potato, you will not need to add any beetroot juice for colouring.
- The smoked snoek can be replaced with smoked angelfish, mackerel or any other smoked fish or your choice.

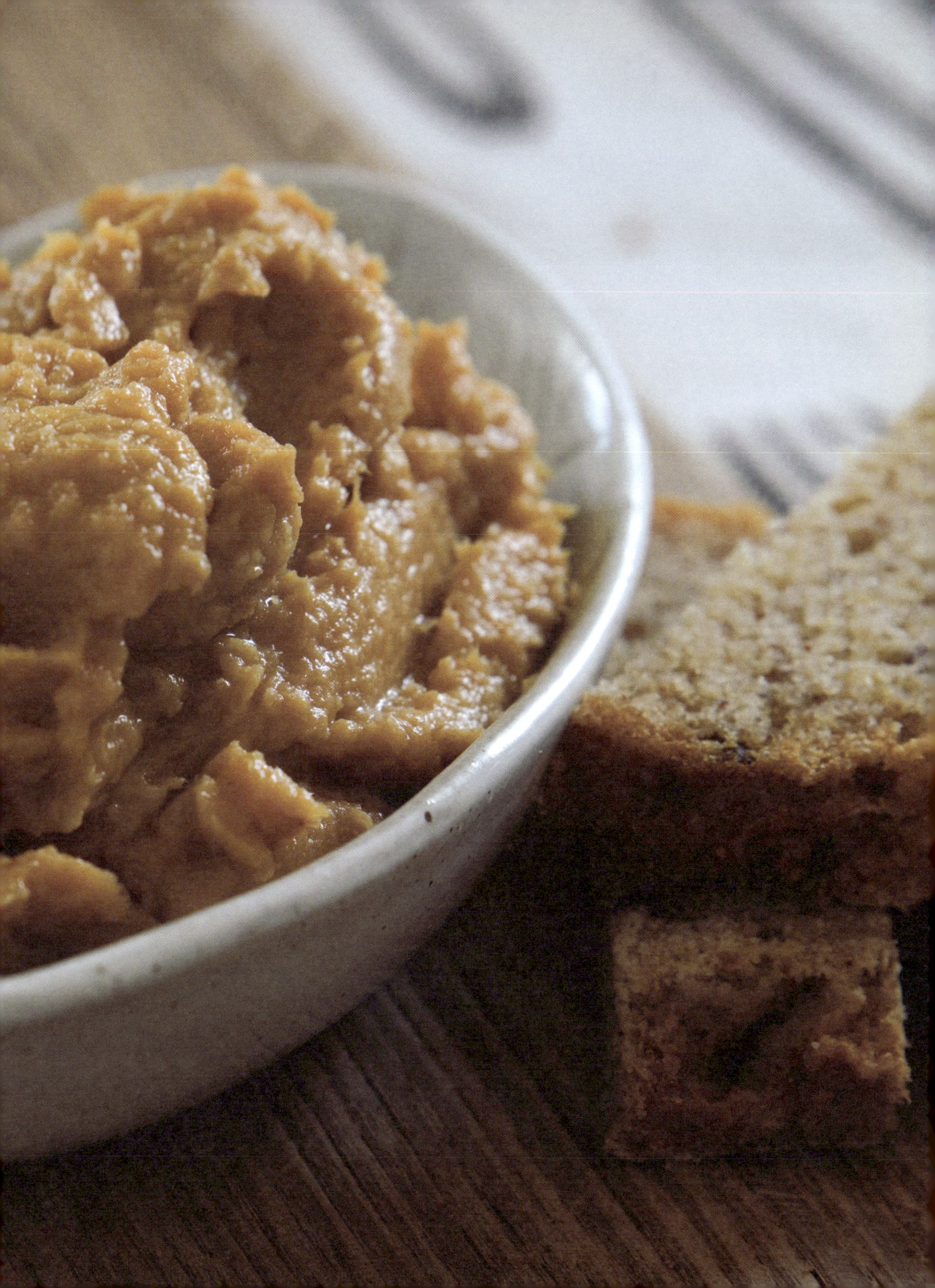

Recipes: Dip Dips & Spreads

GUACAMOLE

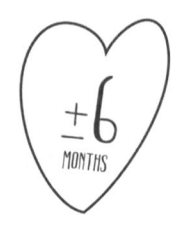

±6 MONTHS

raw; vegetarian; vegan; egg-free; grain-free; for adults too; great for lunchboxes

Avocado was one of the first foods I introduced to Mila. She has always loved it – and I love how easy it is to prepare!

Sometimes called "nature's perfect food" avocados are high in unsaturated fats, which are important for normal growth and development of the central nervous system and brain. They are a good source of bone supportive vitamin K as well as heart-healthy dietary fibre, vitamin B6, vitamin C, and folate. Avocados are also a good source of energy-producing vitamin B5 and muscle-healthy potassium.

Avocados have anti-inflammatory properties; regulate blood sugar levels and support heart and blood vessels.

1 avocado
1 T. lemon juice, freshly squeezed
pinch Himalayan or sea salt
pinch black pepper, freshly ground

Peel and pit the avocado and mash with a fork.

Add the lemon juice, salt and pepper and mix well.

Serve as a dip dip with steamed veggies, or spread it on a cracker. Mila likes to eat it as is!

This is best eaten fresh.

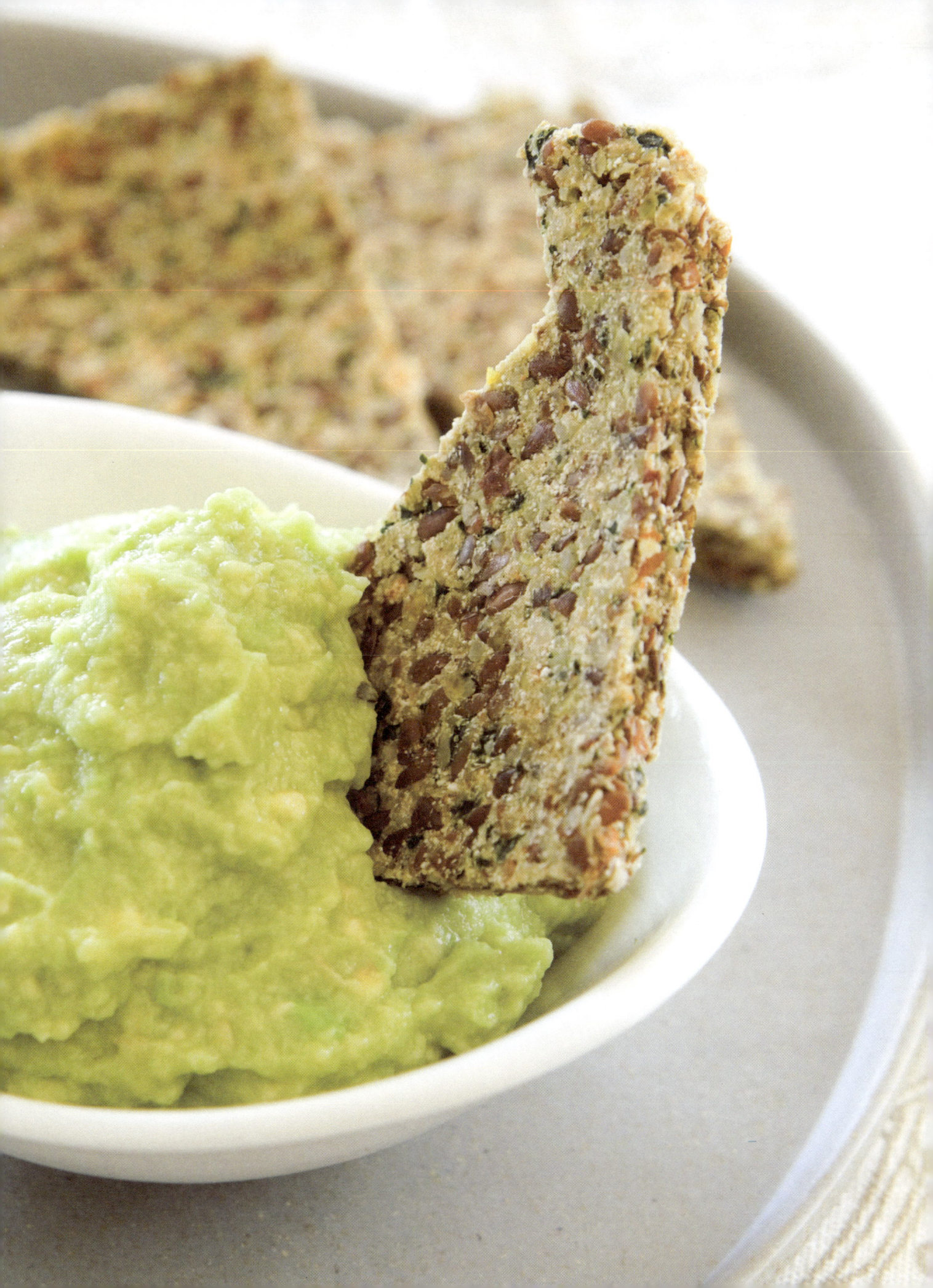

Recipes: Dip Dips & Spreads

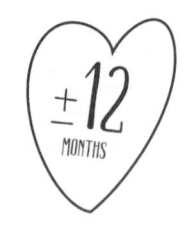

CHOCOLATE SPREAD

± 12 MONTHS

raw; superfood; vegetarian; egg-free; grain-free; for adults too; great for lunchboxes

Makes 500 ml (½ qt.)

• •

Although Mila is on a free-from diet I never want her to feel like she is missing out. As such, foods like this chocolate spread work well as a delicious and nutritious sweet treat.

Tahini is a paste made from ground sesame seeds. It has an earthy, nutty flavour that is subtler and more understated than other nut butters. It is a nutritionally dense food and a great way to boost the nutrients in any of your little one's dishes. Tahini is an excellent source of calcium and protein; healthy unsaturated fat, fibre, vitamins B and E, phosphorus, magnesium, potassium, copper and iron. It makes a useful addition to any dairy-free diet due to its high calcium content and its a great source of iron and protein for vegans or vegetarians – and little ones who are not big meat eaters like Mila.

Sesame seeds (and therefore tahini) can cause a severe allergic reaction in some people. It is important to apply the 3-day wait rule when introducing them and to watch for any signs of a reaction.

2 cups tahini *(or nut butter)*
¼ cup raw cacao powder
½ cup raw honey
¼ cup coconut oil, melted
1 t. vanilla extract *(sugar-free, colourant-free and alcohol-free)*
pinch of Himalayan or sea salt

Blend all the ingredients together until smooth.

Store in a sealed glass jar in the fridge.

CHOC-NUT SPREAD

± 12 MONTHS

raw; superfood; vegetarian; egg-free; grain-free; for adults too; great for lunchboxes

Makes 500 ml (½ qt.)

• •

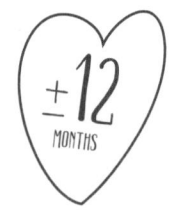

Having grown up on a steady diet of Nutella myself, this is a great alternative for your sugar-free little one.

This spread is great on pancakes, toast or simply straight off the spoon! It can also be used as an icing for cakes and cupcakes.

1 cup hazelnuts, soaked
90 ml filtered water
2 T. raw cacao powder
¼ raw honey
2 T. coconut oil, melted
½ t. vanilla powder
pinch of salt

Blend all the ingredients together until smooth.

Store in a sealed glass jar in the fridge.

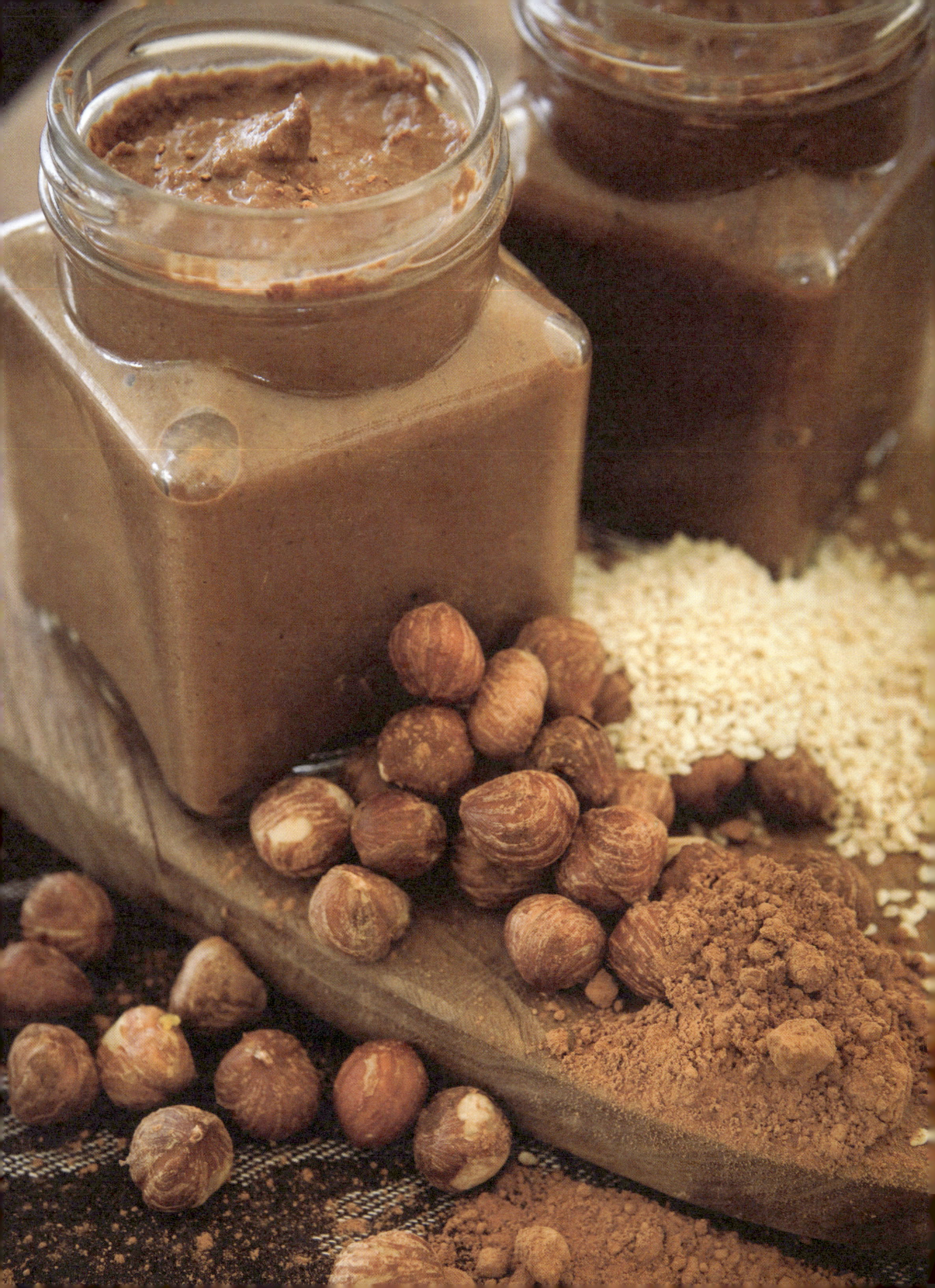

Recipes: Dip Dips & Spreads

DATE JAM

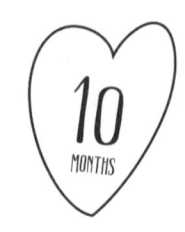

10 MONTHS

raw; vegetarian; vegan; egg-free; grain-free; for adults too; great for lunchboxes

Makes 250 ml (¼ qt.)

Date jam is use as an ingredient in some other recipes in this book – but it is also a great alternative to the highly sweetened and artificially coloured jams you find in the supermarkets.

Dates have been referred to as an "almost perfect food," based upon their nutritional content and health benefits. They contain many essential nutrients including vitamin A, B6, and K, niacin, folate, choline, calcium, iron, magnesium, phosphorus, potassium, sodium, zinc, copper, and manganese. Added to all this, they are a source of protein and over 23 different amino acids.

1 cup dates, pitted
water to cover

Cover the dates with water and allow to soak for a couple of hours or overnight.

In a food processor or blender, blend the dates with 4 T. of the soak water until smooth.

Store in a glass jar in the fridge. The jam will last for 2 weeks.

Variations:
- Add ¼ cup of fresh mint leaves for an all natural, raw mint sauce condiment.

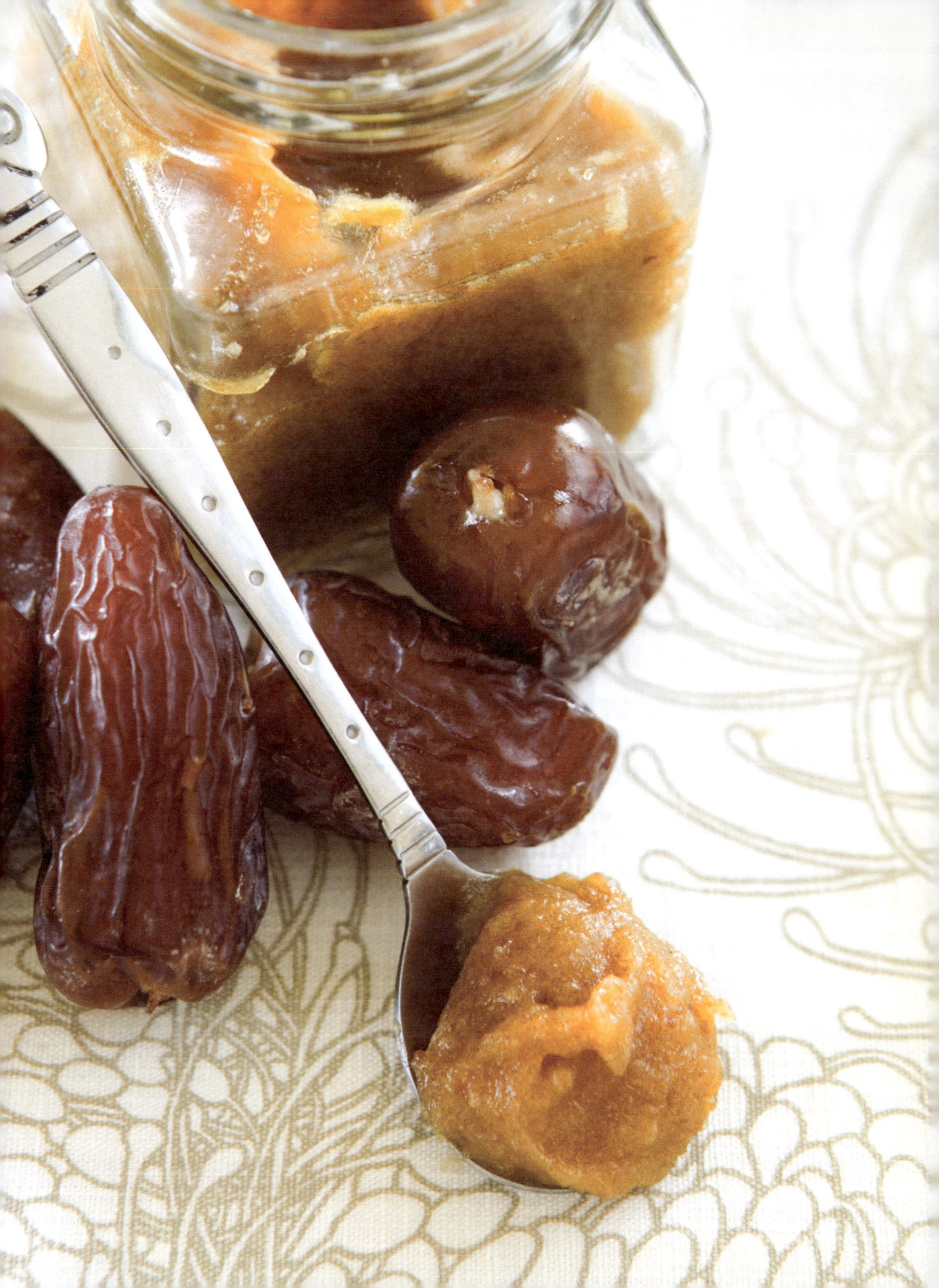

Recipes: Dip Dips & Spreads

STRAWBERRY JAM

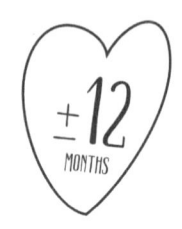

±12 MONTHS

raw; vegetarian; vegan; egg-free; grain-free; for adults too; great for lunchboxes

• •

2 cups fresh strawberries *(or any other berry of your choice)*
½ cup dates, pitted and chopped
¼ cup water
2 T. chia seeds, ground
1 T. beetroot juice, freshly presssed *(optional)*

Place the dates in a bowl and cover with the water. Allow to soak for a couple of hours or overnight.

Place the dates, soak water, berries and chia seeds into a food processor or blend and process until smooth (or until you have the consistency you desire).

Add the beetroot juice if you want a brighter red colour – the jam will then look more like the one you find in the supermarkets. (Mila did not approve of the light pink colour of this strawberry jam!)

Scoop the jam into a glass jar, seal and place in the fridge for 30 minutes to allow the chia seeds to thicken the jam.

Serve on toast, pancakes or crackers.

Store in a glass jar in the fridge. The jam will last for 3- 4 days.

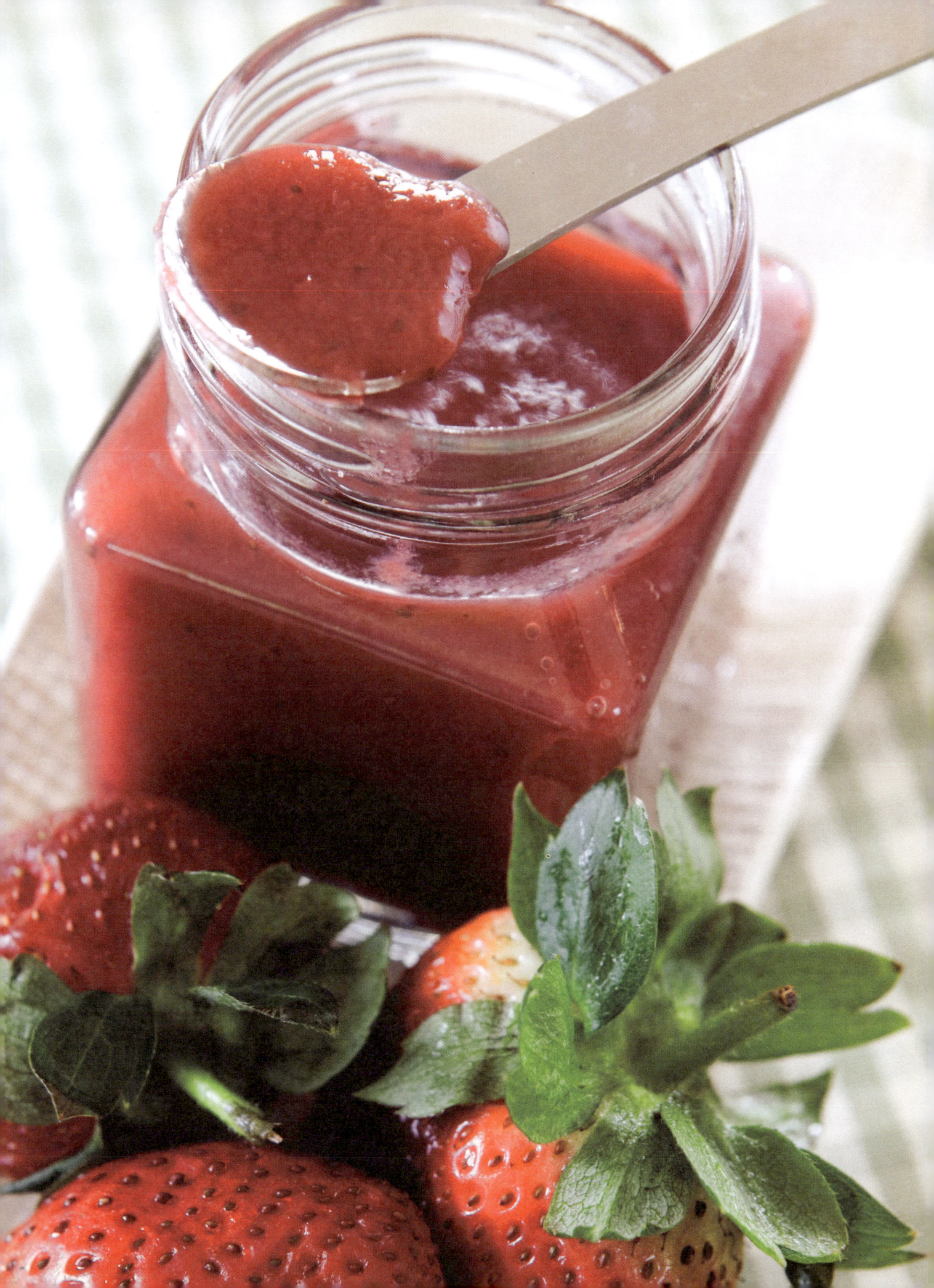

Recipes: From the Fork (or spoon)

Some food is just better eaten with the help of utensils!

Recipes: From the Fork

SCRAMBLED EGGS
GREEN EGGS → 304
ORANGE EGGS → 306
IMMUNE BOOSTER EGGS → 306

EGG FRIED RICE → 308

CRUSTLESS QUICHE → 310

COTTAGE PIE → 312

LAMB CASSEROLE → 314

CHICKEN CURRY → 316

Recipes: From the Fork

SCRAMBLED EGGS

vegetarian; grain-free; for adults too

Makes 1 toddler sized portion

Mila went through an egg phase - she wanted eggs for dinner pretty much every night for a few months! I had to come up with different ways of cooking them to add a variety of nutrients into her diet. As for eating so many eggs – well eggs are one of nature's perfect foods – as long as they are from organic, pasture fed chickens that is.

Eggs whites are one of the top 8 allergenic foods. While recent research indicates that waiting to introduce allergenic foods to your baby does not necessarily delay or prevent an allergic reaction, it is important to watch your little one closely for possible reactions when introducing these foods. If your family has a history of egg allergy it is best to wait until your little one is 12 months old before introducing whole eggs (even in baked goods).

GREEN EGGS

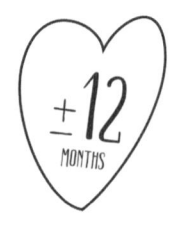

+12 MONTHS

1 egg yolk *(you can use the whole egg if your little one is older than a year)*
½ T. Mila's Meals pesto
pinch of Himalayan or sea salt
pinch of turmeric
Coconut oil for frying
pinch of dulse flakes *(optional)*

Place the egg, pesto, salt and turmeric in a small mixing bowl and whisk with a fork.

Heat some coconut oil in a small frying pan and pour in the egg mixture.

Stir continuously with a wooden spoon until cooked through.

Allow to cool, sprinkle with some dulse flakes and serve.

Although many books recommend avoiding salt until your little one is a year old, it is necessary for digestion and unrefined salt contains many beneficial trace minerals. Add a pinch to some foods however, it is not advisable to get your little one used to eating very salty food.

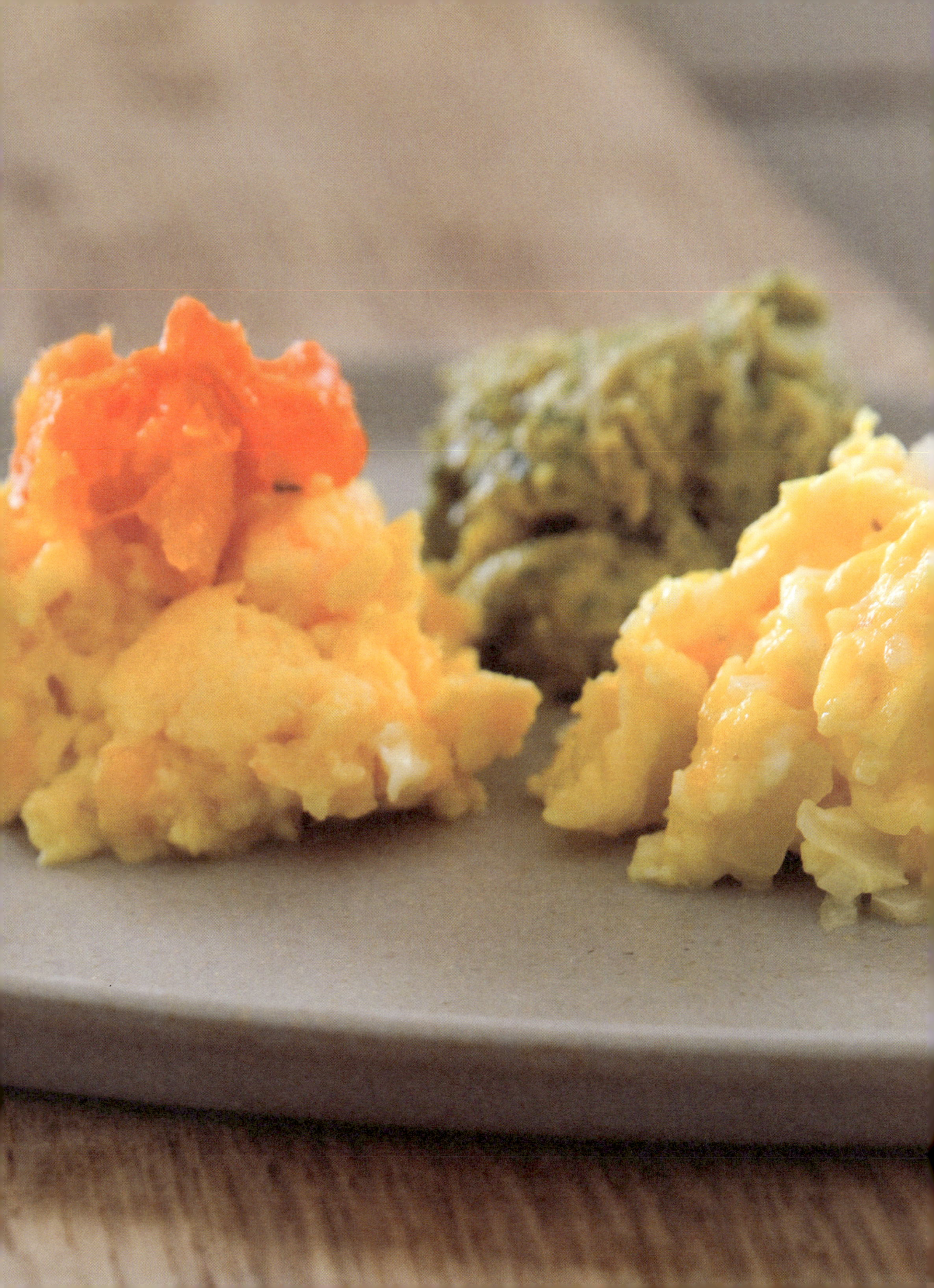

Recipes: From the Fork

ORANGE EGGS

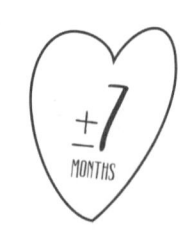

±7 MONTHS

1 egg yolk *(you can use the whole egg if your little one is older than a year)*
1 T. butternut, cooked and mashed
pinch of Himalayan or sea salt
pinch of turmeric
Coconut oil for frying
pinch of dulse flakes (optional)

Place the egg yolk, butternut, salt and turmeric in a small mixing bowl and whisk with a fork.

Heat some coconut oil in a small frying pan and pour in the egg mixture.

Stir continuously with a wooden spoon until cooked through.

Allow to cool, sprinkle with some dulse flakes and serve.

Dulse is an edible seaweed that has a long history of use in different Asian cultures. It is high in vitamins and minerals – specifically Vitamins B6, B12, A, iron, potassium, phosphorus, iodine and manganese. It is also high in calcium, fibre, and protein. It has many purported health benefits including healing poor digestive systems, rebuilding and maintains all glands in the body, cleansing the body of heavy metals, supporting healthy brain function and heals and enhancing the liver. It has a spicy salty flavour that enhances the flavour of many meals. It is such an easy, convenient nutrition enhancer to add to a meal before serving.

IMMUNE BOOSTER EGGS

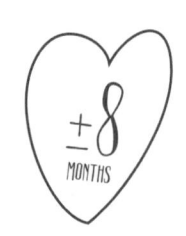

±8 MONTHS

1 egg yolk *(you can use the whole egg if your little one is older than a year)*
1T. onion, finely chopped
1t. garlic, crushed and left to stand for 10 minutes
pinch of Himalayan or sea salt
pinch of turmeric
Coconut oil for frying

Heat some coconut oil in a small frying pan gently fry the onion and garlic over low heat until the onion is translucent (approximately 5 minutes).

Place the egg yolk, salt and turmeric in a small mixing bowl and whisk with a fork.

Pour the egg mixture into the frying pan and stir continuously with a wooden spoon until cooked through.

Allow to cool and serve.

Mila was sick for the very first time when she was 11 months old. She had a fever with no other symptoms. As we were away on holiday with no access to a homeopath or GP, I used food to help her system fight off the virus. Both garlic and onion are natural antibiotics. After eating these scrambled eggs, she was better within a day.

Turmeric is a powerful medicinal food that has long been used in the Chinese and Indian systems of medicine as an anti-inflammatory agent to treat a wide variety of conditions. It also adds a bright yellow colour to the eggs.

Recipes: From the Fork

in this house
we are a family & we dream **BIG**
we are happy and respectful
we use kind words
we always tell the truth
we give (big) hugs and kisses
we say "i love you", "please" and "thank-you"
we make mistakes and learn from them
we say I'm sorry
we keep our promises
we dance and cook (alot!)
we giggle and are silly
we do our best
We share
we seize the moment
we make memories
we forgive quickly
we laugh (alot.) and love deeply
we believe in ourselves
we try new things
WE LISTEN
we enjoy the little things
we embrace our inner weird
we are grateful
we imagine
we blow bubbles
WE KEEP CALM, AND CARRY ON

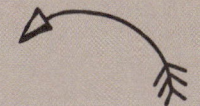

Mila and Mama's house rules

Recipes: From the Fork

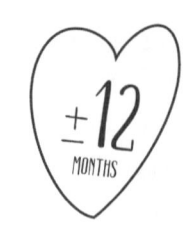

±12 MONTHS

EGG FRIED RICE

vegetarian; for adults too; great for lunchboxes

Makes 1 toddler sized portion

This is another really easy-to-make egg recipe to which you can add various ingredients each time you make it.

I usually cook a large portion of rice, and freeze it in meal size portions. It is then ready to add to meals as and when I need it.

Be sure to buy non-GMO, organic rice.

1 T. onion, finely chopped

½ t. garlic, crushed and left to stand for 10 minutes

1 egg yolk *(you can use the whole egg if your little one is older than a year)*

¼ cup rice, soaked and cooked *(Thai red rice is delicious as is brown Basmati rice)*

pinch of Himalayan or sea salt

1 T. baby marrow, finely grated

Coconut oil for frying

Melt the coconut oil in a frying pan and add the onion and garlic. Fry on low heat for approximately 5 minutes or until the onions are translucent.

Place the egg in a mixing bowl and whisk with a fork. Add the egg to the frying pan and then the rice and salt.

Turn the heat up to medium and fry while stirring for 2 – 3 minutes (or until the eggs are cooked through).

I add the baby marrow at the end – although you can add it with the egg and rice if you would like it to cook.

Allow to cool slightly and serve.

Variations:
- *You can add other ingredients such as: finely grated ginger, sesame oil, red peppers, carrot, spring onions, crushed nuts, corn, and tomatoes.*

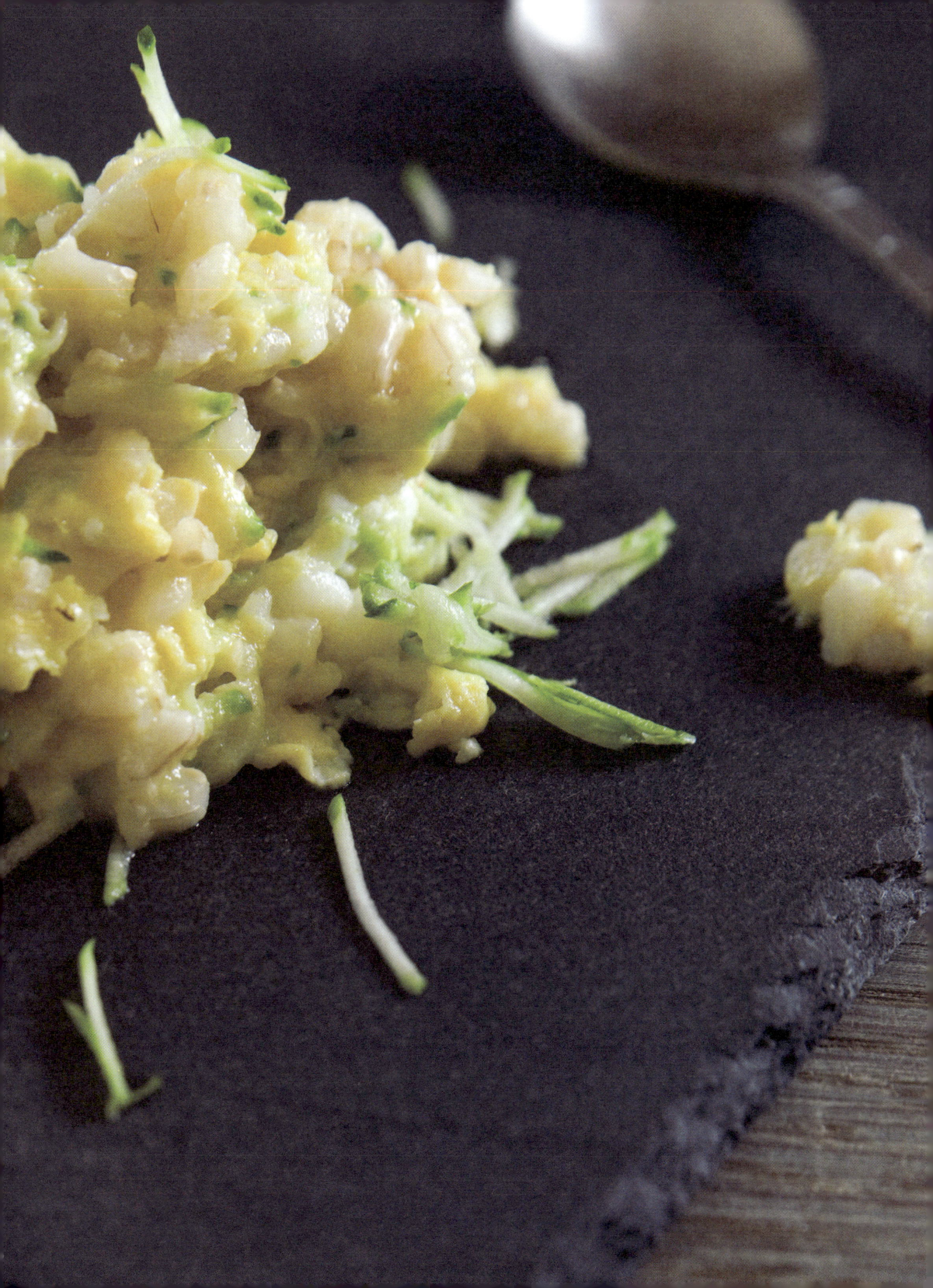

Recipes: From the Fork

The introduction age here is 12 months due to the tomatoes. Try a different combination of vegetables if you'd like to serve your little on quiche earlier. See the variations below.

+12 MONTHS

CRUSTLESS QUICHE

vegetarian; grain-free; for adults too

Makes 6 adult portions

This is a great way of using left-over cooked vegetables to create a whole new beautiful meal for breakfast, lunch or dinner!

It is easy-to-prepare meal that the whole family can enjoy. This recipe makes a big quiche that can serve 6 adults.

You can make quiche with a gluten-free base, I prefer to eliminate the traditional base altogether – it makes the preparation that much quicker!

8 eggs
400ml goat's milk or any dairy-free milk alternative
8 baby tomatoes
handful fresh basil
pinch of Himalayan or sea salt
pinch of freshly ground black pepper

Heat the oven to 180°C (350°F).

Beat the eggs and the milk in a large mixing bowl.

Season with salt and pepper.

Dice the baby tomatoes and shred the basil. Place them in a flan or casserole dish.

Pour the egg mixture over the tomatoes and basil.

Bake the quiche for 40 - 50 minutes, or until it has risen slightly and is firm to the touch.

Allow to cool slightly and serve.

Leftover quiche can be kept in the fridge for a couple of days.

Variations:
- You are only limited by your imagination when it comes to quiche! Use any left-over roast vegetables or try some of the following combinations:
  - *Sautéed spinach, artichoke and goat cheese,*
  - *Sautéed onion, roasted butternut and sage,*
  - *Baby marrow, and cooked sweet potato.*

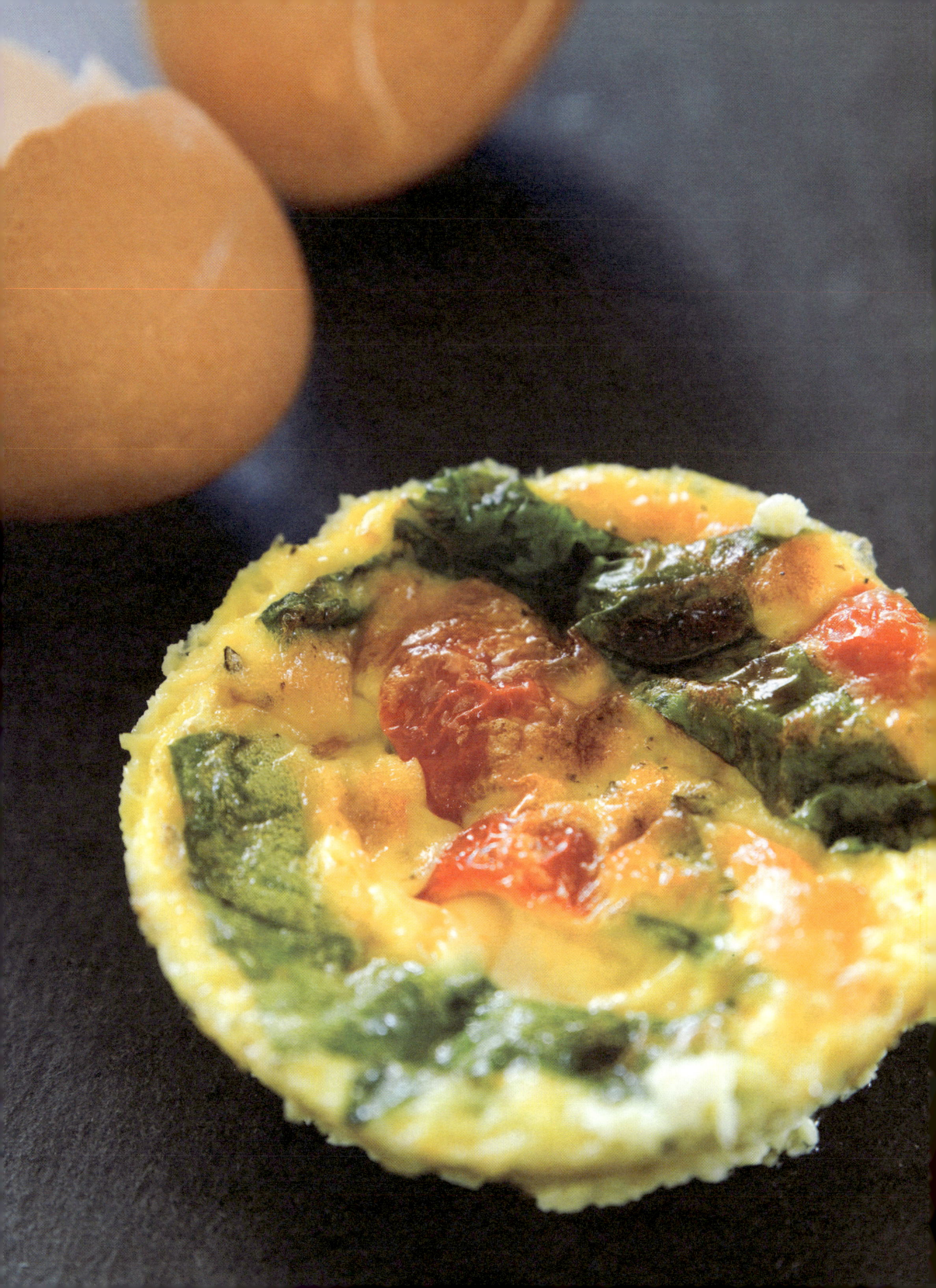

Recipes: From the Fork

COTTAGE PIE

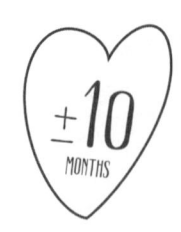

±10 MONTHS

egg-free; for adults too

Makes 1 large casserole dish plus 4 individual ramekins

This is one of the more time consuming recipes to make. But you can bake it in individual ramekins and freeze for easy future dinners. It is a great meal for the whole family to enjoy.

Mila has been eating this since she was 10 months old – she enjoys it more the older she gets and appreciates the novelty of having her own ramekin to eat out of.

This is an excellent way to sneak the nutrient-dense vegetables in as they are barley noticeable in the final dish. The homemade beef stock also adds to the high nutritional value of this meal.

- 2 T. coconut oil, butter or ghee
- 1 onion, finely chopped
- 1 garlic clove, finely chopped and left to stand for 10 minutes
- 1 carrot (50 g), peeled and finely chopped or grated
- 2 courgettes (50 g), finely chopped or grated
- 500 g (1lb) ground beef, lamb, kudu or ostrich
- 1 t. Himalayan or sea salt
- ½ t. ground cumin
- 1 t. ground coriander
- 1 t. mixed dry herbs
- 4 T. Mila's Meals All Good Tomato sauce
- 1 cup Mila's Meals beef stock
- 6 medium sized potatoes, peeled and chopped
- water or bone broth *(stock)*
- 1 T. coconut oil, butter, or ghee
- ½ t. Himalayan or sea salt
- ½ cup coconut milk *(or any other dairy-free alternative)*

Heat the oven to 180°C (350°F).

Bring a pot of water or bone broth to the boil and add the potatoes. Boil for 30 minutes, or until they are tender. Drain.

While the potatoes are cooking, melt the coconut oil (butter or ghee) in a frying pan. Add the onion, garlic, carrot and courgette and fry gently for 5 minutes (or until the onions are translucent).

Turn the heat to high, add the ground meat and fry stirring continuously to brown the meat evenly.

Turn the heat to medium, add the salt, cumin, coriander, herbs and tomato sauce and stir well. Allow to simmer for a couple of minutes.

Add the beef stock and stir well. Cover and simmer on medium to low heat for 15 minutes.

My mom-in-law would be horrified at this cooking time! She slow cooks her mince the whole day. So, you can at this stage transfer the mixture to a slow cooker turned onto low and continue with the meal preparation later in the day.

Place the cooked potatoes in a pot over low heat and add the coconut oil (butter or ghee), milk and salt. Mash until smooth and creamy.

Spoon the meat mixture into a casserole dish or individual ramekins until they are two thirds full.

Spoon some mashed potato over the meat mixture.

Bake in the oven for 30 minutes, or until golden on top.

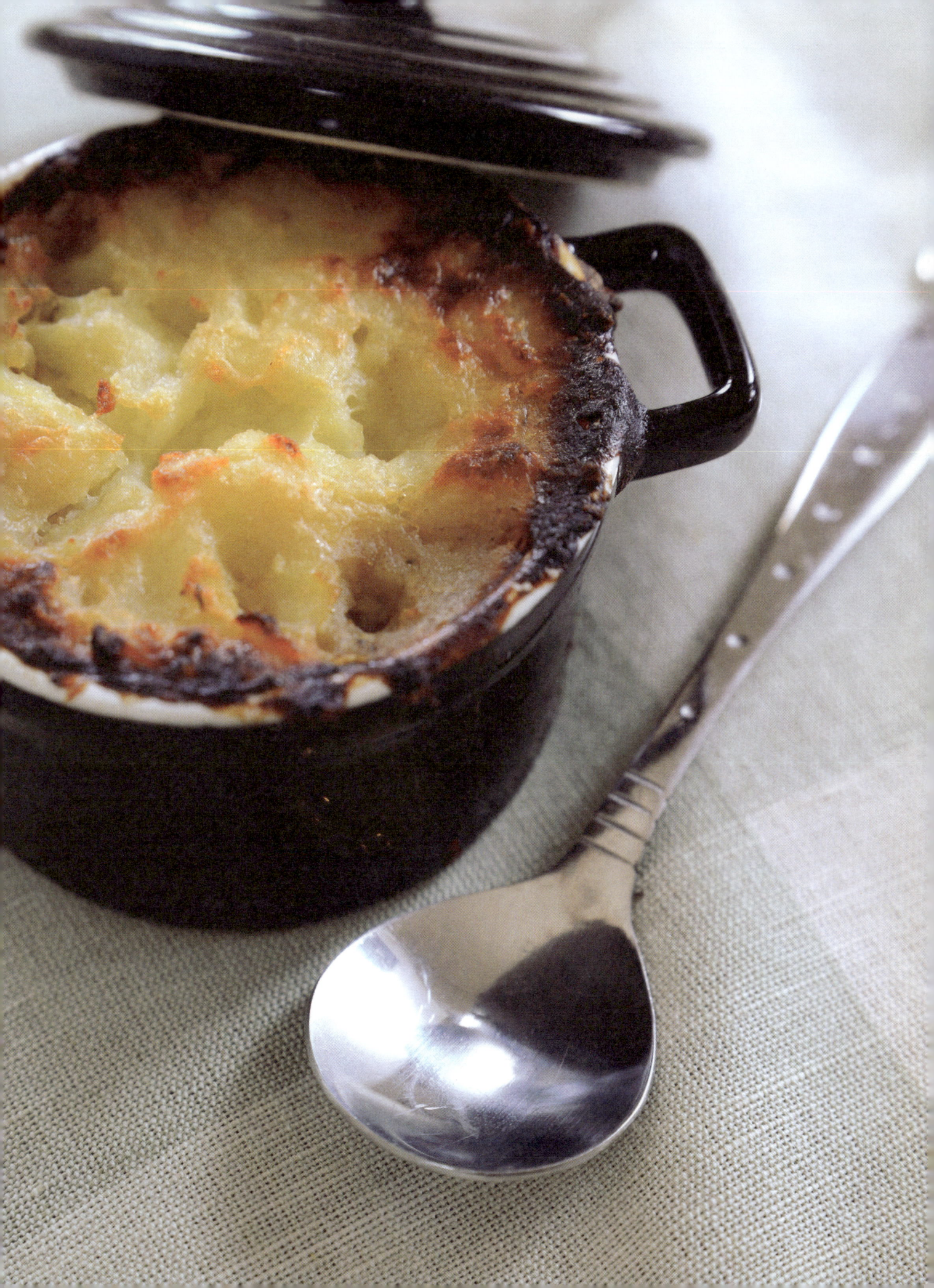

Recipes: From the Fork

LAMB CASSEROLE

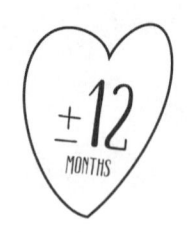

± 12 MONTHS

egg-free; for adults too

Makes 4 adult sized portions

• •

Slow cookers are, in my opinion, one of the best inventions ever! Not only does the low heat preserve many valuable nutrients that would otherwise be lost by cooking in the oven at a higher heat, but also being able to do the prep in the morning and having the meal ready at dinner time, frees up your time at 'crazy hour' when children need to be bathed etc. I also love having a complete meal in one pot - no need to prepare additional side dishes.

Grass-fed lamb is a highly nutritious food. It is a great source of vitamin B12, protein, selenium, niacin, zinc, iron and phosphorus. It also provides a significant amount of omega-3 fatty acids.

The secret to slow cooking meat which is tender and juicy is to use cuts which still have the bone in them. Lamb neck has the added benefit of the bone marrow which is exceptionally nutritious.

Remember to keep the bones for making broth at a later stage.

If your little one, like Mila, does not enjoy eating vegetables she can identify as vegetables, simply purée some casserole sauce with some of the vegetables. Pour this sauce into a serving bowl with the meat. We call this "shlurpie" – and Mila loves it!

This casserole is delicious served over spiralised veggie noodles, rice or gluten-free pasta.

• •

1 kg (2 lbs) lamb neck or chops
2 t. ground coriander
2 T. coconut oil *(or ghee)*
2 t. Himalayan or sea salt
2 onions, finely chopped
8 carrots, peeled and chopped
4 stalks celery, finely sliced
3 potatoes or sweet potatoes, peeled and chopped
2 cloves garlic, crushed and left to stand for 10 minutes
½ t. freshly ground black pepper
1 T. apple cider vinegar
2 cups Mila's Meals vegetable, chicken or beef broth
2 cups green lentils, soaked (optional)
2 bay leaves
2 stems fresh rosemary

Turn your slow cooker on to low.

Season your lamb with the ground coriander on both sides.

Melt the coconut oil or ghee in a frying pan over high heat and add your lamb pieces, browning and seasoning with salt on both sides. Transfer to the slow cooker – leaving the fat in the frying pan.

Place the onions, carrots, celery, potatoes and garlic in the frying pan and sauté over medium heat. Season with salt and pepper. Continue to sauté for 10 minutes.

Add the apple cider vinegar, broth, lentils and bay leaves and bring to the boil. Pour the vegetable mixture over the lamb in the slow cooker. Add additional water to make sure the lamb is covered by liquid.

Cook on low for 8 hours or on high for 4 hours.

In the last half an hour add the fresh rosemary allowing it to infuse its flavour. Remove before serving.

Scoop some casserole from the slow cooker, removing the meat from the bone for your little one.

Allow to cool and serve.

Left over casserole can be kept in the fridge for a couple of days or frozen in individual portions for up to 2 months.

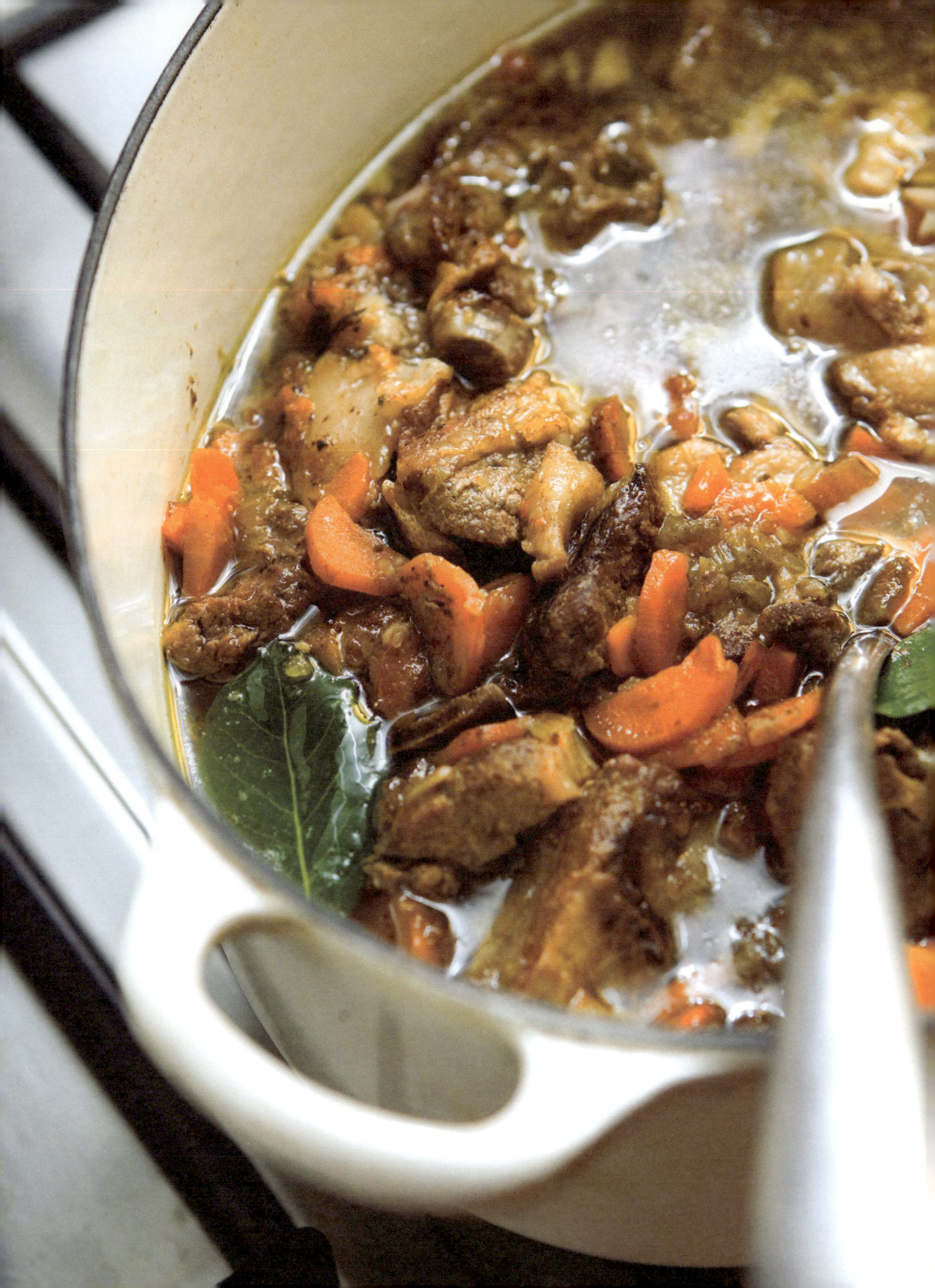

Recipes: From the Fork

CHICKEN CURRY

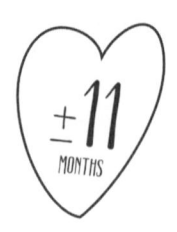

+11 MONTHS

egg-free; grain-free; for adults too

Makes 4 adult portions

• •

I really did not think an 11-month old would enjoy a curry, but I was pleasantly surprised! I think the sweetness of the dried fruit helped a lot.

This casserole is delicious served over spiralised veggie noodles, rice or cauliflower rice.

• •

2 T. coconut oil

1 kg (2 lb) organic or free-range chicken thighs

2 t. Himalayan or sea salt

1 onion, finely chopped

2 cloves garlic, minced and left to stand for 10 minutes

2 T. arrowroot powder

3 T. mild curry powder

1½ cups sweet potato, peeled and chopped

1 cups carrots, peeled and chopped

¾ cup mango (fresh or dried), dried apricots or apple, chopped

1 zucchini, chopped

2 cups Mila's Meals chicken stock

200ml coconut milk *(preservative-free)*

Turn your slow cooker on to low.

Melt 1 T. coconut oil in a frying pan over high heat. Add the chicken and brown on both sides. Season with salt on the cooked side.

Transfer the chicken pieces to the slow cooker.

Add the remaining 1 T. coconut oil to the frying pan with the onion and garlic and sauté over medium heat until the onion is translucent.

Add the arrowroot and curry powder and stir to combine. Sauté for another minute.

Add the sweet potatoes, carrots, fruit and zucchini and stir fry for 5 minutes or until the vegetables begin to soften. Add the chicken broth and bring to the boil.

Transfer to the slow cooker ensuring that all the chicken is covered with liquid – adding more boiling water if necessary.

Cook on low for 5½ hours or on high for 2½ hours.

Add the coconut milk and stir to combine. Cook for another 20 minutes.

Remove a piece of chicken, cut the meat from the bone, add some of the sauce and vegetables and serve.

The remaining curry can be frozen in individual portions or served to the rest of the family.

The curry will keep in the fridge for a couple of days or in the freezer for 3 months.

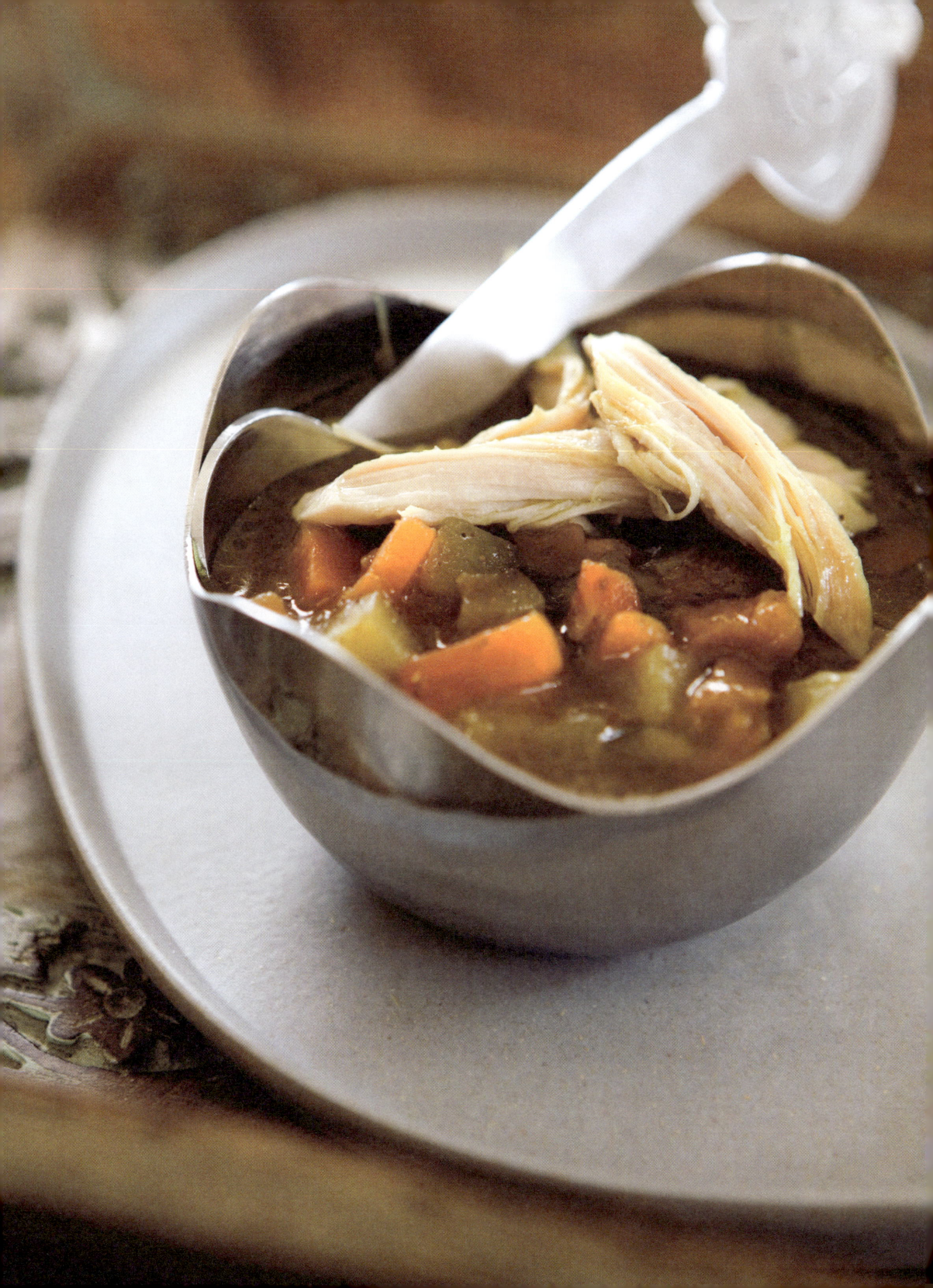

Recipes: Party Food & Something Sweet

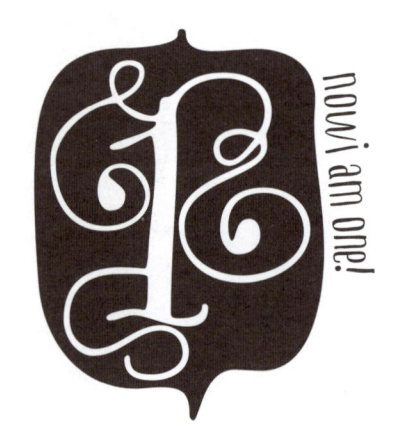

now i am one!

Birthday parties are generally a sweet affair with sugar-fuelled children running around like lunatics! Not Mila's – much to my mother's dismay.

At the time of Mila's first birthday party I was still very new to the whole gluten-free, sugar-free baking thing. My mom asked me how I could feed "that food" to people – at the time the criticism upset me, but in hindsight (and looking back at the photos) I have to admit… she was right! I have come along way since then, and have proven (to myself and my mom) that free-from parties can be a delicious treat - for both children and adults alike!

The greatest benefit of putting so much effort in to preparing a 'free-from' party is that the whole day is enjoyable – there are no sugar-highs and crashes, there are no lunatic kids, there are no temper tantrums.

One word of advice – start preparing the food a few days in advance! You do not want the actual birthday to be overshadowed by the cooking and the stress of preparation. For Mila's first birthday party, I made the mistake of trying to make everything 'fresh' and on the day - by the time everyone had arrived I just wanted to go and hide in my bedroom!

The great thing about these 'party foods' is that they are so nutritious they can be served as part of a meal, or as a meal on their own! What child gets to eat chocolate fudge for dinner and ice-cream for breakfast? Who says free-from kids are deprived?

Recipes: Party Food & Something Sweet

CHOC-NUT FUDGE → 320
CHICKPEA FUDGE → 322
DATE BALLS → 324
CHOCOLATE MOUSSE → 326
ICE CREAM BASE → 328
NANA-CHOC ICE CREAM → 330
RAW ICE CREAM CUPS → 332
ICE LOLLIES → 334
CHOCOLATE (OR VANILLA) CUPCAKES → 336
CARROT CUPCAKES → 338
STICKY CHOCOLATE LAYER CAKE → 340
ICINGS → 342-344
CUPCAKE AND CAKE DECORATIONS → 346

Recipes: Party Food & Something Sweet

CHOC-NUT FUDGE

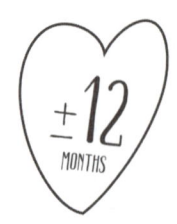

±12 MONTHS

raw; superfood; vegetarian; vegan; egg-free; grain-free; for adults too; great for lunchboxes

Makes: 30 (2 cm x 2 cm) fudge squares.

Mila had her first taste of fudge on her first birthday and it is now one of our favourite treats. It makes for a great party food too - I always take some along to birthday parties Mila goes to, as a substitute for the sweets that are on offer there.

The fudge is packed with nutrients and has antioxidant, anti-inflammatory, antifungal, antibacterial, antimicrobial and general body nourishing properties. It is a great source of healthy fats, calcium, iron, potassium, zinc, protein, iron, fibre, copper, magnesium, manganese, phosphorus, vitamins A, B's, C and K, folate, and choline.

This recipe can be used as an icing for cakes or cupcakes. Simply add an additional ¼ cup water and omit the nuts.

- **1 cup dates, soaked and pitted**
- **1 cup coconut oil, melted**
- **½ cup cashew nuts, activated**
- **¼ cup raw cacao powder**
- **1 t. vanilla powder**
- **1 t. green powder**
(chlorella, spirulina, barley and wheatgrass mix)
- **a pinch of Himalayan or sea salt**
- **½ cup water**

Place all the ingredients (except the water) in the food processor and process with an S-blade for a couple of minutes.

Gradually add the water while the processor is running until the mixture is smooth. You want to make sure it is not too runny as it will not set – the amount of water you need to add depends on how long you soak your dates for. The longer they have soaked (and the more water they are retaining), the less water you need to add to the mixture.

Scoop the mixture into a shallow dish lined with baking paper.

Place in the fridge and allow to set – this takes approximately 1 hour.

Cut the fudge into squares and serve.

(Please note due to the nature of coconut oil, the fudge will soften when it stands at room temperature.)

If there is any left over, you can store it in an airtight container in the fridge for up to 3 weeks.

Preparation tips:
- Soak the dates by placing them in a bowl and covering with water. Warm water will work quicker.
- Melt the coconut oil by placing it in a bowl, and then placing that bowl in a bowl of hot water.

Party Tip:
- *This can be made a day or two in advance and kept in the fridge.*
- *This fudge will soften if it is left out of the fridge in summer due to the nature of coconut oil. Only place it on the party table when it is time to eat.*

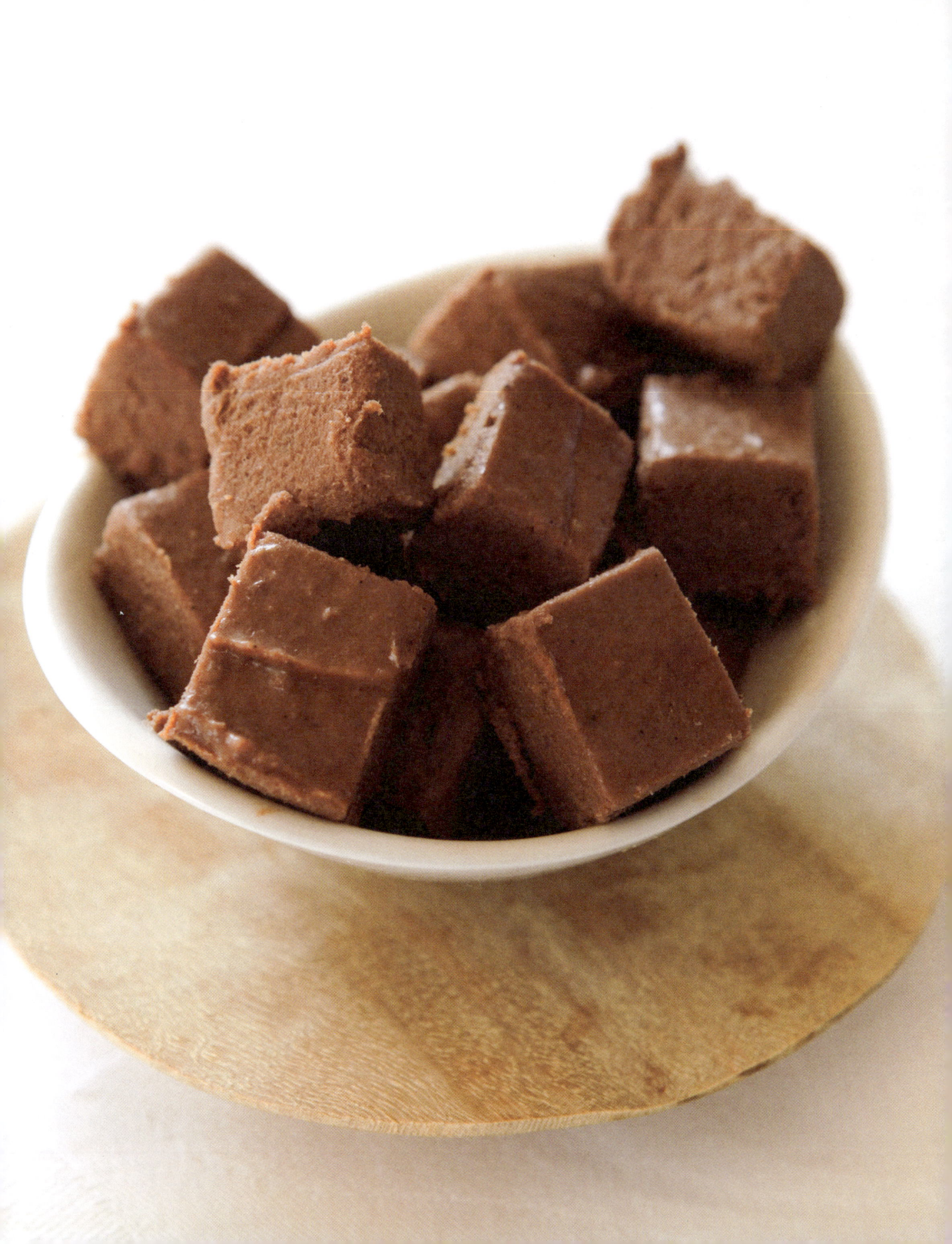

Recipes: Party Food & Something Sweet

CHICKPEA FUDGE

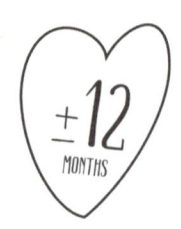

+12 MONTHS

raw; vegetarian; egg-free; for adults too; great for lunchboxes

Makes 18 toddler size fudge pieces

This recipe is drawn from Indian cuisine and is traditionally served as a sweetmeat during the festival of Diwali.

Mila's Aunt Jane craved this fudge throughout her pregnancy - not a bad thing to crave considering its nutritional value! Chickpea flour is an excellent source of protein and folate – both of which are essential during pregnancy. It is also provides vitamin B6, iron, magnesium and potassium. The fats provided by the ghee will help slow down the release of the sugar from the honey into the blood, ensuring there is no high-and-low, or wild-child behaviour!

Did you ever think fudge could be medicinal?

Cardamom is considered one of the most valuable spices in the world. It has antiseptic, antiviral, antispasmodic, and antioxidant properties. It is an excellent spice for the respiratory system and works as a natural expectorant in relieving congestion and phlegm from the lungs and sinus passages. Cardamom is also great for the digestive system - it stimulates the appetite; eases constipation, gas, nausea, indigestion, and colic.

The honey and nutmeg also have anti-inflammatory and antibacterial properties.

- ¾ cup ghee
- 1½ cups chickpea flour
- ¼ cup honey or maple syrup
- 2 T. almond nut butter
- ½ t. ground cardamom *(if you grind your own cardamom – you will need 5 pods)*
- ¼ t. ground nutmeg

Melt the butter or ghee in a heavy-based saucepan over medium heat.

Add the chickpea flour and stir continuously for 10 minutes. The mixture should be golden (not brown).

Remove the saucepan from the heat and stir in the remaining ingredients.

Scoop the mixture onto a greased baking tray (or one lined with baking paper). Spread the mixture evenly to ensure it is about 2 cm (3/4") in height.

Place the fudge in the freezer for an hour to allow it to set then cut into squares using a hot knife.

If you are not serving it immediately it is best to store it in a sealed container in the fridge, or freezer.

The fudge can be frozen for up to a month.

♥ **Party Prep Tip:** *This can be made a day or two in advance and kept in a sealed container in the fridge or freezer.*

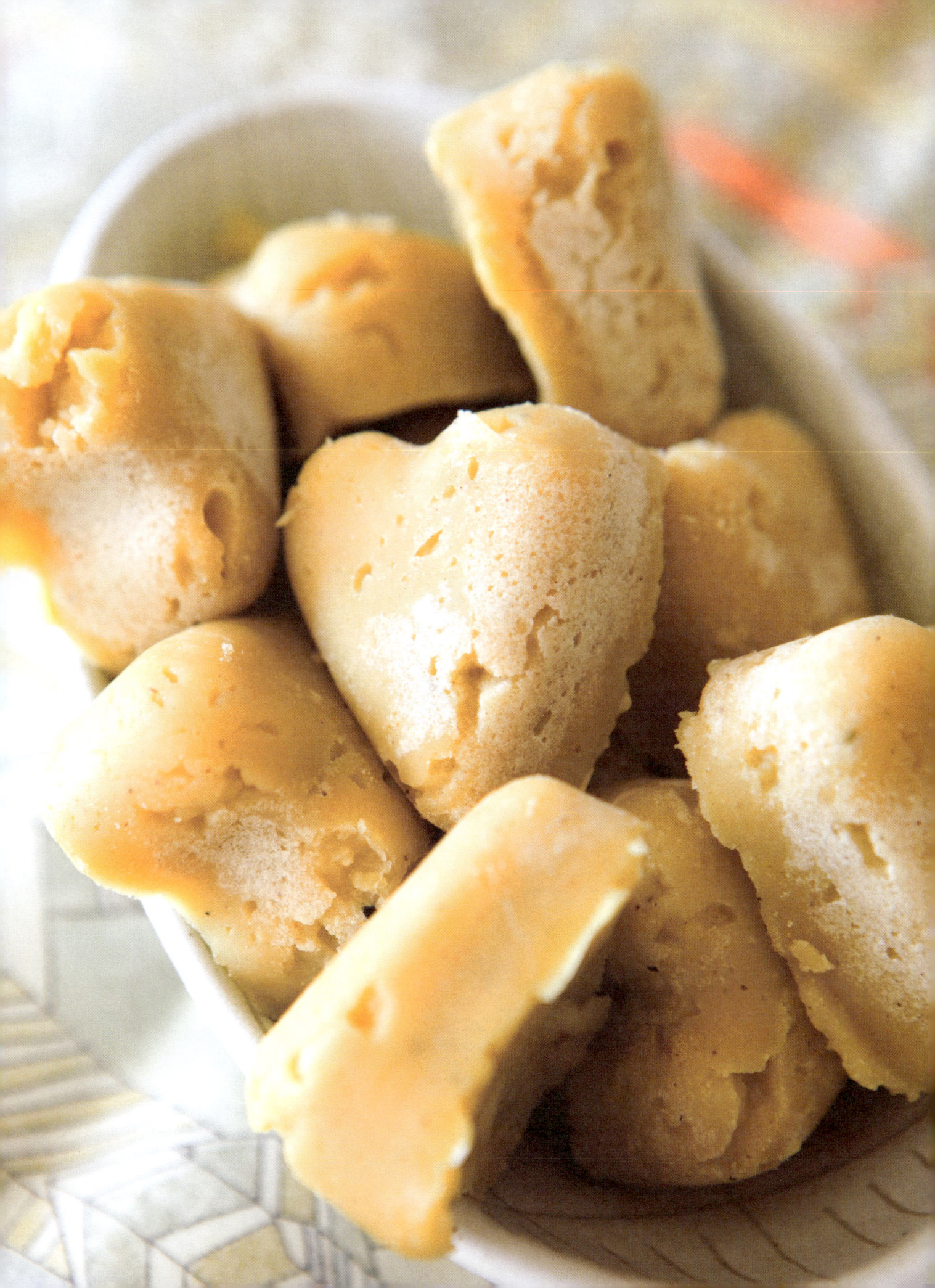

Recipes: Party Food & Something Sweet

DATE BALLS

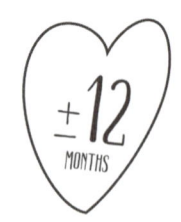

+12 months

raw; superfood; vegetarian; vegan; egg-free; grain-free; for adults too; great for lunchboxes

Makes 40 toddler sized date balls

• •

These are a really great quick-to-make addition to any birthday party treat table. They are also a great addition to school lunchboxes or as an any day snack.

The date balls are full of essential nutrients, vitamins and minerals. Dates do have a high natural sugar content, but due to their high fibre content, they are filling too so your little one will not be tempted to eat too many of them - as opposed to regular sweets!

These will provide a boost of energy so perhaps best not to serve before bedtime!

• •

1 cup dates, pitted
1 cup warm water
½ cup almonds or cashew nuts, activated and ground
½ cup desiccated coconut
¼ cup sunflowers seeds, activated and ground
¼ cup flaxseeds, ground
1 T. raw honey
1 t. green powder *(a blend of chlorella, spirulina, barley and wheatgrass)*
1 t. ground cinnamon
1 t. vanilla powder
coconut oil for rolling

Soak the dates in the water for an hour. If you do not have time to wait for the dates to soak, you can soak them in boiling water instead. This will take approximately 10 minutes.

Place the dates and the rest of the ingredients in a food processor and process until well blended (the younger your little one is, the smoother you need this paste to be).

Coat your hands will coconut oil (to prevent the date ball mixture from sticking to your hands when you roll the balls).

Take a teaspoon of mixture at a time and roll into a ball. Place the prepared ball on a plate while you make the rest.

Place the date balls in the fridge for half an hour before serving – to harden them slightly.

Date balls can be frozen in a sealed container for a month. Defrost by leaving out at room temperature.

Variations:

- *You can experiment with many other flavours and ingredients such as chia seeds, raw cacao powder, goji berries, sesame seeds, nutmeg, pecan nuts, macadamia nuts and oats.*
- *Roll the dates balls in desiccated coconut or raw cacao powder*

♥ *Party Prep Tip: These can be made a day or two in advance and kept in a sealed container in the fridge or freezer.*

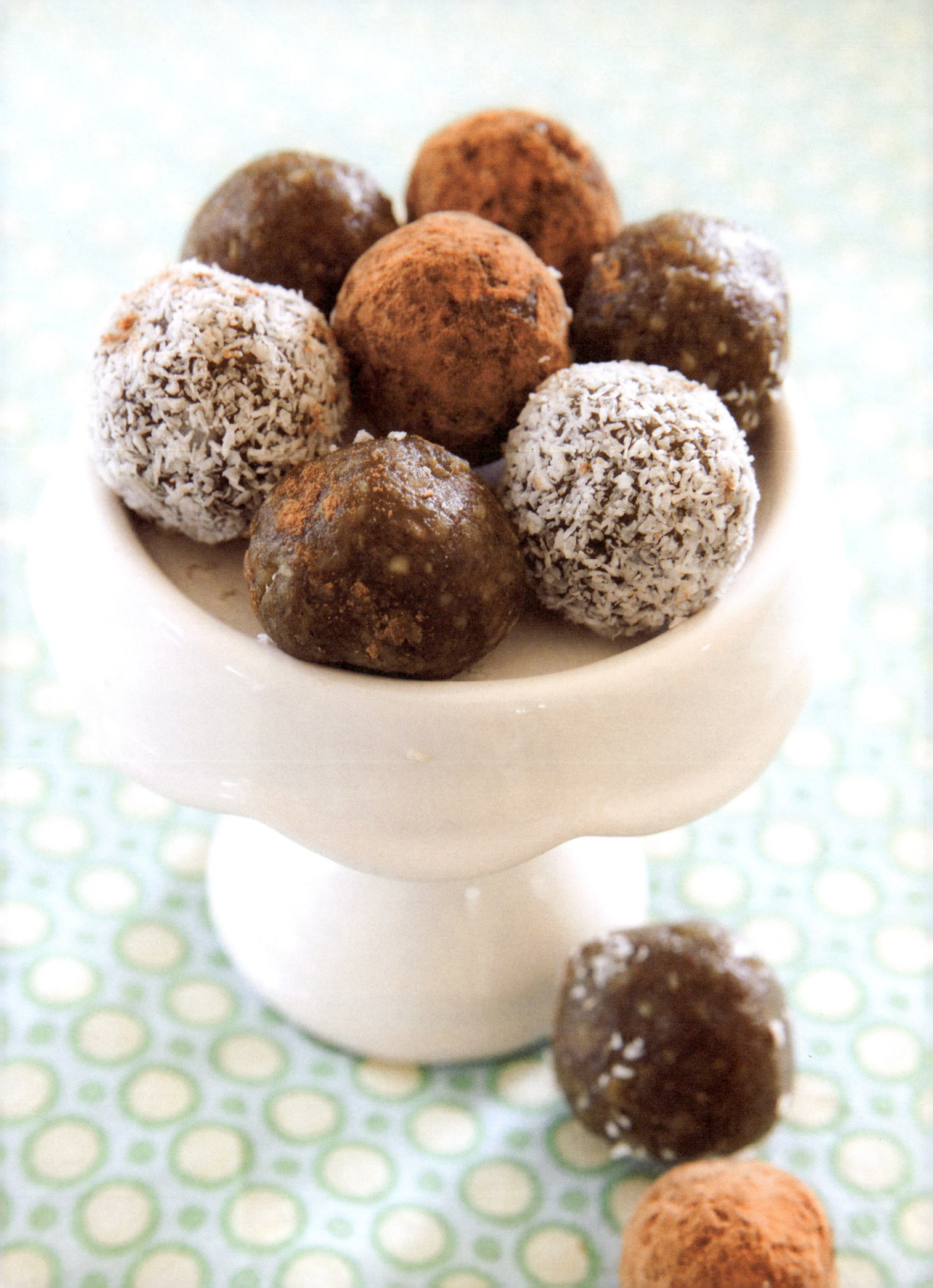

Recipes: Party Food & Something Sweet

CHOCOLATE MOUSSE

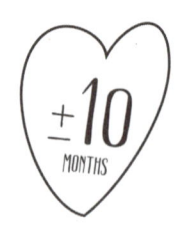

±10 MONTHS

raw; superfood; vegetarian; vegan; egg-free; grain-free; for adults too; great for lunchboxes

Makes approximately 4 little people servings.

What is conventionally considered a dessert is now a wholesome meal! This is currently Mila's go-to school lunch, and here's why:

♡ Avocado is a nutrient-dense food. It is high in unsaturated fats, which are important for normal growth and development of your little one's central nervous system and brain. It is a good source of vitamins B, C and K, fibre, folate and potassium. Avocados have anti-inflammatory properties; regulate blood sugar levels and support heart and blood vessels.

♡ Chia seeds are an excellent source of omega 3 fatty acids, fibre, protein, calcium, magnesium and iron. Gram for gram, they have more calcium than dairy and more omega 3 fatty acids than salmon!

♡ And then there's raw cacao powder – which you will see features quite often in this book! Raw Cacao is pure chocolate – the cacao bean, from the cacao tree, in its unprocessed, raw state.

♡ Besides the fact that it is delicious, it has been shown to be the food with the highest levels of antioxidants of any food on earth as well as having the highest concentration of several key nutrients, including iron and magnesium. Raw cacao also contains essential fatty acids, vitamin C, fibre, calcium, protein potassium, phosphorus, copper, and zinc. Additionally, it is naturally sugar-free and unlikely to cause an allergic reaction.

♡ It has anti-inflammatory and antioxidant benefits; it provides digestive support; and, supports healthy development of bones.

This chocolate mousse is the definition of delicious and nutritious!

1 avocado

3 dates, soaked

1 T. chia seeds, ground

3 T. raw cacao powder

1 T. coconut oil, melted

1 t. green powder *(blend of spirulina, chlorella, wheatgrass and barley grass)*

1 t. vanilla powder

Soak the ground chia seeds in ¼ cup water for 15 minutes.

Place the soaked seeds and water with the rest of the ingredients in a food processor and process until smooth and creamy.

Serve in little bowls or in a Mila's Meals ice cream cup.

It can be stored in a sealed container in the fridge for up to 3 days.

♥ **Party Prep Tip:** *This can be made a day in advance and kept in a sealed container in the fridge.*

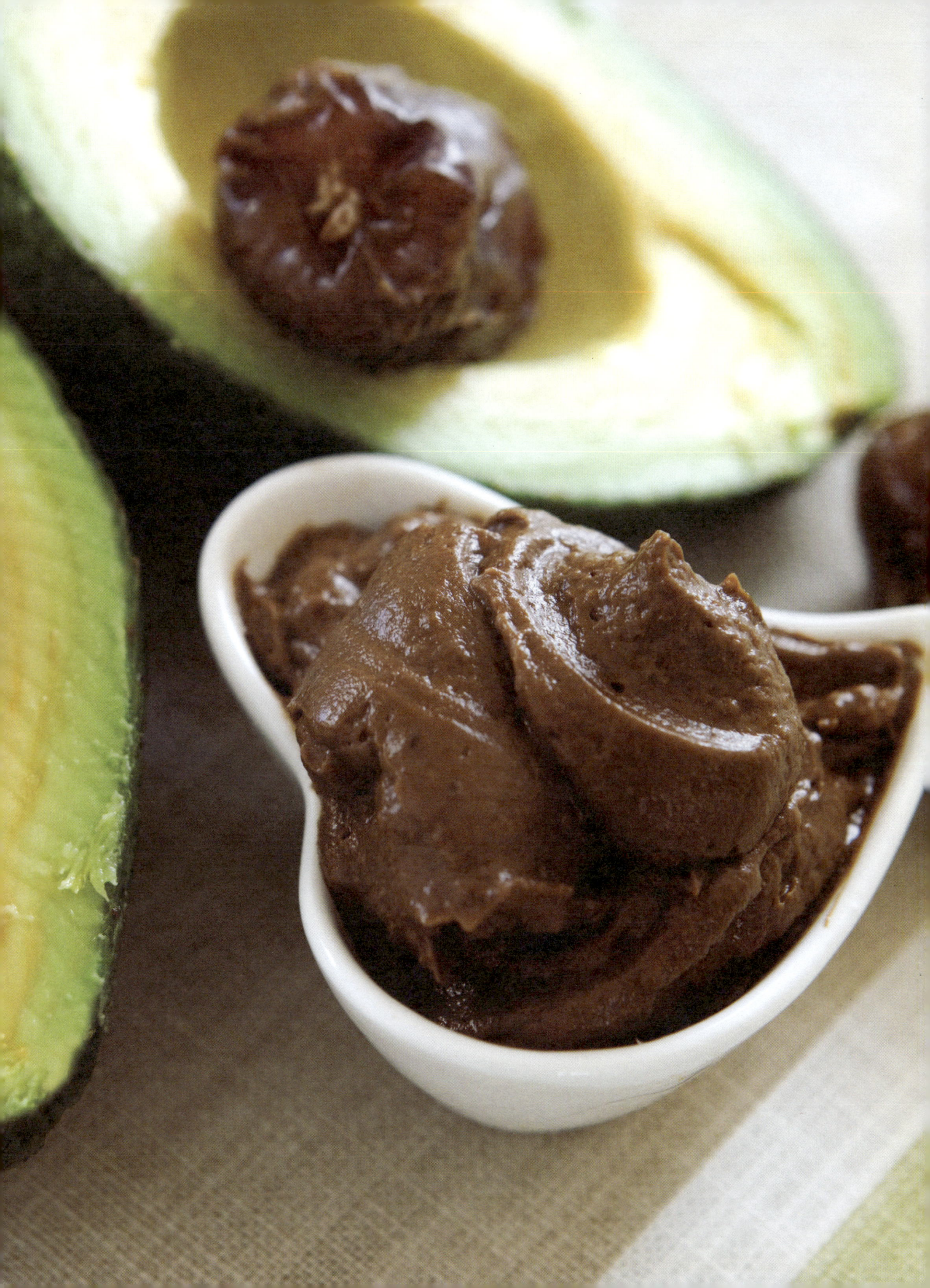

Recipes: Party Food & Something Sweet

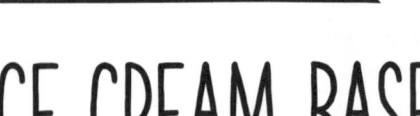

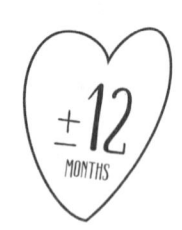

ICE CREAM BASE

±12 MONTHS

raw; vegetarian; vegan; egg-free; for adults too; great for lunchboxes

Makes 1 l (1 qt.) and serves 6 to 8 adults

While conventional ice cream is considered a dessert or a sweet treat, I feel compelled to share why I avoid it at all costs. It is not because of the dairy!

Store-bought ice cream has to be one of the most processed artificial foods available on the market today. Some of the 'ingredients' commonly include: **Calcium Sulphate** (a common lab and industrial chemical); **Polysorbate 80** (negatively affects the immune system and fertility); **Magnesium hydroxide** (can be used as a deodorant, a whitener in bleaching solutions and it even has smoke-suppressing and fire-retarding properties); **HFCS** (GMO); **Potassium Sorbate** (a suspected carcinogen); **Transfats**; **Soy Lecithin** or **Soya Lecithin** (a GM waste product containing solvents and pesticides); **Carrageenan** (has been found to destroy human cells and are linked to various human cancers and digestive disorders).

Then there are the flavourings… here is a partial list of some "flavouring" ingredients found in store-bought ice cream:
- **Diethylglycol** - a chemical used instead of egg yolks. It is also used in antifreeze and paint removers.
- **Piperonal** - it is used in place of vanilla – and to kill lice.
- **Butyraldehyde** - a nut flavouring. It is one of the ingredients in rubber cement.
- **Amylacetate** - a banana flavouring. It is also used as an oil paint solvent.
- **Benzyl Acetate** - a strawberry flavour. It is a nitrate solvent.
- **Castoreum** - a smelly, oily secretion that is found in two sacks between the anus and the external genitals of beavers. It is also used to flavour candies, drinks, and desserts.

Once you know what is actually in this sweet 'treat' – preventing and restricting its consumption should be the priority of any parent concerned with the health of their child.

Homemade ice cream is something completely different! I sometimes offer it to Mila for breakfast! And no, not as a treat… but as a wholesome meal!

Besides the fact that there are no synthetic ingredients or high quantities of genetically modified sugars, the main ingredient in this ice cream (coconut milk) has anti-inflammatory, antiviral, antifungal and antibacterial benefits. It contains high amounts of beneficial fat – including lauric acid, a type of fat rarely found in nature, which can only otherwise be found in breast milk! Other nutrients found in coconut milk include: vitamins B, C and E, iron, selenium, sodium, calcium, magnesium, and phosphorus.

800 ml (2 cans) preservative-free coconut milk
2 T. arrowroot powder
½ cup xylitol, or honey
2 t. alcohol-free vanilla extract, or seeds of 1 vanilla pod
4 T. kefir (optional)

Place the coconut milk and arrowroot powder in a saucepan over medium heat and stir to combine. Bring the mixture to the boil while stirring continuously. Cook for an additional 2 minutes to allow the mixture to thicken – it should be the consistency of thick syrup.

Add the xylitol or honey and vanilla and stir until it has all combined well.

Add any additional flavours at this stage.

Transfer the ice cream mixture to a mixing bowl, cover and allow it to cool (this could take up to 4 hours in the fridge, so perhaps do this overnight).

Transfer the mixture to an ice cream maker, add the kefir if using and follow the manufacturer's instructions.

Serve immediately in bowls, Mila's Meals ice cream cups or transfer to a freezer-safe container and keep frozen until ready to serve.

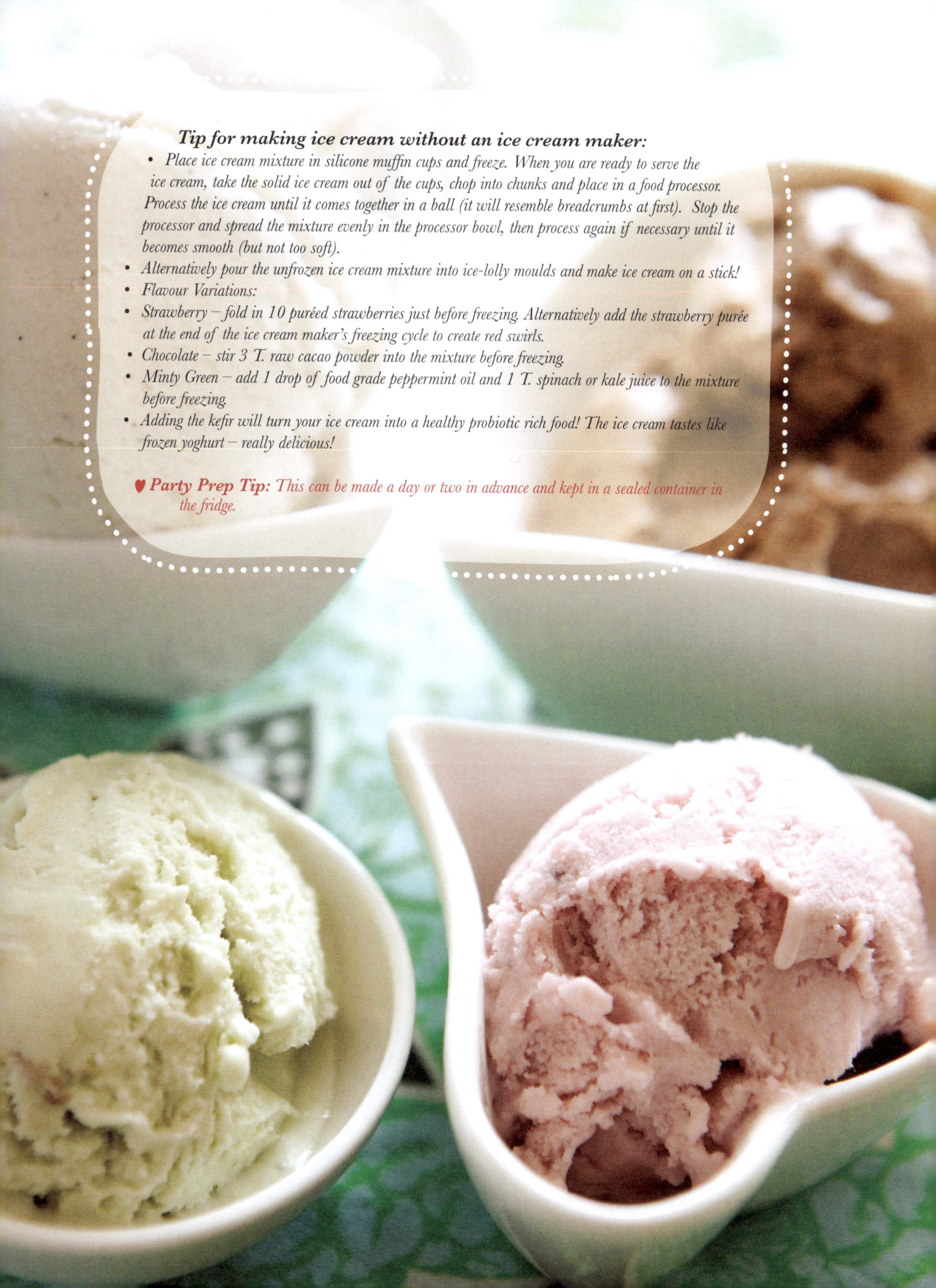

Tip for making ice cream without an ice cream maker:

- *Place ice cream mixture in silicone muffin cups and freeze. When you are ready to serve the ice cream, take the solid ice cream out of the cups, chop into chunks and place in a food processor. Process the ice cream until it comes together in a ball (it will resemble breadcrumbs at first). Stop the processor and spread the mixture evenly in the processor bowl, then process again if necessary until it becomes smooth (but not too soft).*
- *Alternatively pour the unfrozen ice cream mixture into ice-lolly moulds and make ice cream on a stick!*
- *Flavour Variations:*
- *Strawberry – fold in 10 puréed strawberries just before freezing. Alternatively add the strawberry purée at the end of the ice cream maker's freezing cycle to create red swirls.*
- *Chocolate – stir 3 T. raw cacao powder into the mixture before freezing.*
- *Minty Green – add 1 drop of food grade peppermint oil and 1 T. spinach or kale juice to the mixture before freezing.*
- *Adding the kefir will turn your ice cream into a healthy probiotic rich food! The ice cream tastes like frozen yoghurt – really delicious!*

♥ **Party Prep Tip:** *This can be made a day or two in advance and kept in a sealed container in the fridge.*

Recipes: Party Food & Something Sweet

NANA-CHOC ICE CREAM

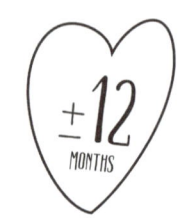

±12 MONTHS

raw; superfood; vegetarian; vegan; egg-free; grain-free; for adults too

Makes 5 toddler sized servings

A quick and easy way to make an ice cream! Perfect for a mid-afternoon snack.

You can freeze the bananas with the peels on. This will prevent them from discolouring. When you are ready to use them, use a knife to top and tail the banana, score the skin lengthwise and peel the skin off.

- 2 bananas, cut into chunks and frozen
- 3 dates, soaked, pitted and chopped
- 2 T. nut butter
- 1 T. raw cacao powder

Place the bananas and dates in a food food processor. Process until relatively smooth.

Add nut butter and cacao powder and process again.

Pour the mixture into serving dishes or freezer container and freeze for half an hour.

Serve as is if you froze it in a serving dish, or scoop it into a Mila's Meals ice cream cup.

Ice cream can be stored in a sealed container for a couple of months.

♥ *Party Prep Tip: This can be made a day or three in advance and kept in a sealed container in the freezer.*

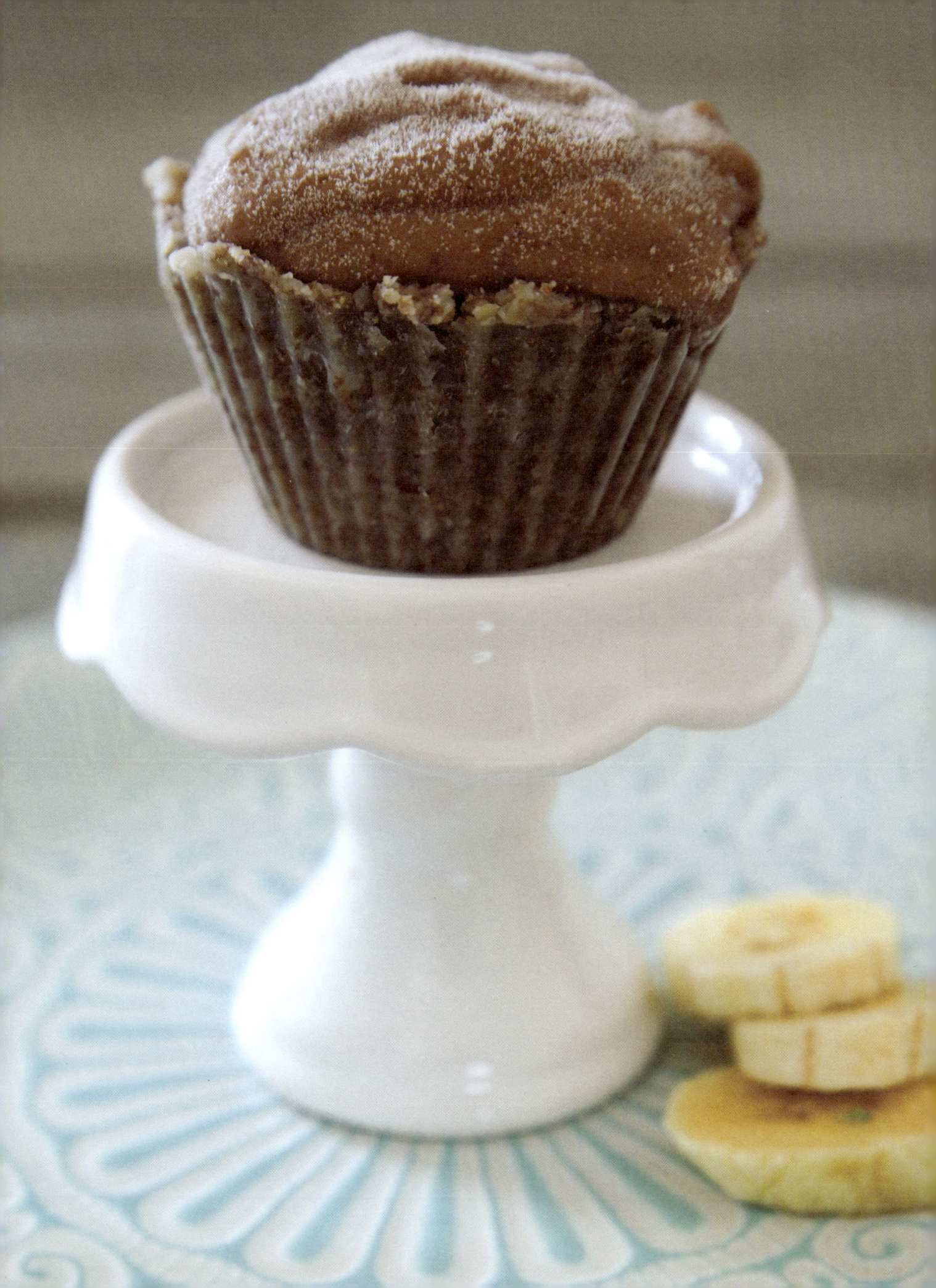

Recipes: Party Food & Something Sweet

RAW ICE CREAM CUPS

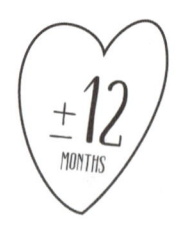

+12 MONTHS

raw; superfood; vegetarian; vegan; egg-free; grain-free; for adults too

Makes 6 cups

I was determined to find a healthy alternative to those neon pink and yellow ice cream cones you buy in the supermarket - I shudder to think what those are actually made of!

This was an experiment that turned out perfectly the very first time I tried it!

For a savoury alternative, simply omit the honey. Savoury cups can be filled with Mila's Meals Guacamole, Hummus or Veggie Spread.

- 1 cup flax seeds, ground
- ½ cup sunflower seeds, activated and ground
- ½ cup coconut oil, melted
- ¼ cup raw honey or maple syrup

Place all the ingredients in a food processor and pulse until well combined.

Scoop a tablespoon of mixture into a silicone muffin cup mould and, using your thumb, press the mixture into the base and the sides of the cup. Wet your hands to prevent the mixture from sticking to them.

Place all the cups on a tray and allow to set in the fridge. This will take approximately 1 hour.

When you are ready to serve your ice cream, pop the ice cream cups out of the silicone moulds and scoop in your ice cream.

Serve immediately.

These cups are also great containers for the Mila's Meals Chocolate Mousse.

Left over cups can be kept in the freezer (without any fillings in them). Allow to stand at room temperature for approximately half an hour to defrost – or serve frozen for extra crunch!

They will keep in the freezer for a couple of months.

- ***Please note:*** *due to the nature of coconut oil, these will get very soft if left out at room temperature on a hot day.*
- ***Party Prep Tip:*** *These can be made a day or three in advance and kept in a sealed container in the freezer.*

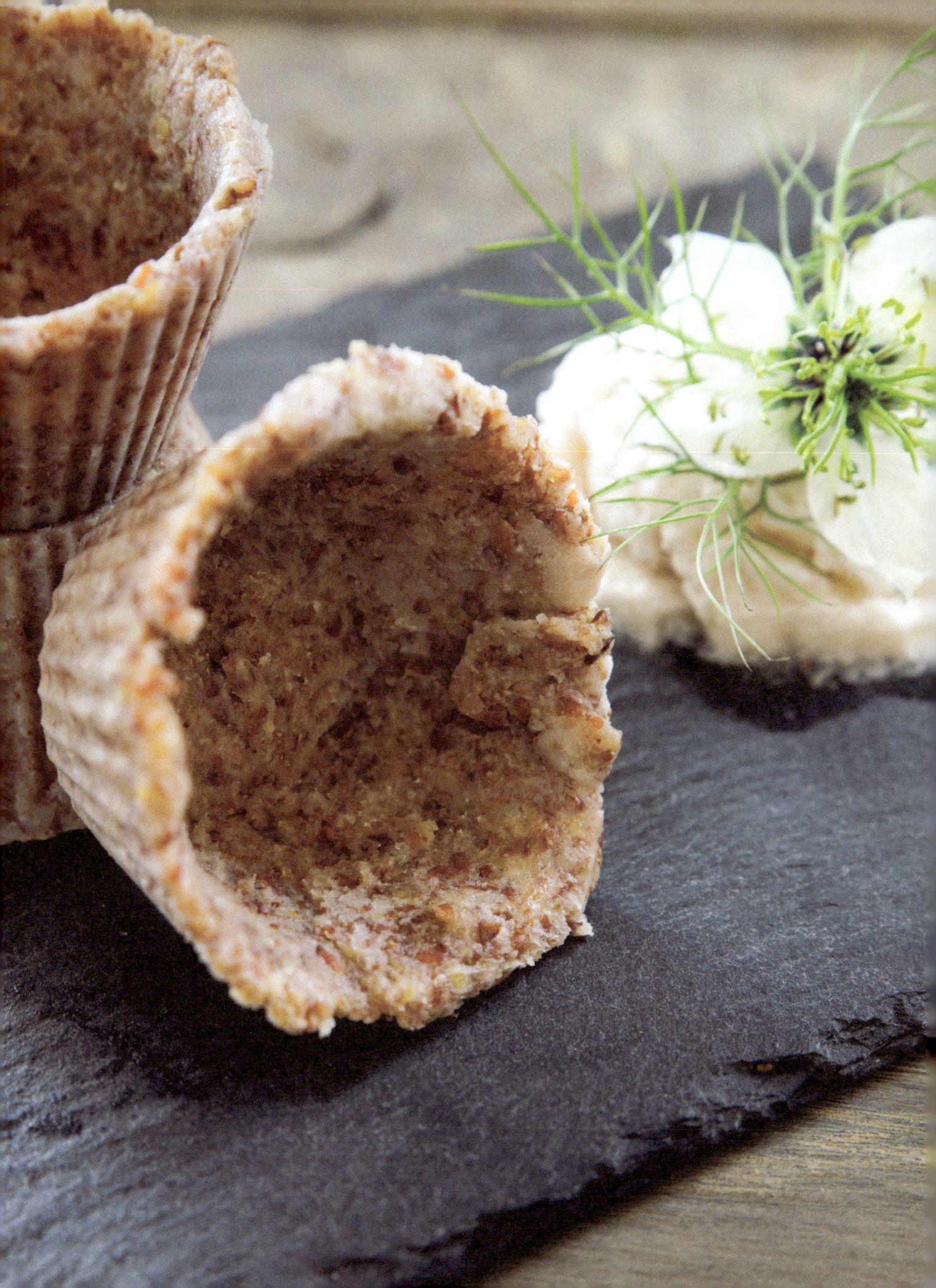

Recipes: Party Food & Something Sweet

ICE LOLLIES

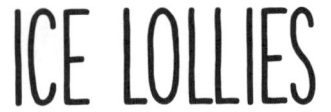

±10 MONTHS

raw; vegetarian; vegan; egg-free; grain-free; for adults too

I remember freezing fruit juice in a cup as a child. I would spend an hour scraping out the iced juice and loving every minute (and mouthful) of it. Today there are ice-lolly moulds available that have turned ice lolly making into something of an art form!

These are some ideas for basic (but delicious and beautiful) fruit lollies using the whole fruit as opposed to just the juice. It works out cheaper that way (you use less fruit) and there is the added benefit of including all the fibre from the fruit.

Ice lollies are a great remedy for sore gums when your little one is teething. They can also help to bring a temperature down – as will any ice cold drink.

1 cup fruit of choice

± 100 ml liquid *(freshly squeezed apple or orange juice, water or herbal tea)*

1-2 t. raw honey or maple syrup *(optional - depending on how naturally sweet the fruit is)*

Add the fruit to a food processor or blender and pulse.

Add the liquid and honey and process or blend until smooth.

Should there be any pip shreds that you think your little one may not like, you can sieve the mixture into a jug.

Pour the mixture into lolly moulds, add the sticks and lids and freeze for at least 4 hours (it is better to freeze overnight).

Run the ice-lolly mould under hot water to loosen the lollies and serve immediately.

Some of Mila's favourite ice-lollies:

- *Mixed Berry* - (simply buy a packet of frozen mixed berries and defrost before blending). You should sieve this mixture.
- *Strawberry* - You should sieve this mixture.
- *Kiwi Fruit* - You should sieve this mixture and you may need to add more honey as the kiwi fruit can be quite tart.
- *Watermelon* - The watermelon has a high water content so you will not need to add additional liquid. Blend the fruit with the seeds and then sieve out the shreds, as the seeds are full of nutrients including fatty acids, essential proteins, vitamins and minerals.
- *Rainbow Lolly* - For a quicker way to make a layered lolly, simply layer purée fruit. Use puréed strawberries, apricot, peach or mango, kiwi fruit and blueberry. Using this method will require you to freeze each layer for before adding the next, as the puree might be too thin to hold the weight of another layer.
- *Lychee and Coconut* - Peel and pit the lychees and use coconut milk as the liquid.

Quick and easy ice lollies:

- *When you prepare your morning veggie juice, make a slightly sweeter version and use that for ice lollies. While this will have less fibre than the recipe above, it is still highly nutritious – and you only have to wash your juicer once that day! Mila's favourite flavour is pineapple and beetroot juice – it is naturally sweet enough so there is no need to add honey and it has a brilliant cerise colour which Mila loves!*
- *You can also freeze any smoothie into an ice lolly. Mila is texture sensitive to some foods – she will not drink a smoothie, but as soon as I make an ice lolly out of it, she loves it!*
- ***Party Prep Tip:*** *This can be made a day or three in advance.*

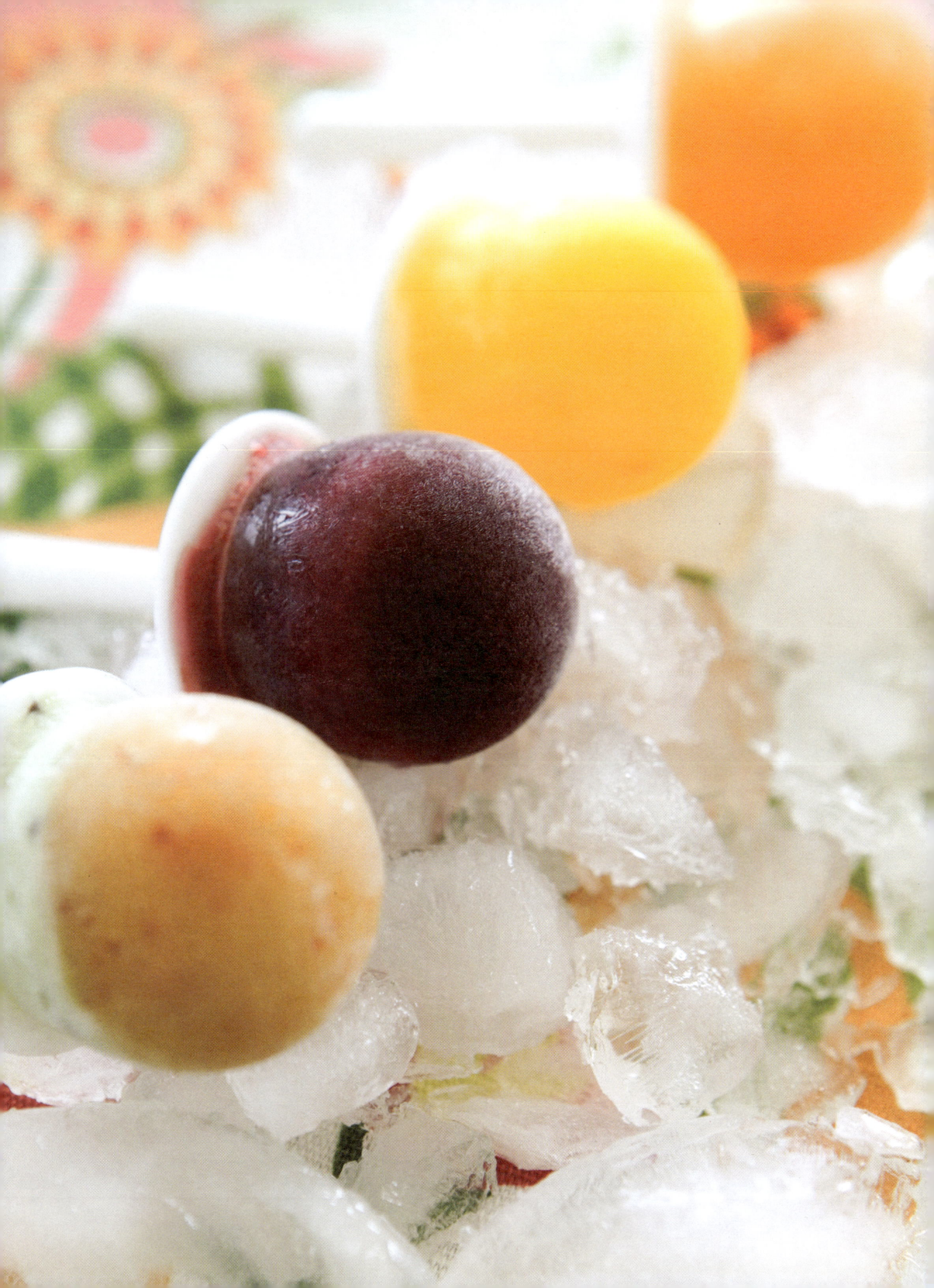

Recipes: Party Food & Something Sweet

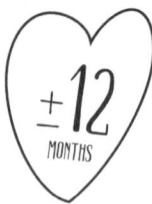

+12 MONTHS

CHOCOLATE (OR VANILLA) CUPCAKES

superfood; vegetarian; grain-free; for adults too; great for lunchboxes

Makes 12 cupcakes

These cupcakes are loved by everyone who tastes them and I am often told they taste even better than regular cupcakes – and they have a vegetable in them!

The sweet potato creates a softer, spongier texture and adds to the sweetness of the cupcake – reducing he amount of sweetener needed.

The trick to using almond flour successfully is to beat it with the eggs for 2 minutes before adding any other ingredients. This allows the rather dry flour to soften before being cooked and prevents the cupcakes from being dry and crumbly.

Please see the end of this chapter for some decoration ideas.

- 2 cups almond flour
- 3 organic eggs
- 2 T. coconut oil, melted
- 1 cup coconut milk *(at room temperature)*
- 3 T. raw honey or maple syrup
- 2 t. vanilla powder or alcohol-free vanilla essence
- ¼ t. Himalayan or sea salt
- ½ t. baking soda
- 1 t. aluminium-free baking powder
- ½ cup sweet potato, cooked, skin removed and mashed *(at room temperature)*
- 3 T. raw cacao powder *(optional)*

Preheat the oven to 180°C (350°F).

Line a muffin tray with paper cupcake liners.

Beat the flour and the eggs with an electric beater for 2 minutes.

Add the coconut oil, coconut milk, honey, vanilla extract and salt and beat for another 30 seconds.

Add baking powder, baking soda, sweet potato and cacao and beat until mixed.

Immediately scoop the batter into the paper cups. They should be 3/4 full to allow space for rising.

Bake for 20 minutes or until toothpick inserted into the centre comes out clean.

Remove cupcakes from muffin tray and cool on a wire rack.

Once the cupcakes are cool, ice them with any one of the icings on the following pages.

If there are any leftovers, they can be frozen for up to a month.

Variations:
- This recipe would work well as a cake too. Double the recipe and bake 2 separate layers for a layer cake. The filling could be a mixture of the Mila's Meals Chocolate Icing and chopped strawberries (or other seasonal berries).

♥ *Party Prep Tip: These are best made on the day of the party.*

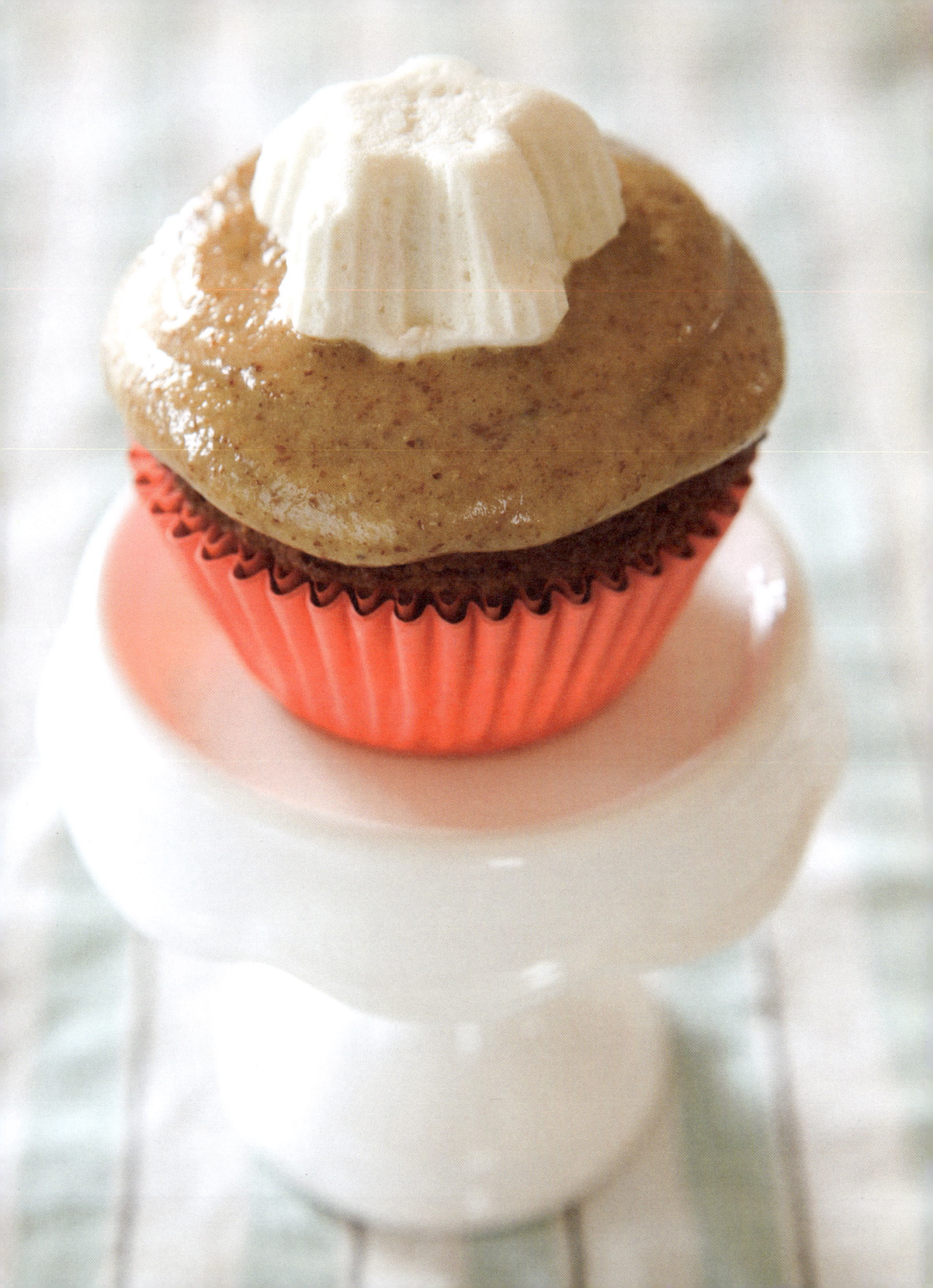

CARROT CUPCAKES

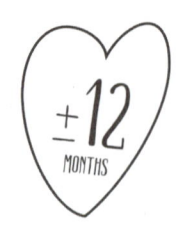

+12 months

vegetarian; grain-free; for adults too; great for lunchboxes

Makes 12 cupcakes

This recipe came about as a way to use up some of the pulp from Mila's morning juices instead of putting it all into the compost bin. It also makes use of cooked sweet potato which you may have leftover from dinner or from another recipe. You can also add some of the other juice pulp such as beetroot, pineapple and apple.

I used to feed Mila these as an afternoon snack when she woke up from her afternoon nap – they are full of vegetables making them a quick-and-easy nutritious snack. I would take one out of the freezer after she had gone to sleep – by the time she woke up it was defrosted and ready to eat.

The Mila's Meals Vanilla Icing or Nut Butter Icing works well on these cupcakes. Alternatively, leave the icing off and call it a muffin – great for breakfast or school lunchboxes.

1¾ cups almond flour

3 organic eggs

¼ t. Himalayan or sea salt

½ t. baking soda

1 t. aluminium-free baking powder

½ T. cinnamon

1 t. vanilla powder or alcohol-free essence

2 T. coconut oil, melted

¼ cup raw honey or maple syrup

1 cup freshly grated carrots, or carrot pulp from your morning juice

½ cup sweet potato, cooked, peeled and mashed

Preheat the oven to 160°C (320°F).

Line a muffin tray with paper cupcake liners.

Beat the flour and the eggs with an electric beater for 2 minutes.

Add the salt, baking soda, baking powder, cinnamon, vanilla powder, coconut oil and honey and beat to mix.

Add the carrots and sweet potato and mix in well with a spoon.

Scoop the batter into the cupcake cups. They should be 3/4s full to allow space for rising.

Bake for 20 minutes or until toothpick inserted into the centre comes out clean.

Remove cupcakes from muffin tray and cool on a wire rack.

Once the cupcakes are cool, ice them with any one of the icings on the following pages.

If there are any leftovers, they can be frozen for up to a month.

♥ *Party Prep Tip: These are best made on the day of the party.*

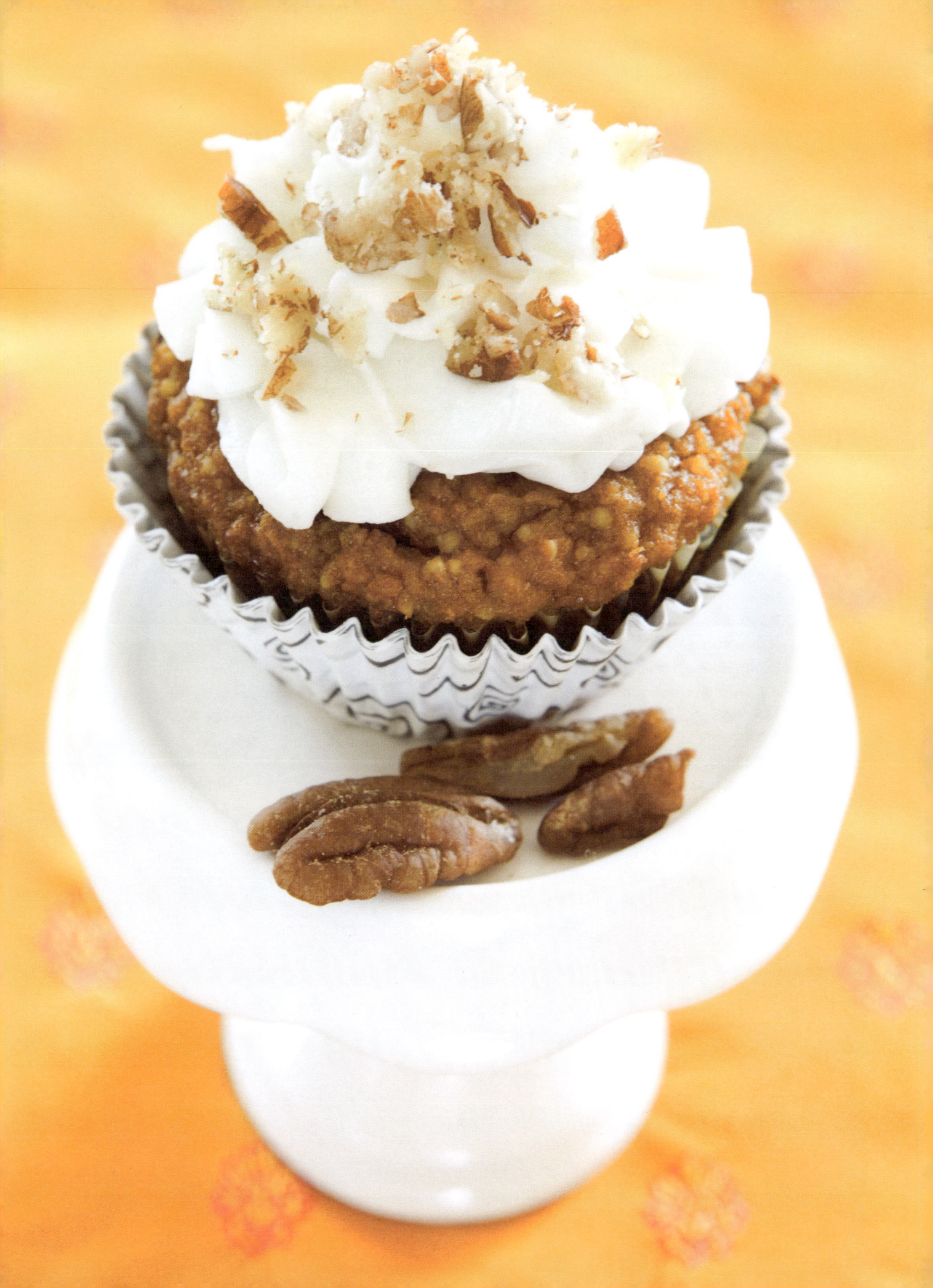

Recipes: Party Food & Something Sweet

STICKY CHOCOLATE LAYER CAKE

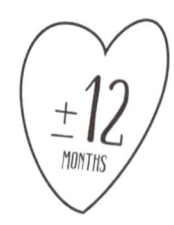

+12 months

superfood; vegetarian; vegan; egg-free; for adults too; great for lunchboxes

This is a great alternative to the previous cupcake recipes should your little one have a nut or egg allergy. It makes for quite a dense, sticky cake – so do not expect a light and fluffy one!

The Mila's Meals Chocolate Icing recipe works really well with this cake. The filling could be a mixture of the chocolate icing and chopped strawberries (or other seasonal berries).

Please see the end of this chapter for some decoration ideas.

1 cup chickpea flour
½ cup brown rice flour
2 T. raw apple cider vinegar
1½ cups warm water
1 cup dates, pitted
½ cup coconut oil, melted
¼ cup honey or maple syrup
1 T. vanilla powder or alcohol-free essence
1 cup tapioca flour
½ cup raw cacao powder
1½ t. baking soda
1½ t. guar gum
¼ t. Himalayan or sea salt

Place the chickpea flour, brown rice flour and apple cider vinegar in a mixing bowl and stir in the warm water. Add the dates to the bowl.

Cover with a dish towel and allow to soak for 8 hours or overnight.

Preheat the oven to 180°C (350°F).

Grease two round cake tins (approximately 20 cm/9").

Place the soaked flours, dates and soak water in a blender or food processor. Add the coconut oil, honey and vanilla powder and blend until smooth.

Place the tapioca flour, raw cacao powder, baking soda, guar gum and salt together in a mixing bowl and mix with a whisk.

Add the dry ingredients to the wet mixture and blend well.

Pour the cake batter into the prepared cake tins and bake for approximately 20 minutes, or until a toothpick inserted comes out clean.

Transfer the cakes to a wire rack to cool.

Allow to cool completely before icing.

Left over cake can be stored in the freezer for up to a month.

Variations:
- Due to the dense, sticky texture of this cake it would make a great chocolate brownie too. Simply bake in a square baking tray and once cool, cut into squares.

♥ *Party Prep Tip: This is best made on the day of the party.*

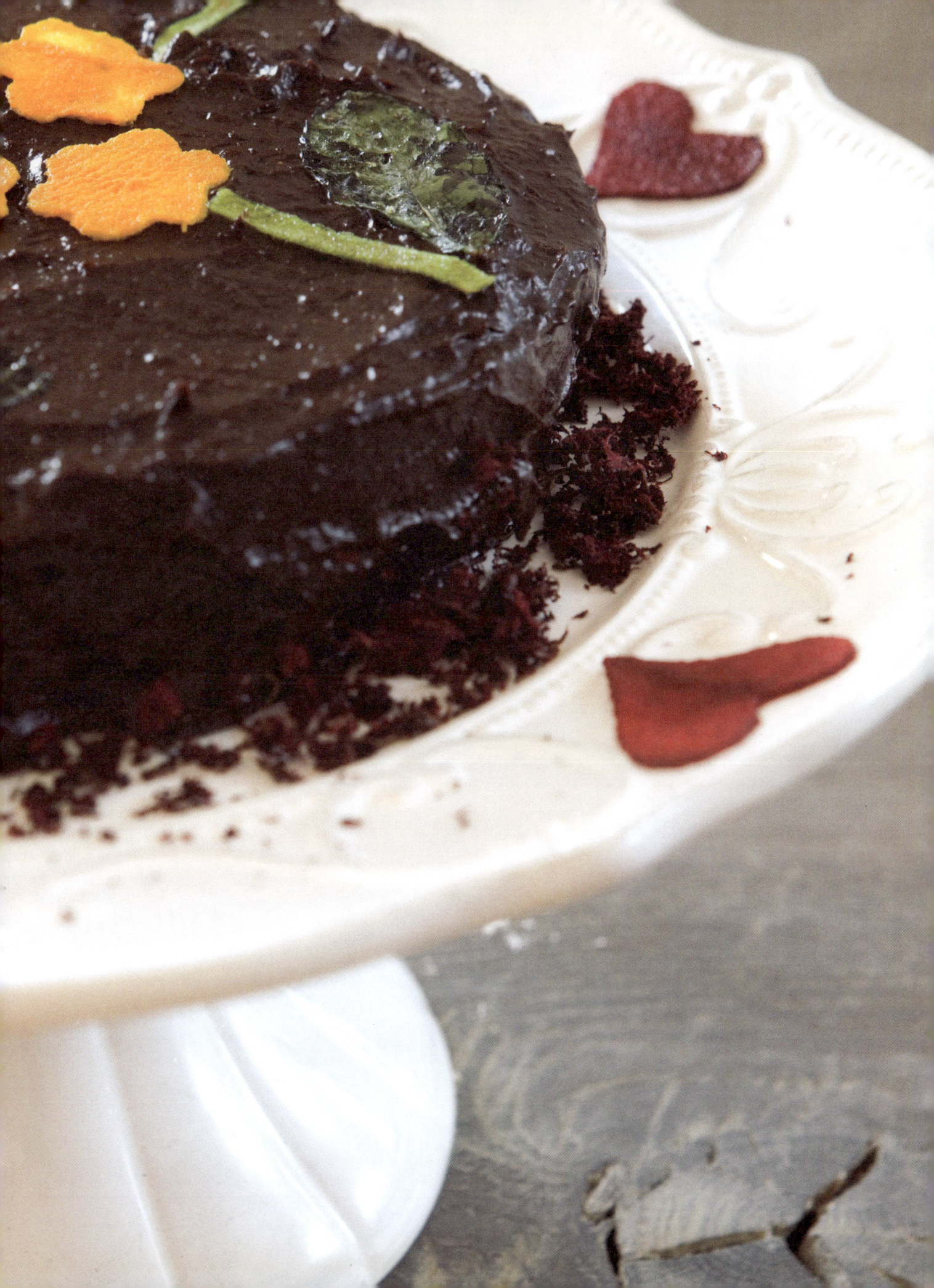

Recipes: Party Food & Something Sweet

ICINGS

♥ *Party Prep Tip:* These are best made on the day of the party.

CHOCOLATE ICING

raw; superfood; vegetarian; vegan; egg-free; grain-free; for adults too

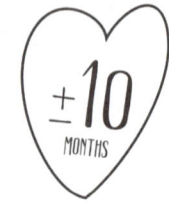

± 10 MONTHS

2 avocados
¼ cup raw honey or maple syrup
4 dates, pitted and soaked for 2 hours
3 T. raw cacao powder
3 T. coconut oil, melted
1 t. vanilla extract

Place all the ingredients in a food processor and process until smooth.

Ice the cakes or cupcakes then place them in the fridge to allow the icing to set.

Notes:
- The icing will 'melt' in hot weather. If your little one's party is in summer, keep the iced cupcakes / cake in the fridge until you need them.
- The Mila's Meals Chocolate Fudge recipe can also be used to make an icing.

• •

VANILLA ICING

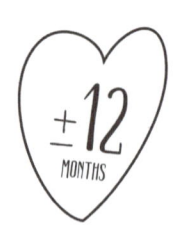

raw; vegetarian; vegan; egg-free; grain-free; for adults too

± 12 MONTHS

1 cup cashew nuts, soaked
¼ cup warm water
2 T. coconut oil, melted
2 T. raw honey or ½ T. stevia
seeds from 1 vanilla pod
1 t. lemon juice, freshly squeezed

Place all the ingredients in a food processor and process until smooth.

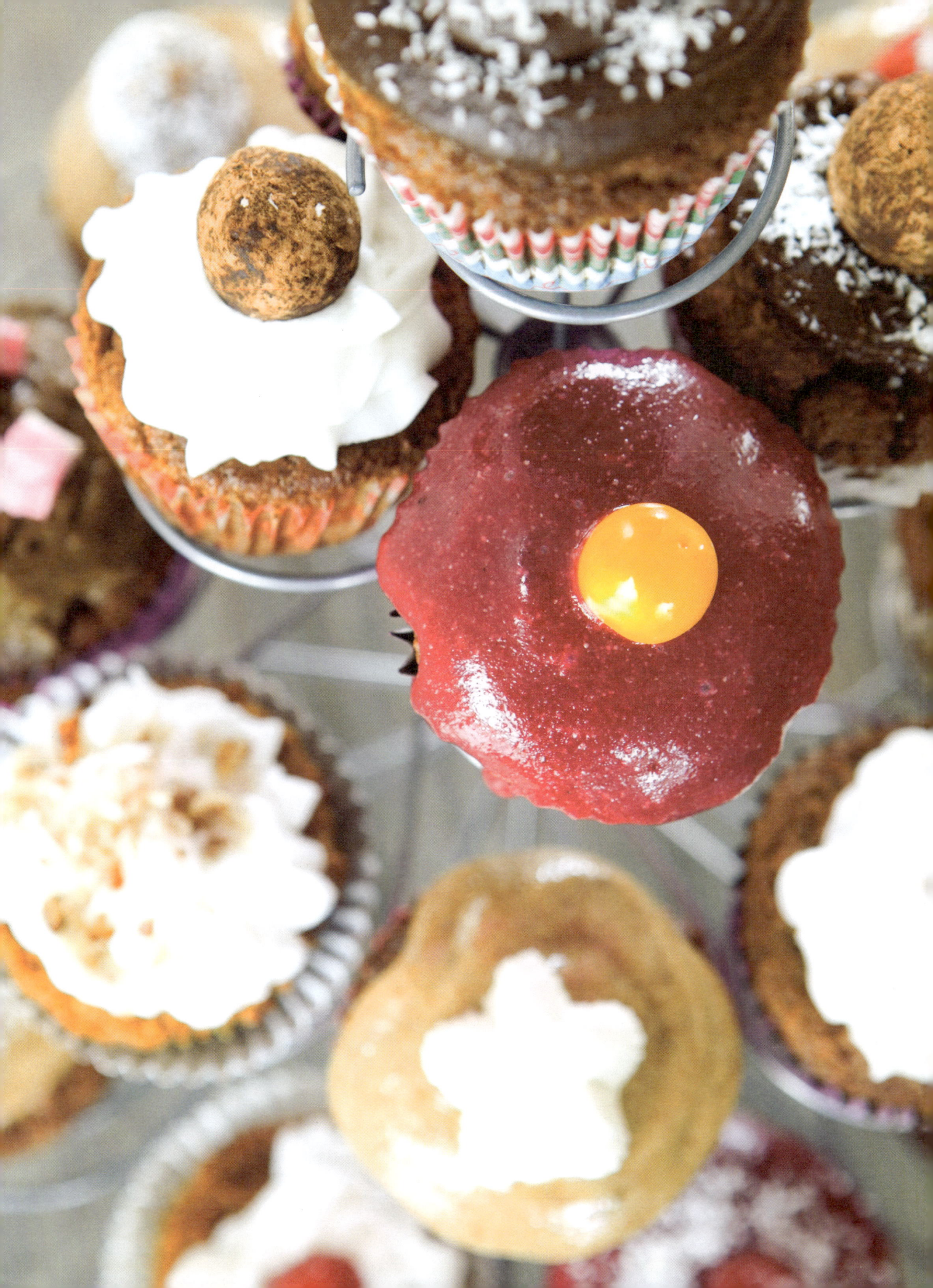

Recipes: Party Food & Something Sweet

± 12 MONTHS

RUBY RED ICING

raw; vegetarian; vegan; egg-free; grain-free; for adults too

½ cup cashew or macadamia nuts, soaked
¼ cup coconut oil, melted
3 T. raw honey or maple syrup
1 - 3 t. beetroot juice

Blend all the ingredients together in a blender or small food processor until smooth starting with 1t. sweetener and adding more as needed.

Chill in the fridge for 5 to 10 minutes (this allows the coconut oil to set).

Variations:
- *For orange icing, use carrot juice instead of beetroot.*
- *For green icing, use spinach juice instead of beetroot (you will not taste it).*
- *You can also flavour the icing with food grade essential oils or extracts such as orange, lemon, peppermint or rose oil.*

NUT BUTTER ICING

raw; vegetarian; vegan; egg-free; grain-free; for adults too

2 cups nut butter *(almond or macadamia butter are great options)*
½ cup honey or maple syrup
¼ cup coconut oil, melted

Place all the ingredients in a food processor and process until well mixed.

COCONUT ICING (& REAL BUTTER ICING OPTION)

raw; vegetarian; vegan; egg-free; for adults too

½ cup xylitol, ground in coffee grinder
1 t. potato or tapioca flour
½ cup coconut oil, solid
½ t. alcohol-free, sugar-free vanilla extract
3 – 4 T. coconut milk *(do not shake the can before opening)*
3 t. any vegetable juice for desired colouring

Open the can of coconut milk and scoop of the solid milk to use in this recipe.

Mix the xylitol and potato or tapioca flour (this makes a sugar-free castor sugar / confectioner's sugar).

Using a handheld or stand mixer, beat coconut oil until smooth.

With the mixer running on low, add the xylitol mix, vanilla and 1 T. of coconut milk at a time, as needed, until the icing reaches a spreadable consistency. You may not need to use all of the coconut milk.

Beat on high for 2 more minutes until light and fluffy.

Add chosen colouring and beat to mix.

Variations:
- *If you are not dairy-free or vegan, you can make a real butter icing using the recipe above – simply replace the coconut oil with butter or ghee.*

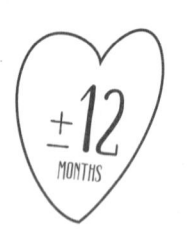

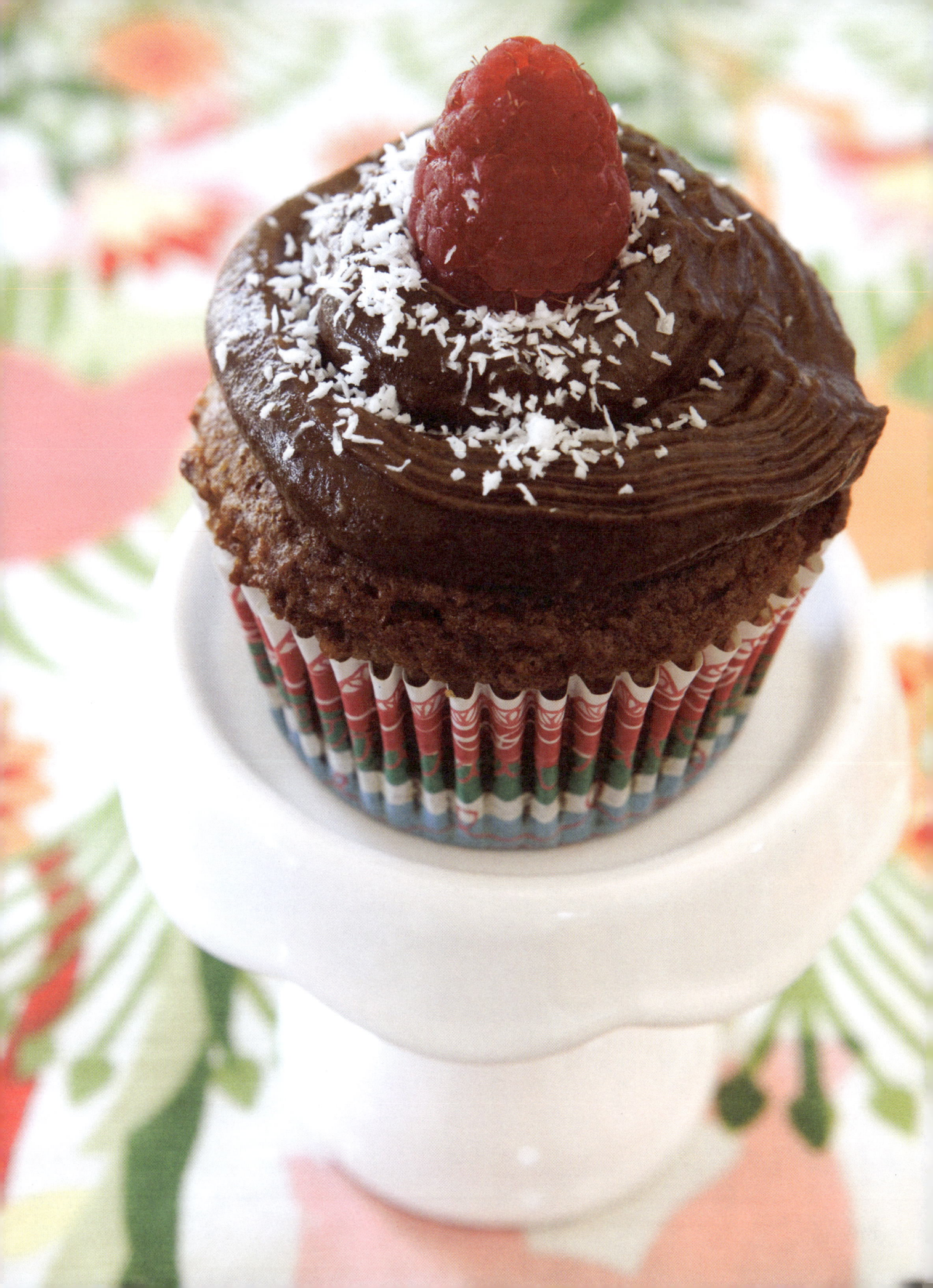

Recipes: Party Food & Something Sweet

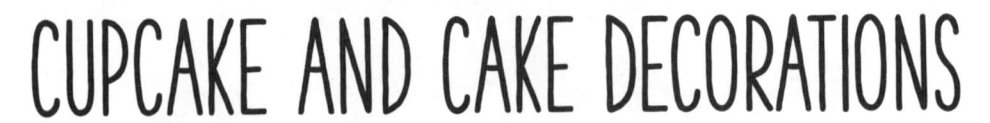

CUPCAKE AND CAKE DECORATIONS

I must say, I do eye out the candy cake decorations in the shops and wish I could sprinkle them on my cupcakes. They really are so pretty and the little ones love them! But I have found some natural alternatives, which work well too.

BALLS

BERRIES

If you are baking in berry season, then there is no easier way to add some colour and décor to your cupcakes and cakes. Simply pop a berry into the centre of your cupcake! Try one of these colourful berries: **raspberries; blueberries; gooseberries; strawberries** (these may have to be sliced if they are too big).

DATE BALLS

Miniature date balls are another way to add ball shaped decorations to your cupcakes. Although fairly time consuming to make, they can be made a day or three in advance. If you are using chocolate icing, roll the date balls in desiccated coconut so that there is a colour contrast. If you are using vanilla icing, dust them in raw cacao powder.

SHAPES

Apples are a very useful fruit for decorating - you can easily cut shapes out of apple slices and the apple flesh absorbs colours from fresh fruit juices – so you can create different coloured shapes.

Simply peel the apples, slice and soak in some lemon water to prevent discolouration. If you are going to dye the apple, simply add lemon juice to your fruit juice dyes.

Try beetroot juice for pink, blueberry juice for purple, spinach or kale juice for green and carrot juice for orange.

Dry the apple slices on kitchen towel and then using cookie cutters or special fondant icing shaping tools, cut out the shapes.

You can also cut shapes out of slices of peaches, nectarines, pineapples and plums – basically any fruit that has a big enough surface area once sliced.

The Mila's Meals Choc-Nut Fudge can also be used to create fun shapes for cupcakes with a vanilla or light coloured icing. Simply make a thin layer of fudge on a baking sheet, and once it has set, cut out your shapes.

STRANDS

Create wispy strands by finely shredding or grating carrots, spinach, beetroot or fresh coconut flesh.

Grated coconut strands can be dyed different colours using vegetable juices such as beetroot, pomegranate, cranberry, blueberry, spinach and carrot.

SPRINKLES

Desiccated coconut, sesame seeds and ground nuts work well on chocolate or any dark coloured icing. Chia seeds, poppy seeds and raisins work well on vanilla or light coloured icing.

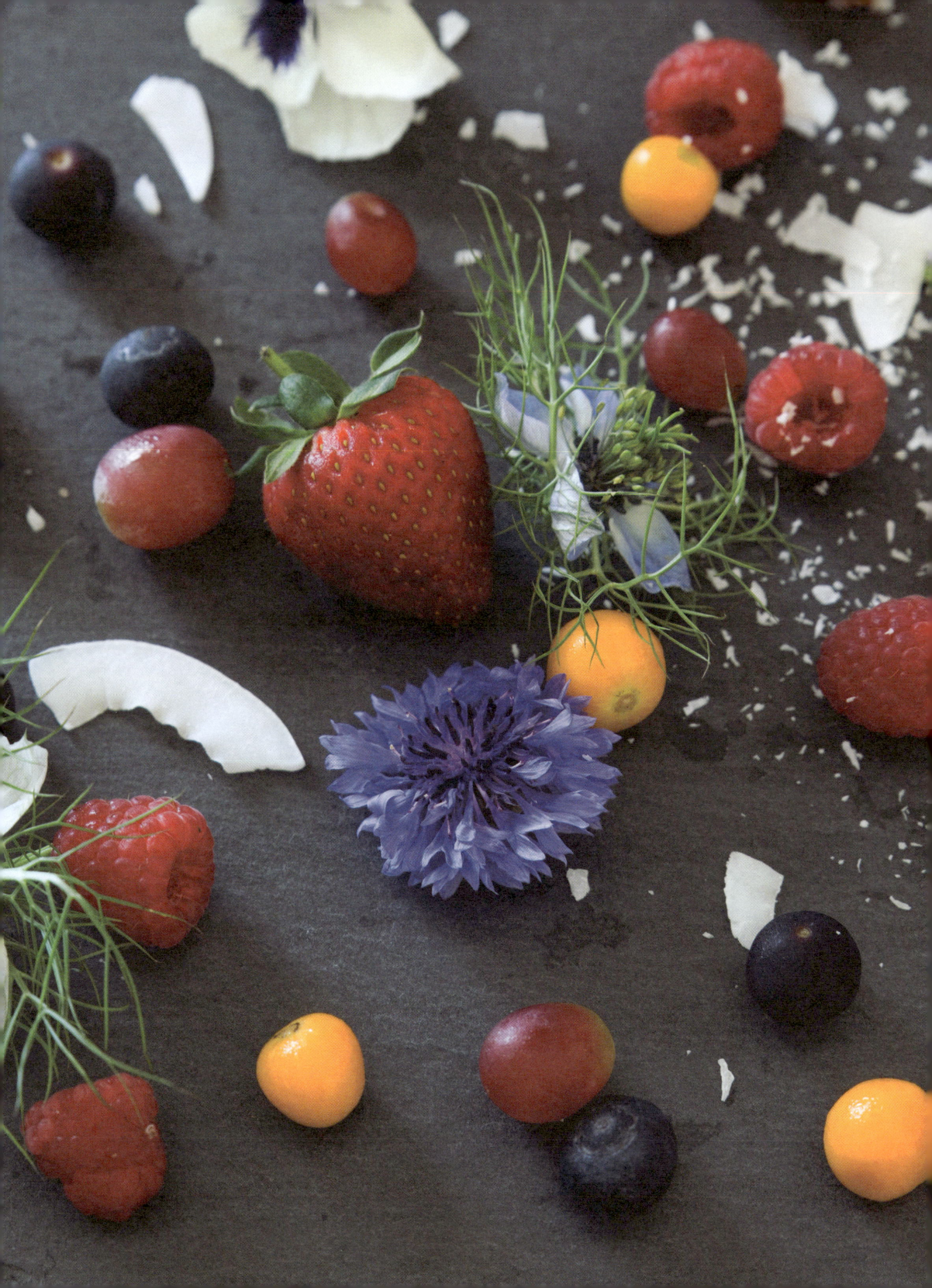

Recipes: Pantry Items

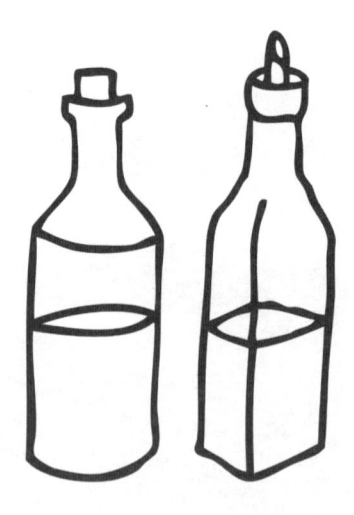

Quite a few recipes in this book require ingredients that need to be made ahead of time. With your time in the kitchen being limited now that you have a little one, it is best to pre-make a large batch of certain basics to save you time when you want to prepare a meal. Included in this section are some of the things I have pre-made in my pantry (or freezer).

Also included in this section are some of the nutritional enhancers that can be added to every meal as well as fermented foods… which should be added to every meal!

Recipes: Pantry Items

APPLESAUCE → 350
BREADCRUMBS → 352
STOCK (BONE BROTHS) → 354
   CHICKEN BONE BROTH (STOCK) → 356
   BEEF BONE BROTH (STOCK) → 358
CULTURED (FERMENTED) FOODS → 360
   DILLY CARROTS → 362
   BUBBLING BERRIES → 364
   FERMENTED APPLE SAUCE → 366
   SAUERKRAUT → 368
   KEFIR → 370
   KEFIR WHEY, YOGHURT & CHEESE → 372
FLOURS → 374
MILKS → 376
GLUTEN-FREE PLAY DOUGH! → 378

Recipes: Pantry Items

APPLESAUCE

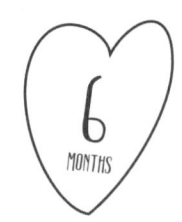

6 MONTHS

vegetarian; vegan; egg-free; grain-free; for adults too; great for lunchboxes

General rule of thumb: 450 g of apples will make 1 cup of applesauce.

• •

Apple sauce is an ingredient used in a couple of recipes in this book so it is convenient to make a big batch and keep it in the freezer to have ready for when you need it.

It also makes a great first food for your little one.

Naturally sweet apple varieties include Gala, Golden Delicious, Fuji and Pink Lady.

Apples are on the Dirty Dozen list so either buy organic, or be sure to wash them in a hydrogen peroxide or vinegar water solution.

• •

5 – 10 apples *(depending on how much applesauce you would like to make)*
½ t. cinnamon or nutmeg
1 cup water

Peel, core and chop the apples in to large chunks.

Place in a steamer and sprinkle with cinnamon or nutmeg. Steam for 20 minutes or until the apple is soft all the way through.

Alternatively place the apple and spices in a pot on the stove top, add the water and bring to the boil. Once the water is boiling, reduce the heat, cover the pot and simmer for 30 minutes or until the apple is soft all the way through.

Reserve the cooking liquid and place the apple pieces in a blender. Blend until smooth using some of the cooking water to thin the applesauce if necessary.

Transfer to containers or ice cube trays for freezing.

Applesauce can be refrigerated for up to 1 week and will keep in the freezer for 8 months.

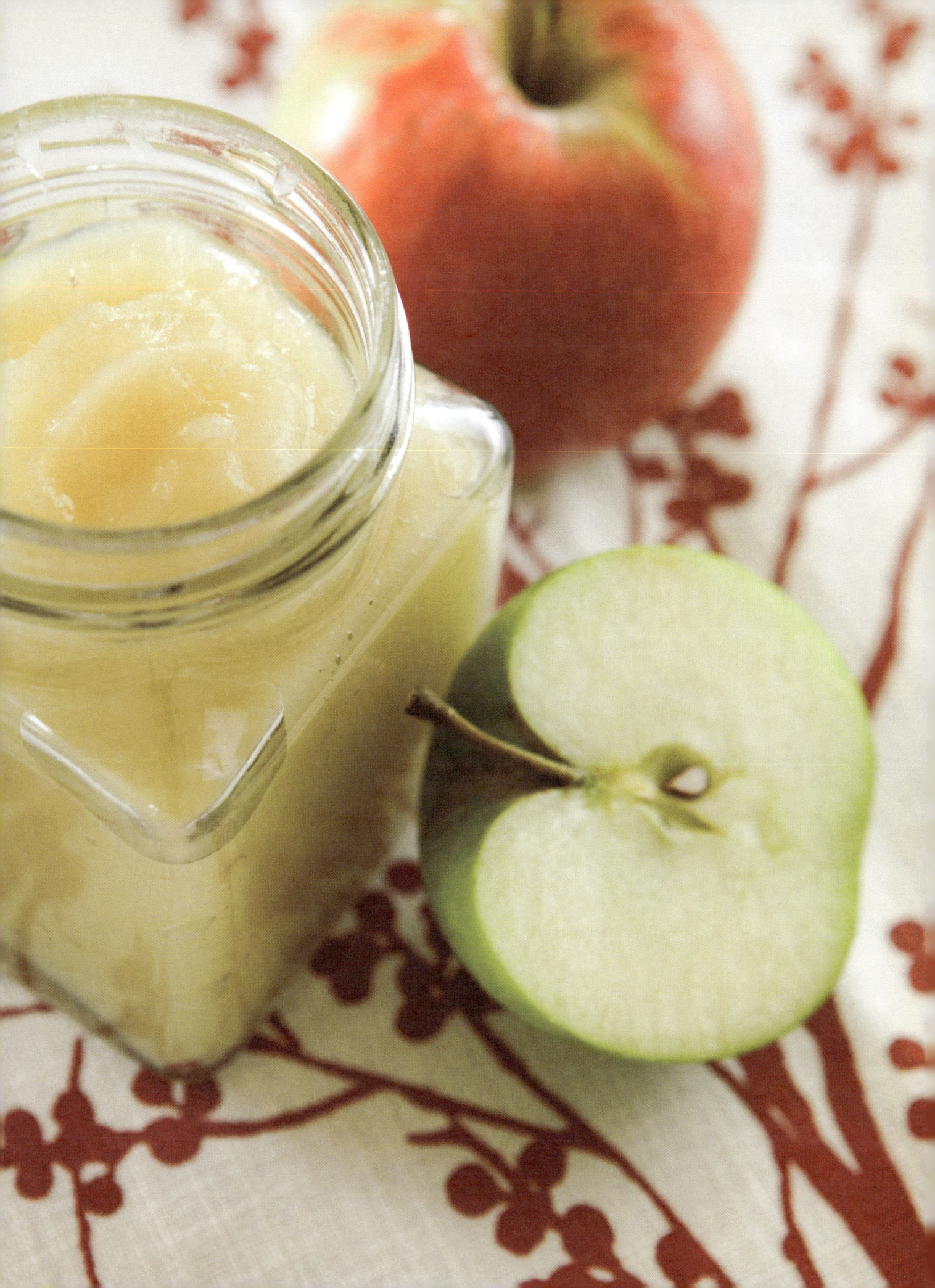

Recipes: Pantry Items

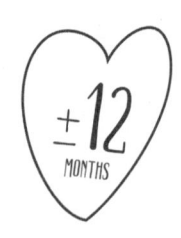

±12 MONTHS

BREADCRUMBS

A couple of recipes in this book call for breadcrumbs. They are easy to make and freeze well – so keep a Ziploc bag of them in the freezer for when you need them.

When you are making breads or pizza bases that do not turn out the way you want them to – turn them into breadcrumbs! You can also save the crusts and ends of the bread if your little one, like Mila, prefers not to eat these.

2 cups Mila's Meals Sweet Potato Bread or Mila's Meals Pizza Base
½ t. Himalayan or sea salt *(optional)*
dried Italian herb mix *(to taste)*
1 T. olive oil, or coconut oil

Preheat your oven to 160°C (325°F).

Break up your bread or pizza bases into chunks. Place in a food processor and process until you have coarse crumbs.

Add the seasoning and oil and pulse again until combined and you have the desired grain size.

Pour the crumbs onto a baking sheet and place in the oven for 5 minutes.

After 5 minutes stir the crumbs and bake again for another 5 minutes.

Remove from the oven and allow to cool. Transfer to a Ziploc bag and freeze until needed. There is no need to defrost the crumbs before using them.

The crumbs will keep in the freezer for a couple of months.

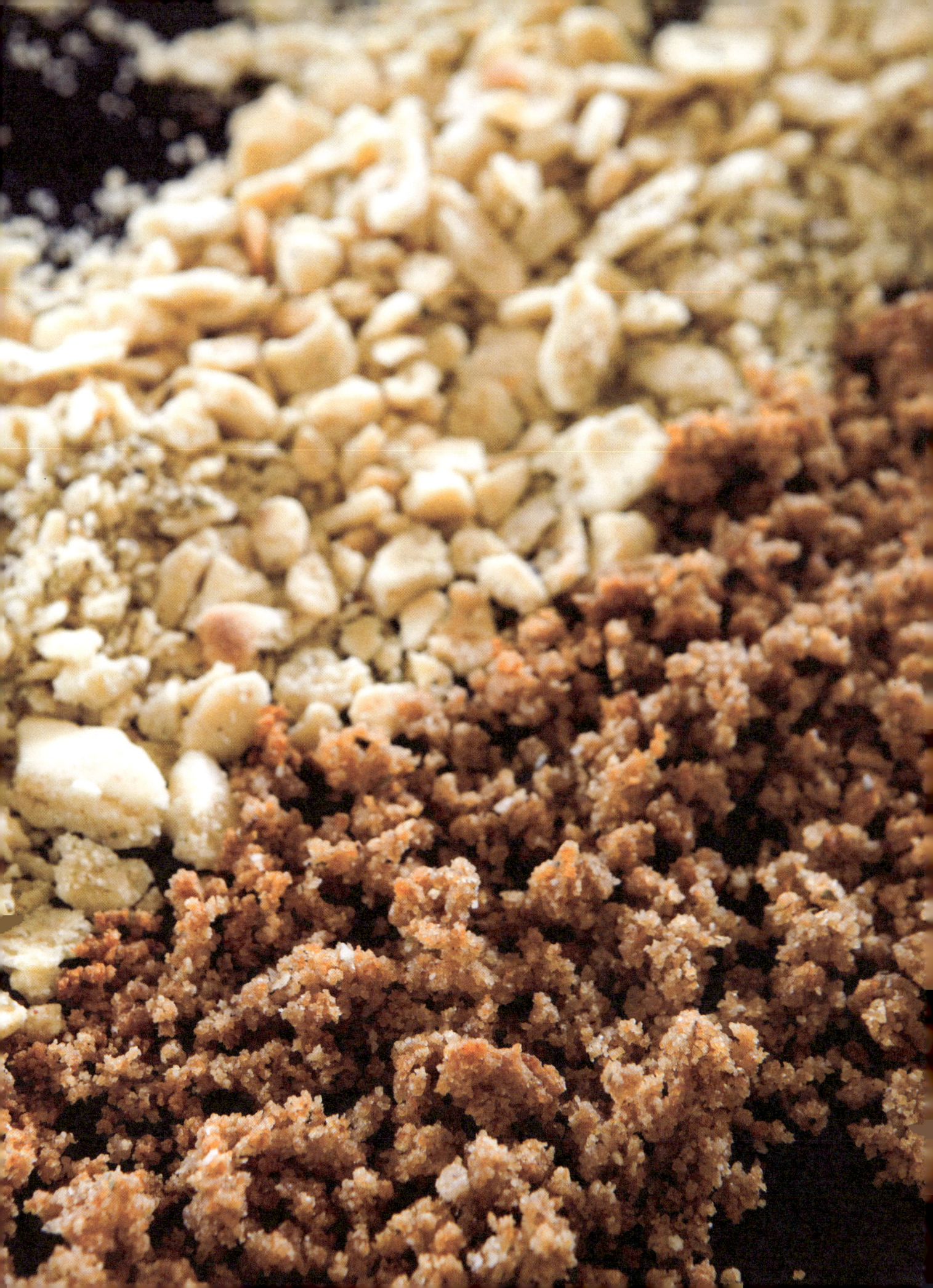

STOCK (BONE BROTHS)

Stock is used as an ingredient in many dishes in this book but, the stock cubes that you buy in the shops are a big No No! They are loaded with salt, hydrogenated oil (a source of trans fats) and, quite often, MSG.

This is an excellent example of how the food industry has taken a traditional, healing, nutrient dense food and processed it for our convenience. In doing so they have stripped away all of its healing properties and turned it into something quite harmful to your health.

Making your own stock is a great way to add not only flavour, but also many nutrients to your little one's meals making them "delicious and nutritious" as Mila would say!

'Broth', 'stock' and 'bone broth' are words that are often used interchangeably, however, there are slight differences in each one.

They all have the same foundation: water, meat or bones (or both), vegetables and seasonings that are cooked over a period of time. The liquid is strained to separate it from the solids and what remains is 'broth', 'stock' and 'bone broth'. The differences are:

- Broth is cooked using meat and a small amount of bones and is simmered for a short amount of time (45 minutes to 2 hours) and is light in flavour, thin in texture and rich in protein.
- Stock is made with bones, only a small amount of meat and is simmered for 3 – 4 hours and is rich in minerals and gelatine.
- Bone Broth is made with bones, a small amount of meat and is simmered for 24 - 48 hours to remove as many nutrients and minerals from the bones as possible. It is an extremely nutrient dense food – high in minerals (like calcium, magnesium and phosphorus), amino acids and gelatine. Bone broths help detoxify the body, stimulate digestion and support overall digestive health.

In this book, when I refer to stock or broth – I mean bone broth.

Bone broths are so easy to make and are a really affordable way to include nutrient dense foods in your little one's diet. They are an immune boosting, rich source of easily absorbed calcium, magnesium, phosphorous and other trace minerals that support the adrenal glands and the growth of strong bones and teeth. The gelatine which leaches from the bones is a good source of protein. It supports the body's connective tissues, promotes healthy hair, skin, teeth and nails, improves digestion, allergies, immune health, brain health, and much more.

I am particularly excited by the fact that they can be made from food that you, or the butcher, would otherwise throw away. Whenever you have a roast chicken, a lamb stew or any other meal that includes meat with a bone – keep the bones in a Ziploc bag in your freezer. When you have approximately 2kg's of bones, put them in a slow cooker and make a large pot of bone broth. Alternatively ask your local butcher for a bag of bones – they are incredibly cheap!

You can also use bones with the meat still on (like a whole chicken) which will make a really rich bone broth – and there will be ready-cooked meat for you to add to other meals.

Once the bone broth is made, you can store it in the fridge for 5 days or in the freezer for up to 6 months. I freeze some in ice cube trays so I can easily add a few cubes to boiling water when making vegetables, pasta or grains for Mila.

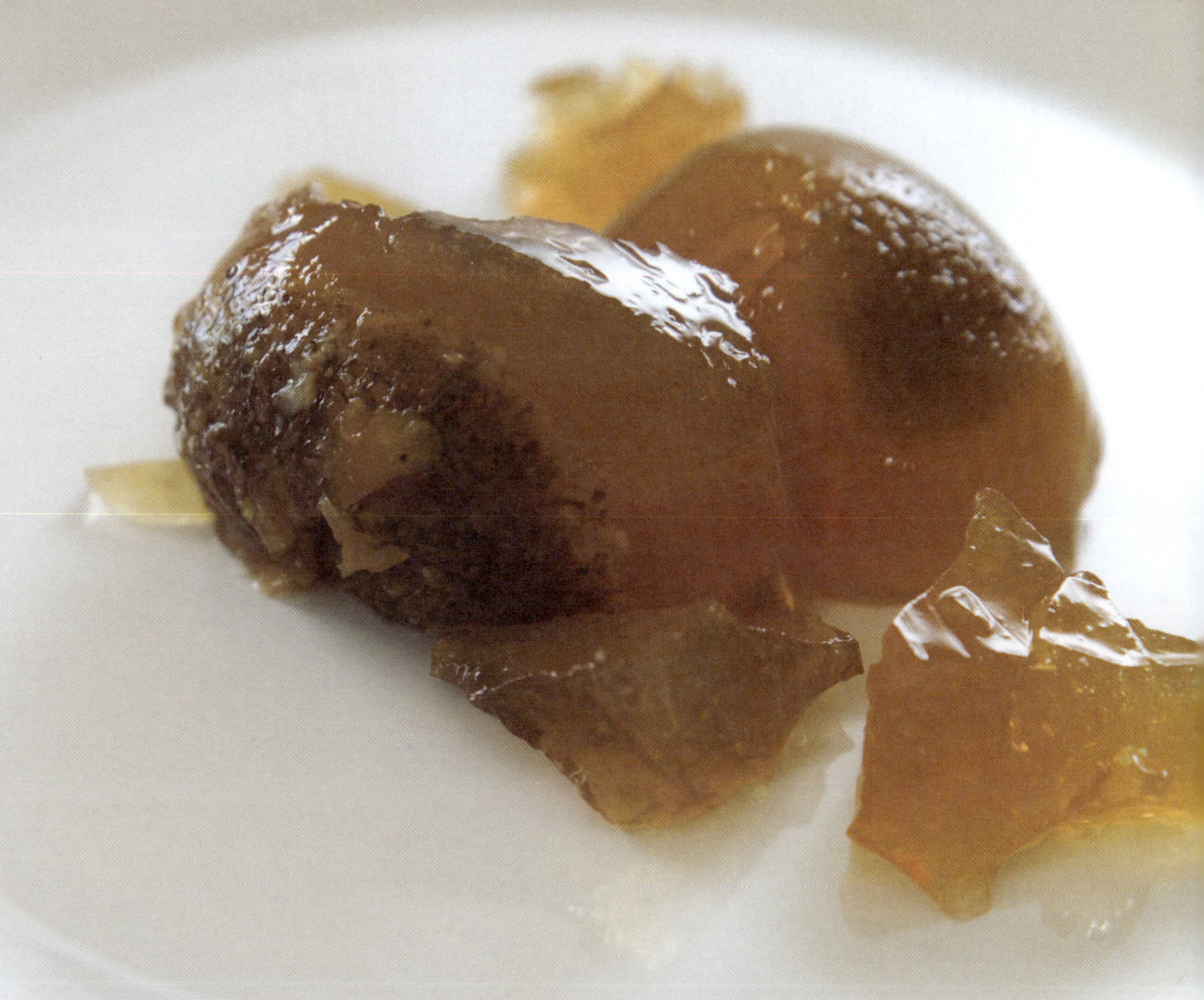

Bone broth is currently being hailed as a magical elixir – and I tend to agree!

Bone broth contains minerals in a form the body can absorb easily - like calcium, magnesium, phosphorus, silicon, sulphur and trace minerals as well as amino acids like glycine and proline.

When collagen from the bones is broken down during cooking it produces gelatine. According to Sally Fallon Morell this "is the glue that holds the body together." Collagen strengthens all the connective tissues in the body; it lubricates the joints; supports the skin and internal organs; helps skin retain firmness, suppleness and elasticity; builds a barrier that prevents the spread of pathogens, toxins and cancerous cells. It also heals and seals a damaged gut lining.

The healing benefits of bone broth:
- ♥ Helps heal and seal your gut, and promotes healthy digestion.
- ♥ Inhibits infection caused by cold and flu viruses, etc.
- ♥ Reduces joint pain and inflammation.
- ♥ Eases the symptoms of autoimmune disorders.
- ♥ Fights inflammation.
- ♥ Has calming effects, which may help you sleep better.
- ♥ Promotes strong, healthy bones.

If you want to know more about the healing qualities of Bone Broth, I encourage you to read Natasha Cambell-Mcbride's book 'Gut and Psychology Syndrome' as well as Sally Fallon Morell's books 'Nourishing Broth' and 'Nourishing Traditions'.

Recipes: Pantry Items

CHICKEN BONE BROTH (STOCK)

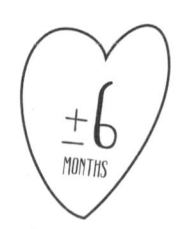

±6 MONTHS

egg-free; grain-free; for adults too

Makes 6 l. (6 qt.)

•••

While I made and used homemade chicken stock in my cooking when Mila was a baby, I only learnt about bone broths and their value when I went on the GAPS diet when Mila was 2 years old. How I wish I had known about them earlier.

Broth/stock can be used as the liquid when making soups, stews, gravies and sauces. It can be used to sauté or roast vegetables or as a marinade for meat. You and your little one can also drink it on its own – this is especially useful when they are unwell and refusing to eat anything. According to the Sally Fallon Morell, bone broth can be introduced as a cooking ingredient and as a drink when your little one is 6 months old.

These measurements are based are for a 6.5 liter slow cooker.

•••

1 whole organic or free-range chicken OR 2kg's chicken bones and parts from cooked or raw chicken
¼ cup apple cider vinegar
filtered water
½ onion, peeled and chopped
2 carrots, peeled and chopped
3 celery sticks, chopped (you can include the leaves too)
2 bay leaves
2 sticks kombu seaweed
½ T. Himalayan or sea salt
Spices *(all optional, but they add to the medicinal qualities of the broth):*
½ t. turmeric powder
½ t. coriander seeds
½ t. black cumin seeds
½ t. fennel seeds
½ t. caraway seeds
5 peppercorns, cracked
3 cardamom seeds, cracked

4 cloves of garlic, roughly chopped and left to stand for 10 minutes *(or more)*
handful of herbs *(thyme, rosemary, oregano, parsley or a combination of these)*
filtered water

Place the chicken, chicken parts or bones into the slow cooker, cover with water and add the apple cider vinegar. Allow to soak for 1 hour. This gives the apple cider vinegar time to draw out the minerals from the bones.

Turn your slow cooker onto high. Add the onion, carrots, celery, bay leaves, kombu, salt, and choice of spices to the slow cooker.

Cover with more cold filtered water if needed to ensure that all the ingredients are covered. Once the liquid starts to boil, turn the heat down to low.

Check on the slow cooker once or twice during the first 2 hours of cooking. There may be some scum (frothy foam) on the surface. This should be skimmed off.

If you are using whole chicken or bones with meat on, remove them after 6 hours of cooking. Remove the chicken meat from the bones, allow it to cool and then refrigerate or freeze for use in other meals. Return the bones to the slow cooker and continue cooking for a further 18 hours.

Be sure to check on the pot occasionally to make sure there is still enough liquid in the pot. Add more if necessary.

Half an hour before the end of the cooking time, add the herbs and garlic to the slow cooker. This will allow the flavour to infuse without destroying their health benefits from over cooking.

After 24 hours total cooking time, strain the liquid through a sieve. You should have a dark golden liquid – "liquid gold" I like to call it!

Fill glass jars to the ¾ mark and freeze for future use. Be sure to fill and freeze some ice cube trays with the stock to add to boiling water when preparing vegetables, grains or pasta for your little one.

Once cooled a layer of fat will form on the top of the broth. You can remove this and use it for high heat cooking, or leave it in the broth – it is nutrient dense, has immune boosting properties and adds a rich flavour to any meal.

Broth can be refrigerated for up to 5 days or keep in the freezer for up to 6 months.

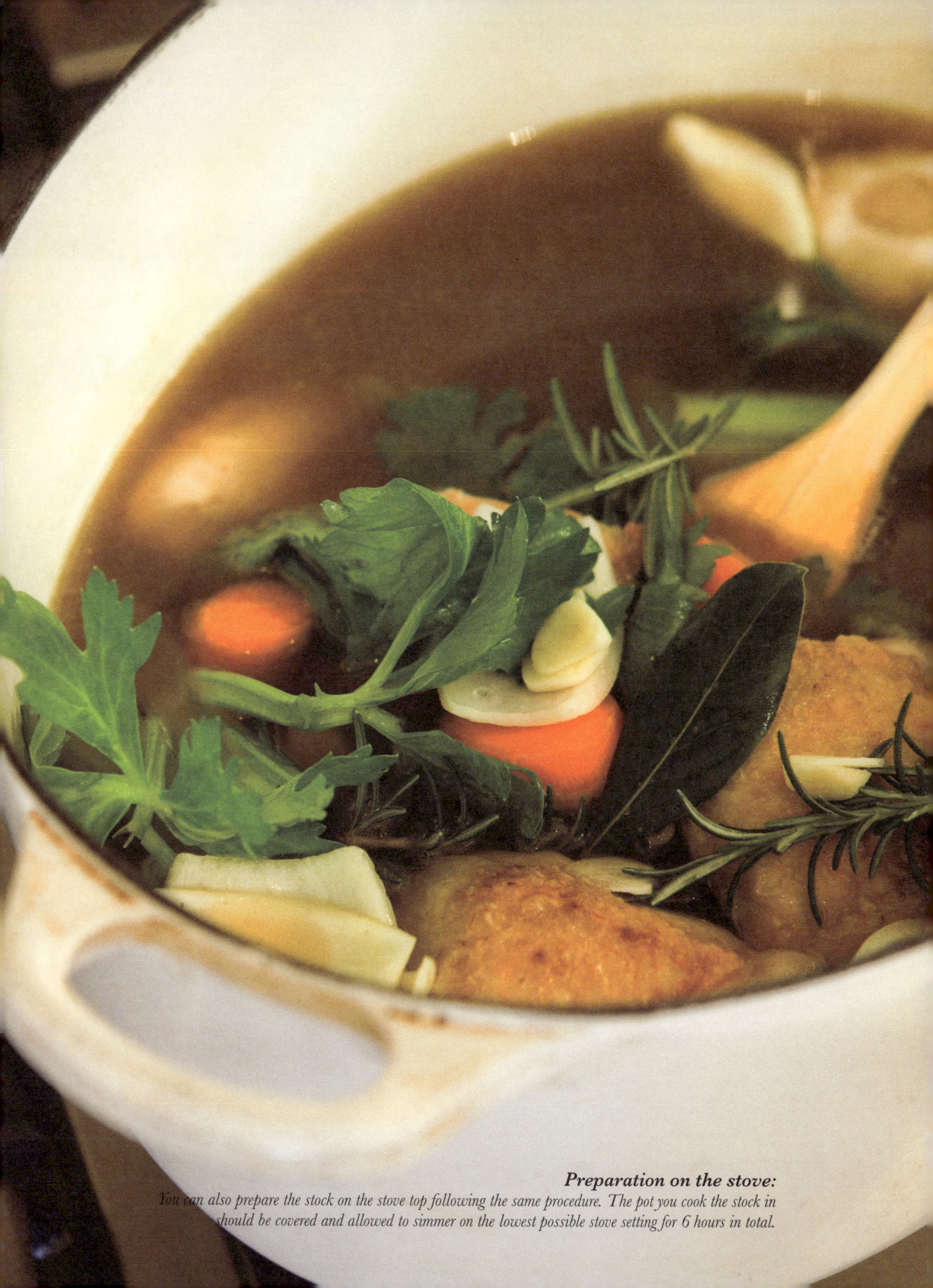

Preparation on the stove:
You can also prepare the stock on the stove top following the same procedure. The pot you cook the stock in should be covered and allowed to simmer on the lowest possible stove setting for 6 hours in total.

Recipes: Pantry Items

BEEF BONE BROTH (STOCK)

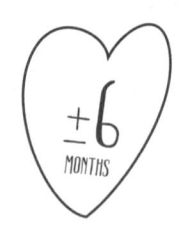

egg-free; grain-free; for adults too

Makes 6 l. (6 qt.)

♡ +6 MONTHS

• •

Preparation on the stove: *You can also prepare the stock on the stovetop following the same method as above. Cook at a slight simmer with the lid askew or off for 12 – 24 hours.*

Tips: *While you may be tempted to speed this preparation up by skipping some steps, they all serve an important purpose.*
- *When making beef bone broth it is important to roast the bones before hand as this develops the taste of the broth.*
- *It is also necessary to soak the bones in a vinegar-water solution. The vinegar helps draw the minerals out of the bones. This can only be done when the bones are cold, as the pores of the bones close when they are hot – thus preventing the minerals from leaching out. So you will have to wait for the roasted bones to cool before moving onto the soaking step.*

Variations: *You can also make this stock with lamb bones.*

• •

2 kg grass-fed, organic or free-range beef marrow, oxtail and/or knuckle bones

1 kg grass-fed, organic or free-range beef rib or neck bones

1 T. Himalayan or sea salt

filtered water

¼ cup apple cider vinegar

2 onions, peeled and chopped

3 carrots, peeled and chopped

3 celery sticks, peeled and chopped *(you can include the leaves too)*

2 bay leaves

2 sticks kombu seaweed

4 cloves garlic, roughly chopped and left to stand for 10 minutes *(or more)*

bunch of herbs *(thyme, rosemary, or oregano - or a combination of these)*

Heat your oven to 200°C (400°F).

Place your bones in one or two large roasting dishes – ensuring they are spread out in a single layer. Season with salt. Roast for ½ - 1 hours until the bones are well browned and fragrant.

Allow the bones to cool completely. Place them (and the fats from the bottom of the roasting dish) in the slow cooker (which must be turned off), cover with water and stir in the apple cider vinegar. Place the lid on the slow cooker and allow the bones to soak for 1 hour.

Turn the slow cooker on and add the onions, carrots, celery, bay leaves and kombu.

During the first couple of hours of cooking check the slow cooker to see if any scum has risen to the top. Skim this with a spoon.

After 12 hours remove the bones with meat on it and strip the meat from the bones. Allow it to cool and then refrigerate or freeze for use in other meals. Return the bones to the slow cooker and continue cooking for a further 36 – 60 hours.

Half an hour before the end of the cooking time, add the herbs and garlic to the slow cooker. This will allow the flavour to infuse and prevent the health benefits from being destroyed due to over-cooking.

Remove the bones and vegetables with a slotted spoon and pour the liquid through a sieve.

Fill glass jars to the ¾ mark and freeze for future use. Be sure to fill and freeze some ice cube trays with the stock to add to boiling water when preparing vegetables, grains or pasta for your little one.

Once cooled a layer of fat will form on the top of the broth. You can remove this and use it for high heat cooking, or leave it in the broth – it is nutrient dense, has immune boosting properties and adds a rich flavour to any meal.

When the broth cools, it will be gelatinous - that is, full of gelatine with the consistency of jelly – this is what you want!

Broth can be refrigerated for up to 5 days or keep in the freezer for up to 6 months.

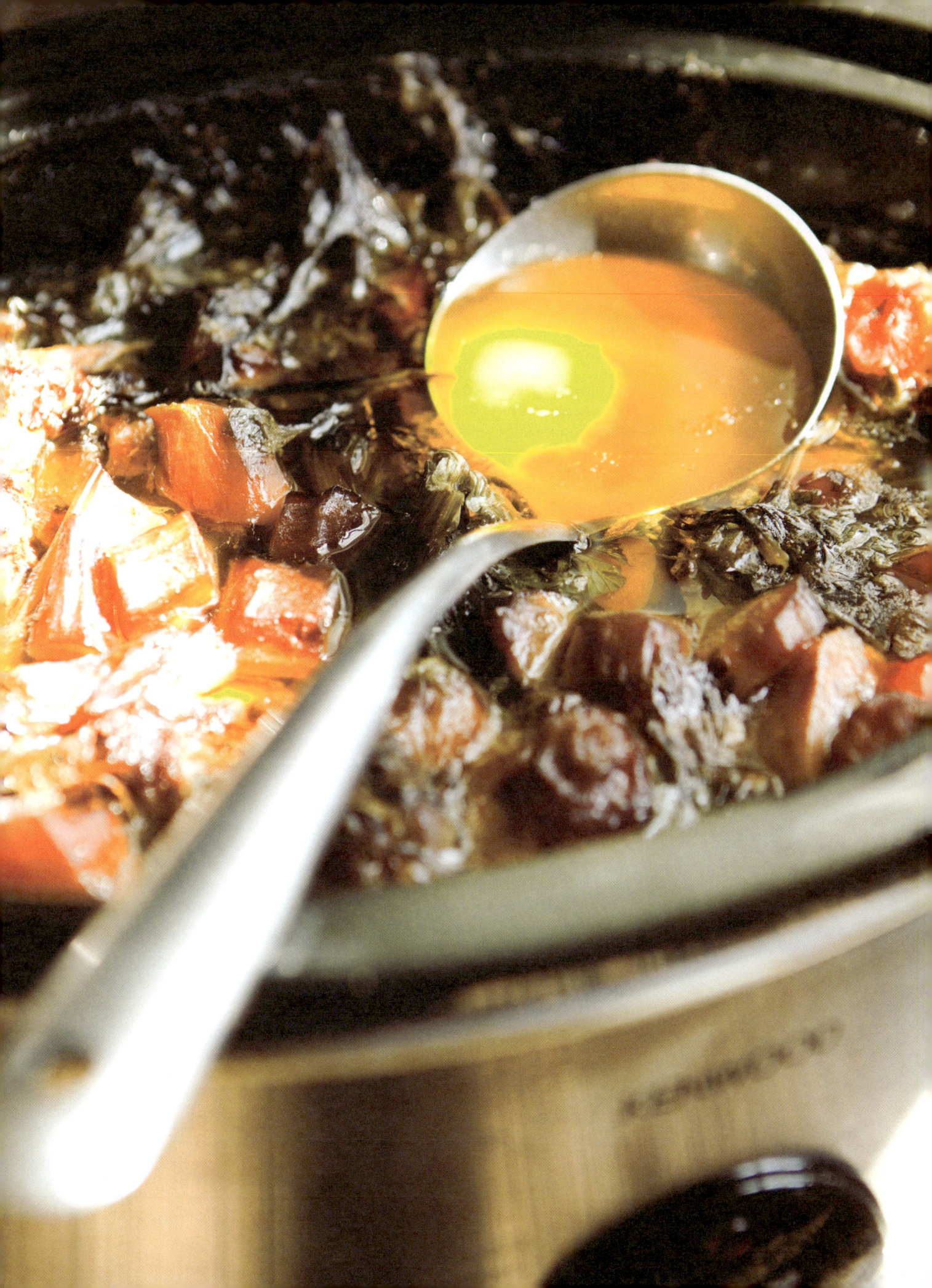

Recipes: Pantry Items

CULTURED (FERMENTED) FOODS

It was not until I went on the GAPS diet, when Mila was 2 years old, that I learnt about these amazingly beneficial foods. While many people know of and regularly eat pickles (gherkins) and some may have heard of sauerkraut, store bought varieties are another example of the food industry taking a traditional superfood, processing it and rendering it nutritionally bankrupt.

WHAT ARE FERMENTED FOODS?

Fermented foods are foods that have been through a process of lacto fermentation in which natural bacteria feed on the sugar and starch in the food creating lactic acid. This process preserves the food, and creates beneficial enzymes, b-vitamins, omega-3 fatty acids, and various strains of probiotics.

"Fermented foods have been around for thousands of years. For people living without modern medicine and refrigeration, fermentation has always been not only a simple means of food preservation, but also a way to imbue foods with health-promoting properties, an essential tool for maintaining the gut health.

It's estimated that roughly 70% – 80% of your immune system is in your gut. Feed it poorly and your gut will be left with few defences, easily overwhelmed by bad bacteria, wide open to disease-triggering inflammation and plagued by gastrointestinal ills like IBS-type symptoms (i.e., gas, bloating, constipation, diarrhoea, etc.). In your weakened state, you may also be more susceptible to colds and flu. But, if you introduce good bacteria into the gastric mix via fermented foods, you'll enable your gut to crush opportunistic invaders and disease-triggering inflammation, long before they can gain the upper hand. Simply put: A healthy, balanced gut can send illness packing."

- Dr. Frank Lipman, South African founder and director of the Eleven Eleven Wellness Centre in New York City

Fermented foods balance your gut bacteria and stomach acids, release enzymes to help ease and improve digestion and make it easier for your body to extract and absorb more nutrients from the foods you eat. They are powerful detoxifiers, helping to break down and eliminate heavy metals and other toxins from your body. The proliferation of good bacteria boosts the immune system and the high bacteria and enzyme content in fermented foods have been shown to assist with the treatment of baby colic.

Besides a diet completely lacking in good bacteria (thanks to pasteurisation), the balance of good and bad bacteria in the gut can be disrupted by the use of antibiotics, excessive alcohol use, excessive sugar intake, stress, diseases and toxins. All of these allow harmful bacteria to thrive. To rebalance the scales, good bacteria (or probiotics) are needed to repopulate the gut.

Homemade fermented (or cultured) vegetables provide billions of beneficial bacteria and probiotics – far more than any supplement can, and at a fraction of the cost.

Introducing fermented foods to your little one not only reinforces the concept that food can be your medicine, but also introduces a new taste profile to their palate – as fermented foods are sour. It is important to broaden your little one's range of taste beyond that of sweet and salty.

According to Donna Gates from the Body Ecology food protocol, your little one can be introduced to fermented foods (fruits and vegetables) as early as 4 days old. Start dipping your finger into the fermented vegetable juice and letting your little one suck it off. He/she will likely pull a face due to its sour taste, but keep offering it everyday.

You can continue offering the fermented vegetable juice on a spoon and when your little one starts solids, mix it into a purée as a nutritional enhancer. Later add fermented vegetables to his/her purée, or offer a whole fermented vegetable (they soften as they ferment to the same texture as a cooked vegetable).

If your little one is older and has not ever been introduced to fermented foods (like Mila, who was only introduced to them when she was 2 years old), you can hide the fermented vegetable juice in smoothies or vegetable juices. Alternatively introduce fermented foods to your 'big' little one with fermented fruits - as some of the fruit's sweetness is retained in the final product.

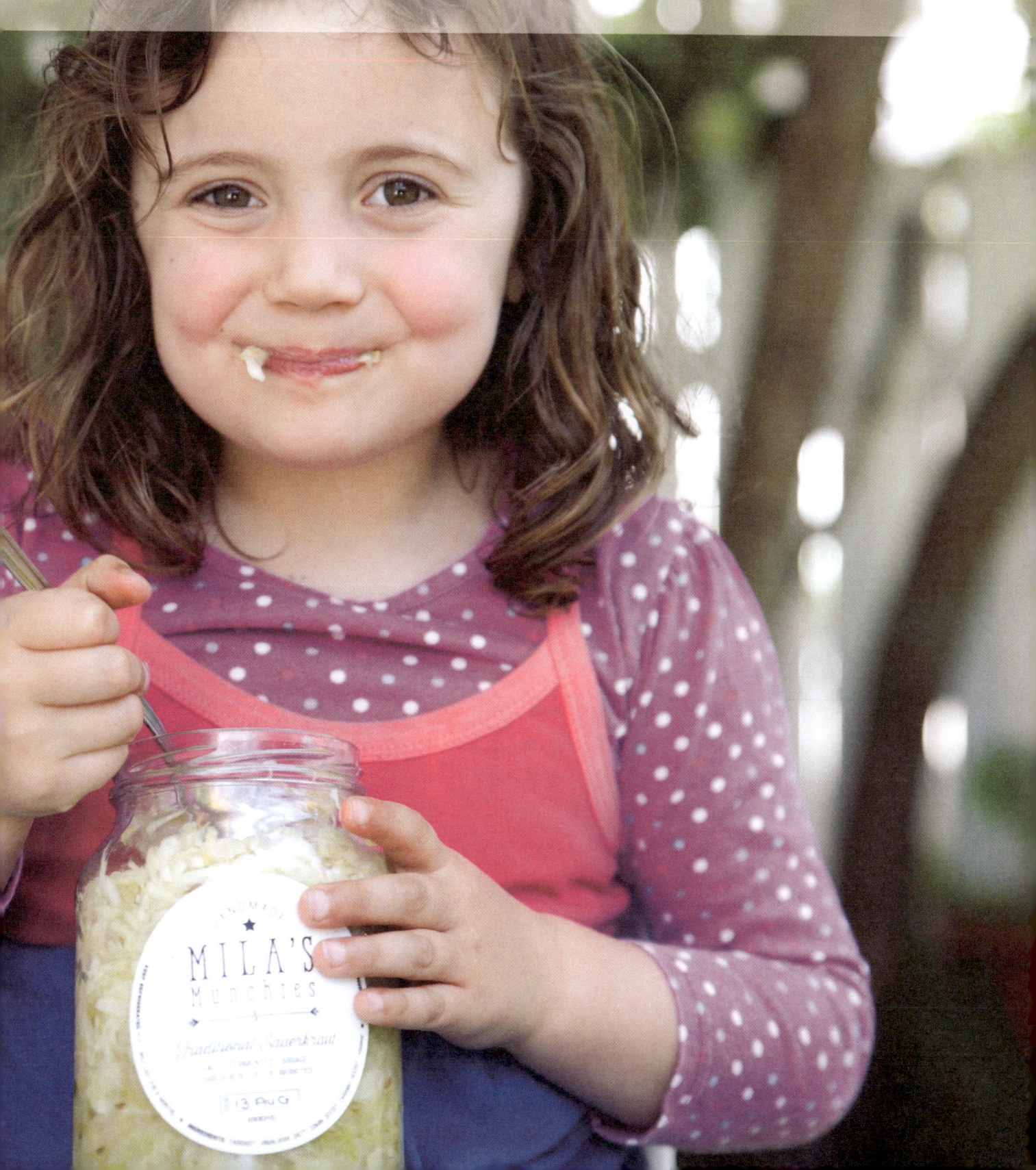

Recipes: Pantry Items

DILLY CARROTS

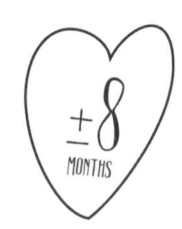

±8 MONTHS

raw; vegetarian; egg-free; for adults too; great for lunchboxes

Makes 1 l. (1 qt.)

•••

These are so easy to make and so delicious! They are a great introductory fermented food and can be introduced to your little one as soon as he/she is starting finger foods and is chewing well. The fermentation process softens the carrots a great deal – so while they are raw, they are far easier to chew and digest.

Alternatively, add some of the fermented carrots, or brine to any purée you are making.

•••

- 2 cloves garlic, peeled and halved
- 1 T. fresh dill, chopped
- 6 carrots (peeled if they are not organic), sliced
- 1 T. whey or contents of 1 probiotic capsule
- ½ T. Himalayan or sea salt
- 2 cups filtered water
- 1 cabbage leaf

Fermenting foods requires an extremely clean environment! Make sure that all utensils and your hands have been washed thoroughly.

Place the garlic and dill at the bottom of a 1 l. (1 qt.) glass/mason jar.

Pack the carrots above the garlic and dill. Ensure that they are at least 3 cm (1½") below the neck of the glass jar (as the liquid must cover them completely).

Make your brine by dissolving the salt in the water. Stir in the whey. Pour the brine into the jar – make sure the carrots are completely covered, but leave a 2 cm (1") air pocket between the liquid and the rim of the glass jar.

Fold the cabbage leaf over the carrots to hold them down.

Put the lid on the glass jar and close tightly.

Leave the jar in a cool, dark place at room temperature for 4 -10 days (fermenting will go quicker in summer when the ambient temperature is higher).

'Burp' the jar everyday by just barely unscrewing the lid until you hear the gas escape and then sealing tightly again.

Once there are no more bubbles forming in the brine the fermentation is complete. Place them in the fridge where they will keep for a couple of months.

The longer you leave the carrots at room temperature the softer and the sourer they will become.

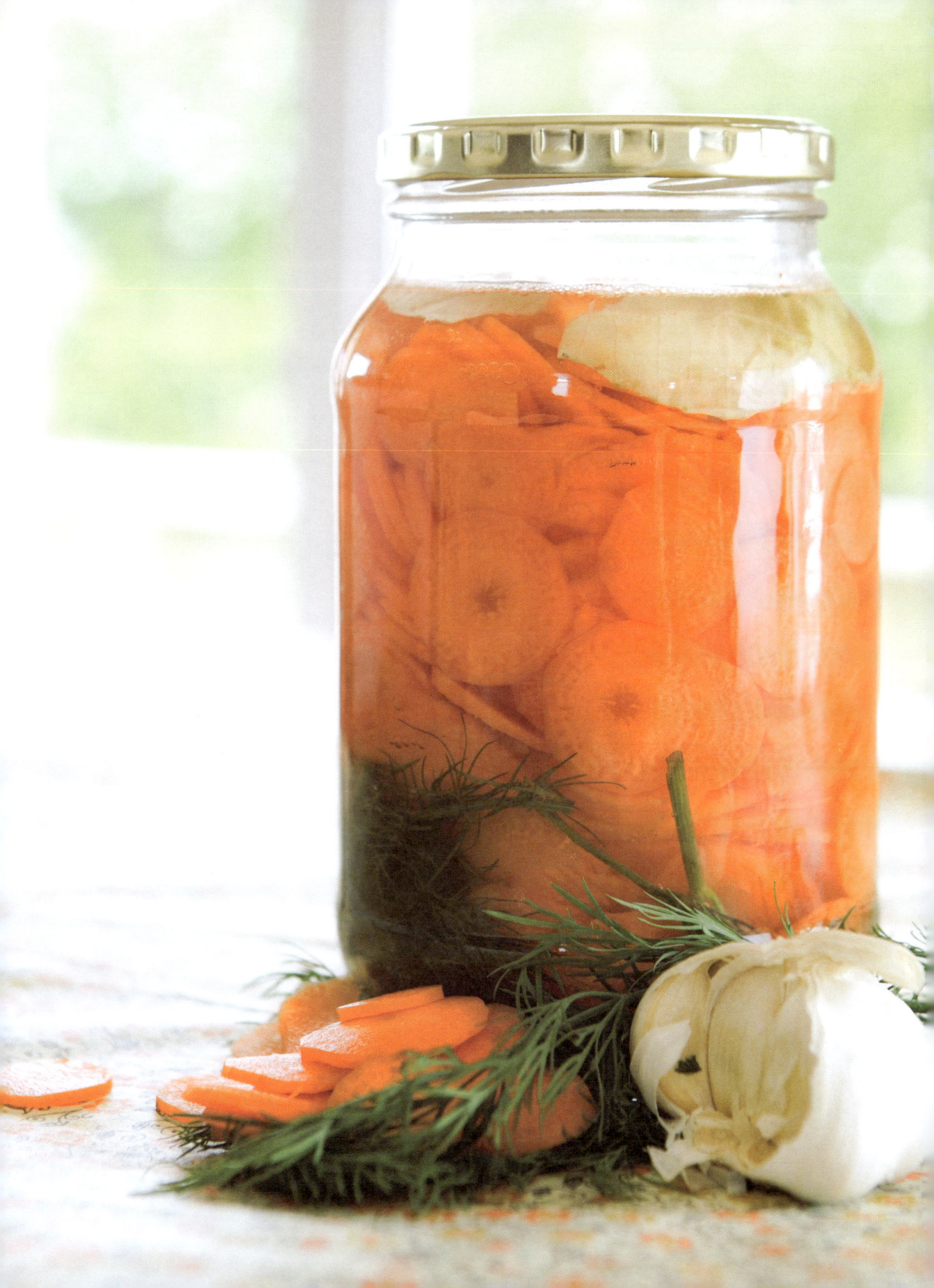

Recipes: Pantry Items

BUBBLING BERRIES

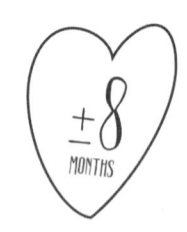

±8 MONTHS

raw; vegetarian; egg-free; for adults too; great for lunchboxes

Makes a 375ml (¾ qt.) jar

•••

While strawberries and raspberries can cause an allergic reaction, blueberries are not a common allergen and can be introduced from 8 months.

They are, however, one of the Dirty Dozen so try to find organic ones or wash them in a hydrogen peroxide or vinegar water solution before using.

Blueberries are an exceptionally phytonutrient-dense fruit. They are also a very good source of vitamins C and K, manganese, fibre and copper.

These Bubbling Berries are delicious eaten on their own but make a great addition to a smoothie too. They are a great finger food and are easily 'gummed' by your toothless little one! Alternatively, they can be added to any purée you may be making for your little one.

•••

2 cups organic blueberries

2 T. raw honey *(or organic maple syrup if your little one is younger than a year old)* – this is optional, but a little sweetness may be more enticing for your little one

2 T. whey *(or contents of 2 probiotic capsules)*

¼ t. Himalayan or sea salt

2 cups filtered water

Wash the berries well and place in a 1l (1 qt.) glass/mason jar. Squash them down so that they are quite tightly packed and will not float in the brine.

Make your brine by mixing the honey, whey (or probiotics), salt and 2 T. filtered water together.

Pour the brine over the berries and top up with the remaining water until the berries are completely covered, but leave a 2cm (1") air pocket between the liquid and the rim of the glass jar.

Using a wooden spoon, push the berries down again to make sure the brine fills any air pockets.

Seal the glass jar tightly and leave at room temperature for 2 days.

'Burp' the jar everyday by just barely unscrewing the lid until you hear the gas escape and then sealing tightly again.

After 2 days, place the berries in the fridge and use within 2 months.

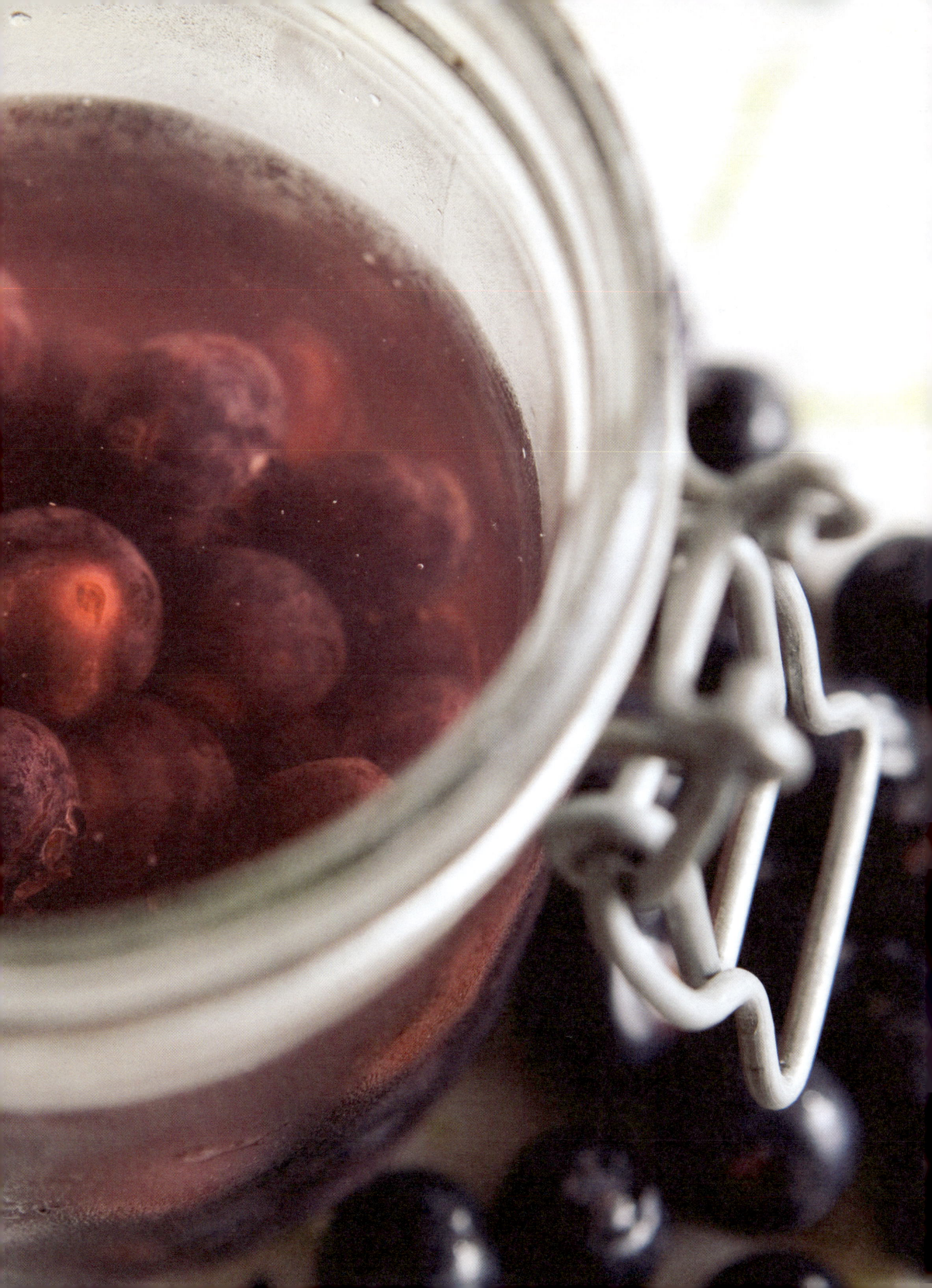

Recipes: Pantry Items

FERMENTED APPLE SAUCE

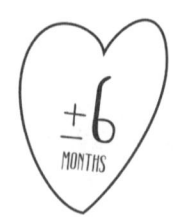

± 6 MONTHS

raw; vegetarian; egg-free; for adults too; great for lunchboxes

Makes a 375ml (¾ qt.) jar

•••

Apples are on the Dirty Dozen list so either buy organic, or be sure to wash them in a hydrogen peroxide or vinegar water solution prior to peeling them.

Add a teaspoon of this to any other purée you are making for your little one – or let him/her eat it as is. This would also make a great filling for pancakes.

Do not use this applesauce as a replacement for non-fermented applesauce in recipes which require cooking – heat destroys the enzymes and beneficial bacteria. It may, however, be used in fruit leather prepared in a dehydrator at 45°C (110°F).

•••

6 organic apples, peeled and cored

2 T. whey *(or contents of 1 probiotic capsule)*

1 t. cinnamon

½ t. Himalayan or sea salt

Place the apples in a blender or food processor and process until you have your desired consistency.

Add the whey, cinnamon and salt and stir well to combine.

(If you are using a probiotic capsule, empty the contents into a ¼ cup of filtered water. Stir well to combine and add this to the apples with the cinnamon and salt.)

Pour the mixture into a glass jar leaving a 2 cm (1") air pocket between the mixture and the rim of the glass jar.

Seal the glass jar tightly and leave at room temperature for 2 days.

After 2 days, place the applesauce in the fridge and use within 1 month.

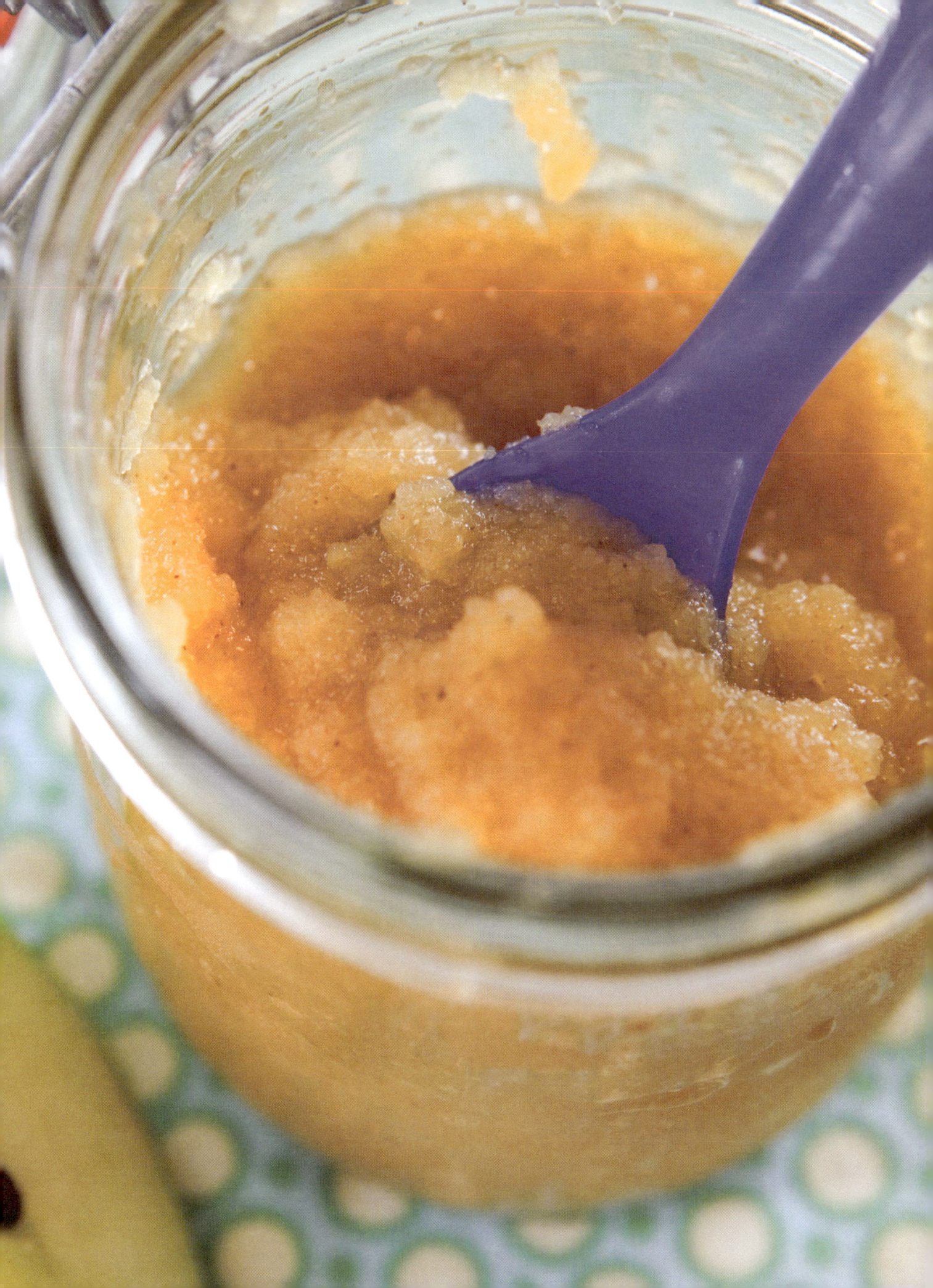

Recipes: Pantry Items

SAUERKRAUT

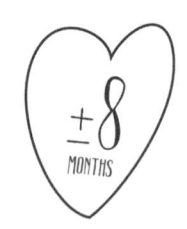

±8 MONTHS

raw; vegetarian; vegan; egg-free; grain-free; for adults too; great for lunchboxes

Makes 1 l. (1 qt.)

• •

I have added this recipe especially for my niece and nephew – Lily and Matthew. Two incredible children who eat everything – even sauerkraut straight out of the jar!

I only learnt about the benefits of fermented foods long after I had weaned Mila. As such it was more difficult for me to introduce them to her – she immediately thought of them as something 'strange'. I do, however, manage to sneak it into her morning veggie juice!

Sauerkraut was said to have originated in China over 2,000 years ago and later brought over to Europe. It could perhaps be one of the most vital things you could add to your diet. To nourish your gut, is to nourish your body and mind. Sauerkraut works wonders for your digestion, producing amazing amounts of probiotics and other disease-preventing compounds.

• •

1 t. cumin seeds
1 t. caraway seeds
½ cup filtered water
1 cabbage, shredded (save one big leaf)
1 T. Himalayan or sea salt, ground

Place the seeds in ½ cup filtered water to soak.

Shred the washed cabbage in a food processor then place in a large bowl.

Sprinkle the salt over the cabbage and start rubbing! After 10 minutes of massaging the salt into the cabbage you will notice a lot of juice being released. This is good!

Mix in the seeds.

Transfer the cabbage to sterilised glass jars and pound down to release any air bubbles. If the cabbage is not submerged in its own juice, add some of the seed soak water and additional filtered water.

Place the big cabbage leaf over the shredded cabbage to hold it down.

Put the lid on and leave the jar in a cool, dark cupboard.

Everyday for the first three days open the jar and pound down the cabbage again. If there is liquid spilling out the top, that's okay (good in fact). Just clean it up.

Leave the jars in a cupboard for 10 days to allow the fermentation to develop. After 10 days your sauerkraut is ready to eat and can be transferred to the fridge.

Sauerkraut can be stored in the fridge for up to 6 months.

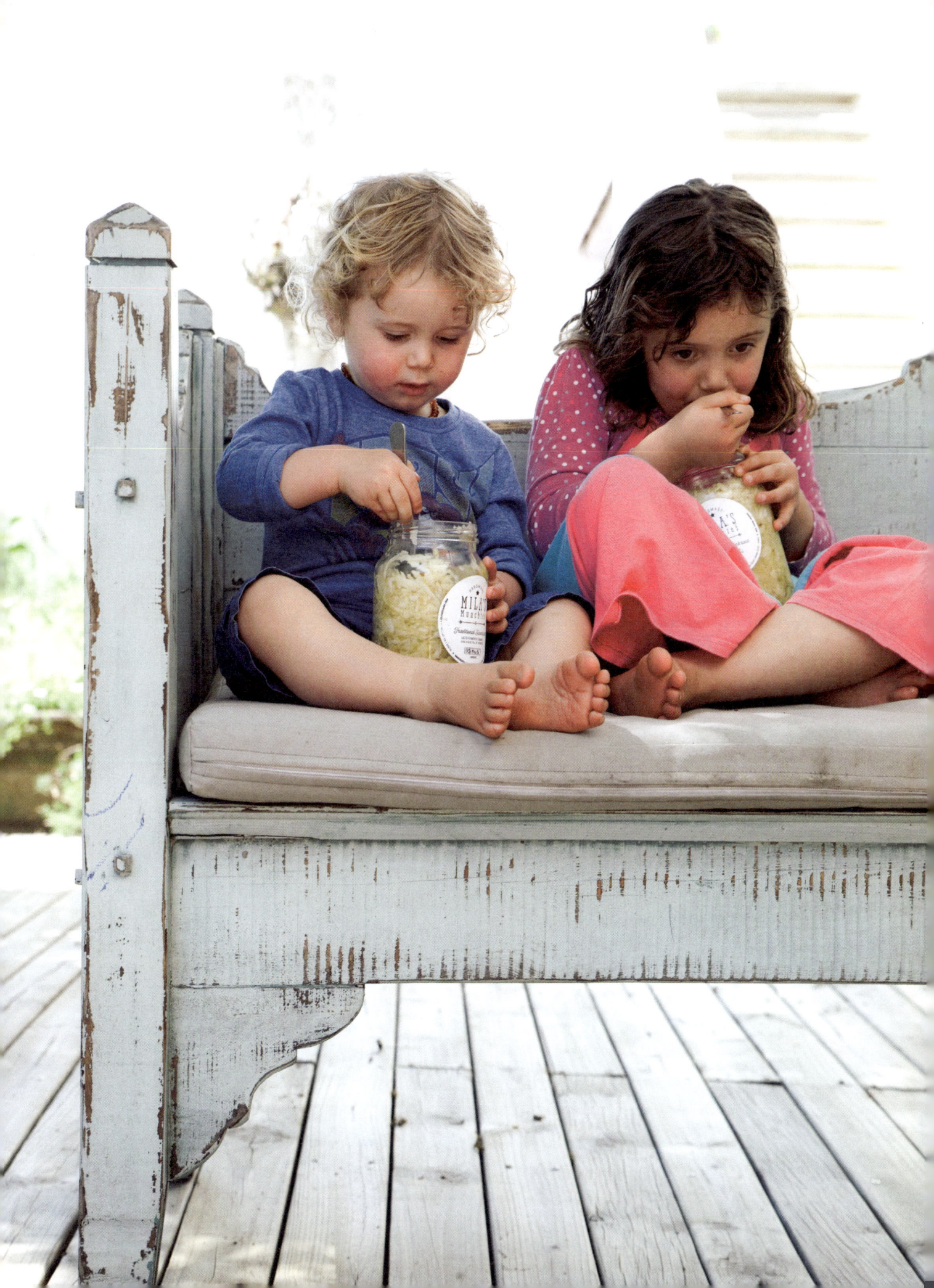

Recipes: Pantry Items

KEFIR

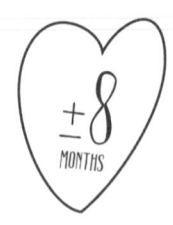

±8 MONTHS

Kefir is a fermented milk product with a slightly sour taste. Kefir 'grains' are used to culture the milk. These gelatinous white or yellow particles are not actual grains, but a grain-like matrix of proteins, lipids, sugars, bacteria and yeasts. They look like pieces of coral or small clumps of cauliflower. The grains ferment the milk, incorporating their friendly organisms to create the cultured milk. The grains are then removed with a strainer before you drink the kefir and are added to a new batch of milk to repeat the process.

Kefir milk is one of the most potent probiotic foods available.

Mila suffered from colic and constipation from birth. If only I had known then what I know now!

Your little one is born with an almost sterile gut – that is to say, it is populated with a very limited amount of bacteria. As a baby passes through the mom's birth canal it takes on whatever microflora (gut bacteria) the mother has – good or bad.

Having suffered from Candida for most of my adult life, it stands to reason that Mila's gut was populated with many pathogens and a very limited number of good flora when she was born. This imbalance obviously contributed to her colic and constipation. While I did supplement her with a probiotic powder – I wish I had known about fermented foods and kefir as they are a far superior source of probiotics. According to Dr. Mercola "providing abundant probiotics in the form of fermented foods is one of the most powerful ways to restore your baby's beneficial gut flora". Kefir is also a far more economical way of providing your little one with essential probiotics.

Importantly to those who are lactose intolerant, after 24 hours of fermentation the beneficial yeast and bacteria provide lactase, an enzyme which is required to digest lactose. Not only does it digest the lactose in the culturing milk (so the kefir in very low in lactose), but it also assists your little one in digesting the lactose from breast milk or formula.

Kefir can be introduced in small amounts when you start introducing solids. Although I have also read reports of mothers to premature babies giving it to their babies from birth. It is a good idea to introduce it as early as possible, not only for the probiotics, but so your little one can get used to the slightly sour taste.

. . . .

Recipes: Pantry Items

MILK KEFIR

raw; vegetarian; egg-free; for adults too

Makes 1 l. (1 qt.)

2 T. real kefir grains
½ l. (1 qt.) raw goat's milk, or coconut milk

* Only use plastic, glass or wooden utensils with the kefir grains.

Place the kefir grains in a glass jar and cover with raw goat's milk, or coconut milk.

Cover the jar with some muslin cloth and leave in a dark place at room temperature for 24 hours - or longer if you would like a thicker consistency and stronger flavour. The longer you leave the kefir to ferment, the less lactose and the more probiotics are in the end product.

Once the kefir is ready, strain through a plastic colander or sieve and place the grains into a clean glass jar with more fresh milk to prepare the next batch. This process is simply repeated.

The strained kefir milk should be kept in the fridge.

Add kefir to homemade formula, smoothies, muesli or make a milkshake by blending it with some fruit, raw cacao or other superfoods.

WATER KEFIR

raw; vegetarian; egg-free; for adults too

Makes 1 l. (1 qt.)

2 T. hydrated kefir grains
½ l. (1 qt.) young green coconut water, or filtered sugar water (add ¼ cup sugar to 1 l./1 qt. water)

* Only use plastic, glass or wooden utensils with the kefir grains.

Place the kefir grains in a glass jar and cover with coconut water or filtered water.

Cover the jar with some muslin cloth and leave in a dark place at room temperature for 24 - 48 hours. It is not recommended to leave water kefir to ferment for longer than 48 hours.

Once the kefir is ready, strain through a plastic colander or sieve.

Place the grains into a clean glass jar with more fresh coconut water or filtered water to prepare the next batch. This process is simply repeated.

Coconut water kefir can be drunk as is. Water kefir would need to be flavoured with something like juice or a flavour extract (such as vanilla essence, orange essence etc.).

You can make a fizzy drink by mixing the water kefir with some fruit juice, sealing in a glass jar and allowing it to rest for a couple of days. Otherwise, the strained kefir water should be kept in the fridge.

KEFIR WHEY, YOGHURT AND CHEESE

Whey is a source of the eight essential amino acids (which is why it is sold in powdered form as a protein shake) and contains potassium, calcium, magnesium & phosphorous. It is a great source of electrolytes, is very hydrating and regenerates the intestinal flora.

While it may not taste great, it can be hidden in smoothies and juices.

Whey is used as the starter culture when making fermented fruit and vegetables and it can be used to soak your grains in before cooking them.

Kefir whey, yoghurt and cheese have all the health benefits of kefir milk.

....

Milk Kefir

Place a piece of muslin cloth in a glass bowl making sure it is big enough to fold over the edges.

Pour your milk kefir into the cloth.

Gather the edges of the cloth and suspend it over the bowl. I do this by placing my bowl in the sink and tying the cloth to the tap above it.

Allow the kefir to drain through the cloth for 2 – 24 hours.

After 2 hours what is left in the cloth will resemble yoghurt and can be eaten as such. Eat as is or add puréed fruit or a flavour extract (like vanilla essence) and some maple syrup or honey.

After 24 hours of straining, more whey would have drained from the kefir and what remains in the cloth is kefir cream cheese. Eat it as is spread on toast or crackers; or, add spices and herbs to make an appetising dip.

Both the yoghurt and the cheese can be kept in an airtight container in the fridge for 2 weeks.

The opaque liquid left in the bowl is whey. This can be stored in a sealed glass jar in the fridge for up to 6 months. Add whey to smoothies and juices; use it to soak your grains in; and, make fermented fruits and vegetables.

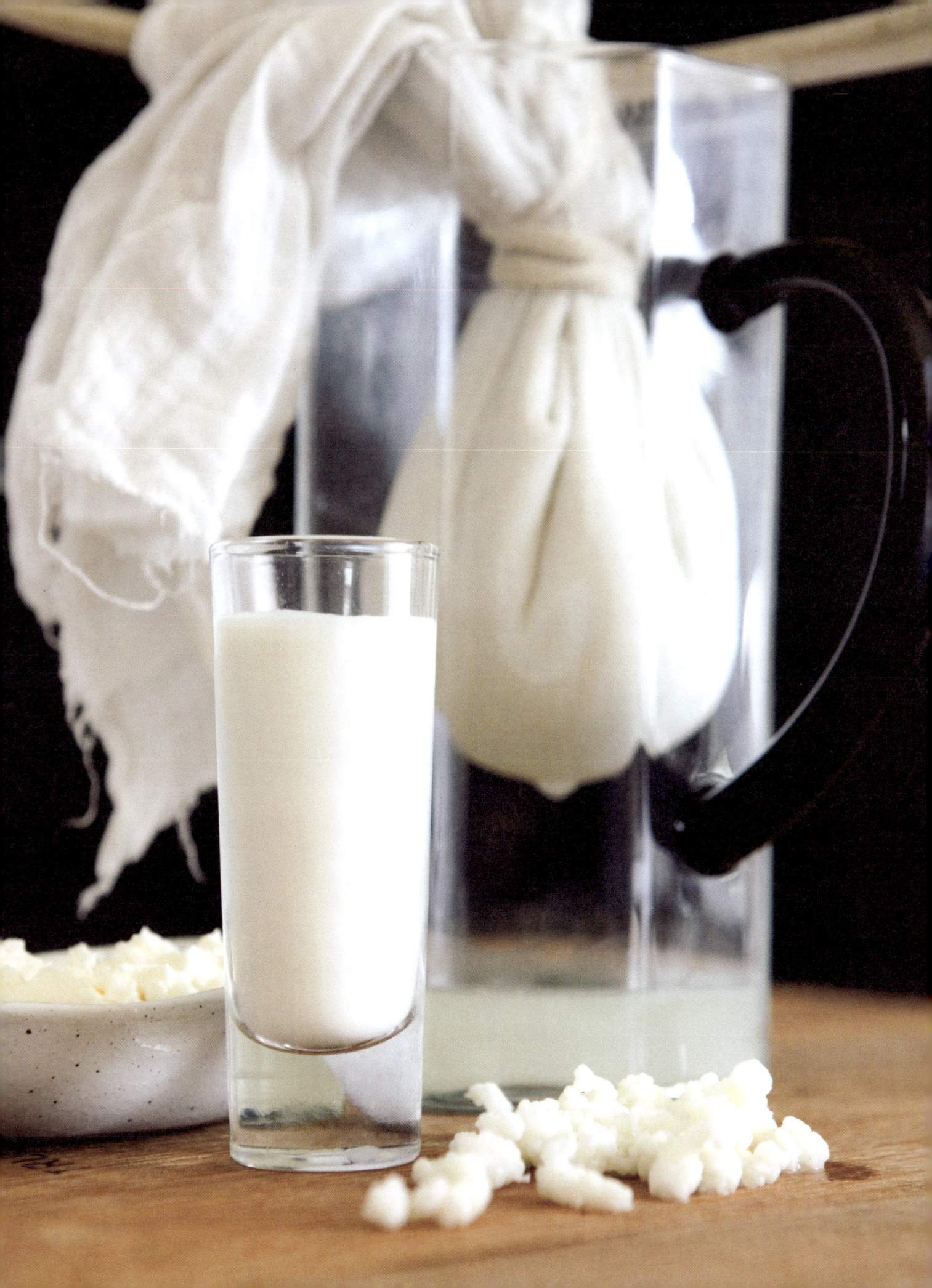

FLOURS

The benefits of making your own flours are that freshness is guaranteed and the anti-nutrients have been released so the flours will be more nutritious and easier to digest.

RICE FLOUR

Cover the rice with warm water and an acid medium (whey, lemon juice or apple cider vinegar). The ratio of rice to acid should be ½ T. acid for every 2 cups of rice. Soak for twelve to twenty-four hours (or overnight), then drain and rinse. To remove more phytates, you can add a tablespoon of buckwheat grains to the soaking bowl (this increases the phytase necessary for the breaking down of phytate.)

Dehydrate the rice at 45°C (110°F) for 12 – 15 hours.

Once dry, grind the kernels in a coffee grinder or food processor. Pour through a sieve to remove any bigger particles.

QUINOA FLOUR

Cover the quinoa with warm water and add an acid medium (whey, lemon juice or apple cider vinegar). The ratio of quinoa to acid should be ½ T. acid for every 2 cups of quinoa. Soak for twelve to twenty-four hours (or overnight), then drain and rinse.

Dehydrate the rice at 45°C (110°F) for 12 – 15 hours.

Once dry, grind the kernels in a coffee grinder or food processor. Store extra flour in a sealed container in the fridge.

ALMOND FLOUR

The process of soaking nuts is called "activation". Activated almonds are easier to digest and have a higher nutritional content.

To activate your almonds, cover the whole raw almonds with salt water (1 T. salt to 4 cups almonds). Leave to soak for 12 - 24 hours. Rinse, and then dehydrate in a dehydrator or in your oven (set to its lowest temperature). Dehydration will take 6 – 24 hours. Ensure your nuts are completely dry to prevent mould from growing.

To make your own almond meal, simply grind the activated almonds in a food processor. This will have a coarser texture than almond flour.

To make almond flour, remove the skins from your soaked almonds before dehydrating them. Then grind in a food processor.

Alternatively, dehydrate the almond pulp left over from making almond milk. Grind this briefly in a food processor.

CHICKPEA FLOUR

1 bag dry chickpeas
water
lemon juice / apple cider vinegar / whey

THE LONG OPTION

Preparing the flour this way has all the benefits of soaking and a milder flavour due to the chickpeas being cooked.

Place the dry chickpeas in a bowl and cover with plenty of water (they will swell, so keep checking on them to make sure they are still covered with water).

Soak the chickpeas in water with 1 T. lemon juice, apple cider vinegar or whey for every cup of water added. Stir, then cover with a tea cloth and allow to soak for 12 – 24 hours.

Rinse the soaked chickpeas thoroughly, then place in a pot with plenty of fresh water. Bring to a boil, and then reduce to a simmer. Cook for 2 hours.

Drain the cooked chickpeas and place them in a blender or food processor. Grind the chickpeas to a paste. Transfer the paste to dehydrator sheets and dehydrate at 60°C (140°F) for 4 – 5 hours until dry and crumbly.

(Alternatively, spread out on baking trays and dehydrate in the oven at 60°C/140°F).

Place the dry, crumbly mixture back into the food processor and process for another minute. Ta da! Homemade, fine, healthy chickpea flour.

Store in an airtight container in the fridge or freezer.

THE QUICKER OPTION

(Quicker, with the benefits of soaking and a stronger flavour than the cooked version above.)

Place the dry chickpeas in a bowl and cover with plenty water (they will swell, so keep checking on them to make sure they are still covered with water).

Soak the chickpeas in water with 1 T. lemon juice, apple cider vinegar or whey for every cup of water added. Stir, then cover with a dish towel and allow to soak for 12 – 24 hours.

Rinse the soaked chickpeas thoroughly, place in the dehydrator or oven and dry at 60°C/140°F until dry. Transfer to a food processor, blender or coffee grinder and grind until smooth.

Store the chickpea flour in a closed container in your refrigerator or freezer.

MILKS

RICE MILK

Place 1 cup cooked rice into a blender and add 4 cups of filtered water. Blend until smooth. Strain through cheesecloth or nut milk bag. Store in the refrigerator and enjoy cold. Shake before using.

You can add a pinch of vanilla powder or cinnamon for extra flavour, and a date or two for sweetness.

ALMOND MILK

Blend 1 cup soaked almonds with 3 cups water, then strain through cheesecloth or nut milk bag. Store in the fridge for up to 3 days. You can sweeten the milk by adding 4 pitted dates to the mix, and flavour with vanilla powder, cinnamon or raw cacao.

HEMP MILK

Blend 1 cup hemp seeds and 1 T. coconut oil with 3 cups warm water, then strain through cheesecloth or nut milk bag. Store in the fridge for up to 3 days. You can sweeten the milk by adding 4 pitted dates to the mix, and flavour with vanilla powder, cinnamon or raw cacao.

QUINOA MILK

Blend ½ cup cooked white quinoa with 2 cups water, then strain through cheesecloth or nut milk bag. Store in the fridge for up to 1 week. You can sweeten the milk by adding 4 pitted dates to the blender mix, and flavour with vanilla powder, cinnamon or raw cacao.

COCONUT MILK

Blend 1 cup of unsweetened, dried coconut flakes with 2 cups of boiling water, then strain. Store in the fridge for up to 1 week.

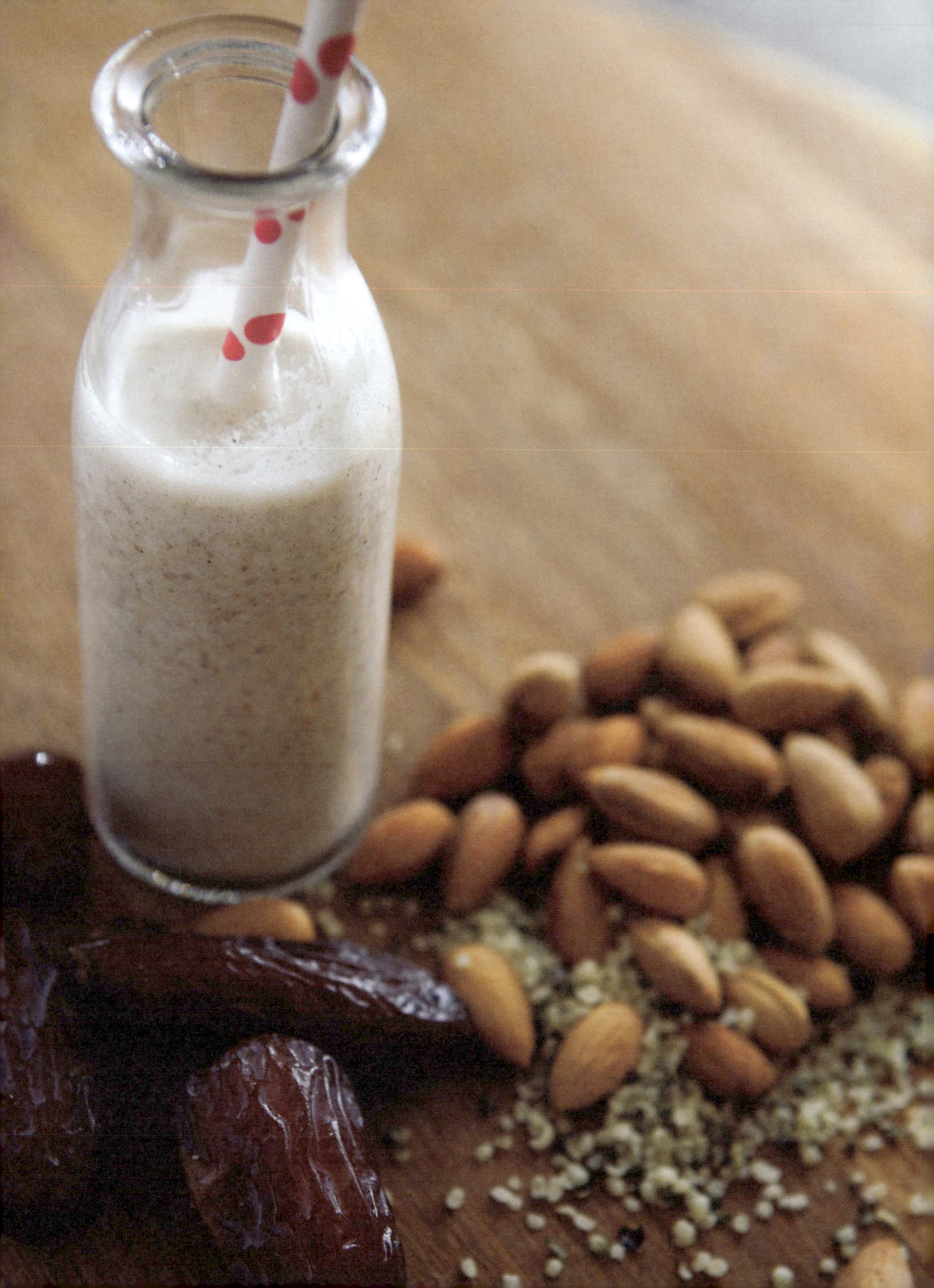

Recipes: Pantry Items

And last, but by no means least....

GLUTEN-FREE PLAY DOUGH!

½ cup rice flour

½ cup non-GMO corn starch or potato flour

½ cup salt

2 t. cream of tartar

1 T. extra virgin olive oil

1 cup water and natural food colouring (see below)

Optional: a few drops of essential oils for fragrance. Citrus oils like orange, lemon and lime are good choices that are safe for small children.

Mix flour, corn starch or potato flour, salt and cream of tartar in a medium-sized pot

Add the olive oil and coloured water and stir until ingredients are well blended. Add the fragrance at this time.

Place pot on the stove over low-medium heat. Cook the dough – stirring often – until begins to pull away from the sides of the pot (about 3 - 5 minutes)

Allow the dough to cool a little and then knead for a minute or so.

Store in an airtight container

Natural food colouring:

- **Red:** *beetroot juice*
- **Orange:** *carrot juice*
- **Yellow:** *turmeric powder*
- **Green:** *spinach juice*
- **Blue:** *purple cabbage juice*
- **Purple:** *blueberry juice*
- **Brown:** *raw cacao powder*
- **Black:** *powder from activated charcoal capsules*

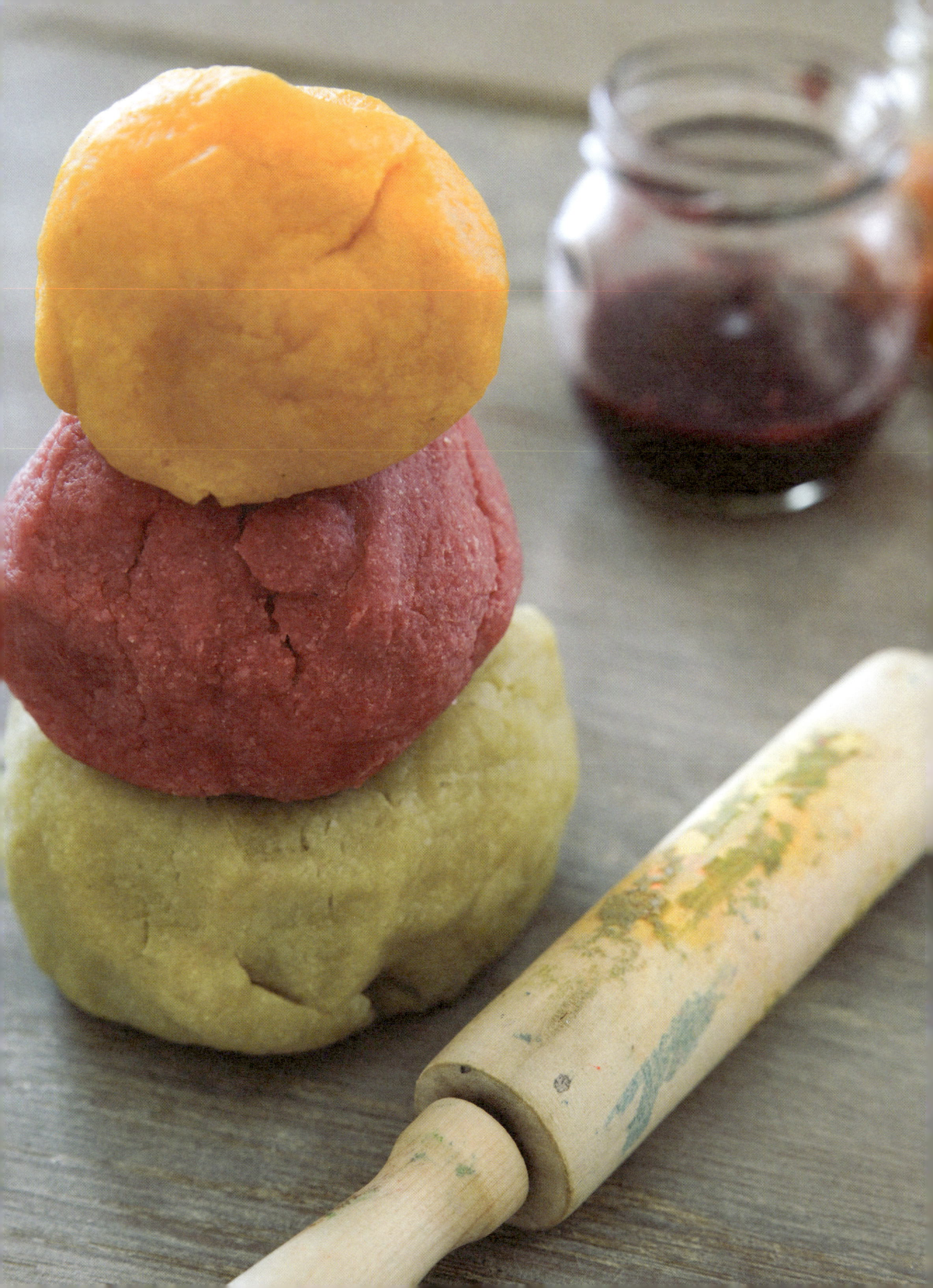

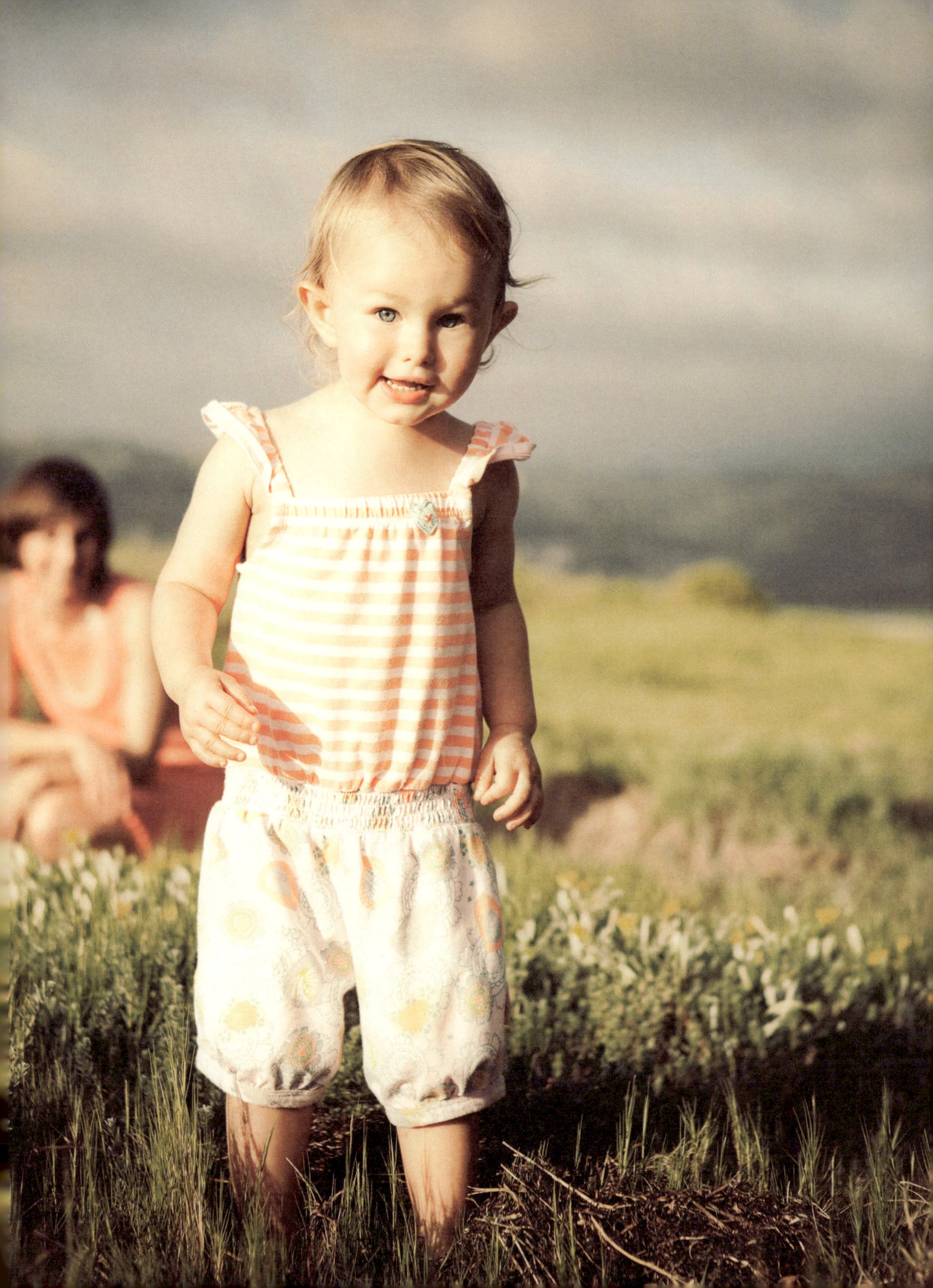

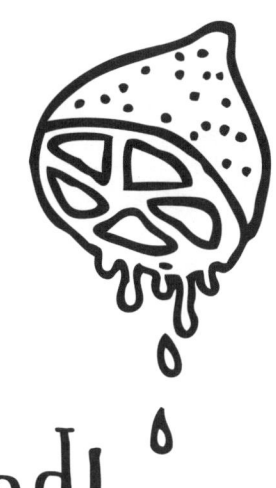

Don't Just Eat Food!

What you put on your body is just as significant as what you put in your body.

Don't Just Eat Food

Since you are putting so much effort into your and your little one's health by eating a natural wholefood diet and avoiding carcinogenic, synthetic additives, pesticides and hormones it only makes sense to avoid putting these ingredients on your skin too.

Your skin is the largest organ of your body and since it is porous, it absorbs whatever you put on it. If the products you use (both on your skin or around your house) contain harmful ingredients such as harsh, toxic chemicals, colours, and fragrances, those ingredients make their way into your body, your blood and lymphatic system. Essentially, if they are on your skin, you are eating them - which is how and why things like hormone patches and topical pain relievers work!

The skin absorbs approximately 60% of whatever formulation you apply to it. On average 200 chemicals are being absorbed through the skin everyday. Think about it… add up your daily 'consumption' of the chemical ingredients commonly found in shampoo, toothpaste, soap, deodorant, hair conditioner, lip balm, sunscreen, body lotion, shaving cream, makeup, and bum cream.

After analysing 2,983 chemicals used in personal care products, the National Institute of Occupational Safety and Health in the US found that 884 were toxic. According to the Environmental Working Group (EWG) "89% of 10,500 ingredients used in personal care products have not been evaluated for safety by the CIR, the FDA, nor any other publicly accountable institution."

The majority of mainstream body care and house cleaning products contain a cocktail of chemicals which are known or suspected carcinogens, neurotoxins and hormone disruptors, allergens, and irritants.

"Putting chemicals on your skin is actually far worse than ingesting them, because when you eat something the enzymes in your saliva and stomach help break it down and flush it out of your body. When you put these chemicals on your skin, however, it is absorbed straight into your blood stream without filtering of any kind, so there's no protection against the toxin." – EWG.

The same motto for food applies to anything that comes into contact with you and your little one's body…. if it has ingredients in it that you cannot pronounce or have only seen in chemistry class, do not use it!

Visit the Environmental Working Group's Skin Deep website for more information www.ewg.org/skindeep/

The 'Dirty Dozen' of skin care

These are the product ingredients which should be avoided.

- **Sodium Lauryl Sulphate:** used to create foam in products such as shampoos, cleansers and bubble bath.
- **Parabens:** a preservative used in many moisturisers and cosmetics.
- **BHA and BHT:** preservatives, mainly included in moisturisers and makeup.
- **Coal Tar Dyes:** in hair dyes and coloured makeup.
- **DEA-Related Ingredients:** found in creamy and foaming products, such as moisturisers and shampoos. Look out also for related chemicals MEA and TEA.
- **Dibutyl phthalate:** used as a plasticiser in some nail care products.

Don't Just Eat Food

- **Formaldehyde-releasing preservatives:** DMDM hydantoin, diazolidinyl urea, imidazolidinyl urea, methenamine and quarternium-15 are used in a variety of cosmetics.
- **Parfum** (fragrance): artificial fragrance ingredients are used in many cosmetics and beauty products.
- **PEG Compounds:** found in the cream base of many cosmetics.
- **Petrolatum:** used for shine in some hair products and as a moisture barrier in many lip balms, lip sticks and moisturisers.
- **Siloxanes:** silicon-based chemicals used to soften, smooth and moisten many cosmetics, hair products and deodorant creams.
- **Triclosan:** an antibacterial included in products such as toothpaste, cleansers and antiperspirants

Use the fact that skin is so absorbent to your advantage. The healing benefits of many foods can be gained by simply applying it to the skin: for example, onions or garlic in your little one's socks at night will help fights colds and flu, as will oreganum oil; and, a few drops of aromatherapy oils in the bath can be used for a wide variety of complaints.

To avoid this unnecessary toxic burden on your little one's tiny body (and yours), choose certified organic and natural skin care and household cleaning products. Or look for solutions in your pantry cupboard!

The ingredients used in this book are not just for eating! Many of them have uses that extend beyond the kitchen and into the bathroom or beyond.

Don't Just Eat Coconut Oil

I have a tub of coconut oil in every room of my house. Here are some of the ways I use it:

- **Bum cream** - Coconut oil makes a great bum cream since it is naturally antibacterial and anti-fungal. It is also effective in soothing and healing nappy rash.
- **Body Lotion** - Coconut oil is quickly absorbed – so there is no sticky film clogging your or your little one's pores. It also soothes psoriasis and eczema.
- **Sunscreen** - Coconut oil as a body lotion has an added benefit of being a natural sunscreen too! It has an SPF of about 5, which means it will protect the skin and underlying tissues from the damage excessive sun exposure can cause, while still allowing UVB rays through – which is necessary for vitamin D synthesis. (Remember while sun exposure is vital for good health, you must protect your little one from the harsh midday sun using long sleeved swim suits and sun hats).
- **Cradle Cap remedy** - Massage onto the affected area on your little one's head, leave on for a few minutes and gently rinse with a warm wash cloth.
- **Antifungal** - Apply topically to kill yeast or yeast infections.
- **Lice remedy** – Rinse the hair with apple cider vinegar, and leave it in until it dries. The vinegar dissolves the 'glue' which sticks the eggs to the hair follicles. When the hair is dry, pour coconut oil into the hair, making sure you get complete coverage. Cover the hair with a shower cap leave it on for the whole day - the coconut oil smothers and kills the lice. Comb the hair with a fine comb to get as many of the eggs and lice out as possible and then shampoo as normal.
- **Ear infection remedy** – Due to its antimicrobial and anti-viral properties melted coconut oil

Don't Just Eat Food

makes an effective ear drop. Place a couple of drops of coconut oil into each ear canal.
- **Sore throat remedy** - A tablespoon melted into a cup of warm tea can help sooth a sore throat.
- **Deodorant** – this is my deodorant of choice. Simply rub some coconut oil under each arm. You can add a sprinkle of bicarbonate of soda for extra odour fighting properties.

Don't Just Eat Olive Oil

- **Cleaning** - Olive oil is an effective way to clean a baby after he/she is born. The vernix covering a baby's skin after birth dissolves in oil – this is a better way of cleaning your newborn than harsh soaps. Meconium (a newborn baby's first stool) is difficult to remove from babies' bottoms. Diaper wipes and warm soapy wash clothes just smear the substance around. Olive oil is the best substance for removing meconium, and it also leaves a protective barrier on the baby's bottom, which makes future meconium clean up easier. Olive oil's high level of antioxidants and its protective factors against damage from UV rays also made it an ideal choice as a first 'soap'. In African tradition it is believed that olive oil helps offer early spiritual protection for the baby.
- **Moisturiser** - Olive oil has been used for centuries for moisturising skin, partly because of its linoleic acid. Apply it directly on the skin, or add a bit to a warm bath for a good soak.
- **Massage oil** - Add a couple of drops of aromatherapy oil and se the mixture to massage your little one before bed.
- **Nappy rash remedy** - Use 2 parts of olive oil to 1 part of water, beat briskly and apply.
- **Cradle cap remedy** - Massage into the affected area, leave for a few hours, then comb the hair. Shampoo as normal to remove oily residue.

Don't Just Eat Honey

A natural anti-viral, anti-bacterial and anti-fungal, raw honey is useful as a:

- **Topical treatment for wounds:** Honey has natural antiseptic properties that ward off bacteria and prevent infections making it a useful and effective treatment for staph infections, burns, cuts and grazes. It also has compounds which accelerate healing. Always use raw honey, and for additional benefits use Manuka Honey.

Manuka honey, produced in New Zealand by bees that pollinate the Manuka bush, is one of the most unique and beneficial forms of honey in the world. It has a considerably higher level of enzymes than regular honey as well as additional healing components that other honey does not have - referred to as the Unique Manuka Factor (UMF). The in honey enzymes create a natural hydrogen peroxide that works as an antibacterial. Manuka has been used by the Maori people of New Zealand for many centuries.

- **Common cough and cold remedy:** Due to its antioxidant compounds, honey has withstood the test of time as a reliable cold remedy. It is considered a demulcent - a medicine that sooths inflamed mucous membranes. Some honey added to herbal tea provides relief for cold symptoms and is very soothing for sore throats. Half a teaspoon before bed can also alleviate irritating night-time coughing.

Honey and thinly sliced onion makes an effective cough mixture. Allow the mixture to 'brew' overnight, remove the onions and give 1 teaspoon of the mixture three times a day.

- **Pink-eye remedy:** The first and only thing that has sent Mila and I running to a conventional GP was pink-eye! For some reason I thought that this was something she really needed western medicine for. The GP prescribed an antibiotic eye ointment, told me it would hurt like hell and that I should bribe Mila with sweets to let me put it in. There and then, I knew I'd come to the wrong place. After returning home and doing some research I found that a warm honey water solution was an effective remedy for pink eye – and a painless one too. Simply dab a piece of cotton wool into the solution and wipe the eye. If some drips down the face – they can just lick it off! It worked like a charm! (Colloidal silver solution works well too.)

HONEY CAN ONLY BE GIVEN TO CHILDREN OLDER THAN A YEAR.

Don't Just Eat Lemon

I could write a whole separate book on the many uses of lemons! Here are a few:

- **Freshen the fridge** - Remove refrigerator odours with ease. Dab lemon juice on a cotton ball or sponge and leave it in the fridge for several hours.
- **Prevent browning of fruits and vegetables** - soak cut fruits like apples and bananas in a lemon water solution; add lemon juice to mashed avo; add a teaspoon of lemon juice to cauliflower and potato cooking water.
- **Refresh cutting boards** - To get rid of the smell and help sanitise your cutting boards (especially after preparing fish, garlic or onions), rub them all over with the cut side of half a lemon.
- **Ant deterrent** - lemon peels along window sills will keep the ants away.
- **Throat infection remedy** - besides gargling with salt water, a cup of warm water with freshly squeezed lemon juice will help fight a throat infection thanks to its antibacterial properties.
- **Moth 'balls'** - take ripe lemons and stick cloves into and all over the skin. The lemons slowly dry with their cloves, leaving a pleasant odour throughout the closets and rooms.
- **Clothes Bleach -** Soak your whites in a mixture of lemon juice and baking soda for at least half an hour before washing.

Don't Just Cook with Bicarbonate of Soda (Baking Soda / Bicarb)

I have a stash of bicarb in my bathroom, my kitchen, my scullery and my laundry room!

- **Detox bath ingredient:** Add 1 - 2 cups of baking soda to a warm bath. It is an effective remedy for swollen glands, sore throat or soreness of the gums and mouth, digestive complaints, vaginal thrush and sunburn. (I generally add something to Mila's bath every night – either Baking soda, Epsom salts, Himalayan salt, seaweed or betonite clay.)

- **Natural oven cleaning:** Baking soda is the most effective natural oven cleaner. Simply sprinkle baking soda on the bottom of the oven, spray or sprinkle with white vinegar and leave for several hours (it will fizz and bubble – very rewarding!). Stuck on grease and burnt on food wipes right off. This works well for very greasy roasting trays too.
- **Deodorant:** Add some bicarbonate of soda to coconut oil for a very effective deodorant.
- **Scouring Powder:** Baking soda, and salt make an effective and natural scouring powder that removes even the toughest stains from baths, pots and floors.
- **Natural antacid:** ¼ t. of baking soda in a glass of water neutralises heartburn and indigestion.
- **Clothes washing powder:** A cup of bicarb with half a cup of salt is sufficient for a normal load (or you can premix a large bath using this ratio). Bicarb cleans, deodorises and softens fabric without damaging the fibres. Salt helps brighten and whiten clothes. You can also add half a cup of white vinegar to the rinse cycle as a natural fabric softener. Your washing will be soft and cared for with a naturally clean fresh smell. (You can add a few drops of essential oil to the soap dispenser for additional natural fragrance.)
- **Nappy soak:** for a cloth nappy soak add ¼ cup of bicarb to five litres of water.
- **Dishwashing powder:** Sprinkle baking soda over the stacked dirty dishes. Add 3% (10 volume) Hydrogen Peroxide into the detergent dispenser and wash! Sparkling clean, sterile dishes at a fraction of the cost!
- **Drain cleaner:** pour ½ cup of bicarb down a blocked drain followed by ½ cup of white vinegar. Let it fizz for a while, then rinse with hot water. No more harsh drain cleaning chemicals!
- **Baby powder:** Mix one part bicarb with six parts organic cornstarch for a safe alternative to baby powders that contain talc. The bicarb deodorises and helps fight infection while the cornstarch absorbs moisture away from the skin. (Don't use this powder if your baby has a yeast infection as the yeast will feed on the carbohydrates in cornstarch.)

Don't Just Drink Rooibos Tea

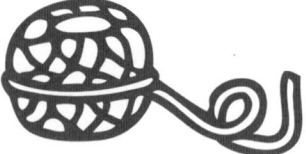

Besides being a delicious, caffeine free drink for your little one, you can use Rooibos tea for the following:

- **Nappy rash:** Mila only ever had nappy rash a couple of times – mostly when I had run out of biodegradable nappies and was using conventional ones instead. At the next nappy change, simply put a dry Rooibos tea bag over the affected area and close up the clean nappy. Repeat whenever you do a nappy change. The rash should disappear within a day or two.
- **Eczema and sunburn remedy:** Add a strong pot of Rooibos tea to your baby's bath to soothe and heal eczema or rashes.
- **Colic remedy:** due to its general anti-inflammatory properties Rooibos tea has long been known as an effective remedy for colic.

Don't Just Eat Cinnamon

Another anti-inflammatory and antibacterial with many uses besides its delicious flavour:

- ♥ **Sandbox:** Add some cinnamon into your little one's sandbox to keep the worms and cat away.
- ♥ **Ant deterrent:** Ants have an aversion to cinnamon. Sprinkle some along windowsills to deter ants.
- ♥ **Athletes foot remedy:** To help kill athlete's foot fungus, soak your feet in cinnamon tea.
- ♥ **Constipation remedy and tummy soother**: a little bit of cinnamon on a teaspoon of honey is a useful remedy to alleviate constipation and sore tummies.

Don't Just Eat All Spice

- ♥ **All spice teething necklace:** Allspice is a natural spice that contains tannin, the tannin slowly enters the system through the skin when wearing an allspice teething necklace. Tannin is said to help gums tighten making it easier for teeth to push through. Allspice teething necklaces also help reduce irritability and fevers and help baby to sleep better. Soak the all spice berries over night. In the morning thread them onto some beading thread or dental floss (super strong). Secure both ends with a magnetic clasp.

Don't Just Eat Sesame Oil

- ♥ **Massage oil:** Sesame oil can be used instead of coconut oil or olive oil for a massage. It is an anti-inflammatory, antioxidant, anti-bacterial, warming and detoxifying oil. Regular massage of your little one leads to: deeper sleep, toned muscles, moisturised and nourished skin, a calm nervous system, decreased stress levels, healthy digestion and healthy bowel movements, balanced weight gain and growth, and improved circulation. Sesame oil is a traditional Ayurvedic oil, and is considered to be the "king of oils" because of its warming and nourishing qualities.

Don't Throw Away Your Banana Skin

- ♥ **Remedy for mosquito bites:** rub the inside of a banana peel onto a mosquito bite to relieve the itch.
- ♥ **Splinter removal:** Tape a piece of banana peel, white side down, over the wound and leave it on for 30 minutes. The enzymes in the peel will seep into the skin and encourage the splinter to move toward the surface for easy plucking.
- ♥ **Wart remedy:** Simply rub a piece of inside of a ripe peel over the wart each night before bed and watch it fade away.

Hydrogen Peroxide (H_2O_2)

Hydrogen Peroxide 3% (10 volume) has been a staple in medicine cabinets and first aid kits for generations. Besides being an effective fruit and vegetable wash, it has the following uses:

- **Cleaning and healing wounds:** A 3% solution helps clean wounds when applied directly, and it also removes dead tissue, stops bleeding in small blood vessels and prevents open wounds from oozing or bleeding. It also helps heal infections.
- **Household disinfectant:** Mix a solution in a spray bottle and use it to disinfect your kitchen and your bathroom. I derive a great sense of satisfaction watching the unseen filth fizz under the spray! It has been shown to kill E. coli and salmonella bacteria on these surfaces.
- **Dishwashing:** put it into the soap dispenser of your dishwasher (instead of dishwashing powder) for sparkling clean dishes.
- **Sinus relief:** when you are all blocked up with a sinus infection, put a drop or two in your ears, one at a time. Let it fizz – tip your head in the opposite direction to let it run out and then repeat in the other ear. (Thank you to my brother for this one!)
- **Disinfect toothbrushes:** Soak toothbrushes in hydrogen peroxide to kill staph. bacteria and other germs common to the bathroom environment.
- **Clean tile surfaces:** Spray hydrogen peroxide directly onto tiles to remove dirt, stains and mould.
- **Soak dish towels & sponges:** Drop dirty towels and cleaning sponges into hydrogen peroxide and let them soak for 15 – 30 minutes to disinfect.

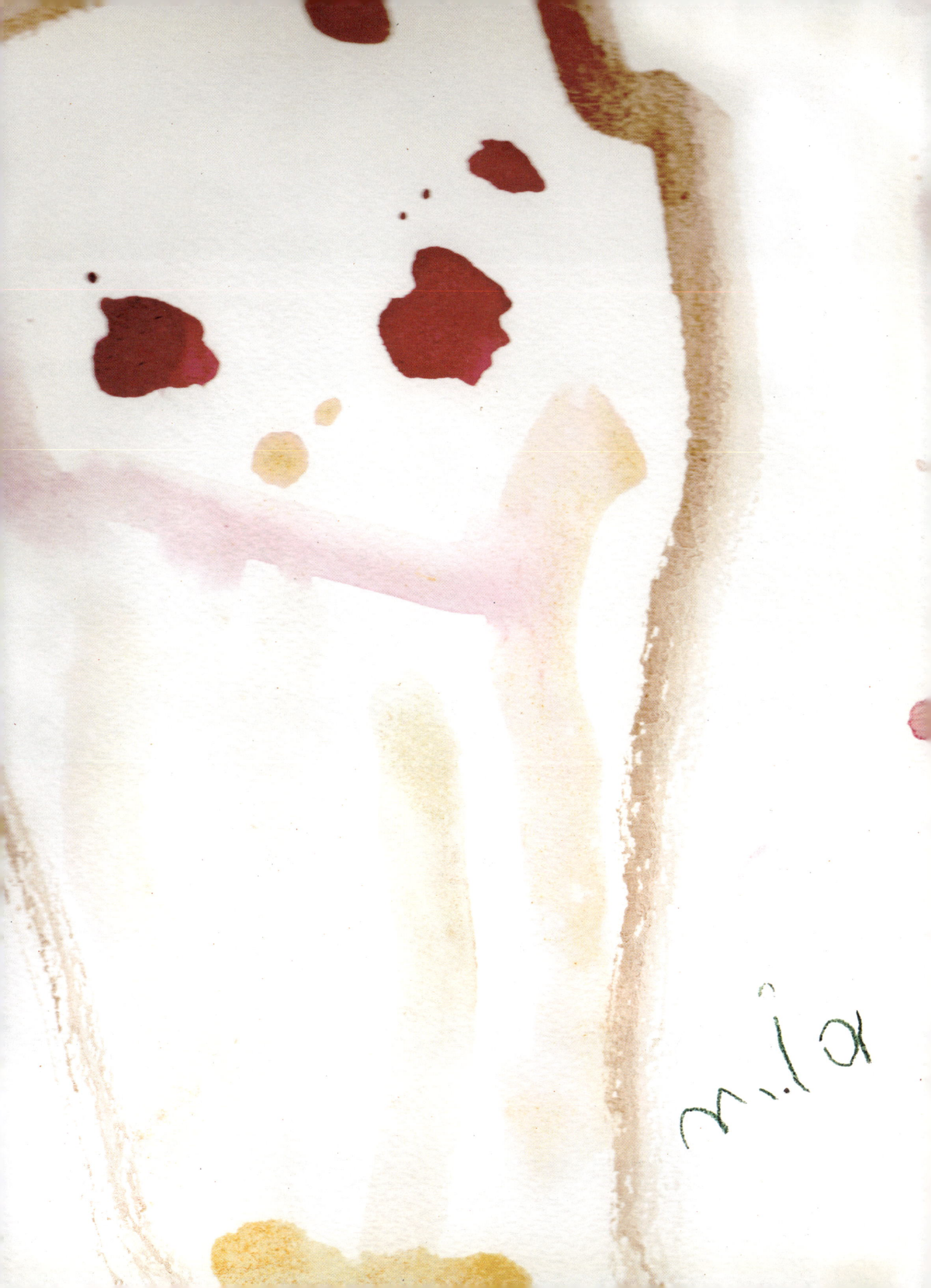

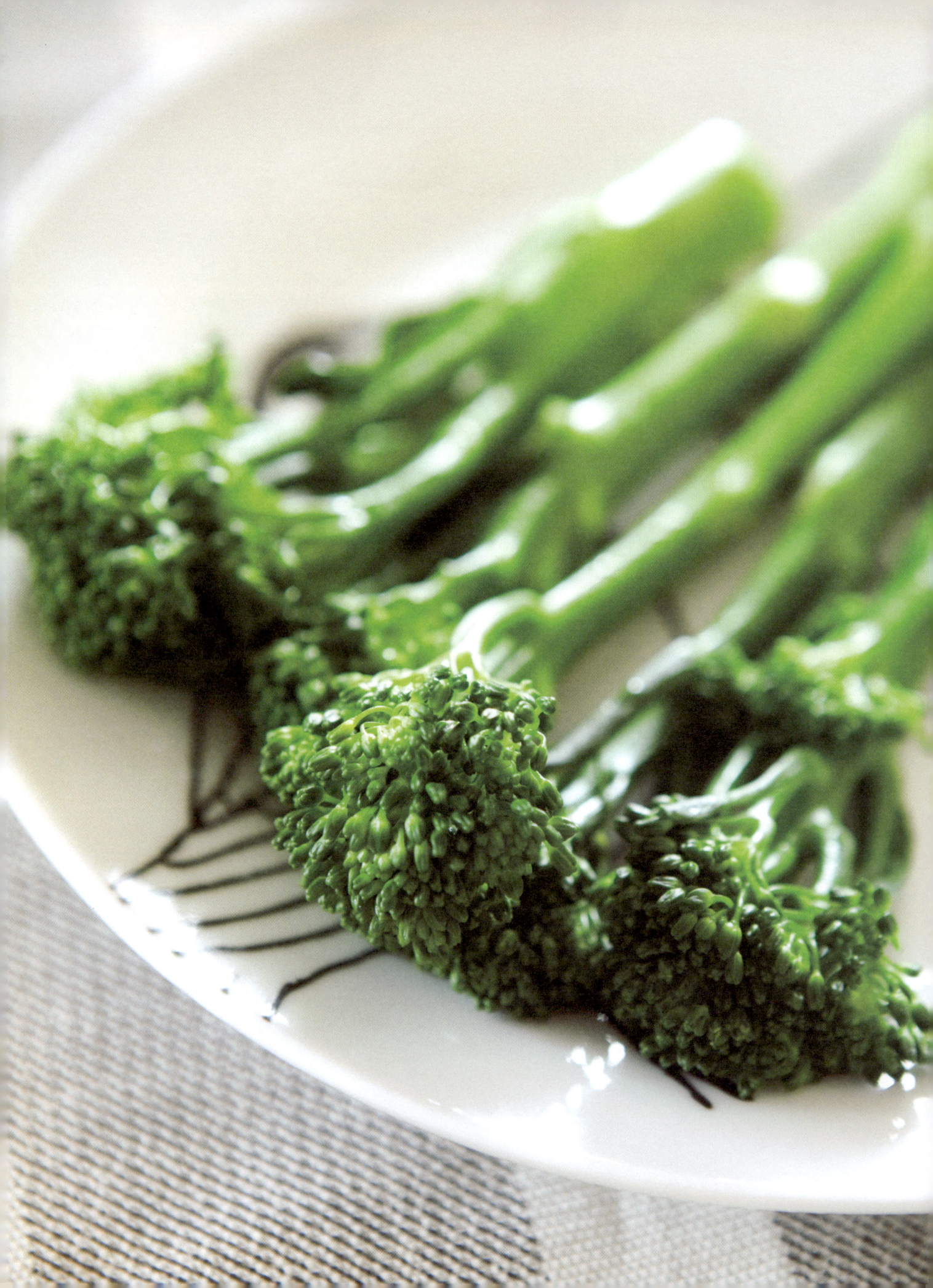

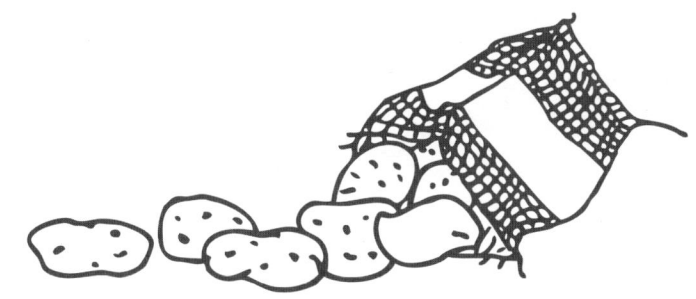

Glossary of Ingredients
All 156 of them!

Glossary of Ingredients

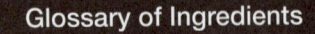

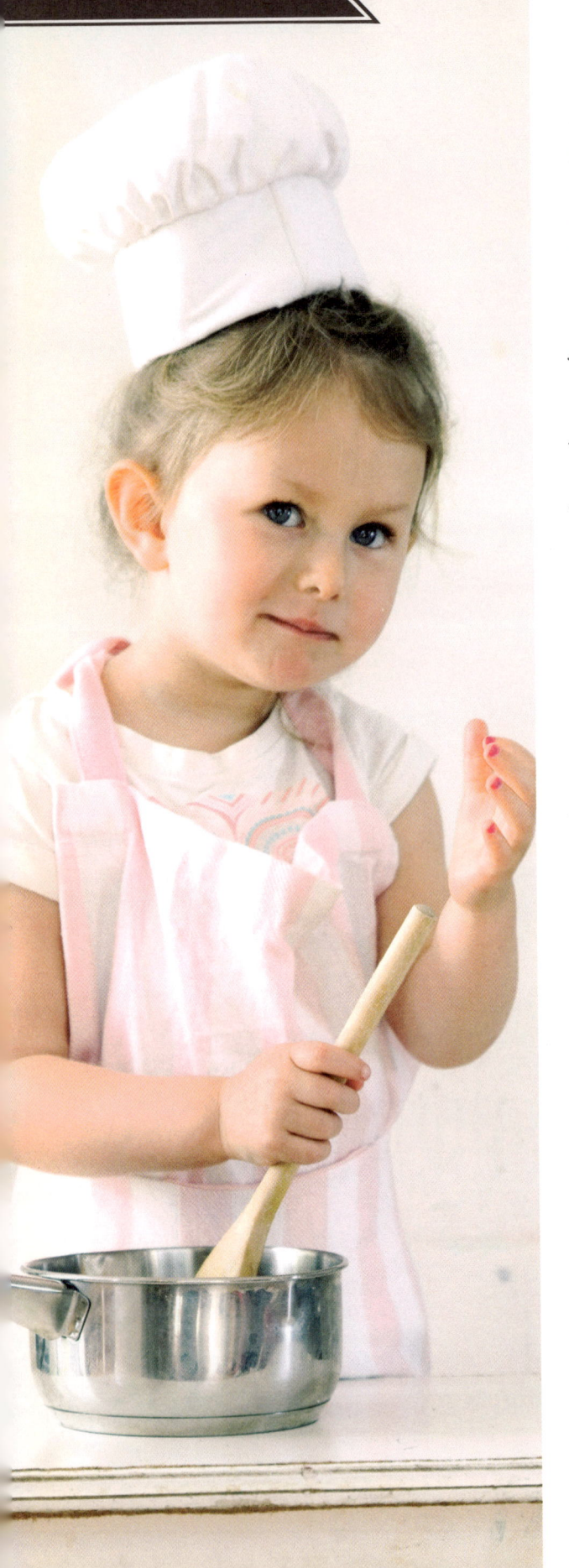

When I started following a gluten-free diet I had not ever heard of many of the ingredients required for gluten-free baking but I had become a bit of a food detective (suspiciously checking all food labels). As such, I spent many hours researching information on each of these foreign ingredients — because I needed to know where they came from and what their nutritional information was before I was going to put them in my body, or Mila's. If this is a new way of eating for you, I trust this section will be a great resource in your food discovery journey.

Another reason for including such in-depth information is that if you, like me, are passionate about feeding your little one as nutritious a diet as possible, then simply knowing that "vegetables are food for you" will not be enough. I am interested in knowing exactly what vitamins, minerals and other compounds are in each food, how they are used, and why they are needed by the body.

When avoiding certain foods (such as dairy) I feel it is very important to substitute those foods with others that have a similar nutritional value. Dairy, for example, is a source of calcium, fat and protein. These are all needed by your growing child. When dairy was not an option for Mila, I discovered that foods such as baobab powder, hemp powder, coconut oil and eggs are great sources of calcium, fat and protein and by including them in her diet, I eliminated the nutritional need for dairy.

This glossary can also serve as a useful reminder of the incredible variety of foods that are available. It is a great idea to introduce a wide variety of flavours to your little one as early as possible to encourage him/her to be an adventurous eater later on.

The majority of the information from this section has been sourced from The George Mateljan Foundation for The World's Healthiest Foods website (www.whfoods.com). The foundation develops and shares scientifically proven information about the benefits of healthy eating and the nutritional content of a wide range of ingredients.

Every single ingredient used in this book is listed alphabetically in this section.

Some health benefits of foods may be more applicable to the mama's and papa's (like cholesterol lowering and heart disease prevention) …. They have been added so that as you become familiar with healthy foods for your little ones, you may find some that can benefit you too.

Glossary of Ingredients

All Spice (Jamaican Pepper or Pimento)

All spice is a dried, unripe fruit and is one of the more widely used spice ingredients in Mexican and other Central American food. Ground allspice has a strong spicy taste and aroma that closely resembles a mixture of black pepper, nutmeg, cloves, and cinnamon.

Allergen: yes

Choking hazard: yes, unless ground

Introduction: 8 months

Selection: Available year round. Choose the whole corns to ensure freshness and flavour. Always buy spices that have not been irradiated.

Storage:
Whole corns ⇢ sealed container ⇢ room temperature ⇢ many years.

Ground spice ⇢ airtight, glass container ⇢ refrigerator ⇢ used as soon as possible.

Nutritional Value:
Good: vitamins A, B2, B3, B6 and C, potassium, manganese, iron, copper, selenium, and magnesium

All spice has anti-inflammatory, warming and soothing and anti-flatulent properties and is known to aid digestion. Traditionally, this spice has been used to treat bacterial and fungal infections as well as coughs, chills, bronchitis, colic and depression. It can be a useful remedy for teething difficulties. The tannin in the allspice helps gums tighten making it easier for teeth to push through. Allspice teething necklaces help reduce irritability, helps your little one to sleep better, and may even eliminate teething fevers.

Almonds

An almond nut is the seed found inside the fruit of the almond tree. Almonds have a delicate, buttery flavour and are one of the most nutritious nuts available.

Allergen: yes

Choking hazard: yes. Alternatively, your little one can eat them in the form of nut butter.

Introduction: 1 year. Grains, nuts and seeds require certain digestive enzymes in order to be digested properly. These enzymes are not present in large enough quantities in your little one's immature digestive system until they are a year old – and only really when they are two years old.

Selection: Always choose raw whole almonds. Many of the beneficial nutrients of an almond are in the skin. Almonds that have been roasted or blanched would have lost many of their nutrients.

Storage:
Activated almonds ⇢ sealed container ⇢ cool, dark place ⇢ several weeks

Soaked almonds ⇢ sealed glass jar ⇢ refrigerator ⇢ 1 week.

Preparation/Use:
So to prevent sore tummies and to get most nutritional benefit from these little superfoods, it is important to prepare them it such a way that reduces the phytic acid, neutralises the enzyme inhibitors and increases the **bio-availability** of the nutrients.

The process of soaking nuts is called "activation". Activated almonds are easier to digest and have a higher nutritional content.

To activate your almonds, cover the whole raw almonds with salt water (1 T. salt to 4 cups almonds). Leave to soak for 12 - 24 hours. Rinse, and then dehydrate in a dehydrator or in your oven (set to its lowest temperature). Dehydration will take 6 – 24 hours. Ensure your nuts are completely dry to prevent mould from growing.

Alternatively, simply soak the almonds and rinse. Store in a glass container in the fridge for no more than 1 week.

Nutritional Value:
Very good: dietary fibre, vitamin E, omega-3 fatty acids, manganese, biotin, and copper

Good: magnesium, riboflavin (vitamin B2), folate, calcium, protein and phosphorus

Almonds are said to contain all the nutrients that the brain needs for optimal development.

Almonds have been used to provide relief from coughs, respiratory disorders, impotency, anaemia and diabetes. They are also found to have great effects on skin care, hair care and dental care. They are rich in mono-unsaturated fatty acids that decrease bad cholesterol (LDL) and increase good cholesterol (HDL).

Almond Flour

Almond flour is made by grinding blanched, skinned almonds. It is an excellent grain-free, gluten-free flour, highly nutritious, easy to use and readily available. It is low GI, high in protein, low in carbohydrates and low in sugars. It should not be eaten in excess almonds have a high amount of Omega-3 fatty acids (which are good), but they are also high in Omega-6 fatty acids (which are essential

Glossary of Ingredients

to your health, but inflammatory if they exceed the amount of Omega 3's in your diet).

Allergen: yes

Introduction: 1 year. Grains, nuts and seeds require certain digestive enzymes in order to be digested properly. These enzymes are not present in large enough quantities in your little one's immature digestive system until they are a year old – and only really when they are two years old.

Selection: Almond flour is susceptible to oxidation (that is, going rancid). Be sure to source almond flour that is as fresh as possible.

As mentioned previously in the section about almonds contain anti-nutrients and, as is the case with all nuts, they should be soaked before eating them. Almond flour that you purchase in the shops would not have been soaked and is therefore be higher in phytic acid than homemade almond flour made from soaked nuts.

Storage:
Airtight, glass container ·· refrigerator ·· 6 months.

Airtight, container ·· freezer ·· 1 year. Be sure to defrost it thoroughly before baking or cooking with it.

Preparation/Use:
To make your own almond meal, simply grind activated almonds in a food processor. This will have a coarser texture than almond flour.

To make almond flour, remove the skins from your soaked almonds before dehydrating them. Then grind in a food processor.

Alternatively, dehydrate the almond pulp left over from making almond milk. Grind this briefly in a food processor.

If using purchased almond flour, use the liquid in the baking recipe as a soaking medium. Soak for a couple of hours before baking.

Nutritional Value:
See Almonds

Amaranth

Amaranth is an ancient grain-like seed cultivated by the Aztecs 8,000 years ago and still a native crop in Peru. It is now grown throughout the world and is gaining popularity, as it is naturally gluten-free.

Amaranth can be popped like popcorn, made into porridge, cooked in a similar way to rice or pasta, or ground into flour. Amaranth flour is very dense and must be combined with other gluten-free flours when baking. It can be used as a thickener (and nutritional enhancer) for sauces, soups, stews, and even jellies.

Allergen: no

Introduction: 1 year. Grains, nuts and seeds require certain digestive enzymes in order to be digested properly. These enzymes are not present in large enough quantities in your little one's immature digestive system until they are a year old – and only really when they are two years old.

Storage:
Whole grains ·· airtight container ·· cool, dark place ·· 4 months.

Whole grains ·· airtight container ·· freezer ·· 8 months.

Amaranth flour ·· airtight container ·· refrigerator ·· 2 months

Amaranth flour ·· airtight container ·· freezer ·· 4 months

It will become bitter if exposed to sunlight and heat.

Preparation/Use:
Amaranth (like other seeds and grains) should be soaked before cooking. Rinse well, cover with water, add 1 tablespoon lemon juice, vinegar, kefir or whey and allow to soak for 8 – 24 hours. Rinse and cook as desired.

To boil use 2 cups water (or stock) to 1 cup amaranth grains. Cook for approximately 20 minutes (cooking time will vary depending on soak time – soaking reduces cooking time).

To make your own flour, soak as above, and then dehydrate the seeds. Once dry, grind them into a flour using a coffee grinder or food processor.

Nutritional Value:
Excellent: amino acids (such as Lysine), manganese, magnesium and potassium.

Very Good: vitamin E, iron, calcium, phosphorous, fibre. Similar vitamin E content to olive oil.

Amaranth is a nutrient-dense food - it is higher in minerals, such as calcium, iron, phosphorous, and carotenoids, than most vegetables. Amaranth is a complete protein (which means it contains all of the essential amino acids). It is an excellent plant source of high quality proteins – with more protein than both oats and rice and a protein content comparable to that of milk. The types of proteins found in amaranth are more digestible than those found in wheat.

Apple

Apples are a crunchy, oval shaped fruit with off-white to cream pulp. The peel colour is either green, light yellow or red depending on apple variety and the flavour can vary

Glossary of Ingredients

from sweet to tart.

Allergen: no

Introduction: 6 months

Being easy to digest, easy to prepare and versatile, apples are a great first food for your little one.

Selection: Apples are one of the Dirty Dozen foods so it is preferable to buy organic. Apples are available all year round.

Storage:
Room temperature ⇢ a few days

Refrigerator ⇢ 2 to 3 weeks

Preparation/Use:
If you cannot find organic apples, soak and wash them in a hydrogen peroxide or vinegar-salt water solution and peel them.

Apples can be eaten raw, steamed, stewed or baked. To introduce them to your little one, blend raw or cooked apples into a purée. Spices such as cinnamon, cloves, vanilla and nutmeg work very well with apples. Soak raw apple in some lemon water to prevent the apple from discolouring.

A rough cooking time guideline

Steam or boil chunks for 5 - 10 minutes (or until just soft).

Bake whole apples at 180°C (350°F) for 30 minutes.

Nutritional Value:
Excellent: phytonutrients (that function as anti-oxidants), vitamin C, insoluble and soluble fibre (namely pectin) and boron.

Apples have antioxidant and anti-cancer properties and are able to regulate blood sugar.

Apple Cider Vinegar

Apple cider vinegar (ACV) is created by fermenting apples. During the fermentation process bacteria break down the sugars and yeast, transforming them first into alcohol and then into vinegar. Apple cider vinegar has been used around the house (for cleaning and disinfecting), as a cooking ingredient and a medicinal remedy for centuries.

Organic, unfiltered apple cider vinegar contains the 'mother' - strands of proteins, enzymes and friendly bacteria that give the product a murky, cobweb-like appearance (and its health benefits).

Allergen: no

Introduction: 6 months (as an ingredient in recipes)

Selection: Always purchase raw, unfiltered apple cider vinegar – it should be cloudy and still have the mother in it.

Storage:: Sealed bottle ⇢ cool, dark place ⇢ use before the expiration date.

It is not necessary to refrigerate an open bottle of apple cider vinegar.

Arrowroot Powder

Arrowroot powder is an easily digestible starch obtained from the rhizomes (underground fleshy stems) of the Maranta arundinacea plant. The plant is considered a herb and is native to the Caribbean.

Arrowroot has a neutral taste, is grain-free and gluten-free, freezes well, tolerates acidic ingredients and dissolves at low temperatures. It is a thickening agent that can be used instead of corn-starch and wheat flour.

Allergen: no

Introduction: 6 months

Storage:: airtight container ⇢ cool, dark place ⇢ use by the expiration date on the packaging.

Preparation/Use:
To thicken with arrowroot, mix it with an equal amount of cold water, then whisk into a hot liquid for about 30 seconds. One tablespoon thickens one cup of liquid.

Nutritional Value:
Very Good: B-complex vitamins

Good: folate

Moderate: copper, iron, manganese, phosphorous, magnesium, and zinc.

Artichoke (Globe Artichoke)

Artichoke is the flower bud of a large thistle. It has spine-tipped leaves with edible bases and an edible 'heart'.

Allergen: no

Introduction: 9 months

Selection: Fresh artichokes are available in spring and summer. Canned and marinated artichokes are available throughout the year – these may have undesirable ingredients added to them, and canned foods contain BPA.

Choose fresh artichokes with compact, dark green leaves. Avoid the very large globes, as they are tough and unappetizing.

Storage:

Glossary of Ingredients

Sealed, plastic bag ⇢ refrigerator ⇢ 1 week.

It is best to eat artichokes as soon as possible after purchase.

Preparation/Use:

Artichokes can be steamed, boiled or roasted.

To prepare the artichokes for cooking soak in a hydrogen peroxide or vinegar water solution then rinse under cold running water. Trim the stem, leaving about 2,5 cm (1") from the base. Remove the lower layers of leaves, as they do not contain any edible flesh. Using a pair of scissors, trim the thorny ends from the remaining leaves. Cut about 2 cm (¾") off the artichoke's top end. Rub a lemon slice over the cut areas in order to prevent them from discolouring.

Boiling: Boil in salt water with some added lemon juice until soft.

Roasting: Tuck a few garlic cloves into the leaves, spray with olive oil and lemon juice and a pinch of sea salt, and wrap in tin foil. Bake at 220°C (425°F) for 1¼ hours.

To eat, simply peel away the leaves, allowing your little one to scrape the soft edible flesh off the bottom of each leaf with her teeth (or gums). Once you reach the heart, remove the furry part, and let them enjoy! You can add this to purées if your little one has not started chewing foods yet.

Nutritional Value:

Very Good: antioxidants in the form of vitamin C and phytonutrients, dietary fibre, vitamin K and folate

Good: magnesium, manganese, copper, potassium, and phosphorus

Artichokes help lower cholesterol, protect and support liver function, increase bile production and prevent gallstones.

Aubergine (Eggplant / Brinjal)

See Eggplant.

Avocado

Avocados are a fruit with a creamy texture and mild, delicate, nut-like flavour. Avocados owe their creamy texture to their high fat content. There are over 50 different commercial varieties of avocado.

Allergen: yes – for those with a latex allergy.

Introduction: 6 months. Avocados make a great first food.

Their mild flavour and high nutrient content make avocados a perfect food for your little one. Sometimes called "nature's perfect food", I think of them as 'mom's perfect food' since they are easy to prepare and do not require any cooking!

Selection A ripe, ready-to-eat avocado is slightly soft and should have no dark sunken spots or cracks. Most avocados you buy in the shops need to be ripened at home. Simply wrap them in newspaper and leave them in your vegetable drawer for a couple of days.

Storage:

Whole ⇢ refrigerator ⇢ 7 – 10 days

Cut ⇢ sealed container ⇢ refrigerator ⇢ 1-2 days

Preparation/Use:

Avocados are best eaten raw.

As a first food you can peel them, remove the flesh and mash it with a fork. As your little one grows, you can it cut into slices.

Sprinkle lemon juice on cut avocado to prevent it from discolouring. Discoloured flesh can be cut away – the rest of the avo will be fine to eat.

Nutritional Value:

Good: phytonutrients, pantothenic acid, dietary fibre, vitamins B6, C, E and K, copper, folate, potassium

Avocados are high in unsaturated fats, which are important for normal growth and development of the central nervous system and brain.

They have anti-inflammatory properties; regulate blood sugar levels and support heart and blood vessels.

Baby Marrow (Courgette / Zucchini)

The baby marrow is a summer squash that resembles a cucumber but is 15-20 cm (6-8") in length. It has a smooth skin, tender crunchy flesh with small edible seeds and a delicate flavour. It has a high moisture content.

Allergen: no

Introduction: 6 months

When first introducing baby marrows, it is best to purée them as the skin may be hard to digest.

Selection: Available throughout the year, but at their best in spring and summer. Choose small to medium-sized baby marrows with shiny, bright green skin, that feel firm and heavy in hand.

Storage:: dry and unwashed ⇢ airtight container ⇢ refrigerator ⇢ 1 week

Preparation/Use:
Baby marrows must be washed thoroughly and may even need to be scrubbed to loosen the dirt. Top and tail the marrows before cooking. They should not be peeled before cooking as the flesh will turn to mush if not held together by the skin (due to its high moisture content).

Baby marrows can be eaten raw, steamed, baked, roasted, grilled and sautéed. Cooking time will depend on cooking method and size, but they generally do not need very long to cook.

Nutritional Value:
Excellent: copper and manganese.

Very good: vitamins B6, C, and K, magnesium, dietary fibre, phosphorus, potassium, folate.

Good: vitamins B1 and B2, zinc, omega-3 fatty acids, niacin, pantothenic acid, calcium, iron, choline, and protein.

Baby marrows have both anti-inflammatory and anti-oxidant properties.

Baking Powder

Baking powder is used as a leavening agent – that is, it lightens texture and makes baked goods rise. It works by means of a chemical reaction that releases carbon dioxide bubbles into the wet batter. These bubbles expand and texturise the batter.

Baking powder be can fast acting, slow acting, or both. Slow acting baking powders start working once the batter is in the warm oven. Fast acting baking powders start working immediately once in the batter (even at room temperature). Most commercial baking powders are double acting – an assurance for success.

Note: if your recipe includes an acid such as yoghurt, kefir, buttermilk, lemon juice or vinegar, there is no need to use baking powder. Just use baking soda - the acidity included as an ingredient in the recipe will activate the baking soda to provide the desired leavening effect.

Allergen: no

Selection: Only purchase aluminium-free baking soda.

Most commercial baking powders contain aluminium in the form of sodium aluminium sulphate or sodium aluminium phosphate. Aluminium is a heavy metal and its consumption has been linked with the development of Alzheimer's Disease. It also tends to add a metallic or 'tinny' flavour to your baked goods.

Choose an aluminium-free baking powder, but be sure that it is GMO-free too. Typically, the starch that is added to aluminium-free baking powders is corn-starch that is likely to be genetically modified.

Alternatively, you can make your own baking powder. This will ensure the purity of the ingredients as well as freshness. Baking powder is not effective unless it is fresh.

To make your own baking powder, simply mix 1t. baking soda (bicarbonate of soda) with 2t. cream of tartar to make a full tablespoon of baking powder.

Storage:: airtight container ⇢ cool, dark place ⇢ 9-12 months

To test if your baking soda is still fresh, stir a teaspoon into a small cup of hot water – if it bubbles it is still usable.

Baking Soda (Sodium Bicarbonate / Bicarbonate of Soda)

Baking soda is one of the safest and most versatile substances around. It is useful not only for baking but for so many medicinal and household purposes I could write a separate book about it!

In its natural form, baking soda is known as nahcolite, which is part of the natural mineral natron. It is identified by the initials E 500 and has a slightly salty flavour. Naturally occurring nahcolite is commercially mined using leach techniques and reconstitution through a natural cooling crystallisation process.

Alternatively baking soda is produced by combining sodium, hydrogen, carbon and oxygen. These elements undergo a chemical reaction to form baking soda.

Baking soda can also be obtained from trona ore. The trona is then heated until it turns to soda ash. Then the soda ash is treated with carbon dioxide to produce baking soda.

In baking, it is used as a leavening agent.

Medicinally, baking soda can be used to: treat colds and flu; remove splinters; soothe sunburn; and relieve itchy insect bites. It is an effective deodorant, toothpaste, tooth whitener, foot soak, exfoliator, and a relaxing and detoxifying bath salt.

Around the house, baking soda can be used to: clean your bathroom and kitchen; safely clean baby toys; unclog your drains by mixing it with vinegar; soften and brighten your laundry; clean your carpets; polish your silver and deodorise your shoes!

Selection: Try find baking soda which is mined from naturally occurring nahcolite.

Storage:: sealed container ⇢ cool, dark place ⇢ indefinitely, but check the use by date on the packaging

Glossary of Ingredients

Banana

Bananas are an easy-to-digest creamy, rich, sweet fruit wrapped in an inedible peel (although the peel has many uses).

Allergen: yes, for people with a latex allergy.

Introduction: 6 months (ideal first food)

Selection: Bananas are picked when they are still green. Allow them to ripen at room temperature. They are best eaten when the skins are yellow and have started to develop black spots.

Storage:
Unripe ⇢ cool, dark place. Unripe bananas should not be stored in the fridge as they will not be able to ripen.

Ripe ⇢ cool, dark place or refrigerator ⇢ 9 days. The skin may turn black in the refrigerator, but the flesh will still be edible.

Ripe ⇢ freezer ⇢ 2 months. Simply peel, plunge into lemon water (to prevent discolouration), place in a plastic bag and freeze.

Preparation/Use:
For your little one… simply peel, mash and serve!

Nutritional Value:
Very good: vitamins B6

Good: manganese, vitamin C, potassium, dietary fibre, potassium, biotin, and copper.

Bananas a good source of pectin, a soluble fibre that can regulate bowel movements. Unripe bananas, however, can cause constipation – as can eating too much banana in one sitting.

While bananas are a sweet fruit and contain a fair amount of natural sugars, they do not cause a blood sugar spike (they have a low GI rating). This is due to their fibre content that slows down the conversion of carbohydrates into simple sugars – therefore regulating the release of sugar into the blood stream.

Bananas are a prebiotic – that is, they feed the friendly bacteria in our guts, and this supports overall digestive health.

Baobab Powder

Baobab powder is found inside the melon-like fruit of the Baobab tree – a tree native to sub-Saharan Africa - where it has been used as a health and beauty aid for centuries. The powder is unprocessed… the inside of the woody-shelled fruit literally contains powder! The powder is simply removed, milled and packaged.

Baobab powder has a sweet, tangy, pear-like flavour.

Allergen: no

Introduction: 6 months

Selection: Baobab powder is available in most health food stores.

Storage:: sealed glass jar ⇢ cool, dark place ⇢ 24 months

Preparation/Use:: Simply add to purées and smoothies.

Nutritional Value:
Baobab powder is said to have: six times more vitamin C than an orange; twice as much calcium as a glass of milk; more iron than a steak; three times more anti-oxidants than blueberries; and, six times more potassium than a banana. It is also a very good source of magnesium, potassium, and B vitamins - all known to benefit general health.

Due to its easily digestible calcium content it is an excellent addition to your little one's diet if you are avoiding dairy.

Baobab protects against free radical damage, builds strong bones, boosts the immune system, soothes tummy upsets, relieves constipation and supports liver detoxification. Baobab is an effective prebiotic.

Basil

Basil is a herb with highly fragrant green leaves that are used as a seasoning for a variety of foods and as the main ingredient in pesto.

As with other herbs, basil has medicinal benefits that could benefit your little one and is a far healthier way to flavour his/her food than sweeteners or artificial flavourings.

Allergen: no

Introduction: 6 months

Selection The leaves of fresh basil should look vibrant and be deep green in colour. They should be free from darks spots or yellowing. When purchasing dried basil, select organically grown basil as this would not have been irradiated (among other potential adverse effects, irradiating basil may lead to a significant decrease in its vitamin C and carotene content.)

Storage:
Fresh ⇢ place the ends in a glass of water ⇢ counter ⇢ 5-9 days

Fresh ⇢ airtight container ⇢ refrigerator ⇢ 5-9 days

Frozen ⇢ whole or chopped, covered with olive oil or water ⇢ airtight container ⇢ 4-6 months

Dried ⇢ tightly sealed glass container ⇢ cool, dark place

⇢ 1 year

Alternatively, grow some in a small pot on your windowsill.

Preparation/Use:
Basil is best eaten raw (fresh). If you add it to one of your cooked meals, make sure you add it near the end to preserve the oils and flavour.

Nutritional Value:
Excellent: vitamin K

Very good: iron, calcium and vitamin A.

Good: dietary fibre, manganese, magnesium, vitamin C and potassium.

Basil has anti-inflammatory and anti-bacterial properties and is able to protect human cells from radiation and oxygen-based damage.

Bay Leaves

One of the most well recognised leaf-spices, the bay leaf has been used for centuries to season soups and stews and for medicinal purposes.

Freshly dried bay leaves have a herbal floral smell, which is infused into any slow-cooked meal. The smell of the spice is more noticeable than the taste – but due to its medicinal qualities I add it at every opportunity. The leaves are removed before serving.

Bay leaves should not be eaten in excess if you are pregnant.

Allergen: no

Introduction: 6 months

Selection You can use fresh or dried bay leaves. Choose non-irradiated dried leaves.

Storage::
Fresh leaves ⇢ sealed container ⇢ fridge ⇢ 2 weeks

Dried leaves ⇢ airtight, glass container ⇢ cool, dark place ⇢ 1 year

Nutritional Value:
Excellent: vitamins A, B's and C

Very good: folate

Good: copper, potassium, calcium, manganese, iron, selenium, zinc and magnesium.

Bay leaves can be used to treat coughs and colds, aches and pains, colic, fevers, digestion and even diabetes.

Beef

Beef is available in a wide variety of cuts that can fulfil many different recipe needs. The different cuts differ in texture and tenderness as well as in fat content. The leanest cuts of beef include eye of round, top round, bottom round, strip steak and flank steak. Fattier cuts include rib, rib-eye, spare rib, T-bone, sirloin, and brisket.

Allergen: no

Introduction: 6 months

Selection: Always source organic, grass-fed beef to avoid the cruelty, hormones and antibiotics used in factory feeding farms.

The meat should be red or purplish in colour (not brown).

Storage:
Once purchased, your beef should be placed in a refrigerator a soon as possible. If you have errands to run after shopping, keep your meat in a cooler box until you get home.

Different cuts of beef while have different **Storage:** times (larger pieces will have a longer shelf life.).
Ground beef ⇢ sealed container ⇢ refrigerator ⇢ 2 days

Ground beef ⇢ sealed container ⇢ freezer for 2-3 months.

Steaks ⇢ sealed container ⇢ refrigerator ⇢ 2 days

Steaks ⇢ sealed container ⇢ freezer ⇢ 2 days

Preparation/Use:
The different cuts can all be prepared in a variety of ways.

Beef is always more tender when slow-cooked, on the bone – this is particularly relevant when cooking for your little one and making purées, or finger food.

Nutritional Value:
Beef from cows who have grazed in pasture year-round, rather than being fed a processed diet for much of their lives, is richer in omega-3 fats, vitamin E, beta-carotene, and CLA (a beneficial fatty acid).

While beef has come under fire lately for being high in saturated fat and cholesterol - this only applies to factory-farmed cows. Grains are not a natural food for cattle (especially genetically modified grains). The grain-based diet used in factory farms largely contributes to the negative aspects of eating beef. Grass-fed cows produce beef which has an omega 6:3 ratio of 0.16 to 1 - science suggests this is the ideal ratio for our diet (and is about the same ratio that fish has). Grass-fed beef usually has less than 10% saturated fat.

Besides the nutrients mentioned above:

Excellent: vitamin B12

Glossary of Ingredients

Very good: protein, niacin, vitamin B6, selenium, zinc, and phosphorus.

Good: choline, pantothenic acid, iron, potassium, and vitamin B2.

Beetroot (Beets)

Beetroot is an ancient food that originally grew naturally along coastlines in North Africa, Asia, and Europe. Traditionally, it was the beetroot greens that were consumed; the sweet red root that most people think of as a "beetroot" today were only cultivated later. Nowadays, people tend to only consume the root and as such, the supermarkets sell them without the stalks and leaves attached. The leaves and stalks are, however, highly nutritious and work well in juices and broths and can be sautéed or boiled in a similar way to spinach.

Raw beetroot has a crunchy texture that turns soft and buttery when cooked. Beet leaves have a lively, bitter taste similar to chard.

Beetroot is incredibly versatile - beetroot juice makes an excellent food colouring for desserts and party food; whole beetroots are an earthy addition to vegetable juices; they ferment well; and, are delicious raw or cooked.

Today, sugar beets (a different variety to those that are sold in supermarkets) are a common raw material used for the production of sugar in place of sugar cane. Be cautious as these are often genetically modified.

Allergen: no

Introduction: 8 - 10 months

Beetroot is relatively high in nitrates that could make your little one nauseous if introduced too early.

Selection: Choose beetroots that are firm, smooth-skinned and deep in colour and avoid any which have spots, bruises or soft, wet areas. Choose beet greens that appear fresh, tender, and have a lively green colour.

Storage:
Roots and leaves ↦ separate sealed bags ↦ refrigerator ↦ 2 weeks

Cooked beetroot ↦ sealed container/freezer bag ↦ freezer ↦ 12-18 months

When storing beets, the leaves should be separated from the roots - leave approximately 5 cm (2") of the stem attached the to the roots – to prevent the beetroot from 'bleeding'.

Preparation/Use:
Wash the roots gently taking care not to tear the skin as this hold the nutrients inside while cooking. Cut into quarters, leaving the stems attached. Beet roots can be steamed or roasted. They are sensitive to heat so steaming for 15 minutes is recommended. They are cooked when you can easily insert a fork through them. Once cooked, rub the skins off with kitchen towel. If your hands become stained during the preparation, rub them with some lemon juice.

Salt added before cooking will drain the colour from the roots, so best to add it after they are cooked. Adding an acidic ingredient like lemon juice prior to cooking will brighten the red colour of the cooked root.

Once your little one is older and chewing well, raw grated beetroot makes for a great (although messy) snack.

Nutritional Value:
Excellent: folate

Very good: manganese, potassium, and copper.

Good: dietary fibre, magnesium, phosphorus, iron, vitamins B6 and C,

Beets are high in antioxidants, have anti-inflammatory and anti-cancer properties and support detoxification of the body (by neutralising toxins and making them sufficiently water-soluble for excretion in the urine).

Bell Pepper (Red Pepper, Yellow Pepper, Green Pepper)

Red, green and yellow sweet peppers are collectively known as Bell Peppers. They are crunchy, plump, bell-shaped vegetables featuring either three or four lobes. Green and purple peppers have a slightly bitter flavour, while the red, orange and yellow peppers are sweeter and almost fruity. Bell peppers are not 'hot'. They are members of the nightshade family, which also includes potatoes, tomatoes and eggplant. Although they are available throughout the year, they are most abundant and tasty during the summer and early autumn months.

Allergen: no

Introduction: 7 months

Selection: Bell Peppers are one of the EWG's Dirty Dozen so it is important to buy organic ones.

Choose peppers that have deep vivid colours, tight wrinkle-free skin, and that are free of soft spots, blemishes and darkened areas. Their stems should be green and fresh looking. Peppers should be firm enough so that they will only yield slightly to a small amount of pressure.

Storage:
Unwashed, uncut ↦ airtight container ↦ refrigerator ↦ 7 to 10 days.

Unwashed, uncut → airtight container → freezer → 2 months

Preparation/Use:
Soak the bell peppers in a salt water, vinegar water or hydrogen peroxide water solution for 20 minutes then rinse under running water.

Use a knife to cut around the stem and then gently remove it. Cut the pepper in half lengthwise, clean out the core and seeds, and then, after placing the skin side down on the chopping board, cut it into the desired size and shape. Alternatively, after removing the stem, scoop out the seeds and leave the pepper whole to make a stuffed roast pepper. The white pulp inside the bell pepper can be eaten.

As the skin of the pepper may be difficult for your little one to chew and digest, it is best to remove it until he/she is a little older. To remove the skin, place the slices of pepper skin side up on a roasting tray. Place the tray under a hot grill until the skin starts to bubble and turns black. Remove the roasting tray from the oven and cover it with a dish towel. Leave the peppers to cool. Once cool, simply peel off the thin layer of skin. You can now add the pepper to purées and dips.

When your little one is older, raw strips of bell pepper make for a great finger food with a variety of dips.

Nutritional Value:
Excellent: variety of antioxidant and anti-inflammatory phytonutrients, vitamins A (in the form of carotenoids), B6 and C

Very good: folate, molybdenum, vitamins B2, B6, and E, dietary fibre, niacin, and potassium;

Good: vitamins B1 and K, manganese, phosphorus, and magnesium.

Bell Peppers have as much as six times the amount of vitamin C as oranges!

They have antioxidant and anti-cancer benefits; can help lower cholesterol and prevent blood clot formation.

Black Pepper

One of the most popular spices and often referred to as "King of Spice". The peppercorn is a dried berry obtained from the pepper plant originally found in South India, before spreading to the rest of the world. The different coloured peppercorns are the same berry - picked at different stages of maturity. Except for the pink peppercorn, which a berry from the Peruvian peppertree.

It is a versatile spice used in virtually in all kinds of savoury cooking.

Allergen: No for black pepper, but pink peppercorns are members of the cashew family - they may cause allergic reactions (including anaphylaxis) for persons with a tree nut allergy.

Introduction: 6 months

Selection: Available all year round. Choose whole peppercorns and grind just before using, as opposed to the powdered or ground pepper. Always buy spices that have not been irradiated.

Storage:
airtight, glass container → cool, dark place → 2 years

Nutritional Value:
Excellent: B vitamins

Good: potassium, calcium, zinc, manganese, iron, magnesium, vitamin A and C

Pepper has been in use for centuries for its anti-inflammatory, anti-oxidant, anti-carcinogenic, carminative and anti-flatulent properties.

Blackstrap Molasses

Blackstrap molasses is a sweetener that is actually good for you! It is the dark liquid by-product of the process of refining sugar cane into table sugar. It has a strong almost bittersweet flavour and a little bit goes a long way.

Blackstrap molasses is a great flavour enhancer for cookies, gingerbread, chicken or turkey and any of your little one's purées or porridges.

Allergen: no

Introduction: 9 months

Selection: Look for unsulphured blackstrap molasses - sulphur is used as a processing chemical. Unsulphured molasses is chemical-free and has a cleaner, more clarified flavour.

Storage:: Opened → sealed container → refrigerator → 6 months

Nutritional Value:
Very good: manganese, copper, iron, calcium, potassium, magnesium, vitamin B6, and selenium.

It can be useful in alleviating constipation (but too much will cause diarrhoea).

Blackstrap molasses is a great way to boost your little one's iron intake.

Glossary of Ingredients

Blueberries

Blueberries are a small purple fruit with flavours that range from mildly sweet to tart and tangy. They were originally native to North America, Europe, the Mediterranean and Asia. They are as delicious as they are nutritious – being one of the best sources of antioxidants. Blueberries are at their best when in season – which is spring and early summer. They freeze well, so can be enjoyed year round. Recent research indicates that the bio-availability of some of the antioxidants found in blueberries actually increases once they have been frozen.

Allergen: no

Choking hazard: yes

Introduction: 8 months

Selection: Blueberries are unfortunately one of the Dirty Dozen – which means they are usually heavily contaminated with pesticides. It would be best to purchase organic (or grow your own at home). Organic blueberries also have a higher nutritional content than conventionally grown ones.

Choose blueberries that are firm and have a lively, uniform colour with a whitish bloom (this is a natural protective coat). Shake the container they are in to ensure that the berries move freely – the berries tend to clump together if they are mouldy, soft or damaged – or if they have previously been frozen.

Storage:
sealed container ↪ fridge ↪ 5-10 days

sealed container ↪ freeze ↪ 6-8 months

Do not wash the berries before storing them as this will remove the protective coating and cause them to spoil sooner.

Preparation/Use:
Blueberries are best eaten raw as their vitamins, antioxidants, and enzymes are damaged during the cooking process.

They make a great out-and-about finger food, are delicious in smoothies and are the main ingredient in Mila's all time favourite – purple fruit leather!

Blueberry juice makes a great purple food colouring.

Nutritional Value:
Blueberries are an exceptionally phytonutrient-dense fruit.

Very good: vitamin C and K, and manganese

Good: fibre and copper

Blueberries provide whole body antioxidant support as well as having: cardiovascular benefits (balancing blood fats, lowering total cholesterol, raising of HDL cholesterol, and lowering of triglycerides); cognitive benefits (improving memory and motor function); blood sugar benefits (acting as a low GI fruit and regulating blood sugar levels); providing they eyes with protection from oxidative and sunlight exposure; providing anti-cancer benefits; protection against heavy metals.

Brinjal (Eggplant / Aubergine)

See eggplant.

Broccoli

Broccoli is a vegetable that is a member of the cabbage family, and is closely related to cauliflower. It was originally cultivated in Italy. The whole broccoli can be eaten and as such, provides a range of tastes and textures from soft and flowery (the florets) to fibrous and crunchy (the stem and stalk). The colour can range from dark green to purplish-green, depending on the variety.

Allergen: no

Introduction: 8 months

As with other cruciferous vegetables, broccoli may cause gas. Start with small amounts of the florets at first and gradually increase the amount if it is well tolerated, introducing the stems last. Adding grated ginger or ginger powder to the broccoli will aid digestion and reduce gas.

Selection: Choose broccoli that is not bruised, yellow or slimy. The stalks and stems should be firm and the leaves should be vibrant in colour and not wilted.

Storage:
Raw ↪ Sealed bag ↪ fridge ↪ 10 days

Cooked ↪ sealed container ↪ 1 week

Cooked ↪ sealed container ↪ up to a year

The Vitamin C content degrades shortly after the broccoli has been picked, so it is best to eat it as fresh as possible.

Preparation/Use:
Soak the broccoli in a salt water, vinegar water or hydrogen peroxide water solution for 20 minutes then rinse under running water. Cut to desired sizes and leave to stand for 10 minutes. The **Nutritional Value:** of broccoli increases if it is left to stand after cutting and before cooking (much the same as garlic).

Steam broccoli for a short time (5 minutes) to maximum flavour and nutrition. The stems may need a couple of minutes longer.

To blanche, place the cut broccoli in a colander and pour a kettle full of boiling water over the florets.

Broccoli can also be enjoyed raw, in juices or dehydrated.

Broccoli seeds make delicious and nutritious sprouts that have high concentrations of Vitamin C.

Nutritional Value:
Excellent: vitamins C and K, chromium, and folate

Very good: dietary fibre, vitamins A (in the form of beta-carotene), B1, B6, and E, manganese, phosphorus, choline, potassium, and copper

Good: magnesium, omega-3 fatty acids, protein, zinc, calcium, iron, niacin, and selenium.

Both the iron and calcium are bio-available to your little one due to the high vitamin C content (vitamin C helps the body absorb calcium and iron).

Broccoli is an incredibly healing and healthy food. It has anti-inflammatory nutrients, antioxidant nutrients, detox-support nutrients, and anti-cancer nutrients. Recent research has shown the ability of a specific nutrient in broccoli to lessen the impact of allergy-related substances on our body – making it a good addition to any hypo-allergenic diet.

Buckwheat (Kasha)

Despite its name, buckwheat is not a variety of wheat – it's not even a grain (although commonly grouped with other whole grains). Buckwheat is, in fact, a seed (like quinoa) and is gluten-free. (I will refer to it as a grain because it categorised as such from a culinary perspective.)

Buckwheat kernels are of a similar size to wheat kernels and have a unique triangular shape. In order to be edible, the outer hull of the kernel must be removed.

Energising and nutritious, buckwheat is available throughout the year, roasted (known as Kasha) or raw, whole or milled into flour. Unroasted buckwheat has a soft, subtle flavour, while roasted buckwheat has more of an earthy, nutty taste. Its colour ranges from tannish-pink to brown. Buckwheat makes an excellent gluten-free alternative to porridge, muesli or as part of a flour mix in gluten-free baking.

Buckwheat was originally native to Northern Europe and Asia.

Allergen: no

Introduction: 12 – 24 months

It is now widely recommended that grains, nuts and seeds only be introduced to your little ones after they are a years old, or when their first molars arrive. This is when their bodies begin producing sufficient amounts of the enzyme needed to digest grains (namely, amylase). Undigested grains (nuts and seeds) can cause havoc on your little one's immature gut and lead to a condition known as Leaky Gut which then leads to food intolerances, allergies and eczema.

I did not know this when Mila was a baby – I feel much of her colic could have been avoided had I not given her grains (nuts and seeds) before she was a year old.

Selection: Buy buckwheat in small individual bags rather than from the bulk section bins to ensure freshness. Make sure there is no moisture in the packet.

Storage:
Whole buckwheat kernels ↪ an airtight container ↪ cool dark place ↪ up to one year.

Buckwheat flour ↪ an airtight container ↪ refrigerator ↪ several months.

Preparation/Use:
Place the buckwheat in a glass bowl and cover with a filtered water and acid solution - 1 T. of either lemon juice, kefir or apple cider vinegar for every cup of buckwheat. Cover the bowl with a dish towel and allow to soak for 12 – 24 hours. After soaking, rinse thoroughly - the soak water will be very slimy! You can now either cook or sprout the buckwheat.

(The flour can also be soaked in whatever liquid is used in the baking recipe, or in water prior to making porridge. Alternatively, make porridge from ground soaked kernels).

To cook: add one-part buckwheat to two-parts boiling water or broth. After the liquid has returned to a boil, turn down the heat, cover and simmer for about 30 minutes.

To sprout: place the buckwheat in sprouting jars. Rinse every morning and night. The sprouts are ready when you can see little white tails (generally after 2 days) – be sure to stop the sprouting process before green leaves appear.

Nutritional Value:
Very good: manganese

Good: copper, magnesium, dietary fibre, and phosphorus

Additional: iron, niacin, folate and vitamin K

The protein in buckwheat is a high quality protein, containing all eight essential amino acids, including lysine.

The buckwheat is better at controlling blood sugar than wheat, it satisfies hunger better than wheat, has an array of antioxidants, and as a "whole grain" may reduce the risk of childhood asthma.

Glossary of Ingredients

Butternut

The butternut squash is shaped like a large pear, has tan skin and light-orange flesh that is sweet with a velvety texture.

Allergen: no

Introduction: 6 months (ideal first food)

Selection: Recent agricultural trials have shown that butternut is an effective intercrop for use in remediation of contaminated soils. That is, they seem to pull contaminants out of the soil. As such, it may be beneficial to choose organic.

Choose butternut that is firm, heavy for its size and have dull, not glossy, skins.

Storage:

Raw, whole ↔ cool, dark place ↔ 1-3 months

Raw, cut ↔ sealed container ↔ refrigerator ↔ 2 days

Cooked ↔ sealed container ↔ refrigerator ↔ 5-7 days

Cooked ↔ sealed container ↔ freezer ↔ 6-8 months

Preparation/Use:
Wash the butternut in a hydrogen peroxide or vinegar water solution, even if you plan on peeling it.

Peeling a butternut can be very frustrating! Make sure you use a sharp knife or, cook the butternut with the skin on and scrape the cooked flesh out once cooked.

The butternut seeds make a nutritious snack (for mama and papa) - they contain nine minerals, 13 vitamins, 18 amino acids and healthy oils. After scooping the seeds from the flesh of the butternut, rinse them and blot dry. Place the seeds in a single layer on a baking sheet, lightly coat with some olive oil and roast them in the oven at 75°C (160-170°F) for 15-20 minutes.

Butternut can be boiled, steamed or baked.

Nutritional Value:
Excellent: vitamin A (in the form of beta carotene) and vitamin C

Very good: manganese, dietary fibre

Good: folate, omega-3 fatty acids, vitamins B2, B6 and K, magnesium, potassium, copper and vitamin K.

Cabbage

Cabbage is a member of the cruciferous vegetable family. It has a round shape formed by superimposed leaf layers. The three most common types of cabbage are green, red, and Savoy. Green cabbage has smooth leaves that range from pale to dark green. Red cabbage has smooth leaves that are either crimson or purple with white veins running through it. Red cabbage contains additional health benefits not found in green cabbage. The leaves of Savoy cabbage are more ruffled and yellowish-green in colour with a more delicate taste than the red and green cabbage.

Bok Choy and Chinese (Napa) cabbage are two other varieties of cabbage. Bok Choy has a mild flavour and a high concentration of vitamin A. Chinese cabbage, with its pale green ruffled leaves, is great to use in salads.

Allergen: no

Introduction: 8 months

As cabbage can cause gas, it is best to introduce in small amounts. Fermented cabbage (as in sauerkraut) will be less likely to cause gas and is easier to digest. It is a great idea to introduce your little one to fermented foods and their bitter taste profile as early as possible. Be sure to have the camera ready to get a photo of their face! Keep offering it regularly so he/she grows accustomed to it.

Selection: Choose cabbage heads that are firm and dense with shiny, crisp, colourful leaves free of bruises, and blemishes. There should be only a few outer loose leaves attached to the stem – these are removed when preparing the cabbage. As with other vegetables and fruit - avoid buying it pre-cut, since once cabbage is cut, it begins to lose its vitamin C content.

Storage:
Red and green, whole ↔ sealed container/ bag ↔ fridge ↔ 2 weeks

Savoy, whole ↔ sealed container/ bag ↔ fridge ↔ 1 week

Preparation/Use:
Soak the individual cabbage leaves in a salt-, vinegar- or hydrogen peroxide water solution for 20 minutes. Rinse the leaves and cut or shred to size.

Allow the cabbage to stand for 10 minutes after cutting it as this activates certain enzymes that increase the cabbage's healing properties.

The best methods of cooking cabbage include lightly steaming or sautéing – 5 minutes is ideal. It can also be eaten raw, fermented and added to juices (although this it creates a slightly burny flavour – so do not add too much).

Nutritional Value:
Cancer prevention tops all other areas of health research with regard to cabbage and its outstanding benefits. Its role in preventing (and treating cancer) is due to its richness in anti-oxidant and anti-inflammatory nutrients. Cabbage is also beneficial and healing to the stomach and intestinal linings. It feeds the good bacteria in the gut and eases digestion.

Cabbage is an excellent source of vitamin K, vitamin C, and vitamin B6. It is also a very good source of manganese, dietary fibre, potassium, vitamin B1, folate and copper. Additionally, cabbage is a good source of choline, phosphorus, vitamin B2, magnesium, calcium, selenium, iron, pantothenic acid, protein, and niacin.

Cacao (Raw)

Raw Cacao is pure chocolate – the cacao bean, from the cacao tree, in its unprocessed, raw state.

It is being marketed and sold as a superfood by raw food pioneers such as David Wolfe and Gabriel Cousens.

There is however another school of thought (led by Jeremy Safron – supposedly the true originator of raw cacao within the health movement) which believes that this nutritionally rich and chemically complex food could be toxic. Their argument centres on the chemical Theobromine, which is a stimulant found in raw cacao. Theobromine is similar to caffeine except that it is a cardiovascular stimulant which is metabolised (detoxified) far quicker by your body. David Wolfe counter argues this by stating that Theobromine is in fact a powerful antifungal and antibacterial.

People have reported side effects after eating raw cacao such as anxiety, inability to fall asleep, depression, mood swings, nightmares and paranoia.

My stance on this comes more from a psychological perspective than a purely nutritional one. Mila has friends that eat sugar and other conventional sweets, chocolates, wheat and dairy – so she is aware of these foods, even though we do not have them at home. I do not feel comfortable denying Mila the excitement and joy of 'sweet treats'. To be able to offer her a healthy (but still sweet and exciting) treat is an important part of how I am raising her – I do not want her to feel different or or like she is missing out because of how I have chosen to feed her. As such, I see the benefits in raw cacao. I must say that I have not had any side effects from the raw cacao, and upon observing Mila after she eats it, neither has she. In fact, I noticed that she slept better after having a piece of Choc-Nut Fudge after her dinner! (This may be due to the high levels of magnesium in the raw cacao.)

I believe moderation is key. I regard it as a treat – not as a food group.

Allergen: rare

Introduction: 12 months

Selection: It is very important to buy high quality and organic raw cacao to ensure there are no mycotoxins present (mycotoxins are produced by mould). These toxins are present in cocoa, coffee and cereal grains and their concentration greatly depends on correct harvesting, fermentation and storage.

Raw cacao comes in the form of powder, nibs, beans and butter.

Storage:

sealed container ·· a cool, dry place ·· 1-3 months

sealed container ·· refrigerator ·· 6 months

Preparation/Use:: Raw cacao can be added to smoothies or used to make raw chocolates and chocolate desserts.

Nutritional Value:
Raw cacao has been shown to have the highest levels of antioxidants of any food on earth.

Excellent: iron and magnesium.

Good: vitamin C, fibre, calcium, protein potassium, phosphorus, copper, and zinc.

Additional benefits of raw cacao are that: it is naturally sugar-free; it is unlikely to cause an allergic reaction; it contains important essential fats and it has less of an effect on blood sugar than nearly any other food (as discovered by Dr. Cousens).

Cantaloupe (Spanspek)

See Spanspek

Cardamom

Cardamom is a seed pod used for both its culinary and medicinal properties. Cardamom is considered one of the most valuable spices in the world due to its rich aroma and therapeutic properties. It is often used in Indian cooking, and is one of the main ingredients of Garam Masala. As it relieves digestive problems induced by garlic and onion it is more than just a flavour enhancer when used in dishes containing these ingredients.

There are two cardamom varieties – a small, light green pod and a larger dark brown pod. The pods are cracked open to release the seeds – these are then crushed and added to the dish. Whole pods can be used to flavour savoury dishes.

Allergen: no

Introduction: 6 months

Selection: Fresh cardamom pods and powder are available year round. Always buy spices that have not been irradiated.

Storage:

Glossary of Ingredients

whole pods → airtight, glass container → cool, dark place → 2-3 years

ground → airtight, glass container → cool, dark place → 1 year

Nutritional Value:
Excellent: iron and manganese

Good: potassium, calcium, magnesium, dietary fibre, vitamins B2, B3 and C

Cardamom is used as an antiseptic, antispasmodic, carminative, digestive, diuretic, expectorant, stimulant, stomachic and tonic. It is used to treat bad breath, tooth and gum decay, sore throats, constipation, indigestion, colic, and may help prevent hormone-induced cancers.

Carrots

Carrots are a root vegetable that are available all year round but are most flavourful when in season in summer and autumn. Carrots have a crunchy texture and a sweet taste, while their green stems and leaves (which are also edible) are fresh tasting and slightly bitter. The most common carrot is the orange variety, although they also come in white, yellow, red, or purple.

Allergen: no

Introduction: 6 months (although they can be constipating)

Selection: Carrot roots should be firm, smooth, and bright in colour (the brighter orange they are the more beta carotene they contain). If the leaves are still attached, they should be brightly coloured, feathery and not wilted. As the sugars are concentrated in the core of the carrot – the larger the core, the sweeter the carrot.

Do not be fooled by the 'baby carrots'! Baby carrots are usually full sized older carrots that have been mechanically shaped into a 'baby carrot'. These mechanically produced carrots are often washed in a chlorine solution to prevent them from turning white. Real baby carrots will still have their skins on and their leaves and stems attached.

Storage:
Raw, root → sealed container/bag → refrigerator → 2 weeks

Stems (separated from the roots) → sealed container/bag → refrigerator → 5 days

Preparation/Use:
Soak the carrots in a salt-, vinegar-, or hydrogen peroxide water solution for 20 minutes then scrub them under running water. If the carrots are not organic, it is best to peel them. When feeding them to your little one, it is best to peel them anyway, as the skins are difficult to digest.

Carrots are delicious either raw or cooked, and make a great finger food for your little one. The beta-carotene found in carrots is actually more bio-available when the vegetable is cooked as opposed to raw. The healthiest way to prepare cooked carrots is to steam them until just soft – this maintains the **Nutritional Value:**.

Nutritional Value:
Excellent: array of phytonutrients, vitamin A (in the form of carotenoids).

Very Good: biotin, vitamins B6, C and K, dietary fibre, molybdenum, and potassium

Good: manganese, niacin, vitamins B1, B2 and E, panthothenic acid, phosphorus, folate, and copper

Carrots are a good source of antioxidants and have cardiovascular benefits, anti-cancer benefits and support the development of healthy eyes.

Cashew Nuts

Cashew nuts are seeds of the cashew apple - the fruit of the cashew tree - which is native to the coastal areas of north-eastern Brazil. The kidney-shaped cashew 'nut' is delicate in flavour with a firm, but slightly spongy texture.

Allergen: yes (more likely if there is a family history)

Chocking Hazard: yes. Alternatively, your little one can eat them in the form of nut butter.

Introduction: 12 months

Grains, nuts and seeds require certain digestive enzymes in order to be digested properly. These enzymes are not present in large enough quantities in your little one's immature digestive system until they are a year old – and only really when they are two years old.

Selection: It is preferable to buy small amounts of pre-packaged cashew nuts rather than buying in bulk from bulk-bins where you cannot be sure of the freshness of the nuts. Make sure that there is no evidence of moisture or insect damage and that they are not shrivelled.

It is always better to buy whole, raw nuts as opposed to the roasted and salted ones - commercially roasted nuts are flash-fried in cheap, rancid oils, while dry roasted nuts are exposed to exceedingly high temperatures that denature the nutrients and cause an unhealthy breakdown of fats. You can always gently roast and season your own nuts at home.

Storage:
Sealed container → refrigerator → 6 months

Sealed container → freezer → 12 months

Cashew nut butter → refrigerator once opened → follow

expiry date

Homemade cashew nut butter ⇢ refrigerator ⇢ 2 weeks

Preparation/Use:
Whole grains, nuts and seeds contain anti-nutrients: enzyme inhibitors and phytic acid.

So to prevent sore tummies and to get most nutritional benefit from these little superfoods, it is important to prepare them it such a way that reduces the phytic acid, neutralises the enzyme inhibitors and increases the bio-availability of the nutrients.

The process of soaking nuts is called "activation". Activated cashews are easier to digest and have a higher nutritional content.

To activate your cashews, cover the nuts with salt water (1T. salt to 4 cups nuts). Leave to soak no longer than 6 hours to prevent them from becoming slimy and developing a not-so-nice flavour! Rinse, and then dehydrate. Cashews can be dehydrated at a higher temperature than other nuts, or even roasted, as their enzymes have already been destroyed during the processing before you bought them. Dehydrate at 100°C (200°F) for 12 – 24 hours. Ensure your nuts are completely dry to prevent mould from growing.

Alternatively, simply soak the cashews and rinse. Store in a glass container in the fridge for no more than 1 week.

Nutritional Value:
Cashews are a very good source of monounsaturated fats and copper, and a good source of magnesium, manganese, and phosphorus. They have a lower fat content than most other nuts. Approximately 75% of their fat is unsaturated fatty acids, plus about 75% of this unsaturated fatty acid content is oleic acid, the same heart-healthy monounsaturated fat found in olive oil.

Cashew nuts have antioxidant properties, are great for energy production and promote cardiovascular health.

Cauliflower

Cauliflower is a cruciferous vegetable in the same plant family as broccoli, kale, cabbage and collards. The compact head (called a 'curd') is composed of undeveloped flower buds. The flowers are attached to a central stalk. When broken apart into separate buds, cauliflower looks like a little tree, something that may intrigue your little one. Most cauliflower is white, however it can also be found in light green, orange and purple colours.

Cauliflower can be eaten raw or cooked. Raw cauliflower has a slightly bitter flavour, while cooked cauliflower has a mildly sweet, almost nutty flavour.

Cauliflower is becoming a popular ingredient in grain-free recipes for pizza bases, wraps and pasta. Cauliflower 'rice' and mash are also increasingly popular and a healthier option than white potatoes or white rice.

Allergen: no

Introduction: 8 months

As with other cruciferous vegetables, it may cause gas, so it is best to start with small amounts, watch for any reaction and gradually increase.

Selection: Choose a cauliflower that has a clean, creamy white, compact head. Avoid spotted or dull-coloured or flowering cauliflower and choose heads protected by think green leaves.

Storage:
Raw ⇢ a paper or plastic bag ⇢ refrigerator ⇢ 1 week.

Cooked cauliflower ⇢ sealed container ⇢ refrigerator ⇢ 2 days.

Cooked cauliflower can be frozen, however it may be watery when thawed.

Preparation/Use:
Soak the cauliflower in a salt-, vinegar- or hydrogen peroxide water solution for 20 minutes then rinse under running water. Remove the hard outer leaves and slice the florets from the stem. (The stem and leaves can be added to soups and broths.) Allowing the cauliflower to rest for 10 minutes after cutting will enhance its nutrient value.

Cauliflower is best steamed or sautéed until just soft (approximately 5 -10 minutes).

Nutritional Value:
Excellent: vitamins B6, C and K, folate, and pantothenic acid

Very good: choline, dietary fibre, omega-3 fatty acids, manganese, phosphorus, and biotin.

Good: vitamins B1, B2, and B3, protein, and magnesium.

As with all cruciferous vegetables, cauliflower provides detox and digestive support, has antioxidant benefits, and anti-inflammatory benefits.

Cayenne Pepper

The Cayenne pepper is variety of chilli pepper with a very hot, spicy flavour. The peppers are left to fully ripen on the plant, hand picked and left to dry. They are then ground into a fine powder.

Allergen: no

Introduction: 12 months

Glossary of Ingredients

I would suggest holding off on the Cayenne pepper until your little one is a bit older as it is VERY hot! When you do start introducing it (in chicken livers, for example,) start with just a tiny pinch.

Selection: Cayenne pepper is available year round. If buying the ready ground one, ensure that is does not contain other fillers and additives. Also make sure your ready ground spices have not been irradiated.

Alternatively buy the whole dried Cayenne pepper and grind it in a coffee grinder.

Storage:
Ground ⇢ airtight, glass container ⇢ cool, dark place ⇢ 1 year

Nutritional Value:
Very good: vitamins A, B's and C, iron, copper, zinc, potassium, manganese, magnesium and selenium.

Cayenne pepper has potent anti-oxidant and anti-inflammatory properties and can be used to improve circulation, aid digestion, stimulate the appetite, reduce inflammation, relieve gas, colds, and chills. It is good for the kidneys, lungs, spleen, pancreas, heart, and stomach.

Celery

Celery is a pale green vegetable with firm, solid stalks and leafy ends. The leaves, stalks, roots, and seeds are all edible and have **Nutritional Value:**.

Allergen: no

Introduction: 8 months

Selection: Celery is on the Dirty Dozen list so it is best to buy organic.

Choose celery that looks crisp and snaps easily when pulled apart. It should be relatively tight and compact and the leaves should be pale to bright green in colour and free from yellow or brown patches.

Storage:
Raw celery ⇢ sealed plastic bag ⇢ refrigerator ⇢ 1 week

Cooked celery ⇢ sealed container ⇢ refrigerator ⇢ 1 week

Freezing raw celery is not advisable as it will wilt – but it will be fine if included as an ingredient in other meals.

Preparation/Use:
Pull the stems apart and soak the celery in a salt-, vinegar- or hydrogen peroxide water solution for 20 minutes, then rinse under running water.

While celery is not commonly given to children to eat on its own, it can be an interesting finger food.

To cook, simply cut to size and steam for 10 minutes.

Once your little one is chewing well, raw celery can make a delicious and nutritious snack (on its own, or for eating dips). The ribs can be peeled and the channel filled with nut butter.

It makes a great addition to purées, broths, stews and soups.

Nutritional Value:
Excellent: phytonutrients, vitamin K and molybdenum

Very good: folate, potassium, dietary fibre, manganese, and pantothenic acid

Good: vitamins A, B2, B6 and C, copper, calcium, phosphorus and magnesium

Celery provides antioxidant, anti-inflammatory and cardiovascular support and it helps protects the stomach and digestive tract.

Chia Seeds

Chia is a flowering mint species of plant native to Guatemala and Mexico. The tiny mild tasting, mottled grey-brown and white seeds are the edible part of the plant. They can be ground or used whole in drinks, bread, crackers and puddings. Due to their gelatinous nature when they come into contact with liquid, they are often used as an egg replacement in baking or as a thickener in sauces, puddings or smoothies.

Allergen: no

Introduction: 8 months

Please note that the seeds swell considerably when placed in liquid (they can absorb up to 9 times their weight in water), so a small amount goes a long way - 1 teaspoon a day will be plenty for your little one.

Selection: Due to their essential oils containing natural insect repellents, the plants are grown without the use of harmful chemicals and pesticides so there is no need to look for organic ones.

Storage:
Whole seeds ⇢ sealed container ⇢ cool, dry place ⇢ 2 years

Whole seeds ⇢ sealed container ⇢ fridge/freezer ⇢ 4 years

Chia gel ⇢ sealed container ⇢ fridge ⇢ 2 weeks

Preparation/Use:
You can grind and pre-soak chia seeds when first introducing them to your little one. Later, you can simply add them whole or ground to puddings, smoothies,

porridge and purées.

Chia has no taste or smell and is easy to include in any meal. It is best to grind the seeds in a coffee grinder and then add it to a purée, as your little one's digestive system may not yet be able to break through the walls of the seed to release its nutrients. As he/ she gets older and is able to gum food, you can simply soak the chia seeds in some liquid to soften them before adding to a purée, pudding or smoothie.

Nutritional Value:
Excellent: omega-3 fatty acids, fibre, protein, calcium, magnesium, manganese, phosphorous and iron.

Good: zinc, vitamins B1, B2 and B3 and potassium

Gram for gram, chia seeds have more calcium than dairy and more omega-3 fatty acids than salmon. Naturally gluten-free, they are being recognised as an exceptionally nutritionally-dense superfood.

Chia seeds are exceptionally high in antioxidants, have anti-inflammatory benefits, provide digestive support due to their soluble and insoluble fibre content, and support healthy development of bones due to their calcium, phosphorous, magnesium and protein.

Chicken

When including any meat into your little one's diet it is important to choose organic, pasture-raised meat.

Non-organic (battery) chickens are subjected to extreme cruelty: thousands of birds are crammed into vast windowless sheds with artificial lights on 24 hours a day; their movements are completely restricted; and, their bodies are pumped full of growth hormones to speed up the production cycle. The food that caged chickens are fed is often genetically modified grains and antibiotics are given as a matter of routine to prevent any diseases rather than administering them if they get sick. Sometimes, the birds grow so fast their legs cannot support their bodies so they spend their short lives sitting in their own waste. As you can imagine, these birds are highly stressed. This is not a good source of food for your little one.

Allergen: no (although an intolerance may show up as eczema)

Introduction: 7 months

Selection: When purchasing chicken, the meat should be solid and plump. Do not be fooled by non-organic value-for-money chickens that look really 'meaty'– these have usually been injected with a saline solution. The skin should be opaque – not spotted. It is preferable to buy fresh chicken and freeze it yourself at home. If you do buy frozen chicken, ensure that there are no freezer burns, icy deposits or frozen liquid in the packaging.

Storage:
The chicken should be in the refrigerator as soon as possible after purchase. Store in the coolest part of your fridge (not the door).

raw chicken ⇢ original packaging or sealed container ⇢ refrigerator ⇢ 2 days

raw chicken ⇢ original packaging ⇢ freezer ⇢ 2 months

cooked chicken ⇢ sealed container ⇢ refrigerator ⇢ 3-4 days

cooked chicken ⇢ sealed container ⇢ freezer ⇢ 4 months

To thaw the chicken, place it on a plate in the fridge. Whole chickens may take up to 2 days to fully thaw in this way, while boneless breasts should thaw overnight. Once the chicken thaws, it should be kept in the refrigerator no more than a day before cooking it.

You can use previously frozen chicken in your little one's food then freeze the prepared meal.

Preparation/Use:
When handling raw chicken prevent it coming into contact with other foods, especially those that will be served uncooked. Wash the cutting board, utensils, and even your hands very well with hot soapy water after handling chicken.

Chicken can be steamed, poached, cooked in the slow cooker, baked or roasted.

Nutritional Value:
Excellent: vitamin B3.

Very good: protein and selenium.

Good: vitamin B6, phosphorus, choline, pantothenic acid, zinc, iron and vitamin B12.

Chickpeas (Garbanzo Beans)

Chickpeas are a round legume with a mild nut-like taste and buttery texture.

Introduction: 12 months

Legumes require certain digestive enzymes in order to be digested properly. These enzymes are not present in large enough quantities in your little one's immature digestive system until they are a year old – and only really when they are two years old.

Selection: Ensure there is no evidence of moisture or insect damage and that the chickpeas are whole and not cracked. Canned chickpeas should be avoided due to the

Glossary of Ingredients

BPA in the can lining.

Storage:
Dry → airtight container → cool, dry and dark place → 12 months

Cooked chickpeas → airtight container → refrigerator → 3 days

Cooked chickpeas → airtight container → freezer → 6 months

Preparation/Use:
Chickpeas contain anti-nutrients, enzyme inhibitors and phytic acid.

So to prevent gas and to get most nutritional benefit from chickpeas, it is important to prepare them it such a way that reduces the phytic acid, neutralises the enzyme inhibitors and increases the bio-availability of the nutrients.

Cover the chickpeas with hot water and add an acid medium (whey, lemon juice or apple cider vinegar) and a teaspoon of baking soda. Soak for twelve to twenty-four hours (or overnight), changing the soaking water at least once during this time. Drain, rinse and cook.

Cover the chickpeas with boiling water or broth (make sure there is twice as much liquid to chickpeas). After the liquid has returned to a boil, turn down the heat, cover and simmer for 1½ hours.

As the preparation of dried chickpeas takes a long time, I usually cook the whole bag, use what I need and then freeze the rest for the next recipe that requires them. That way, I am not tempted to use the canned ones!

Nutritional Value:
Excellent: manganese and protein

Very good: folate and copper

Good: dietary fibre, phosphorus, protein, iron, and zinc.

Chickpeas provide a concentrated source of protein, which makes them a useful addition to your little one's diet if he/she is not a big meat eater. They also contain a wealth of phytonutrients, which function as antioxidants, and many also function as anti-inflammatory nutrients.

Chickpea Flour (Gram Flour, Garbanzo Bean Flour, Besan)

Chickpea flour is made from ground raw or roasted chickpeas. It is a staple ingredient in Indian, Pakistani, Nepali and Bangladeshi cuisines. Chickpea flour is naturally gluten-free and as such is often used in a gluten-free flour mix. Beyond it's health benefits (see above), chickpea flour is remarkably versatile and has a subtle flavour, which makes it ideal for cooking savoury dishes as well as for baking sweet treats.

Allergen: no

Introduction: 12 months

Selection: Chickpea flour can be found in most health stores or Indian food stores. As with all ground flours, it is best to buy flours that are as fresh as possible (from a shop with a high turnover). Ensure that they have been stored away from direct sunlight.

Alternatively, you can make your own. The benefit of doing this is that you can soak/ferment the beans overnight that will help release the phytic acid - making the flour easier to digest and more nutritious. Although time consuming, this flour will be more cost effective than the store bought one.

Storage:
Sealed container → dark, cool place/fridge → 4 months

Nutritional Value:
Chickpea flour has double the amount of protein than whole-wheat flour and six times more than all-purpose flour. It's an excellent source of folate, and also provides vitamin B6, iron, magnesium and potassium.

Cinnamon

Cinnamon is the brown bark of the cinnamon tree. It is available in its dried stick form or as ground powder. It has a fragrant, sweet and warm taste and has been used as a spice and medicine for centuries.

Allergen: no

Introduction: 6 months

Selection: Cinnamon is available year round. Always buy spices that have not been irradiated.

Storage:
Ground cinnamon → tightly sealed glass container → cool, dark and dry place → 6 months

Cinnamon sticks → tightly sealed glass container → cool, dark and dry place → 1 year

Nutritional Value:
Excellent: manganese and fibre

Very Good: calcium

Additionally: potassium, iron, zinc, magnesium and vitamin A.

Cinnamon is known to have antioxidant, anti-diabetic, antiseptic, local aesthetic, anti-inflammatory, warming, and anti-flatulent properties.

> Glossary of Ingredients

Cinnamon supports digestive function; relieves congestion; relieves pain and stiffness of muscles and joints; stimulates circulation; helps prevent urinary tract infections, tooth decay and gum disease and it is a powerful anti-microbial agent that can kill E. coli, Candida and other bacteria.

Cloves

Cloves are the unopened pink flower buds of the evergreen clove tree. The buds are picked by hand when they are pink and then dried until they turn brown. They have a warm, sweet and spicy, aromatic flavour.

Allergen: no

Introduction: 6 months

Selection: Cloves are available year round. Where possible buy the whole cloves and grind in a coffee grinder as needed. Ground cloves should be refrigerated as they loose their flavour quickly once ground. Always buy spices that have not been irradiated.

Storage:: Airtight, glass container ⇢ cool, dark place ⇢ 1 year

Nutritional Value:
Excellent: manganese

Very good: vitamin K and dietary fibre

Good: iron, magnesium, and calcium

Medicinally, cloves are used for their anti-inflammatory, anti-bacterial and antioxidant properties. They are well known for their ability to relieve tooth and gum pain, but their many other benefits include: a digestive aid (stimulates enzyme production and soothes the intestines); relief from asthma and bronchitis (acts as an expectorant); relief from muscle pain from injuries or arthritis and rheumatism; eliminating intestinal parasites, fungi and bacteria (including Candida); encouraging creativity and mental focus.

Coconut

Coconuts are the fruit of the coconut palm tree. Coconuts provide a nutritious source of meat, juice, milk, and oil that has fed and nourished populations around the world for generations. For millions of people in South and South-East Asia, and the Pacific islands coconut is a staple in the diet and provides the majority of the food eaten. The coconut palm is so highly valued by them as both a source of food and medicine that it is called "The Tree of Life." Nearly one third of the World's population depends on coconut to some degree for their food and their economy.

Allergen: rare

Introduction: 9 months

Selection: When choosing a fresh coconut nut, it should feel heavy for its size. When you shake the coconut you should hear a lot of liquid sloshing around inside - if you do not hear anything at all, it means that the coconut is too ripe and it is likely that it will taste soapy.
Coconuts have three eyes. The 'soft eye' is the one that doesn't have the shell slightly raised round one side of it. Once you find the 'soft eye' check it for any discolouration, it should look clean. There should not be any moisture leaking from the eyes. Overall the coconut should look brown not grey. Avoid any coconuts that are cracked or punctured.

Storage:
Dry nuts in the husks ⇢ cool, dry, and humid-free place ⇢ 6 months

Cut, raw coconut ⇢ sealed container ⇢ refrigerated ⇢ 1 week

Cut, raw coconut ⇢ sealed container ⇢ freezer ⇢ 6 months

Preparation/Use:
Using a hammer and a screwdriver, pierce the soft eye on the coconut shell. Drain off the juice, strain and drink - it is delicious! Wrap the coconut in a towel, use a hammer or axe to crack open the shell (it should loosen and break into pieces). Pick out the white flesh. The dark skin can be taken off with a vegetable peeler.

Nutritional Value:
Excellent: protein, fibre, copper, calcium, iron, manganese, magnesium, potassium, zinc and the B-complex vitamins.

Coconut is classified as a functional food because it provides many health benefits beyond its nutritional content. It has anti-inflammatory, anti-viral, anti-fungal and anti-bacterial benefits. It boosts immunity, helps strengthen bones and supports a healthy digestive system.

Coconut Milk

Coconut milk is made by grinding coconut meat and diluting it with plain water. It is rich in protein and fat, and has a consistency similar to fresh cow's milk.

Coconut milk is lactose-free, and is a great dairy substitute.

Allergen: rare

Introduction: 9 months

Selection: Coconut milk is available in tins, cans, cartons or as a milk-powder. When buying coconut milk it is crucial to look at the list of ingredients on the packaging. Many

Glossary of Ingredients

brands of coconut milk contain sodium metabisulphite (E221) as a preservative which is being reported to be a neurotoxin.

Storage:
Canned milk transferred to a glass container ⇢ refrigerator ⇢ 4-6 days

Homemade milk ⇢ glass container ⇢ refrigerator ⇢ 4 days

Canned milk transferred to a glass container ⇢ freezer ⇢ 2-3 months

Nutritional Value:
Coconut milk contains high amounts of beneficial fat in the form of medium-chain fatty acids (MCFAs). Unlike long-chain fatty acids (LCFAs) primarily found in vegetable or seed oils, MCFAs are easier to break down. They are converted to energy rather than stored as fat. Lauric acid, a type of MCFA rarely found in nature, can be found in coconut milk (and breast milk!)

Other nutrients found in coconut milk include: vitamins B1, B3, B5, and B6, C and E, iron, selenium, sodium, calcium, magnesium, and phosphorus and fibre.

Coconut Oil

This information relates to Organic Virgin Cold Pressed Coconut Oil.

Coconut oil is the oil content extracted from the coconut kernel. It is an excellent fat to include in your little one's diet. Due to its high smoke point, it is the only oil I use in my cooking.

Allergen: no

Introduction: 6 months

Selection: It is important to purchase organic virgin cold-pressed coconut oil as the hydrogenated version does not have the same health benefits.

Storage:
Sealed container ⇢ cool, dark place ⇢ 2 years

Coconut oil is solid at temperatures below 24°C (72°F). It does not need to be stored in the fridge as its unique composition stops it becoming rancid as quickly as other oils.

Preparation/Use:
Recipes most often call for melted coconut oil. To achieve this without compromising its health benefits, place the required amount of coconut oil in a bowl. Place that bowl into a bowl containing boiled kettle water. The coconut oil will melt (gently) in a few minutes.

Nutritional Value:
Coconut oil has previously been thought of as a 'bad' oil due to its high concentration of saturated fats. Recent research has revealed, however, that there are actually different types of saturated fats: long-chain fatty acids (LCFA's) and medium-chain fatty acids (MCFA's), and some types of saturated fats are good for you. Much of the saturated fat in coconuts are not LCFA's, but MCFA's. These are easily digested - as opposed to the LCFA's which are generally stored within the body - and are great source of fuel for your baby. The other great source of medium chain fatty acids is… breast milk!

The MCFAs in coconut oil include: lauric acid, caprylic acid, and capric acid. Lauric acid is known to provide immunity against infection by killing harmful pathogens like bacteria, viruses and fungi. This is what gives coconut oil its anti-oxidant, antifungal, antibacterial, antimicrobial and general body nourishing properties.

The MCFAs in coconut oil are also believed to help with the body's absorption of vitamins and minerals from other foods and have been used for many years as dietary supplements in situations where absorption of nutrients needs improvement - including situations involving premature babies.

Coconut Sugar

Coconut sugar is made from the sap of cut flower buds from the coconut palm.

Due to its low glycaemic index, sweetness and lack of coconut flavour it is a great substitute for conventional sugar and can be used instead of honey when your little one is younger than a year old.

Allergen: no

Selection: Be sure to choose a brand that is created by means of low temperature evaporation as opposed to boiling. This will ensure that the enzymes remain intact.

Storage:: sealed container ⇢ cool dark place ⇢ 2 years

Nutritional Value:
It is a source of vitamins B's and C, potassium, magnesium, zinc, iron, and some amino acids - unlike conventional sugar which is an empty food devoid of any nutrients.

Dried Coconut (desiccated coconut or coconut flakes)

Look at the list of ingredients when buying coconut flakes, shredded, or desiccated coconut. Make sure there are no preservatives or sweeteners added.

Check the expiration date - avoid any packets that are close to, or past that date as the coconut will have no moisture or softness and could have a rancid flavour.

Coriander (Cilantro / Dhania)

Coriander is considered both a herb and a spice since both its leaves and its seeds are used as a seasoning condiment.

Fresh coriander bears a strong physical resemblance to Italian flat leaf parsley. It has a strong flavour that pairs well with hot, spicy dishes making it a common ingredient in Thai, Vietnamese, Indian and Mexican dishes. It is best used fresh and added to food after the cooking process in order to preserve its flavour.

The seeds are yellowish-brown in colour with longitudinal ridges. Coriander seeds are available whole or in ground powder form and have a fragrant flavour that is reminiscent of both citrus peel and sage. They pair well with meat dishes.

Allergen: no

Introduction: 6 months

Selection: Fresh coriander leaves should look vibrantly fresh and be deep green in colour. They should be firm, crisp and free from yellow or brown spots. Whenever possible, buy the whole coriander seeds instead of ground coriander powder since the powder loses its flavour quickly. Coriander seeds can be easily ground with a mortar and pestle. Only buy non-irradiated coriander seeds or powder.

Storage:
Fresh coriander, unwashed ↬ plastic bag/sealed container ↬ fridge ↬ 3 days

Chopped, fresh coriander ↬ ice-cube trays, covered with olive oil, water or stock ↬ freezer ↬ 1 year

Add a cube to purées, stews or soups.

Coriander seeds ↬ sealed glass container ↬ cool, dark place ↬ 1 year

Ground coriander ↬ sealed glass container ↬ cool, dark place ↬ 4-6 year

Preparation/Use:
Soak the coriander leaves in a salt-, vinegar- or hydrogen peroxide water solution for 20 minutes then rinse under running water.

Coriander can be added to veggie juices, smoothies, salsas, salads, guacamole, soups, pesto, tomatoes, beans, and veggie dishes.

Nutritional Value:
Coriander seeds

Very good: dietary fibre

Good: copper, manganese, iron, magnesium, and calcium

Coriander leaves

Very Good: vitamins A, K, & C, iron, calcium, and magnesium.

Coriander has anti-inflammatory, antibacterial benefits and cholesterol-lowering effects. It is a remarkable heavy-metal detoxifier and is able to remove mercury and aluminium from where it is stored in the body's tissues.

Corn

See Sweetcorn.

Cranberry

The cranberry is a glossy, scarlet red, very tart berry, which belongs to the same family as the blueberry.

Allergen: no

Introduction: 8 months.

They are very acidic so introduce slowly in small amounts and watch for any acidic reactions like a rash around the mouth or nappy rash.

Selection: Choose fresh, plump cranberries, deep red in colour, and quite firm to the touch. Dried cranberries are sold in many grocery shops and may be found with other dried fruit.

Fresh cranberries ↬ sealed container ↬ refrigerator ↬ 2 weeks

Fresh cranberries ↬ sealed container ↬ freezer ↬ 10 months

Preparation/Use:: Soak the fresh berries in a salt-, vinegar- or hydrogen peroxide water solution for 20 minutes then rinse under running water. If you are using frozen berries, do not thaw them before adding them to your recipe in order to retain maximum flavour.

Nutritional Value:
Excellent: vitamin C

Very good: dietary fibre and manganese

Good: vitamin E and K

Cranberries have long been valued for their ability to

help prevent and treat urinary tract infections. Now, recent studies suggest that this Native American berry may also promote gastrointestinal and oral health, lower LDL and raise HDL (good) cholesterol, aid in recovery from stroke, and even help prevent cancer.

Cucumber

Cucumbers are long cylindrical fruits. Most commonly they have a smooth, dark green, tough (but edible skin) and light green flesh containing soft, edible seeds. You can also find white, yellow, and even orange-coloured cucumbers, and they may be short, slightly oval, or even round in shape. They have a mild flavour and a very high (90%) water content.

Originally from Southern Asia, they are now grown all across the world. Cucumbers belong to the same botanical family as melons and squashes. Although technically a fruit, they are often perceived, prepared and eaten as vegetables.

Allergen: no

Introduction: 8 months

Selection: Conventionally grown cucumbers were ranked the 12th most contaminated food and the second in cancer risk due to their pesticide content, according to the EWG. Additionally, conventionally grown cucumbers are often waxed after being harvested to withstand the long journey to market unscarred and to protect them during handling. While the wax is supposed to be food-grade and safe, petroleum-based waxes are sometimes used. You could simply peel the cucumber, but that is one of the most nutrient-dense parts of the fruit (the other is the seeds), so finding organic cucumbers is a good idea.

Choose cucumbers that are firm, rounded at their edges, with a bright medium to dark green colour. Avoid cucumbers that are yellow, puffy, have sunken water-soaked areas, or are wrinkled at their tips.

Storage:: Covered ↪ refrigerator ↪ 7 days

Preparation/Use:
Soak the cucumber in a salt-, vinegar- or hydrogen peroxide water solution for 20 minutes then rinse under running water. Removing the skin will also make it easier for your little one to eat if he/she doesn't have any teeth yet.

Cucumbers are eaten raw – simply wash, slice (or grate) and serve! Cucumber sticks make a great finger food for when your little one is ready to start gumming his/her food.

Cucumbers are a great addition to vegetable juices due to their high water content and mild flavour. I use one everyday as a way to increase the volume of juice while adding to the overall nutrient content (adding water would increase the volume but dilute its nutrient content).

Nutritional Value:
Cucumbers are often overlooked when considering nutrient dense foods but they do contain a number of necessary vitamins, minerals and phytonutrients.

Excellent: vitamin K and molybdenum

Very good: vitamin B5

Good: copper, potassium, manganese, vitamins B1 and C, phosphorus, magnesium, silica and biotin

Cucumbers have antioxidant, anti-inflammatory and anti-cancer benefits. Fresh cucumber juice is also an excellent remedy for bringing down a fever in children.

Cumin

Cumin is an annual herb. Cumin seeds are yellow-brown and have a nutty, peppery flavour.

Allergen: no

Introduction: 6 months

Selection: Cumin spice is available year round as whole seeds and ground spice. It is preferable to buy the whole seeds and grind with a pestle and mortar as needed. Ready ground spices tend to loose their flavour quickly and may contain other fillers and additives. Always buy spices that have not been irradiated.

Storage:
Whole cumin seeds ↪ airtight, glass container ↪ cool, dark place ↪ 2 years

Ground cumin ↪ airtight, glass container ↪ refrigerator ↪ 1 year

Preparation/Use:
Lightly roast whole cumin seeds before grinding them to enhance their flavour.

Nutritional Value:
Excellent: iron

Very good: manganese

Good: calcium, magnesium, phosphorus, and vitamin B1

Additionally: dietary fibre, vitamins A, C and E, copper, potassium, selenium and zinc.

Cumin is said to prevent gas, clear jaundice, aid digestion, stop diarrhoea, relieve constipation, strengthen bones, lower blood sugar, relieve colds, fevers and sore throats, detoxify the liver, and reduce seizures. Cumin steeped in warm milk with a splash

of honey is said to increase breast milk supply when taken regularly.

Curry Powder

Curry powder is a generic term describing a blend of spices associated with East Indian food.

A typical curry blend would include: turmeric, dried red chilies, coriander seeds, black peppercorns, cumin seeds, fenugreek seeds, fennel seeds, curry leaves, mustard seeds, cinnamon, cardamom, cloves, nutmeg, ginger and bay leaves.

Curry powders range from mild to hot.

Allergen: no

Introduction: 8 months

Selection: Always buy spices that have not been irradiated.

Storage:: airtight, glass container ⇢ cool, dark place ⇢ 1 year

Nutritional Value:: The nutritional profile and medicinal qualities of a curry powder will depend on its ingredients.

Dates

The date, also known as the date palm, is an edible sweet fruit. Dates have a single seed which should be removed before offering the fruit to your little one.

Allergen: no

Introduction: 10 months

Selection: Dates are sold several different ways: with and without pits, fresh, dried, or cured. Both fresh and dried dates should be glossy and plump, with a little wrinkling on their smooth skins. Their skins should not be broken, cracked, or shrivelled. Avoid fruit with any smell of sour milk or with crystallized sugar on the surface. Dried dates should be firm but not hard.

Storage:
Fresh dates ⇢ airtight container ⇢ cool, dark place ⇢ 1-8 months

Fresh dates ⇢ airtight container ⇢ refrigerator ⇢ 3-12 months

Fresh dates ⇢ airtight container ⇢ freezer ⇢ several years

Preparation/Use:
Dates can be soaked before hand to soften them and cut into wedges if serving them as a finger food.

Dates can be used as a natural sweetener in many sweet treats and desserts.

Nutritional Value:
Dates are sometimes referred to as an "almost perfect food," based upon their nutritional content and possible health benefits.

Very Good: vitamins A, B6, B3 and K, beta carotene, folate, choline, calcium, iron, magnesium, phosphorus, potassium, sodium, zinc, copper, and manganese.

Additionally: a source of protein and over 23 amino acids.

Invert sugars make up about 70-78% of the sugar content. Invert sugars are easily absorbed and assimilated in the body and provide the body with energy within minutes after eating it.

Desiccated Coconut

Desiccated coconut is finely grated and dried flesh from the coconut fruit.

See Coconut.

Dill

Dill is a herb with wispy, fern-like leaves that have a soft, sweet taste. Both the leaves and the seeds are used in seasoning food. The seeds are light brown with an oval shape. They have a similar taste to caraway seeds – aromatic, sweet and slightly bitter.

Dill has traditionally been used to add a tangy flavour to pickles (gherkins), salad dressing and fish dishes and medicinally to soothe upset tummies and to relieve insomnia.

Allergen: no

Introduction: 6 months

Selection: Choose fresh dill whenever possible as it has a far better flavour. If you buy dried dill, make sure it is organic to ensure that it has not been irradiated.

The leaves of fresh dill should look feathery and green in colour. Dill leaves that are a little wilted are still acceptable since they usually droop very quickly after being picked.

Storage:
Fresh dill ⇢ plastic bag ⇢ refrigerator ⇢ 4-10 days

Fresh dill, chopped ⇢ in ice-cube trays and covered with olive oil, water or stock ⇢ freezer ⇢ 4 months

Add a cube to purées, stews or soups.

Dried dill ⇢ sealed glass container ⇢ cool, dark place ⇢ 6 months

Glossary of Ingredients

Preparation/Use:
Soak the dill in a salt-, vinegar-, or hydrogen peroxide water solution for 20 minutes then rinse under running water.

Dill leaves can be added to purées, soups, pickles, scrambled eggs to name but a few.

As with other herbs, you can make a medicinal tea from the leaves - place fresh dill into boiling water, steep for at least 5 minutes, strain, and sip throughout the day. The Ancient Egyptians used this for: calming colicky babies, calming the nerves, and soothing upset stomachs.

Nutritional Value:
Good: vitamin A (in the form of pro-vitamin A carotenoid phytonutrients) and other healing components (monoterpenes and flavonoids)

Additionally: vitamin C, calcium, magnesium, folate and iron.

Dill offers protection against free radicals (as an antioxidant) and carcinogens. It has antibacterial, anaesthetic and antiseptic qualities that have made it highly beneficial for viral, bacterial, yeast, and fungal infections, parasites, pain relief, sleep disorders, cancer prevention, and respiratory disorders.

Eggs (Chicken Eggs)

Allergen: yes

Eggs whites are one of the top 8 allergenic foods. While recent research indicates that waiting to introduce allergenic foods to your baby does not necessarily delay or prevent an allergic reaction, it is important to watch your little one closely for possible reactions when introducing these foods. If your family has a history of egg allergy it is best to wait until your little one is 12 months old before introducing whole eggs (even in baked goods).

Introduction: Egg yolks – 6 months

Selection: When choosing eggs, it is important to opt for eggs from organically fed, free-ranging chickens – so as not to support the cruelty battery chickens are subjected to; because the nutrient content of organic, pasture-raised chickens is much better than the alternative; and, to avoid eating eggs from chickens who have been fed GMO grains.

To check your egg is still fresh:

- ♥ Place the whole egg in a glass of water. If it lies horizontally on the bottom – it is fresh; if it stands upright – it is still good to eat; if it floats – do not use!
- ♥ The egg whites should be white and cloudy. Discard the egg if the egg white has a pinkish tinge.
- ♥ The egg yolk should be rich in colour and hold a round shape.
- ♥ The egg should not smell bad. Trust me – you will smell a bad egg as soon as you break it open!

Storage:
Farm fresh, organic eggs ⇢ cool, dark place ⇢ 30 days

Eggs from battery chickens ⇢ refrigerator ⇢ 3-4 weeks.

Eggs from battery chickens are usually washed with a chlorine mist before packaging. This erodes the natural protective layer surrounded the egg and allows bacteria to enter and multiply. Eggs from these facilities are more likely to be contaminated with bacteria (such as salmonella) due to the crowded conditions in which the chickens are raised. It is important to refrigerate these eggs. Once eggs have been refrigerated, they must not be left out at room temperature – it will result in them sweating, which is an ideal breeding ground for bacteria.

Preparation/Use:
Eggs are so versatile and make a variety of different meals. They can be boiled, poached, fried or scrambled.

Nutritional Value:
Excellent: choline

Very good: selenium, biotin, vitamins B2, and B12, molybdenum, and iodine.

Good: vitamins A, B5, and D, protein, phosphorus

Eggs are a source of high-quality protein and cholesterol. According to Sally Fallon Morrell, "Cholesterol is vital for the insulation of the nerves in the brain and the entire central nervous system. It helps with fat digestion by increasing the formation of bile acids and is necessary for the production of many hormones. Since the brain is so dependent on cholesterol, it is especially vital during this time when brain growth is in hyper-speed."

Eggplant (Aubergine / Brinjal)

Eggplants belong to the nightshade family of vegetables, which also includes tomatoes, sweet peppers and potatoes. The most popular variety has a tear drop shape, a deep purple, glossy skin, a pleasantly bitter taste and spongy texture that becomes creamy once cooked. Eggplants are in season in Summer and Autumn, although they are generally available throughout the year.

Allergen: no

Some people may be sensitive to nightshade vegetables.

Introduction: 8 months. The skin may be difficult to digest and should be removed until your little one is a bit older.

Selection: Choose eggplants that are firm and heavy for their size. Their skin should be smooth and shiny, with a bright colour. They should be free of discolouration, scars, and bruises. The stem and cap should be bright green in colour. To test for the ripeness of an eggplant, gently press the skin with your thumb. If it springs back - the eggplant is ripe.

Storage:
Whole, uncut eggplant ⇢ cool, dark place ⇢ 3 days

Preparation/Use:
Soak the eggplant in a salt-, vinegar-, or hydrogen peroxide water solution for 20 minutes then rinse under running water.

It is advisable to 'sweat' the eggplant before cooking it to reduce its bitter taste and to tenderise it. To do this, cut the eggplant, sprinkle it with salt, and allow it to rest for 30 minutes. Rinse the eggplant slices under running water and cook as desired.

Eggplant takes on the flavours of other foods well and can therefore be mixed with a wide variety of foods. Steamed or tempura eggplant makes a great finger food.

Eggplant can be baked, roasted, fired, sautéed or steamed and is cooked once a fork passes through it easily.

Nutritional Value:
Very good: dietary fibre, vitamin B1, and copper

Good: manganese, vitamin B6, niacin, potassium, folate, and vitamin K.

Eggplant also contains important phytonutrients, many which have antioxidant activity.

Eggplant has anti-oxidant benefits, and has been shown to help lower cholesterol and chelate excess iron.

Fish (not including shellfish)

Fish is a food of excellent **Nutritional Value:**, providing high quality protein and a wide variety of vitamins and minerals, and easily digestible protein. There are, however, three major concerns regarding the consumption of fish:

- ♥ The unsustainable harvest of the world's oceans has led to the depletion, and in some cases collapse, of many of the world's major fish stocks. Choose fish that has been 'line-caught' as opposed to trawled.
- ♥ The Southern African Sustainable Seafood Initiative (SASSI) was initiated by WWF South Africa in order to, amongst other things, shift consumer demand away from over-exploited species to more sustainable options. They have developed a simple 'traffic light' approach to categorising fish species: Green - good to go; yellow – purchase on special occasions; red –do not purchase. For more information on this please visit: http://www.wwfsassi.co.za
- ♥ Most major waterways in the world are contaminated with mercury, heavy metals, and chemicals like dioxins, PCBs, and other agricultural chemicals. These contaminants are consumed by the fish, and then by you when you eat the fish. It is important to check where your fish comes from, and choose fish with a shorter life-cycle – they have a lower contamination risk and higher **Nutritional Value:**. A general guideline is that the closer to the bottom of the food chain the fish is, the less contamination it will have accumulated.
- ♥ Unethical fish farming practices whereby fish are fed an artificial diet of GMO corn and soy, and treated with hormones and antibiotics. Choose fish that it is wild caught – as opposed to farmed.

I have limited the fish descriptions to those used in this book.

Sole (East Coast Sole)

Sole is a lean fish and, as such, is very easy to digest.

Sole is on the SASSI orange list of fish species and as such should only be eaten on special occasions. It can be substituted with angelfish that has similar flat, thin fillets.

Hake

Hake is a lean fish of the same family as cod and haddock.

Hake is an easy fish to prepare as it has few bones. It is on the SASSI green list and one of the more affordable fish options.

Allergen: yes.

Seafood allergy – allergic to both fish and shellfish

Shellfish allergy – allergic to shellfish but can eat fish

People with a fish allergy might be allergic to some types of fish but not others. A fish allergy can cause a very serious reaction, even if a previous reaction was mild. A child who has a fish allergy must completely avoid eating fish. Fish allergy can develop at any age. Even people who have eaten fish in the past can develop an allergy. Some people outgrow certain food allergies over time, but those with fish allergies usually have that allergy for the rest of their lives.

Introduction: 8 months (unless there is a family history of allergy)

Selection: It is always best to buy fresh seafood. The flesh should be firm and shiny and should not have an overly fishy or ammonia-like smell.

Glossary of Ingredients

Choose from the SASSI green list, line- and wild-caught fish with a short life-cycle.

Storage:
Raw fish ⇢ sealed container ⇢ refrigerator ⇢ 2 days

Raw fish ⇢ sealed container ⇢ freezer ⇢ 4 months

Cooked fish ⇢ sealed container ⇢ refrigerator ⇢ 3 days

Cooked fish ⇢ sealed container ⇢ freezer ⇢ 2 months

Preparation/Use:: Fish can be steamed, poached, grilled, baked or fried.

Nutritional Value:
Excellent: high-quality protein, vitamin B12, selenium and phosphorus

Very good: choline

Good: omega-3 fatty acids, vitamin B6, potassium, phosphorus, magnesium, zinc, selenium, iodine and iron.

Flaxseeds (Linseeds)

Seeds of the perennial flax plant come in two basic varieties: brown and golden. In their raw form, flaxseeds usually range from amber/yellow/gold in colour to tan/brown/reddish brown. White or green flaxseeds have typically been harvested before full maturity, and black flaxseeds have been harvested long after full maturity. It is recommended to avoid raw flaxseeds that are white, green, or black in colour.

Allergen: no

Introduction: 12 months

Seeds require certain digestive enzymes in order to be digested properly. These enzymes are not present in large enough quantities in your little one's immature digestive system until they are a year old – and only really when they are two years old.

Selection: When purchasing flaxseeds make sure that there is no evidence of moisture. It is preferable to buy flaxseeds in smaller individual packets, as they are highly perishable and can go rancid. Buying often in smaller quantities will ensure you are getting fresh seeds as opposed to those sold from bulk bins.

Flaxseeds can be purchased either whole or already ground. Once flaxseeds are ground, they are much more prone to oxidation and spoilage and as such have a shorter shelf life than whole flaxseeds. It is a better option to buy whole flaxseeds and grind them yourself, as you need them, in a coffee grinder.

Storage:
Ground flaxseeds ⇢ airtight container ⇢ refrigerator ⇢ 6 weeks

Whole flaxseeds ⇢ airtight container ⇢ refrigerator ⇢ 6-12 months

Preparation/Use:
Flaxseeds can be very difficult to chew (especially for your little one) so grinding the seeds prior to consumption can increase their digestibility. The soluble fibre in flaxseeds will tend to thicken any food they are added to.

Add ground flaxseeds to any of your little one's purées, cereals, smoothies or vegetables. You can even coat diced fruit with ground flaxseeds to give otherwise slippery fruit some grip – making it easier for your little one to pick up.

Flax seeds to not contain the levels of anti-nutrients of other seeds and as such I do not soak them overnight before using them.

Nutritional Value:
Excellent: anti-inflammatory omega-3 essential fatty acids

Very good: dietary fibre, vitamin B1 and manganese

Good: magnesium, phosphorus and copper.

Flaxseeds have both anti-oxidant and anti-inflammatory benefits; anti-cancer benefits and can both prevent and relieve constipation.

The primary source of omega-3 fatty acids in flaxseeds has been found to be stable for at least 3 hours of cooking at oven temperatures of 150°C (300°F) – which makes it available after ground flaxseeds have been added to baked goods like muffins or breads.

Flaxseeds are also a good source of lignans - fibre-like compounds that provide antioxidant protection and are a naturally occurring oestrogen. They also contain 'mucilage' - water-soluble, gel-forming fibre that can provide special support to the intestinal tract.

Flaxseed Oil (Linseed Oil)

Flaxseed oil is an edible oil with a sweet, nutty flavour. It comes from the seeds of the flax plant and is widely used as a nutritional supplement.

Allergen: no

Introduction: 6 months

Selection: Flaxseed oil is extremely perishable and should always be purchased in opaque bottles that have been kept refrigerated.

Storage:

Sealed opaque bottle ⇢ refrigerator ⇢ 3 months

Flaxseed oil should have a sweet nutty flavour – if the flavour is bitter, the oil has gone rancid and needs to be discarded.

Preparation/Use:
Flaxseed oil should never be used for cooking purposes or heated in any way, since it is far too easily oxidized. Add flaxseed oil to foods (after they have been cooked) as a nutrient enhancer.

Nutritional Value:
Excellent: anti-inflammatory omega-3 essential fatty acids

Very good: vitamin B1, and manganese

Good: magnesium, phosphorus, and copper

Due to its high concentration of essential fatty acids, flaxseed oil has anti-inflammatory and anti-cancer benefits. It may also assist with resolving constipation, soothing eczema, lowering cholesterol and controlling high blood pressure.

Garbanzo Beans (Chickpeas)

See Chickpeas.

Garlic

Garlic is a vegetable affectionately called "the stinking rose" thanks to its numerous therapeutic benefits. It is a member of the Lily family and is related to onions, leeks and chives.

Garlic is arranged in a pear-shaped head, called a "bulb", which averages about 5 cm (2") in height and consists of numerous small separate cloves. Both the cloves and the bulb are encased in paper-like sheaths that can be white, off-white, or have a pink/purple colour. Although garlic cloves are firm, they can be easily cut or crushed. The taste of garlic is pungent, subtly sweet and nutty. Elephant garlic has larger cloves, but does not offer the full health benefits of regular garlic.

Allergen: no

Introduction: 8 months

Introduce garlic to your little one, in small amounts, in a food that he/she is already enjoying. Treat it as a new food and use the 3-day rule and watch for any reactions. Garlic can cause gas in your little one – even if a breast feeding mother eats it and then feeds her baby.

Selection: For maximum flavour and nutritional benefits, always purchase fresh garlic. The garlic should be plump with unbroken skin. Gently squeeze the garlic bulb between your fingers to check that it feels firm and is not damp.

Always choose locally-grown garlic. Over 80% of the garlic sold worldwide comes from China. It is: grown with chemicals that are now banned in many other countries; bleached to whiten the bulbs; gamma irradiated to prevent sprouting; and, sprayed with the toxic chemical herbicide Maleic Hydrazide to extend shelf life. Imported garlic may also be fumigated with Methyl Bromide on arrival in the destination country.

Storage:
Fresh garlic ⇢ uncovered or a loosely covered container ⇢ cool, dark place away from exposure to heat and sunlight ⇢ 30 days

Preparation/Use:
Separate the cloves and remove the skin. Chop or crush the garlic to activate its health benefits. Allow it to rest for 10 minutes before cooking or adding it to any high acid ingredient (like lemon). Try adding the garlic as near to the end of the cooking process as possible to preserve its health benefits.

Chopped or crushed garlic will loose its flavour and medicinal benefits overtime – so avoid buying pre-crushed garlic.

Nutritional Value:
Excellent: manganese

Very good: vitamins B6 and C

Good: thiamin (vitamin B1), phosphorus, selenium, calcium, and copper.

Garlic is a potent anti-inflammatory, anti-viral and anti-oxidant and is effective in controlling infection by bacteria, viruses, and other microbes including yeasts/fungi and worms. Garlic is a powerful, natural antibiotic - and it does not kill off our healthy bacteria like antibiotic drugs do.

For garlic to be effective as a healing agent and general antibiotic, it needs to be raw. It should also be crushed and exposed to air for ten minutes before it's consumed to fully activate its key germ-killing compound.

Gem Squash (Little Gem Squash, Rolet Squash, 8-ball Squash)

Gem squash seems to be a unique favourite in South Africa (much like biltong) although it originated in Central America. It is a round vegetable, the size of a large apple, with a dark green thick shell of a skin and sweet, firm,

Glossary of Ingredients

dense, yellowy-orange flesh filled with immature seeds. It falls into the summer squash category, although unlike other summer squashes it has a tough, inedible skin.

Allergen: no

Introduction: 6 months

Gem squash is a perfect first food for your little one. It is not **Allergen**ic, easy to prepare, has a soft texture and mild flavour – and it comes in its own biodegradable serving bowl!

Selection: Choose gem squash that is heavy for its size and has a dark green colour with no bruises or marks on the skin.

Storage:
Whole, raw gem squash ⇢ cool dark place ⇢ 2 weeks

Cooked gem squash ⇢ sealed container ⇢ refrigerator ⇢ 2 days

Cooked gem squash ⇢ sealed container ⇢ freezer ⇢ 2 months

Once cooked, you can store it in the fridge for a couple of days, or freeze it for a couple of months.

Preparation/Use:
Soak the gem squash in a salt-, vinegar-, or hydrogen peroxide water solution for 20 minutes then rinse under running water. Cut the squash in half and steam for 10 minutes, or until the flesh is soft. Scoop out the seeds; add a teaspoon of coconut oil or ghee and a sprinkle of sea salt and serve. Alternatively, you can scoop out the flesh and mash or purée.

Nutritional Value:
Good: vitamin A (in the form of carotenes), vitamin C, vitamin B, potassium and fibre.

Ghee (Clarified Butter, Butter Oil, Drawn Butter)

Ghee is butter that has been melted over low heat and allowed to bubble and simmer until most of the water has been evaporated. The highest-quality ghee is obtained when the long-simmered butter is allowed to cool and only the top-most layer is skimmed off.

It is a nutrient dense fat used in cooking (traditionally in India) and for medicinal benefits within the Ayurvedic system. Ghee is more stable (has a higher smoke point), has a longer shelf life, and is easier to digest than butter… even by those with lactose or casein intolerance since the milk solids and impurities have been removed. Ghee has a unique and flavourful taste and aroma that is different from butter, but it can be used in almost all of the same ways.

Allergen: no

May cause a reaction for people with a dairy/lactose/casein intolerance.

Introduction: 6 months

Selection: Choose ghee that has been made from raw, organic butter source from pasture-fed cows.

Storage:
Sealed container ⇢ cool, dark place ⇢ 2-3 months

Sealed container ⇢ refrigerator ⇢ up to a year

Use:
Ghee has a high smoke point so it is one of the best fats to cook with. You can use ghee instead of butter in all recipes. It can be added to purées and smoothies or melted on top of veggies for a shot of healthy fat and a nutrient boost.

Nutritional Value:
Excellent: vitamins A, D, E, and K, omega 3 fatty acids and CLA (Conjugated Linoleic Acid)

Ghee - like butter - is one of the best sources of butyric acid (butyrate). The cells of the colon feed on butyrate for energy which helps them to produce a healthier intestinal lining. In Ayurveda ghee is a trusted means to increase one's "digestive fire" which will, in turn, improve the assimilation of nutrients and enhance the nutritional value of food. In addition, butyrate has been found to have antiviral and anti-cancer properties. Research shows that adequate production of butyric acid supports the production of killer T cells in the gut, and thus a strong immune system.

Ghee has anti-cancer, antiviral, anti-inflammatory benefits. It protects your gastrointestinal system and is beneficial in the prevention or treatment of cancer, heart disease, asthma, osteoporosis, colitis, and insulin resistance.

Ginger

Ginger is a popular root* herb with an aromatic, pungent, spicy flavour. The flesh can be yellow, white or red in colour, depending on the variety. It is covered with a brownish skin that may either be thick or thin, depending upon whether the plant was harvested when it was mature or young. This thick, knotted root has a wide range of culinary and medicinal uses.

* To be technically correct the fleshy ginger 'root' is in fact a rhizome. Rhizomes are fleshy, horizontal stems that usually grow underground.

Allergen: no

Introduction: 6 months

Selection: Ginger is available year round either fresh,

dried or ground. It is always preferable to use fresh ginger. Fresh roots should feel heavy, be juicy and have a peel that is free from dark spots or mould.

When purchasing ground ginger make sure it has not been irradiated.

Storage:
Whole, fresh ginger root ⇢ refrigerator ⇢ 1 month

Cut fresh ginger ⇢ refrigerator ⇢ 1 week

Ground ginger ⇢ airtight, glass container ⇢ refrigerator ⇢ 1 year

Nutritional Value:
Good: vitamin C, magnesium, potassium, copper and manganese.

Ginger is well known as a remedy for headaches, menstrual cramps, motion sickness, nausea, indigestion, wind, colic, irritable bowel, loss of appetite, chills, cold, flu, bronchitis, poor circulation, and heartburn. Ginger tea is a useful remedy for morning sickness. It boosts the immune system and protects against bacteria and fungi.

Goat's Milk

Allergen: yes (as with cow's milk)

May be better tolerated than cow's milk in people who have a cow's milk allergy.

Introduction: 8 months - in baked or cooked foods

No plain milk other than breast milk (or formula) should be given to your little one before he/she is 12 months old.

Selection: If possible choose raw, organic milk. It is important to find raw milk that has been produced under sanitary and healthy conditions and comes from organic, pasture-fed goats.

I was lucky enough to be able to collect Mila's milk straight from the farm.

Storage:
Raw, unpasteurised ⇢ sealed glass jar ⇢ refrigerator 3 - 5 days

Raw, unpasteurised ⇢ sealed glass jar ⇢ freezer ⇢ 2 months

Nutritional Value:
Some of the health benefits of goat milk include its ability to reduce inflammation, optimize digestion, improve bio-availability of nutrients, strengthen bones, boost heart health, increase immunity, increase your metabolism, prevent toxins from accumulating in the body, protect against weight loss, and benefit the overall environment.

Goat's milk contains relatively high levels of tryptophan, calcium, Vitamin D, phosphorus, Vitamin B2, protein, and potassium. Goat's milk lacks folic acid and is low in vitamin B12, both of which are essential to the growth and development of your little one, so you will need to ensure they are getting these nutrients from other sources.

Goat Cheese

Goat cheese is made from goat's milk. As with other natural cheeses it is a fermented dairy product, made with nothing more than a few basic ingredients — goat's milk, starter culture, salt, and an enzyme called rennet. Salt is a crucial ingredient for flavour, ripening, and preservation.

Goat cheese has a tangy flavour and can be found in semi-soft and hard forms.

Goat cheese is often called chèvre, which means 'goat' in French. Other varieties include the French bûcheron, which becomes firmer and sharper as it ages (although the inside may remain creamy) and brunost, which is a rich, brown type of goat cheese popular in Scandinavia.

Goat cheese contains less lactose than cheese made from cow's milk and due to the different proteins in goat's milk (A2 vs. A1 casein), cheese made from goat's milk is usually better tolerated by those with a lactose intolerance than cheese from cow's milk.

Goat's milk also has a chemical structure that's similar to that of breast milk, and it has smaller fat globules than cow's milk, which tend to make goat cheese easier to digest than cow's milk cheese

Allergen: yes (as with cheese from cow's milk)

May be better tolerated than cow's milk in people who have a cow's milk allergy.

Introduction: 8 months

Be sure to watch for any signs of dairy/lactose intolerance.

Selection: Choose goat cheese that has been made from high-quality milk, ideally raw organic milk, from grass and natural vegetation-fed animals. Read the label to make sure there is no added sugar or any preservatives.

Storage:
Real cheese requires refrigeration - processed cheeses should be avoided.

Use:

Soft goat cheese has unlimited uses: a replacement for cream in a cooked dish; a melted topping for vegetables; a dip or an ingredient in other dips and spreads. The hard

Glossary of Ingredients

cheese is perfect for pizza – it has a stronger flavour than mozzarella so you end up using much less.

Nutritional Value:
Good: protein, calcium, phosphorus, copper, riboflavin, vitamin D, vitamin K, thiamine, and niacin

Soft, raw goat cheeses are a source of probiotics which are important for gut health and digestion.

Gooseberry (specifically Cape Gooseberry, Ground Cherry, Physalis)

Gooseberries are a round, tangy-sweet, juicy, golden yellow fruit with a similar texture and size to cherries. They grow on bushes like little parcels - naturally wrapped in a papery cream coloured husk/cape (looking a bit like a Chinese lantern). The cape turns from green to cream, and the berry turns from green to yellow as they ripen. The capes are often removed for shipping, so you will usually just find the golden berries in the market. Cape Gooseberries are from the same plant family as the tomato, potato and tomatillos.

They are native to South America but get their name from the settlers of the Cape of Good Hope (South Africa). They are easy to grow and are now cultivated in many countries.

You really should grow a gooseberry bush at home – fresh, organic fruit and endless delight for your little one! Mila loves unwrapping them and finding the fruity treat inside!

Allergen: no (not to be confused with the Kiwi Fruit also known as the Chinese Gooseberry which is an **Allergen**)

Cape Gooseberries should be avoided if your little one has an allergy to cherries or berries.

Choking hazard: yes

Introduction: 8 months

Selection: Unripe gooseberries are poisonous and should be avoided! Choose brightly coloured gooseberries with dry capes and no signs of mould or soft spots.

Storage:
Unwashed, whole, raw → sealed container → refrigerator → 5-14 days

Unwashed, whole, raw → sealed container → freezer → 1 year

Preparation/Use:
Soak gooseberries in a salt-, vinegar-, or hydrogen peroxide water solution for 20 minutes then rinse under running water. Gooseberries can be eaten raw or cooked, dried or preserved. They are often used as an ingredient in tarts. The vitamin C content is reduced if they are cooked.

Cut them in half until your little one has enough teeth to get a firm grip on the slippery skin, as they may be a choking hazard.

Nutritional Value:
Excellent: vitamin A and C

Good: vitamin B's, flavonoids (also known as vitamin P), potassium, manganese and fibre.

Gooseberries have antioxidant, anti-inflammatory benefits and digestive benefits. They boost the immune system, lower blood pressure and are good for heart and eye health.

Grapes

Grapes are small round or oval berries that feature semi-translucent flesh encased by a smooth skin – which can be red, purple (black) or green. Some contain edible seeds while others are seedless. Grapes are often covered by a protective, whitish bloom (coating) – this is natural and helps to protect the fruit. There are three categories of grapes: table grapes (those that are eaten as is); wine grapes (used in viniculture) or raisin grapes (used to make dried fruit). Grapes are native to many parts of the world, including regions in Asia, Africa, and North America.

Allergen: no

Choking hazard: yes

Introduction: 8 months

Selection: Fully ripe grapes are the best tasting and have the highest concentrations of antioxidants. They are uniform in colour, plump, free from wrinkles, firmly attached to a healthy looking stem, not leaking juice, bruised or mouldy.

Grapes are listed as one of the EWG's Dirty Dozen. It is very important to buy organic if you want to avoid heavy pesticide residue.

A note about seedless grapes: Just because a grape has no seeds, this does not mean it has been genetically modified. While agricultural researchers are definitely exploring genetically modified grape varieties and while genetically engineered (GE) grapes do exist, they are currently very rare in the marketplace. The seedless grapes are, in fact, a result of natural mutations, pollination being withheld, cross-breeding or grafting. None of these methods involves direct manipulation of the grape plant's genetic material.

Storage:
Unwashed, whole grapes → sealed container → refrigerator → 7 days

Grapes freeze well... in fact, they are DELICIOUS! They

really are like little parcels of natural sorbet! I thank my mom for introducing me to this all-natural treat! In an attempt to get me to eat fewer grapes when I was young, my mom decided to freeze them. She thought they would be less appealing to me, and that perhaps the 'cold factor' would slow me down – it had the opposite affect! While frozen grapes will be a no-no for your little one until they are at least 4 or 5 years old (an extreme **Choking hazard**), they may be something the mama and papa's would like to try? Simply wash the grapes, pat dry, place on a tray in a single layer in the freezer. Once they are frozen you can transfer them to a plastic bag (to take up less space in your freezer).

Preparation/Use:
Soak the grapes in a salt-, vinegar-, or hydrogen peroxide water solution for 20 minutes then rinse under running water.

Whole grapes are a choking hazard - cut the grapes in half so your little one is able to get a grip on them.

Grapes are best eaten raw as cooking destroys their nutrient content.

Diluted grape juice is a great constipation remedy that does not run the risk of cramps like prune juice does.

Nutritional Value:
Excellent: phytonutrients

Very good: vitamins C and K, and copper

Good: vitamin B2 and manganese

Grapes have antioxidant, anti-inflammatory, antimicrobial and cognitive benefits.

Green Onion (Scallion, Spring Onion)

See Spring Onion.

Green Powder

There are many varieties of 'green powders' in health food stores today. They are generally a mix of green foods in powdered form (for example, wheat, barley, alfalfa grasses and spirulina).

Allergen: yes – Chlorella and Spirulina can be **Allergen**s.

Introduction: 8 months

Selection: When purchasing a green powder it is important to choose an organic brand which was processed with protection from UV light, heat, and moisture (which ensures that the chlorophyll and nutrient content is maintained). You should also avoid brands that have 'fillers' such as lecithin, fibres, whole grasses, pectin, rice bran or flax.

Storage:: store in a sealed container in a cool, dark place. Follow expiration date on packaging.

Use: Add to juices, smoothies and raw desserts.

Nutritional Value:
Spirulina

A green algae that has a lot more protein than beef, chicken, pork, and fish. It is a complete protein, which means that it's made up of all the essential amino acids the body needs.

Additional **Nutritional Value::**
- ♥ Good source of omega 3-, 6- and 9 fatty acids and is especially high in omega-3;
- ♥ High amounts of Chlorophyll, which helps remove toxins from the blood and boost the immune system;
- ♥ A very high concentration of bio-available iron;
- ♥ Source of vitamins B1, B2, B3, B6, B9, vitamin C, vitamin D, vitamin A and vitamin E;
- ♥ Good source of potassium, calcium, chromium, copper, iron, magnesium, manganese, phosphorus, selenium, sodium and zinc.
- ♥ High in calcium - with over 26 times the calcium in milk

It is an anti-inflammatory, reinforces your immune system, controls high blood pressure and cholesterol, and helps protect you from cancer.

Wheatgrass

Wheat grass is the young shoots of wheat before stalks form a head with the grain. It contains no wheat gluten. Wheat grass is a superfood thanks to its concentration of chlorophyll, vitamins, minerals, and enzymes.

Wheatgrass is a source of vitamins A, C and E, folic acid, chlorophyll, antioxidants, zinc, iron, calcium, magnesium, amino acids and essential fatty acids. It has antioxidant, anti-inflammatory and anti-bacterial properties.

Barley Grass

Barley grass is sprouted from barley seeds and is very easily digested. It is gluten-free and is, by composition, a superfood. There is very little nutritional difference between wheat grass and barley grass.

Barley Grass has more protein than a sirloin steak, five times the amount of iron as broccoli, seven times more vitamin C than orange juice and 11 times more calcium than milk. Barley grass is full of enzymes, amino acids, vitamins and minerals.

Alfalfa grass

Alfalfa grass is sprouted from the alfalfa seeds - a common flowering perennial plant that originated in Asia.

Glossary of Ingredients

Alfalfa has a high chlorophyll content, and is rich in vitamins A, B1, B6, C, E and K as well as calcium, potassium, iron, zinc and contains 8 amino acids. It has anti-fungal, anti-inflammatory and antioxidant properties.

Guar Gum

Guar gum is a fine powder derived by grinding the seeds of the guar bean, or Indian cluster bean, which grows primarily in India and Pakistan. They look similar to green beans, and are a common vegetable dish in the areas in which they grow.

Guar Gum is used as a thickening and binding agent in gluten-free cooking and baking.

Allergen: no

It can cause gas and bloating in some people (usually those with pre-existing gut conditions).

Introduction: 8 months

Selection: Guar Gum can be found in most health stores, or in the health section of the supermarket.

Storage:: sealed container ⇢ cool, dark place ⇢ follow packaging expiration date.

Use
Guar Gum has eight times more thickening power than corn-starch – a little goes along way! Measure carefully when using guar gum or you may end up with heavy, stringy baked goods.

Foods with a high acid content (such as lemon juice) can cause guar gum to lose its thickening abilities. For recipes involving citrus you will want to increase the amount of guar gum used.

Here are some helpful measurements on how much guar gum to use (although it is not always necessary):

- ♥ Cookies - ¼ - ½ t. per cup of flour
- ♥ Cakes and pancakes - ¾ t. per cup of flour
- ♥ Muffins - 1 t. per cup of flour
- ♥ Breads - 1½ - 2 t. per cup of flour
- ♥ Pizza dough - 1 T. per cup of flour
- ♥ Hot foods (gravies, stews) - 1-3 t. per one litre (or quart) of liquid
- ♥ Cold foods (ice creams, pudding) - 1-2 t. per litre (or quart) of liquid

Hake

See fish.

Hemp (oil, seeds, nuts, milk and powder)

Hemp and marijuana (cannabis) are not one in the same! While they both share the same scientific name (Cannabis sativa), they are two distinct varieties. The marijuana variety has a high THC content (the compound that has psychoactive properties) and a low CBD content (which has medicinal properties). Hemp is the opposite – it is high in CBD and low in THC – meaning, it is going to heal you and your little one, not get you high! This is also why hemp and its products are legal, while marijuana is (generally) illegal, or classified as a drug or controlled substance.

Not only is hemp a highly nutritious food, it can be used to make many products including rope, fabric, paper and even parts for cars!

Hemp seeds, oil and milk have a nutty, slightly sweet flavour.

Allergen: no

Making it an excellent source of protein, calcium and omega fats for anyone who is allergic to nuts, lactose and soy.

Nutritional Value:
In any of its forms (oil, seeds or powder) it is a nutritional superfood. Each seed contains approximately 44% oil (mostly polyunsaturated fat), 33% protein, 12% fibre and carbohydrates as well as vitamins and minerals such as iron, zinc and copper as well as calcium, magnesium, potassium, carotene, thiamin (vitamin B1), riboflavin (vitamin B2), vitamin B6 and vitamin E.

Hemp oil and seeds are an excellent source of essential fatty acids – more than any fish and most fish oil supplements and with the omega 3 and 6 in perfect ratio. Essential fatty acids are essential for a strong and healthy immune system.

Hemp has a high protein content (more than beef, chicken, dairy and eggs) and it contains all of the 21 amino acids – including the 9 essential ones. The protein is easily digested and assimilated into the body. It is a great source of protein for those avoiding dairy, vegans and vegetarians and a simple way to get more essential protein into your little one. Only a handful of the seeds provides the minimum daily requirement of protein for adults!

In additional to the nutrient content mentioned above, hemp seeds are an excellent source of fibre (both soluble and insoluble).

> Glossary of Ingredients

Hemp has anti-cancer, anti-oxidant, anti-depressant, anti-nausea and anti-inflammatory benefits. It also improves the functioning of the immune system; supports brain health; lowers LDL (bad) cholesterol; regulates blood sugar; and soothes eczema and psoriasis.

Hemp Seed Oil

Hemp seed oil is extracted from pressed hemp seeds. It has a slightly green colour and looks similar to olive oil.

For breastfeeding mothers, the essential fatty acids (EFAs) from hemp can be a big help in replenishing the 11 grams of EFAs that are pulled from the mother daily through breastfeeding. The extra EFAs need to come from a food source as the body does not replenish them on its own.

Introduction: 6 months

The best way to introduce hemp as the seeds may be difficult to digest in your little one's immature digestive system.

Selection: Choose cold-pressed, unrefined hemp seed oil. It should be found in the refrigerated sections of the shop. Always taste the oil before giving it to your child. If it is overly bitter, it has gone rancid and needs to be discarded.

Storage:
Dark, sealed bottle ⇢ refrigerator ⇢ 2-4 months

Dark, sealed bottle ⇢ freezer ⇢ 6 months

It will not solidify in the freezer, so you can store it there and pour it without having to defrost it first.

Preparation/Use:
Hemp oil (like flax oil) must not be heated or used as a cooking oil. It can be added to already cooked dishes; as a replacement for olive oils in salads and other dressings; or, as a nutrient enhancer in smoothies and purées.

Hemp Seeds and Nuts

Hemp seeds are the whole unprocessed seed of the hemp plant and are the world's most nutritious seed. The seeds are rounder, softer, and greener than sesame seeds and slightly sweeter than sunflower seeds.

Hemp nuts (or hearts) are hemp seeds which have been hulled.

Introduction: 8 months

You can feed him/her up to three teaspoons per day – but spread that amount out over a few meals, not all in one go.

Storage:
Hemp seeds ⇢ airtight container ⇢ cool, dark place or fridge ⇢ up to a year.

It is recommended, though, to keep them in the fridge or freezer to preserve their nutritional content.

Preparation/Use:
Hemp seeds can be eaten raw, ground into a meal (in your coffee grinder), sprouted, made into hemp milk, made into tea, and used in baking. Try adding some ground hemp seeds to your little one's purées or smoothies. Or use them to coat otherwise slippery fruit pieces – this will enable your little one to get a better grip.

Hemp Milk

Hemp milk is a great option for anyone avoiding dairy.

Introduction: 6 months (in other food)

Breast milk should be your little one's primary source of liquid up till 12 months old but as hemp milk is non-**Allergen**ic it can be added to your little one's food from 6 months of age.

Selection: Be sure to choose a hemp milk which is free from carrageenan, titanium dioxide, synthetic vitamins A and D, refined sugars, soy lecithin, vegetable oils, and other 'natural' flavourings. Alternatively, you can make your own.

Storage:: Once opened, hemp milk must be kept in the fridge. Follow the pack guidelines for **Storage:** times.

Hemp Milk Recipe

Place 1 cup hemp seeds, 2 cups water and 2 teaspoons vanilla powder into your blender and blend. Pour the mixture through a milk bag, or cheesecloth. Store in the fridge for a couple of days.

Hemp Powder

Hemp protein powder is the end stage of the processing of hemp seeds. The whole seeds are pressed for oil, leaving behind a hemp cake. The cake is then ground into a flour, which is used in many products like baked goods. The flour can then be processed further to make the protein powder. Much of the fibre and healthy fats have been removed at this point.

My suggestion would be to rather use freshly ground hemp seeds so that your little one gets all the benefits of the whole food.

Glossary of Ingredients

Honey

Honey is the sweet, delicious syrup that results from honey bees feasting on flowers. The honey bees feed on the naturally occurring nectars found in flowers, allowing the nectar to mix with enzymes in their saliva. The nectar is then regurgitated into beehives in the form of honey.

In addition to being a delicious treat, honey has several health benefits and homeopathic uses. When selecting honey, it is important to choose the purest raw form available in order to maximize these benefits.

Allergen: no

Introduction: 12 months

Honey should never be given to a child under the age of 12 months old. This technically, applies even to honey in baked or processed food goods.

Honey may contain bacteria in the form of Clostridium botulinum which can lead to botulism poisoning. Botulism spores will not be destroyed during and under household cooking methods and temperatures. The intestines of an adult contain sufficient acids to counteract the production of the toxins the botulism bacteria produce. Once your little one reaches the age of a year or older, his/her intestines will have a balance of acids that will help destroy and fight off any toxins that the botulism bacteria produce – thereby making him/her less susceptible to poisoning.

Selection: Only choose certified organic, raw, local, unfiltered honey. By consuming local raw honey, you get a homeopathic dose of pollens from your area that help immunise you against allergies. Commercial honey is not recommended, as it has been filtered, strained, heated and pasteurised thereby killing all the beneficial digestive enzymes and reducing its mineral and vitamin content. It also usually has additional sugar or HFCS added, as well as other undesirables.

Storage:
Sealed container ↔ cool, dark place ↔ lasts pretty much forever!

Nutritional Value:
Honey mainly consists of glucose and fructose but natural whole foods are more than just the sum of their nutrients… They contain various substances that work synergistically to nourish and positively affect health in ways that science has yet to uncover.

Raw, organic honey contains magnesium, potassium, calcium, sulphur, sodium chlorine, phosphate, antioxidants, vitamins B1, B2, B3, B5, B6, and C, digestive enzymes, amino acids, and carbohydrates. Darker coloured honey has more minerals. Honey also contains a type of complex sugar that acts as a prebiotic to support friendly probiotic bacteria populations in the gut.

Raw, organic honey naturally boosts the immune system due to its antifungal, antiviral, anti-inflammatory, anti-allergic and anti-bacterial properties.

For centuries it has been used as in the treatment of burns, eczema, wounds, rashes, gut issues, bronchitis, sore throat, bleeding gums, morning sickness and more. A teaspoon of honey before bed will soothe a sore throat and ease a dry cough (and your little one with love it!).

Kale

Kale is a leafy green vegetable that belongs to the Brassica family (a group of vegetables including cabbage, broccoli, and Brussels sprouts) that have gained recent widespread attention due to their health-promoting, sulphur-containing phytonutrients. There are several varieties of kale all of which differ in taste, texture and appearance:

Curly kale has ruffled leaves and a fibrous stalk and is deep green in colour. When cooked it has a pungent flavour with bitter peppery qualities.

Ornamental kale is a more recently cultivated species that is oftentimes referred to as salad savoy. Its leaves may either be green, white, or purple. Ornamental kale has a more mellow flavour and tender texture.

Dinosaur kale features dark blue-green leaves that have an embossed texture. It has a slightly sweeter taste than curly kale.

Allergen: no

Introduction: 8 months

As with spinach, kale is high in nitrates so it is best to wait until your little one is 8 months old before introducing kale.

Selection: Choose kale with firm, deeply coloured leaves and moist hardy stems. You should find kale in a cool environment of the market since warm temperatures will cause it to wilt and negatively affect its flavour. The leaves should not be wilting, browning or yellowing. Choose kale with smaller-sized leaves since these will be more tender and have a milder flavour than those with larger leaves. Kale is available throughout the year, although it is more widely available, and at its peak, from the middle of winter through the beginning of spring.

Kale is on the EWG's Dirty Dozen Plus list. conventionally grown kale is usually contaminated with a certain type of insecticide that is considered to be highly toxic to the nervous system. Purchase organic kale whenever possible.

Storage:
Whole, raw kale ↔ unwashed ↔ plastic bag refrigerator ↔ 5 days

Kale does not freeze well.

Preparation/Use:
Soak the kale in a salt-, vinegar-, or hydrogen peroxide water solution for 20 minutes then rinse under running water.

Kale is best cooked by lightly steaming or briefly sautéing it. You can purée the cooked kale with some other creamier vegetables or fruits. It can also be added raw to a veggie juice or smoothie. Dehydrated kale chips are one of Mila's all time favourites!

Nutritional Value:
Kale is one of the most nutrient-dense vegetables on the planet and a nutritional superfood in three basic areas: antioxidant and anti-inflammatory nutrients; micronutrients; and, cancer-preventive nutrients.

Excellent: vitamins A (in the form of carotenoids), C and K, copper, and manganese

Very good: vitamins B1, B2, B6, and E, dietary fibre, calcium, potassium, iron, magnesium, omega-3 fatty acids, phosphorus, protein, folate, and niacin.

To really impress upon you why kale is considered a vegetable superfood – 1 cup of kale has 684% of the RDA (recommended daily amount) of vitamin K, 206% of the RDA of vitamin A, and 134% of vitamin C. If that was not impressive enough - it has more calcium by weight than milk, and its calcium is 25% more bioavailable than that in milk!

A special mention must also be made of kale's protein content – like meat, it has all the essential amino acids and 9 non-essential ones (amino acids are the building clocks of protein within the body). With this exceptionally high amount of protein (especially for a vegetable) it has recently been acclaimed as the "new beef" and is a useful addition to any, but especially, a vegetarian diet. The protein is more bioavailable than meat protein and the body has to expend less energy to make use of it.

Mila has never been a big meat-eater – I add kale to her veggie juice every morning and am happy knowing she is getting a healthy dose of protein and omega 3 fatty acids.

Kale's phytonutrients have potent antibiotic, antiviral, and anti-inflammatory properties that work to boost the immune system and provide significant benefits for chronic inflammation and oxidative stress.

Kefir

This information relates to milk kefir.

Kefir (pronounced Ke-Feer, Kee' fir or Keff ' ir) is an ancient fermented (cultured) dairy drink which originated in Russia. Its unique name comes from the Turkish work "keif", which means "good feeling". Well-fermented kefir resembles yoghurt (although thinner), has a sour or tart taste and can be slightly carbonated. It is an enzyme-rich food filled with probiotics (friendly bacteria) that provide health benefits when consumed. In fact, kefir is one of the highest probiotic foods you can eat with up to 35 different probiotic strains.

You get two types of kefir: milk kefir (made from cow, sheep, goat or coconut milk) and water kefir (made from sugary water or coconut water).

Kefir is made by adding kefir 'grains' to milk and leaving it to stand at room temperature for a couple of days. 'kefir grains' are not grains at all, but are a delicate balance of yeast and bacteria. They look a bit like cauliflower florets and are gelatinous in texture. These micro-organisms feed off the lactose (sugar) in the milk. 99% of the lactose in the milk is digested by the kefir grains during the fermentation process so kefir it is generally well tolerated by people with lactose-intolerance.

Allergen: yes (as with cow's milk)

Kefir may be well tolerated by people with lactose intolerance.

Introduction: 8 months

Selection: Choose kefir that has been made from organic, raw grass-fed milk and has no other additives or flavourings.

Storage:
Sealed glass jar ⇢ refrigerator ⇢ 2 weeks

Preparation/Use:
One of the best and least expensive ways to get healthy bacteria into your diet is to make kefir yourself. A litre of kefir has far more active bacteria than you can possibly purchase in any probiotic supplement, and it is very economical - kefir grains get used continuously.

Your little one may not enjoy the slightly sour taste of kefir, but you can flavour it in many ways: add pure honey (preferably raw), pure maple syrup, pure vanilla extract or powder, or organic stevia extract. Also try adding puréed fruit to your plain kefir (like banana or blueberries) to boost the nutrient content even more.

Nutritional Value:
Very good: vitamin B12 (if made from cow's milk), calcium, magnesium, vitamin K2, biotin, folate, phosphorous, protein, enzymes and probiotics.

Kefir has extensive health benefits: it regulates the immune system; promotes production of bile; provides natural protection against diseases; improves blood circulation; regulates cholesterol

Glossary of Ingredients

and sugar levels; regulates blood pressure; provides relief and healing from bronchitis, anaemia, constipation, diarrhoea, irritable bowel syndrome, colitis, leaky gut syndrome, eczema, acne, allergies, psoriasis, and arthritis.

Lamb

This information relates to 100% grass-fed, organic lamb.

Lamb is the meat from young sheep that are less than a year old. It is available in different cuts including: shoulder; rack, shank/breast, loin, leg and the South African staple… chops.

Allergen: no

Introduction: 7 months

As lamb is very high in protein it is best to offer your little one regular, but small amounts of it – very large amounts of protein may put strain on your little one's immature kidneys.

Selection: Currently, lamb is not produced on factory farms – so the lamb you find in the supermarkets is generally organic and pasture-raised without the use of routine antibiotics and growth hormones.

Choose lamb that has firm flesh, is fine textured and pink in colour. Any fat surrounding or marbled throughout the lamb should be white, not yellow.

Storage:
Raw lamb → sealed container/original packaging → refrigerator → 3-5 days

Raw, ground lamb → sealed container/original packaging → refrigerator → 2 days

Raw lamb → two freezer bags → freezer → 6-9 months

Raw, ground lamb → two freezer bags → freezer → 3-4 months

Thawed, lamb → sealed container/original packaging → refrigerator → 3-4 days

Thawed, ground lamb → sealed container/original packaging → refrigerator → 1-2 days

Preparation/Use:
It is advisable to use a separate cutting board and utensils for raw meats as they can contain the E. coli bacteria. Wash all boards and utensils with hydrogen peroxide once you have finished preparing the meat. Do not forget to wash your hands well too!

My favourite method of preparing most lamb cuts is to slow cook it – the lamb is tender and juicy with a beautiful flavour and you get a delicious stock to use in other dishes or purées. Different cuts of lamb are best prepared using different methods:

- ♥ Shoulder: Best slow roasted
- ♥ Shank: Best in the slow cooker
- ♥ Lamb chops: Best grilled or braaied (barbecued)
- ♥ Rack of Lamb: Best roasted
- ♥ Minced Lamb: Best sautéed

Purée lamb with some of the cooking broth or juices and vegetables for a delicious easy-to-digest introduction to meat - puréeing meat breaks down its fibres and connective tissues and vastly improves its digestibility. As your little one develops, you can shred the lamb instead of puréeing it.

Nutritional Value:
Excellent: vitamin B12

Very good: protein, selenium, and niacin

Good: zinc, iron and phosphorus

Additionally: omega-3 fatty acids

Lamb provides support for a healthy heart and can also assist with blood sugar regulation. With regards to your fast growing little one, its main benefit is as a high quality source of protein, iron and zinc – both of which are essential once you reduce breast feeding.

Lemon

Lemons are a sour-tasting, oval citrus fruit with a yellow, texturized outer peel. Like other citrus fruits, their inner flesh is encased in eight to ten segments.

Although lemons are not usually eaten on their own as you would other fruit (although my niece did eat them just like that!), they are helpful in: bringing out the flavour of other foods; preventing certain foods from discolouring; and, their high vitamin C content makes them a useful addition to food and juices.

Allergen: no

Introduction: 6 months

Lemons are not acidic once eaten unlike other citrus fruit which may lead to nappy rashes.

Selection: Conventionally grown lemons may be waxed to protect them from bruising during shipping. Plant, insect, animal or petroleum-based waxes may be used. Other compounds, such as ethyl alcohol or ethanol, milk casein and soaps may also be added to these waxes. Since you may not be able to determine the source of these waxes, it is good idea to choose organically grown lemons.

Choose lemons that are heavy for their size with peels that have a finely grained texture. They should be fully yellow in colour as those that have green tinges will be more acidic (due to the fact that they have not fully ripened). Signs of an over-ripe lemon include wrinkling, soft or hard patches and dull colouring. Fresh lemons are available all year round.

Storage:
Whole lemons ⇢ cool, dark place ⇢ 1 week

Whole lemons ⇢ refrigerator ⇢ 4 weeks

Preparation/Use:
Soak the lemons in a salt-, vinegar-, or hydrogen peroxide water solution for 20 minutes then rinse under running water - so that any dirt or bacteria on the skin will not be transferred to the inside of the fruit when you cut it. This will also wash off some of the pesticide residue and wax if you have not been able to find organic lemons.

Cut the lemon in half and squeeze the juice out using a juicer, orange squeezer or simply by inserting a fork into the centre and squeezing with your hand. Pour the juice through a sieve to remove bits and pips. If you have organic lemons, the entire lemon can be put through a juicer (skin and all!).

To make lemon zest, use the fine side of a cheese grater and grate the outer skin. Be sure not to grate the white pith as this has a bitter flavour.

Lemon juice can be added to any purées and vegetable juices, or squeezed over meat and seafood dishes, for a vitamin C and flavour boost. Warm water, lemon juice and honey is a great remedy for colds and flu. Lemon water is a great thirst quencher (and detoxifier) – I drank litres of it everyday when I was breastfeeding Mila!

Nutritional Value:
Excellent: vitamin C

Good: folate

Additionally: vitamin B, iron, calcium, magnesium, silicon, copper, and potassium.

Vitamin C is vital to the function of a strong immune system. The immune system's main goal is to protect you from illness, so extra vitamin C may be useful in conditions like colds, flu, and recurrent ear infections.

Although lemons have an acidic taste they actually have a very strong alkaline reaction in the body (excess acidity in the body leads to an ideal playground for viruses and other diseases). Lemons are a source of phytonutrients that have both antioxidant and antibiotic effects. They also have anti-cancer benefits.

Lemon essential oil has been shown to have anti-stress and anti-anxiety effects.

Lentils

Lentils are legumes like other types of beans but, they are comparatively quick and easy to prepare. Lentils are the round, oval or heart-shaped seeds of the Lens ensculenta plant. They grow in pods that contain either one or two lentil seeds.

Lentils are classified according to whether they are large or small in size with dozens of varieties of each being cultivated. Two of the more popular varieties are the red and the brown lentils. Red lentils are the quickest to cook, have a delicate sweet flavour and become mushy when cooked. They are easier to digest than other varieties. Brown lentils are the most commonly found and the cheapest. They keep their shape quite well making them a perfect finger food.

Allergen: no

Introduction: 1 year

Legumes require certain digestive enzymes in order to be digested properly. These enzymes are not present in large enough quantities in your little one's immature digestive system until they are a year old – and only really when they are two years old.

Selection: make sure there is no evidence of moisture or insect damage and that the lentils are whole and not cracked.

Storage:
Dry lentils ⇢ sealed container ⇢ cool, dark place ⇢ 12 months

Cooked lentils ⇢ sealed container ⇢ refrigerator ⇢ 3 days

Cooked lentils ⇢ sealed container ⇢ freezer ⇢ 6 months

Preparation/Use:
Legumes contain anti-nutrients: enzyme inhibitors and phytic acid. It is important to prepare them in such a way that reduces the phytic acid, neutralises the enzyme inhibitors and increases the bio-availability of the nutrients.

Cover the lentils with warm water and add an acid medium (whey, lemon juice or apple cider vinegar). The ratio of lentils to acid should be 2 tablespoons acid for every 2 cups of lentils. Soak for twelve to twenty-four hours (or overnight), then drain, rinse and cook.

Add one part lentils to two parts boiling water or broth. After the liquid has returned to a boil, turn down the heat, cover and simmer for about 15 - 25 minutes (depending on the variety).

Glossary of Ingredients

Nutritional Value:

Excellent: molybdenum and folate

Very good: dietary fibre, copper, phosphorus, and manganese

Good: iron, protein, vitamins B1 and B6, pantothenic acid, zinc and potassium

Liver

Note: This information relates to 100% grass-fed organic lamb and beef liver and 100% pasture-fed, organic chicken liver.

Liver is an organ meat, along with heart and kidneys. In the West we are unaccustomed to eating organ meats, but organs from organically raised, grass-fed animals are some of the most nutrient-rich foods you can eat.

Many people object to eating liver as they believe that the liver is a **Storage:** organ for toxins in the body. While it is true that one of the liver's roles is to neutralize toxins (such as drugs, chemical agents and poisons), it does not store these toxins. Toxins the body cannot eliminate are likely to accumulate in the body's fatty tissues and nervous systems.

Allergen: no

Introduction: 6 months

Selection: Choose liver from organic, grass-fed, pasture-raised cows or lamb, or organic, pasture-raised chickens. The liver should be so deeply coloured that it appears almost purple.

Storage:
Highly perishable

Raw liver → sealed container/original packaging → refrigerator → 1-2 days

Raw liver → original packaging and double wrapped in bags → freezer → 3-4 months

Cooked liver → sealed container → refrigerator → 3-4 days

Cooked liver → sealed container → freezer → 3 months

Preparation/Use:
It is advisable to use a separate cutting board and utensils for raw meats as they can contain the E. coli bacteria. Wash all boards and utensils with hydrogen peroxide once you have finished preparing the meat. Do not forget to wash your hands well too!

The Weston A. Price Foundation suggests incorporating liver into your little one's diet by grating some raw, frozen liver into other purées or over a soft boiled egg yolk. The liver must be frozen for a minimum of 2 weeks before using it (fourteen days will ensure the elimination of pathogens and parasites). If this is a little bit too 'out-there' for you (it was for me), please see the recipe for chicken-liver pâté.

Any cooked liver will purée well. Simply sauté the liver with some garlic and onion and a sprinkle of ground coriander and salt in a small amount of broth until cooked through. Add some of the cooking broth to the liver to create a smooth purée or pate.

Nutritional Value:
Excellent: high quality protein, omega 3 fatty acids, vitamin B complex (including choline, B12 and folate), iron, Vitamin D, Vitamin E, pre-formed Vitamin A (retinol), Vitamin K2, copper, zinc and chromium

Good: cholesterol

Cholesterol is vital for the insulation of the nerves in the brain and the entire central nervous system. It helps with fat digestion by increasing the formation of bile acids and is necessary for the production of many hormones. Since the brain is so dependent on cholesterol, it is especially vital during this time when brain growth is in hyper-speed.

A note on vitamin A: Dr. Mercola states, "When people began taking synthetic vitamin A supplements, we began to see vitamin A toxicity. But this does not happen with natural vitamin A from real, whole foods. Therefore, the advice to refrain from organ meats during pregnancy is unfounded. It is best to obtain your vitamin A from natural sources like yellow butter, egg yolks, and organ meats."

Love

"If a woman could see the sparks of light going forth from her fingertips when she is cooking, and the energy that goes into the food she handles, she would realize how much of herself she imbues into the meals that she prepares for her family and friends. It is one of the most important and least understood activities of life that the feelings that go into the preparation of food affect everyone who partakes of it. This activity should be unhurried, peaceful and happy because the energy that flows into that food impacts the energy of the receiver." - Maha Chohan

Lucuma Powder

Lucuma is a fibrous fruit native to Peru, Chile and Ecuador. It was viewed in the ancient Peruvian culture as a symbol of fertility and creation. Traditionally known as the "Gold of the Incas", the orange and yellow pulpy lucuma fruit is naturally sweet and low on the Glycaemic Index.

Lucuma Powder is made from whole lucuma fruit that has been dried at low temperatures and milled into a fine powder. Yellow lucuma powder has a unique, maple-like taste.

Allergen: no

Introduction: 6 months

In Peru this fruit is often baby's first solid food. Just like bananas and sweet potatoes, lucuma is soft, sweet, and extremely easy to digest.

Selection: Lucuma powder can be found in most health shops.

Storage:
Sealed container ⇢ cool, dark place ⇢ up to a year

Use:
Lucuma powder can be used to flavour a variety of dishes in place of regular sugar. The texture is similar to granulated sugar, but the taste is more reminiscent of brown sugar. It can be easily substituted for brown sugar in a 2:1 ratio.

It is an excellent flavouring for ice cream and can also be used in smoothies, oatmeal, and any purées or to sweeten cooked deserts such as cakes, chocolate and pancakes. You can even add it to your little one's tea to get a creamy drink without the milk!

Nutritional Value:
Excellent: carbohydrates, fibre, protein, beta-carotene, niacin and vitamin C

Very Good: iron

Good: calcium, phosphorus and zinc

Lucuma has antibiotic, antimicrobial, antifungal and anti-cancer benefits. It can help stabilize blood sugar, boost the immune system and fertility and speeds up the healing process.

Maca Powder

Maca is a plant that grows in central Peru in the high plateaus of the Andes mountains. It has been cultivated as a vegetable crop there for at least 3000 years. Maca is a relative of the radish and has a fragrance similar to butterscotch. It is a potent, ancient superfood used by indigenous Andean societies as a source of nourishment and healing for thousands of years.

Maca powder is made from the maca roots, which are gently dried and milled at low temperatures. This careful process preserves the complex nutrition of this superfood. It has a malted flavour – much like Horlicks.

Allergen: no

Introduction: 6 months

Selection: Maca can be found in most health food stores in powder form. You may also find it available in capsule, liquid, or extract form. Its best to buy maca that is raw and organic.

Storage:
Sealed container ⇢ cool, dark place ⇢ 24 months

Sealed container ⇢ fridge/freezer ⇢ 2 years

Use:
Maca can be added to any purée, smoothie, dessert and sweet treat.

Since it is so nutrient dense, introduce maca in small amounts. For adults, ½ a teaspoon is a good place to start with 2 tablespoons being an average daily dose. It is also a good idea to rotate this with other superfoods so you are not giving your little one the same ones everyday.

Nutritional Value:
Maca is a complete protein and has over 20 amino acids.

Excellent: vitamins B, C and E

Very good: calcium, zinc, iron, magnesium, phosphorous, potassium, sulphur, copper, selenium and fatty acids.

Traditionally Maca has been used for 'tired blood' (anaemia); chronic fatigue syndrome (CFS); and enhancing energy, stamina, athletic performance, memory, and fertility. Women use maca for female hormone imbalance, menstrual problems, and symptoms of menopause. Maca is also beneficial for osteoporosis, depression, tuberculosis, and to boost the immune system. Today maca is regarded as an adaptogen - meaning it normalises the body and keeps things in homeostasis (at normal levels). Adaptogens allow the body to better respond to internal and external environmental factors such as anxiety, illness and physical injuries.

Macadamia Nuts

Macadamia nuts are native to Australia and are some of the most sought-after nuts in the world. The small, round cream coloured nuts have a subtly sweet flavour and a creamy texture.

Special note: macadamia nuts are toxic to dogs.

Allergen: yes

Macadamia nut allergy is quite a rare occurrence and not as common as other tree nut allergies like cashew, and pistachios.

Glossary of Ingredients

Choking hazard: yes. Alternatively, your little one can eat them in the form of macadamia nut butter.

Introduction: 12 months

Selection: Macadamias can be available year round. They are available shelled, unshelled, raw, salted or roasted. It is preferable to buy organic, raw nuts. Healthy nuts will be compact and uniform in size and feel heavy in hand. The nuts should be free from cracks (other than natural split), cuts, mould, and spots and should not smell rancid.

Storage:
Whole, unshelled ⇢ sealed container ⇢ cool, dark place ⇢ 6 months

Shelled ⇢ sealed container ⇢ refrigerator ⇢ 6 months

Shelled ⇢ sealed container ⇢ freezer ⇢ 9-12 months

Preparation/Use:
Nuts contain anti-nutrients: enzyme inhibitors and phytic acid. It is important to prepare them it such a way that reduces the phytic acid, neutralises the enzyme inhibitors and increases the bio-availability of the nutrients.

The process of soaking nuts is called "activation". Activated macadamia nuts are easier to digest and have a higher nutritional content.

To activate your macadamias, cover the nuts with salt water (1T. salt to 4 cups nuts). Leave to soak for at least 7 hours or overnight. Rinse, and then dehydrate in a dehydrator or in your oven (set to its lowest temperature). Dehydration will take 12 – 24 hours. Ensure your nuts are completely dry to prevent mould from growing.

Alternatively, simply soak the macadamias and rinse. Store in a glass container in the fridge for no more than 1 week.

Nutritional Value:
Very Good: vitamin B1, magnesium, manganese, thiamin, calcium, iron, zinc, selenium and essential fatty acids.

Macadamia nuts have anti-inflammatory benefits.

Maize

See Sweetcorn.

Mango

Mangoes are an egg shaped, sweet, juicy tropical fruit with smooth, soft skin. The skin is usually a combination of green, red, and yellow. The flesh is usually bright orange (although you do get green varieties) with a large, flat pit in the middle. Mangoes originated in Southern Asia, but are now cultivated around the world. Many stories in Indian mythology mention the mango plant, and Buddha is said to have meditated in a mango grove. According to Indian beliefs, mangoes symbolise life and are used in almost every sacred ritual.

Allergen: yes

Mangoes can be an **Allergen** to people who are also allergic to cashews and pistachios.

Introduction: 7 months

Selection: When choosing mangoes give them a gentle push with your finger – the fruit should be slightly soft and fragrant. The skin should be free from bruises and should not have any brown dots on it.

Storage:
Mangoes continue to ripen after they are picked - they can be stored in a cool, dark place to ripen.

Ripe, raw, mango ⇢ refrigerator ⇢ 4-5 days

Ripe, raw, cut mango ⇢ sealed container/freezer bag ⇢ freezer ⇢ 10-12 months

Dehydrated mango ⇢ sealed container ⇢ cool, dark place ⇢ 6-12 months

Dehydrated mango ⇢ sealed container ⇢ refrigerator ⇢ 1-2 years

Dehydrated mango ⇢ sealed container ⇢ freezer ⇢ indefinite

Preparation/Use:
Mangoes are best enjoyed raw. Peel the skin off (with a potato peeler), slice the flesh from the pip, mash for your little one, or cut into cubes for finger food. If the pieces are too slippery, try coating them in almond or coconut flour.

Dehydrated mango slices are absolutely delicious and make a great mess-free out-and-about food as well as a perfect teething food.

Nutritional Value:
Excellent: vitamins A (in the form of beta-carotene), B6 and C, and fibre

Good: magnesium, copper, potassium, iron, protein, vitamins E and K

As with other vitamin C-rich foods, mangoes help your little one absorb more iron from the foods he / she eats.

Mangoes have antioxidant and anti-cancer benefits. They boost the immune system; help prevent heart disease; lower blood pressure; improve indigestion and excess acidity; promote natural efficient digestion; and, are beneficial if your little one is anaemic.

Maple Syrup

Maple syrup is made from the sap of red, black or sugar maple trees. The sap is evaporated, leaving behind a thick syrup. It has been consumed for many centuries in North America. Pure maple syrup contains only evaporated maple tree sap.

Maple syrup grades have nothing to do with quality or nutrition. Instead, they refer to the colour of the syrup, when it was harvested and its flavour. Grade B is the darkest, with the strongest maple flavour and the richest in nutrients.

Allergen: no

Introduction: 6 months

Since honey cannot be used before your little one is a year old, maple syrup is a great alternative.

Selection: Check the ingredients on the maple syrup packaging to confirm that it is 100% pure maple syrup. It should not contain maple "flavour" or high-fructose corn syrup.

Storage:
Unopened, sealed container ↬ cool, dark place ↬ 2 years

Opened, sealed container ↬ refrigerator ↬ 6 months

Use:
Maple syrup gives a wonderful flavour to baked goods, desserts and of course, pancakes! As with other sweeteners, use in moderation.

Nutritional Value:
Good: calcium, iron, magnesium, manganese, phosphorus, sodium, potassium, zinc, thiamin, riboflavin, niacin, and B6

Maple syrup delivers more nutrition than all other common sweeteners. It is primarily sucrose (a complex sugar that your body breaks down to the simple sugars fructose and glucose) but, replacing refined sugar in recipes with an identical amount of maple syrup will cut the total sugar content by a third.

Maple syrup has antioxidant and immune boosting benefits.

Mielie

See Sweetcorn.

Millet

Millet is technically a seed but it is classified as a gluten-free grain in the food world. It is tiny in size and round in shape and can be white, grey, yellow or red. It has a subtly sweet, nutty flavour. The most widely available form of millet is the hulled variety, although traditional couscous made from cracked millet can also be found. Millet can be cooked to be creamy like mashed potatoes or fluffy like rice. It is thought to have originated in North Africa, specifically in Ethiopia, where it has been consumed since prehistoric times. It has also been widely consumed in Asia and India - the Indian flatbread roti / Bajrai is made from ground millet seeds.

Allergen: no

Introduction: 12 months. Grains require certain digestive enzymes in order to be digested properly. These enzymes are not present in large enough quantities in your little one's immature digestive system until they are a year old – and only really when they are two years old.

Selection: Millet is available in its hulled and whole form. When choosing millet make sure there is no evidence of moisture in the packet.

Storage:
Uncooked millet ↬ airtight container ↬ cool, dark place ↬ 2 months

Uncooked millet ↬ tightly wrapped or full container ↬ freezer ↬ 4 months

Cooked ↬ airtight container ↬ refrigerator ↬ 3-5 days

Cooked ↬ airtight container ↬ freezer ↬ 1 month

Preparation/Use:
Whole grains contain anti-nutrients: enzyme inhibitors and phytic acid. It is important to prepare them it such a way that reduces the phytic acid, neutralises the enzyme inhibitors and increases the bio-availability of the nutrients.

Cover the millet with warm water and add an acid medium (whey, lemon juice or apple cider vinegar). The ratio of millet to acid should be ½ tablespoon acid for every 2 cups of grains. Soak for twelve to twenty-four hours (or overnight), then drain, rinse and cook.

Add one-part millet to two parts boiling water or broth. After the liquid has returned to a boil, turn down the heat, cover and simmer for about 15 minutes. The texture of millet cooked this way will be fluffy like rice. If you want the millet to have a creamier consistency, stir it frequently adding additional liquid every now and then.

Millet porridge
If you are making porridge for your little one, I would suggest soaking then dehydrating the grains in bulk. Then whenever you want to prepare porridge, you have soaked grains available and you can simply grind the required amount in a coffee grinder and prepare the porridge with the 'flour'.

When cooking ground millet for homemade baby porridge,

Glossary of Ingredients

use ¼ cup of millet per 1-2 cups of water. The key is to whisk continuously as you are cooking to avoid clumping.

Nutritional Value:
Good: copper, phosphorus, manganese, magnesium.

Additional: B vitamins, potassium, iron, protein, fibre and anti-oxidant phytonutrients.

Due to its high concentrations of magnesium, millet is useful in reducing the severity of asthma, the frequency of migraines, and in lowering blood pressure. Phosphorous plays a crucial role in the development of body tissue and bones.

Millet is considered to be one of the most digestible and non-**Allergen**ic grains available, and it is alkalizing to the body.

Moringa Leaf Powder

Moringa is a plant that is native to India, Bangladesh, Pakistan and Afghanistan where it has long been used as a medicinal plant as well as a nutritional booster. It is referred to as "the miracle tree", the "tree of life", "mother's best friend" and "never die tree." It is a nutritional superfood that is currently being promoted as a solution to malnutrition in Africa. The moringa leaf powder has mild, somewhat spinach-like taste.

Allergen: no

Introduction: 6 months

Selection: Choose organic moringa powder that has no other ingredients or additives.

Storage:
Opaque container ↔ cool, dark place ↔ 6 months

Use:
Moringa works well in smoothies, green juices, soups or sprinkled over almost anything.

A little goes a long way – start with 10 grams/day.

Nutritional Value:
Moringa has anti-aging, anti-cancer, anti-inflammatory and anti-oxidant benefits.

The leaves of the tree contain more than 90 essential nutrients! They are an excellent source of vitamin A, several B vitamins, calcium, iron, vitamin C, potassium and complete protein. Moringa leaves are also one of the few plant sources of omega 3 fatty acids.

Moringa boosts the immune system and can benefit conditions such as anaemia, asthma, arthritis, constipation, cancer, diabetes, epilepsy, diarrhoea, stomach ulcers, gastritis, intestinal ulcers, heart conditions, headaches, high blood pressure, inflammation, kidney stones, thyroid disorders, infections, sex drive, athlete's foot, warts, dandruff, snake bites and gingivitis. Additionally, it is a natural galactagogue – a food that increases breast milk production.

Mustard powder

Mustard powder is derived from the ground seeds of the mustard plant - a member of the Brassicaeae family which includes broccoli, cauliflower, Brussels sprouts and cabbage. There are three main species of mustard plant including black mustard, brown mustard and white mustard (the white mustard seeds are in fact a straw-yellow colour.) Mustard has a hot, pungent flavour.

Allergen: yes

People with a mustard allergy should avoid consuming the seeds and sprouted seeds of other members of the Brassicaeae family as these have the potential to trigger an adverse reaction.

Introduction: 8 months

Selection: Mustard is available as whole seeds and as mustard powder. Choose non-irradiated seeds and powder.

Storage:
Mustard powder ↔ airtight, glass container ↔ cool, dark place ↔ 1 year

Mustard powder ↔ airtight, glass container ↔ cool, dark place ↔ 2 years

Nutritional Value:
This spice is very rich in phytonutrients, minerals, vitamins and anti-oxidants.

Excellent: selenium

Very good: omega-3 fatty acids and manganese

Good: phosphorus, magnesium, copper, and vitamin B1.

Naartjie (Tangerine / Satsuma / Mandarin)

A very South African name for a juicy, sweet fruit also known as tangerine (in America), mandarin orange (in Europe) and satsuma (in Japan).

Naartjies are a variety of orange (citrus fruit) – although smaller in size with a loose, easily-peeled skin and sweeter flesh.

Allergen: no

Introduction: 12 months

As with other citrus fruits, naartjies are acidic and as such may cause nappy rashes and irritate infant reflux.

Selection: Choose naartjies that have glossy, deep orange skins that feel heavy for their size.

Storage:

Unpeeled ⇢ cool, dark place ⇢ 1 week

Unpeeled ⇢ refrigerator ⇢ 1-2 weeks

Preparation/Use:: Simply peel and enjoy!

Nutritional Value:

Excellent: antioxidant flavonoids (vitamin P), and vitamin C

Good: vitamin A, folate, and fibre (pectin)

Additionally: vitamin B, calcium, magnesium, phosphorous and potassium.

Naartjies have antioxidant and anti-inflammatory benefits; digestive benefits and cholesterol-lowering benefits.

Nectarine

See Peach.

Nut Butter

Many adults today have fond childhood memories of peanut butter sandwiches! Today there are far more nutritious nut butter options for your little one such as almond, cashew, macadamia, walnut and tahini – all free from hydrogenated oils, sugar and salt. They are also really easy to make yourself.

Allergen: yes

Introduction: 12 months

Selection: Read the labels – make sure there are no added sugars, HFCS, or vegetable oils.

Storage:

Store bought ⇢ refrigerator ⇢ follow the expiry date on the packaging

Homemade ⇢ sealed, glass jar ⇢ refrigerator ⇢ 3 weeks

Homemade ⇢ sealed, glass jar ⇢ freezer ⇢ 3 months

Use:
Spread nut butters on everything from toastie to apple slices or add them to your little one's smoothies for a protein boost.

Nutritional Value:
Nut butters are rich in healthy fats (both monounsaturated and polyunsaturated fatty acids). They are known to decrease LDL (bad) cholesterol and triglyceride levels, lowering the risk of metabolic syndrome, heart disease, and type 2 diabetes. They are also good sources of protein and fibre.

Almond Butter: mild and silky and the healthiest one of all. Almond butter contains a significant amount of vitamin E, calcium, magnesium, potassium, phosphorous, iron, and more fibre than the other nut butters.

Walnut Butter: walnuts are a great source of omega-3 fatty acids but slightly lower in protein than other nut butters. It is high in antioxidant and anti-inflammatory compounds.

Cashew Butter: creamy with a light flavour. Lower in protein than almond butter. It is a good source of copper, magnesium iron, zinc, phosphorous, and manganese.

Macadamia Butter: the least protein of all the nut butters. Contains high amounts of vitamin B1, magnesium and manganese

Tahini: technically a seed butter. Tahini is a good source of magnesium, iron, calcium, vitamin B1

Nutmeg

Nutmegs are evergreen trees, native to the rain forest on the Indonesian Moluccas Island - also known as the Spice Islands. Nutmeg spice is made from the sun-dried seed taken from the centre of the nutmeg fruit. It is a rich, fragrant spice.

Allergen: no

Introduction: 6 months

Selection: Nutmeg is available all year round as both a powder and whole kernel. It is preferable to buy the whole kernel and grate it with a fine grater, as you need it. Always buy non-irradiated nutmeg.

Storage:

Ground nutmeg ⇢ airtight, glass container ⇢ cool dark place ⇢ 1 year

Whole nutmeg ⇢ airtight, glass container ⇢ cool dark place ⇢ 2 years

Use:
It is best to add nutmeg to a dish towards the end of the cooking.

It pairs well with sweet potato and pumpkin.

Nutritional Value:
Good: potassium, calcium, iron, manganese, vitamins A, B's and C.

Glossary of Ingredients

Nutmeg has a variety of healing properties and is a useful remedy for: insomnia, anxiety, calming muscle spasms, nausea and vomiting, indigestion (gas) and diarrhoea. It has the ability to detoxify the liver and kidneys and acts as an anti-inflammatory and antibacterial.

Nutritional Yeast

Nutritional yeast is a yeast which is grown on molasses and then harvested, washed, and dried with heat to kill or 'deactivate' it. It is sold in the form of flakes or as a yellow powder. It has a strong nutty, cheesy flavour making it a popular dairy-free cheese substitute for vegans and those avoiding dairy.

Allergen: no

Introduction: 7 months

Selection: You will find nutritional yeast in most health food shops.

Storage:
Sealed container ↔ cool, dark place ↔ 1 year

Use:
Just a tablespoon or two can add richness to soups and gravies, or a cheesy flavour to chickpea flatbread, quinoa cakes or popcorn. Larger amounts can be used to make 'cheese' sauces. You can make almond 'parmesan' by blending nutritional yeast with raw almonds.

Start with small amounts because it is a highly concentrated source of B-vitamins. Two of these B-vitamins (niacin and vitamin B6) can cause adverse reactions if given in excess. Recommended amounts for infants are ¼ teaspoon/day mixed with food. You can gradually increase the amount to about ½ teaspoon/day until one year of age and up to 1 teaspoon/day during the toddler years.

Nutritional Value:
Very good: B-vitamins, folate, selenium, zinc, and a complete protein.

It is gluten-free and contains no added sugars or preservatives.

Special note: Because nutritional yeast is inactive, it does not froth or grow like baking yeast does so it has no leavening ability. It also does not aggravate or contribute towards Candida.

Oats

Oats, known scientifically as Avena sativa, are a hardy cereal grain. Although oats are hulled, this process does not strip away their bran and germ allowing them to retain a concentrated source of their fibre and nutrients.

Oats not contain gluten. However, most of the oats that you buy in the supermarket have been processed in an environment that also processes grains such as wheat, rye and barley. Since these grains contain gluten, there will be cross-contamination. As a result, most oat brands available may not be suitable for celiacs and those following a strict gluten-free diet.

Allergen: no

Introduction: 12 months. Grains require certain digestive enzymes in order to be digested properly. These enzymes are not present in large enough quantities in your little one's immature digestive system until they are a year old – and only really when they are two years old.

Selection: Look for certified gluten-free oats. Avoid instant oats as they have added sugars, salt and preservatives.

Storage:
Airtight container ↔ cool, dark place ↔ 2 months

Preparation/Use:
Oats contain anti-nutrients: enzyme inhibitors and phytic acid so it is important to prepare them it a way that reduces the phytic acid, neutralises the enzyme inhibitors and increases the bio-availability of the nutrients.

Cover 1 cup oats with 1 cup warm water and add 1 tablespoon of an acid medium (whey, lemon juice or apple cider vinegar). Soak for twelve to twenty-four hours (or overnight). They can be eaten at this stage, or you can add them to a cup of boiling water and cook for several minutes.

Nutritional Value:
Very good: manganese and selenium

Good: protein, dietary fibre, magnesium, zinc and phosphorus

As a whole grain, oats have diverse nutritional benefits including enhancing the immune response to infection, stabilising blood sugar as well as anti-oxidant benefits.

Olives

Olives are the fruit from the olive tree and are one of the world's most widely enjoyed foods. They are too bitter to be eaten right off the tree and must be cured to make them palatable. Processing methods vary. Some olives are picked unripe, whilst others are allowed to fully ripen on the tree. You get green and black olives – the colour is not necessarily related to the maturity of the fruit. Many olives start off green and turn black when fully ripe, while other varieties stay green when fully ripe, and others start of black and remain black.

Allergen: no

Introduction: 7 months

Selection: Olives can be bought in cans, plastic bags, glass jars or in bulk from salad bars. Glass jars are preferable to ensure freshness and avoid the possible contamination with BPA. Olives should be firm.

Storage:
Unopened glass jars ⇢ cool, dark place ⇢ 1 year

Opened jar ⇢ refrigerator ⇢ 2 weeks (or according to the expiry date on the packaging)

Preparation/Use:
Be sure to remove the pip before giving an olive to your little one until you are sure he/she is able to chew very well. Simply cut the olive in half and pit.

Olives can be added to purées, dips, or as a topping for many other dishes. Alternatively turn them into a spread (olive tapenade) by processing in a food processor.

Nutritional Value:
Excellent: antioxidant and anti-inflammatory phytonutrients

Very good: copper

Good: iron, dietary fibre, and vitamin E.

Olives are considered a high-fat food with 75% of their fat being monounsaturated fat. Remember – fat is good, essential in fact! Especially for your little one.

Fats make up 60% of the brain and the nerves that run every system in the body. It plays an important role in the development of your little one's brain and helps them reach their maximum growth potential. Fat is also used in the body as fuel; helps the body absorb the fat-soluble vitamins, A, D, E and K; is the building block of hormones and insulates all nervous system tissues in the body. Mother Nature knows how important fat is for babies - 50% of the calories in breast milk are from fat.

Olives have anti-oxidant, anti-inflammatory and anti-cancer benefits. As well as supporting optimum brain development in your little one, they also able to help reduce LDL (bad) cholesterol and lower blood pressure.

Olive Oil

Olive oil is made from the crushing and then subsequent pressing of olives. The quality of olive oil production—especially the stage of pressing—really does make a difference when it comes to health benefits. Extra virgin olive oil is derived from the first pressing of the olives and has the most delicate flavour and strongest overall health benefits.

Allergen: no

Introduction: 6 months

Selection: For maximum health benefits, always choose cold-pressed extra virgin olive oil. Olive oil can go rancid from exposure to light and heat. It is important to buy olive oil that is packaged in dark tinted glass bottles.

Storage:
Sealed, dark glass jar/tin ⇢ cool, dark place ⇢ 1-2 months

Rancid olive oil smells like crayons, tastes like rancid nuts, and has a greasy mouth feel.

Use:
Cooking with olive oil is not recommended - its chemical structure and large amount of unsaturated fats make it very susceptible to oxidative damage when used for cooking. Rather drizzle it over already cooked meals, roasted veggies, purées and salads.

Nutritional Value:
Extra virgin olive oil is a particularly valuable source of antioxidant and anti-inflammatory phytonutrients. Olive oil is a unique plant oil in terms of its fat composition, containing about three-fourths of its fat in the form of oleic acid (a monounsaturated, omega-9 fat). It is a good source of vitamin E and also provides valuable amounts of the beta-carotene.

Extra virgin olive oil has anti-inflammatory, anti-cancer and anti-oxidant benefits. It supports a healthy heart; lowers LDL (bad) cholesterol; inhibits the growth of certain unwanted bacteria in our digestive tract (like H. Pylori); and improves cognitive function.

Onion

Onions are a bulb vegetable with a paper-like brown, red or white skin and an intensely flavoured white or purple-tinged flesh.

Allergen: no

Introduction: 8 months (cooked)

Onions have a tendency to cause gas.

Selection: Choose onions that are clean, well shaped, have no opening at the neck, and feature crisp, dry outer skins. Avoid those that are sprouting or have signs of mould.

Conventionally grown onions are often irradiated to prevent them from sprouting, so purchase organically grown ones

Glossary of Ingredients

whenever possible.

Storage:
Whole, raw ↪ well-ventilated space ↪ room temperature, away from heat, bright light and potatoes ↪ 3-4 weeks

Whole, chopped ↪ sealed container ↪ refrigerator ↪ 1 week

Whole, chopped ↪ sealed container ↪ freezer ↪ 2 months

Cooked ↪ sealed container ↪ refrigerator ↪ 3 days

Refrigerate cut onions as soon as possible. Their antibacterial qualities are so strong, that they absorb bacteria from the air. It has been found that people who get food poisoning after eating egg salad at a picnic, have in fact gotten ill, not from the egg left out at room temperature – but from the onion that has absorbed bacteria from the environment!

Preparation/Use:
Most of the onion's nutrients are contained in the outer layers closest to the skin. As such, peel off as little of the fleshy, edible portion as possible when removing the onion's paper-like layer. To reduce irritated eyes when cutting an onion, use a very sharp knife. Let cut onions stand for 10 minutes before cooking them in order to maximise their health benefits.

Onions are often used as an addition or seasoning in other dishes (especially for your little one's food), but sautéed or baked onions are delicious and sweet on their own.

When your little one (or you) have a cold or the flu, place a freshly cut onion next to the bed every night. This has been found to reduce recovery time.

Nutritional Value:
Excellent: polyphenols content (plant compounds recognized for their disease prevention, antioxidant, and anti-aging properties)

Very good: biotin

Good: manganese, vitamins B1, B6 and C, copper, vitamin C, dietary fibre, phosphorus, potassium, and folate

Onions have been revered throughout time for their therapeutic properties. They have potent anti-oxidant, anti-cancer, antibacterial, antihistamine and anti-inflammatory benefits. They strengthen the immune system, brain and nervous system and their sulphur compounds act as a heavy metal detoxifier. Onions are also a great pre-biotic (food which feeds probiotics).

Oranges

One of the most popular fruits in the world, oranges are round citrus fruits with finely-textured skins that are, of course, orange in colour just like their pulpy flesh. The skin can vary in thickness from very thin to very thick and they usually range from approximately 5-8 cm (2-3") in diameter. Oranges originated thousands of years ago in Asia, in the region between southern China to Indonesia.

Allergen: no

Introduction: 12 months

Oranges are quite acidic when eaten and can cause nappy rashes or rashes around the mouth.

Selection: Oranges do not necessarily have to have a bright orange colour to be good quality - oranges that are partially green or have brown russetting may be just as ripe and tasty as those that are solid orange in colour. The skin should be firm and the orange should be heavy for its size. Smaller oranges and those with thinner skins tend to be juicier than others. Avoid oranges that have soft spots or traces of mould.

Oranges are among the top 20 foods in which pesticide residues are most frequently found, buy organic oranges whenever possible.

I was horrified to discover that the uniform colour of non-organic oranges may be due to them being injected with Citrus Red Number 2 (an artificial dye) at the level of 2 parts per million.

Storage:
Whole oranges ↪ cool, dark place/fridge ↪ 2 weeks

Preparation/Use:
Scrub the whole orange with a vegetable brush and a salt-, vinegar-, or hydrogen peroxide water solution. You can either peel the orange and serve cut-up segments to your little one or cut the orange in half and scoop out the flesh with a serrated spoon (thereby avoiding the membranes which will be difficult to gum).

It is so simple and convenient to make fresh orange juice! Simply cut the orange in half, insert a fork into the centre and squeeze. You may want to run the juice through a sieve to remove any 'bits'. Remember to dilute the juice with water.

This is a great constipation remedy which I used on Mila numerous times – it worked better than prune juice, apple juice or grape juice and I was happy that the natural sugar content was lower than the other fruit juices too.

Nutritional Value:
Excellent: vitamin C

Very good: dietary fibre

Good: vitamin B1, pantothenic acid, folate, vitamin A, calcium, copper, and potassium.

Additionally: magnesium and iron.

Oranges provide antioxidant and immune support; have anti-inflammatory, anti-viral, anti-cancer and cholesterol-lowering benefits; relieve constipation and promote healthy digestion; keep bones and teeth strong; and, provide protection against cardiovascular disease and arthritis.

Oreganum (Oregano)

Oreganum is a herb with greyish-green oval leaves and a warm, balsamic and aromatic flavour. It is very popular in Mediterranean cuisine. Its name is derived from the Greek words oros (mountain) and ganos (joy) and it was considered a symbol of happiness by the Ancient Greeks.

Allergen: no

Introduction: 6 months

Selection: Whenever possible, choose fresh oreganum over the dried form of the herb since it has a far better flavour. The leaves of fresh oregano should look fresh and be vibrant green in colour, while the stems should be firm. They should be free from darks spots or yellowing.

If you do buy dried oreganum, ensure that it has not been irradiated.

Storage:
Fresh → plastic bag → refrigerator → 10-14 days

Fresh, chopped → ice-cube tray, covered with olive oil, water or stock → 4-6 months

Dried → sealed, glass jar → cool, dark place → 6 months

Add a cube to purées, stews or soups.

Preparation/Use:
Soak the oreganum in a salt-, vinegar-, or hydrogen peroxide water solution for 20 minutes then rinse under running water.

No pizza or tomato sauce is complete without a sprinkle of oreganum!

As with other herbs, you can make a medicinal tea from the leaves - place some fresh oreganum into boiling water, steep for at least 5 minutes, strain, and sip throughout the day.

Nutritional Value:
Excellent: vitamin K

Very good: manganese

Good: iron, dietary fibre, and calcium.

Oreganum is a highly effective anti-bacterial, antiseptic, antiviral, antifungal and antioxidant. It is known to remove poisons from the body and detox the entire lymphatic system. It helps rid the body of unwanted phlegm in the lungs, reduces fevers, and relieves diarrhoea. It can also aid digestion and help expel trapped gas from the intestines.

Ostrich

Ostrich meat comes from the largest bird in the world and while it is considered poultry, the meat is red. It has a similar taste to beef and is lower in saturated fat and cholesterol than beef, chicken and turkey.

Ostrich meat comes in a variety of forms, including prime steaks, fillets, sausages, burgers, stir-fry, and diced. It can be substituted for beef, pork, lamb, turkey, or chicken in virtually any recipe.

Allergen: no

Introduction: 7 months

As ostrich is very high in protein it is best to offer your little one regular, but small amounts of it – very large amounts of protein may put strain on your little one's immature kidneys.

Selection: Ostrich meat should be firm in texture and dark red in colour - free of any white or pink coloration.

Storage:
Due to this meat's pH balance, it doesn't harbour or attract harmful E. Coli or salmonella bacteria like other meats.

Raw ostrich → original packaging → refrigerator → 7 days

Raw ostrich → original packaging → freezer → 3 months

Thawed, raw ostrich → original packaging → refrigerator → 5 days

Cooked ostrich → sealed container → refrigerator → 5 days

Preparation/Use:
Since ostrich meat is so lean, you need to be careful not to overcook it. The recommended preparation is medium or medium-rare to prevent it from becoming tough and dry.

Ostrich steaks and fillets can be fried (in coconut oil) or grilled for 3 to 4 minutes per side. Ground ostrich can be used to make burger patties or bolognaise – it will not need to be cooked as long as those you make with beef. Ostrich cubes can be used in a stew in place of beef – and then puréed for your little one.

Nutritional Value:
Very good: protein, vitamins B6 and B12, iron, zinc and selenium

Good: thiamin, riboflavin, niacin and phosphorus.

Glossary of Ingredients

Ostrich meat has antioxidant and anti-inflammatory benefits; muscle building benefits; it supports healthy immune and inflammatory function; improves bone mass; and, improves blood sugar regulation.

Papaya

Papaya is a tropical, spherical-shaped fruit with a thin green to yellow skin and a bright orange, yellow or slightly pink coloured flesh. It is deliciously sweet with a butter-like consistency – prompting Christopher Columbus to name it "fruit of the angels". Inside the cavity of the flesh are edible, black, round seeds. Do not be put off by their peppery and bitter flavour – they are an excellent digestive aid and just one teaspoon contains more digestive enzymes than a whole bottle of digestive enzyme supplements. The seeds are also an effective vermicide or worm/parasite remover.

Not only is it delicious but exceptionally nutritious too! Papaya is considered to be one of the most nutrient dense and healing fruits on the planet. It is available all year.

Allergen: yes

Papayas contain substances that are associated with the latex-fruit allergy.

Introduction: 6 months

Selection: There are two major varieties of papayas on the market today: the big football-size Maradol papayas and the small hand-size solo or strawberry papayas. The Maradol variety contains the most nutrition and healing properties and is not GM. The smaller varieties are sometimes genetically modified and should be avoided.

Papayas are ripe when their skin has a reddish-orange colour and are slightly soft to the touch. Leave yellow papayas to ripen at room temperature for a couple of days.

Storage:
Uncut, ripe papayas → refrigerator → 2 weeks

Preparation/Use:
Wash the papaya with a salt-, vinegar-, or hydrogen peroxide water solution (to remove mould and yeasts). Cut in half, scoop out and save the seeds, then scoop out the flesh. Alternatively, you can peel the whole papaya with a potato peeler. If the pieces of papaya are too slippery for your little one to grip, try coating them with almond or coconut flour.

The seeds can be added to a smoothie or to a juice. Only add a few at a time, as the peppery flavour is quite strong. You can also add them to your salad dressing instead of pepper.

Save the remaining seeds by dehydrating them (at 45°C / 110°F to preserve the enzymes' viability). Once dehydrated, put them in a pepper grinder and grind them over your little one's food.

Nutritional Value:
Excellent: vitamin A (in the form of beta-carotene) and vitamin C

Very good: folate

Good: dietary fibre, magnesium, potassium, copper, iron, and vitamin K

Papaya offers protection against heart disease; anti-inflammatory, anti-viral and anti-cancer benefits; immune system support; and protection against eyesight degeneration and arthritis.

Papaya has a soothing, cleansing effect on the digestive tract and gently removes toxic debris while decreasing swelling and inflammation. It is an exceptionally beneficial fruit for helping to heal any type of digestive disorder such as constipation, acid reflux, colitis, irritable bowel syndrome, Celiac disease, H-pylori, diverticulitis, indigestion, bloating, flatulence, and stomach upset.

Paprika

Paprika is a spice made from grinding dried capsicum (bell) peppers into a fine powder. It has a vibrant red colour and a rich, pungent flavour.

Allergen: no

Introduction: 8 months

Selection and **Storage:**: You can get a variety of flavours of paprika – from sweet to smoked. Paprika is already ground so be sure to find the freshest one possible – stale paprika tastes like chalk. Always buy spices that have not been irradiated.

Storage:
Airtight, glass container → fridge → 1 year

Preparation/Use:
Paprika needs to be heated in order for its flavour to be released, so add it to the food while it is cooking.

Nutritional Value:
Excellent: antioxidant and anti-inflammatory phytonutrients, vitamins A, B6, and C

Very good: folate, vitamins B2 and E, dietary fibre, pantothenic acid, niacin, and potassium

Good: vitamins B1 and K, manganese, phosphorus, and magnesium

Parsley

One of the world's most popular herbs with amazing healing properties is, unfortunately, all to often only used as a garnish! Parsley is a dark green, nutrient-dense herb with a fresh, vibrant taste. There are two common types of parsley: Italian flat leaf parsley and curly leaf parsley.

Allergen: no

Introduction: 6 months

Selection: Whenever possible, choose fresh parsley over the dried form of the herb since it has a far better flavour. Choose fresh parsley that is deep green in colour and looks fresh and crisp. Avoid bunches that have leaves that are wilted or yellow as this indicates that they are either over mature or damaged.

If you buy dried parsley, make sure it has not been irradiated (organic dried herbs are not be irradiated).

Storage:
Fresh, unwashed ↦ in a plastic bag ↦ refrigerator ↦ 5-7 days

Fresh, unwashed ↦ chopped in ice-cube trays, covered with olive oil, water or stock ↦ freezer ↦ 5-7 days

Add a cube to purées, stews or soups.

Dried parsley ↦ sealed glass container ↦ cool, dark place ↦ 6 months

Preparation/Use:
Soak the parsley in a salt-, vinegar-, or hydrogen peroxide water solution for 20 minutes then rinse under running water.

Parsley can be added to purées, soups, stews and are a great addition to veggie juices. It should be added towards the end of cooking so it can retain its taste, colour and **Nutritional Value:**.

As with other herbs, you can make a medicinal tea from the leaves – place some fresh parsley into boiling water, steep for at least 5 - 10 minutes, strain, and sip throughout the day. Traditionally parsley tea has been a used to treat urinary tract infection, kidney stones, and liver-, bladder- and prostrate problems.

Nutritional Value:
Excellent: vitamins C and K

Good: vitamin A, folate, and iron

Parsley also has healing volatile oils and flavonoids.

Parsley is considered a chemo-protective food – that is, it helps prevent cancer and neutralise carcinogens. It is a rich source of antioxidants and offers benefits ranging from heart health to protection against arthritis.

Peaches

Peaches are a fragrant, sweet, juicy fruit with a velvety skin. Different varieties mean they come in a range of colours: from pink-blushed to creamy-white, red-blushed, yellow and orange with the flesh either white, yellow or orange.

Interestingly the only difference between peaches and nectarines is the lack of fuzz on the nectarine's skin. Nectarines tend to be redder, smaller and more fragrant than peaches, but their nutritional profile is the same.

They are available from spring through to autumn.

Allergen: no

Introduction: 7 months

Selection: Peaches (and nectarines) are one of the Dirty Dozen. It is important to find organic ones.

Choose peaches that have are fragrant, have no visible bruises or cuts and are as close to ripe as possible. They do not ripen further after being picked, but they will get softer and juicier.

Storage:
Ripe, whole, uncooked, unwashed ↦ refrigerator ↦ 2 days

Preparation/Use:
Soak the peaches in a salt-, vinegar-, or hydrogen peroxide water solution for 20 minutes then rinse under running water. Peaches can be enjoyed raw or cooked. If you are using pieces as a finger food, you can coat them in almond or coconut flour to make them less slippery. They purée well (especially when cooked). The best cooking methods are steaming, poaching or baking. Many of the valuable nutrients are lost during the cooking process. Frozen peach pieces in a feeder are a useful (and nutritious) way to alleviate teething pain.

Nutritional Value:
Excellent: antioxidants, vitamins A and C, and fibre

Good: riboflavin and potassium

Additionally: calcium, phosphorus, magnesium and Vitamins E, vitamin K, thiamin, niacin, pantothenic acid and selenium

Peaches are a natural laxative and diuretic. They have antioxidant and anti-cancer benefits, and help regulate blood pressure, heart rate and gastrointestinal health.

Glossary of Ingredients

Pears

Pears are a sweet, juicy fruit that typically have a rounded body that tapers into a neck of various lengths. They are a member of the rose family of plants. There are many different varieties of pears belonging to the category known as the European Pear. A secondary group of pears known as the Asian Pear includes what we commonly call the pear apple.

Pears are found in a variety of colours, including many different shades of green, red, yellow/gold, and brown.

Allergen: no

Introduction: 6 months (ideal first food)

Selection: Pears are very perishable once they are ripe, so the pears you find at in the supermarket will generally be unripe and will require a few days of maturing at room temperature. Pears should be firm, but not too hard with a smooth skin that is free of bruises or mould. Avoid pears that are punctured or bruised.

Many varieties fail to change colour as they ripen, making it more difficult to determine ripeness. To see if a pear is ripe, press at the top of the pear, near its stem. If that spot gives in to pressure, the pear is probably optimally ripe for eating.

Storage:
Ripe, whole, uncut ↝ refrigerator ↝ 5-12 days

Ripe, cut ↝ refrigerator ↝ 1-3 days

Cooked ↝ sealed container ↝ refrigerator ↝ 3 days

Cooked ↝ sealed container ↝ freezer ↝ 3 months

Pears should be stored away from other strong smelling foods as they tend to absorb smells.

Preparation/Use:
Soak the pears in a salt-, vinegar-, or hydrogen peroxide water solution for 20 minutes then rinse under running water. Since half of their dietary fibre as well as antioxidant and anti-inflammatory phytonutrients are in the skin, it is best to leave the skin on.

Pears are delicious raw and cooked. After washing, simply purée or cut into desired shapes and sizes and serve. To cook lightly steam for 5 – 10 minutes until just soft. Pears can also be baked or poached in a herbal tea.

Nutritional Value:
Very good: dietary fibre (both soluble and insoluble)

Good: copper, vitamins C and K.

Pears have antioxidant as well as anti-inflammatory benefits and assist with decreasing the risk of Type 2 diabetes, cholesterol related heart disease and certain cancers.

Peas (fresh)

Peas are sweet vegetables that are part of the legume family. They one of a few members of the legume family that are commonly sold and cooked as fresh vegetables (the others are more commonly sold in dried form). There are generally three types of peas that are commonly eaten: garden or green peas, snow peas and snap peas. The pods of both snow peas and snap peas are edible, with a slightly sweeter than the garden pea and make for a great dipping food.

Allergen: no

Introduction: 8 months

Selection: Green peas are sold fresh, canned or frozen. Fresh is always best – but if you are unable to find them, frozen peas are preferable to canned ones as they retain a better colour, flavour and texture. They are also not exposed to BPA as the canned ones are. Frozen peas must be consumed within 6 months of their packing date to ensure maximum nutrient content.

When choosing fresh peas, their colour should be a lively medium green. Peas that are especially light or dark, or those that are yellow, whitish or are speckled with grey, should be avoided. Additionally, do not choose pods that are puffy, water soaked or have mildew residue.

Snap peas are on The Dirty Dozen list and you should only purchase organic ones.

Garden Peas are one of the EWG's Clean Fifteen so purchasing organic is optional.

Storage:
Fresh peas should be refrigerated immediately after purchase to prevent the sugars from converting to starch.

Unwashed, fresh, raw ↝ in a bag or sealed container ↝ refrigerator ↝ 7 days

Blanched ↝ sealed container ↝ freezer ↝ 6 months

Preparation/Use:
Soak the pea pods in a salt-, vinegar-, or hydrogen peroxide water solution for 20 minutes then rinse under running water.

Snow peas and snap peas can be eaten raw, pods and all – although cooking them briefly makes them softer and sweeter.

Once the garden pea pods have been washed, you can snap off either end, open the pod and scrape the peas out. These do not need additional washing as they have been encased in the pod.

Peas can be sautéed, steamed or boiled for 3 minutes.

Peas are very easy to grow at home and as they grow, they add nutrients to the soil which benefits your other vegetables and herbs. They are a great way to introduce your little one to where food really comes from – Mila loves finding the ripe pods on the vine, popping them open and eating the peas straight away. She reacts as if she has found treasure! It is, actually, the only way she eats peas.

Nutritional Value:

Excellent: phytonutrients

Very good: vitamins B1, C and K, manganese, dietary fibre, copper, phosphorus, and folate

Good: vitamins B2 and B6, niacin, molybdenum, zinc, protein, magnesium, iron, potassium, and choline.

Green peas have antioxidant and anti-inflammatory benefits and are able to regulate blood sugar (due to their high protein and fibre content).

Pineapple

Pineapple is an exceptionally juicy fruit with a vibrant tropical flavour that balances the tastes of sweet and tart. Pineapple has a wide cylindrical shape, a scaly yellow skin and a crown of spiny, green leaves and fibrous yellow flesh. It is available year round.

Allergen: no

Introduction: 8-12 months

The pineapple's acidity might present a problem for your little one (in the form of nappy rash, or a rash around the mouth where the juices touch the delicate skin). It may also cause acid reflux to flair up – again, due to the acidity.

Selection: Pineapple stops ripening once it is picked, so be sure to buy pineapple that is already ripe. It is ripe when it has a fragrant, sweet smell at the base. Choose a pineapple that is heavy for its size (bigger pineapples are not necessarily better). It should be free of bruises and darkened 'eyes'.

Storage:

Pineapples are very perishable and can only be left at room temperature for 2 days. To increase their shelf-life, remove the green, spiky crown of leaves by wrapping a dish towel around it and breaking it off.

Whole, uncut, raw pineapple ⇢ sealed plastic bag ⇢ refrigerator ⇢ 3-5 days

Cut, raw pineapple ⇢ airtight container ⇢ refrigerator ⇢ 5 days

Preparation/Use:

Top and tail the pineapple, place it base side down then slice off the thick skin. Remove any additional 'eyes' with a knife tip.

Pineapple is best eaten raw, although grilled pineapple is delicious too. Your little one can enjoy this fruit puréed, mashed, cut into bite size pieces or added to juices and smoothies.

Nutritional Value:

Excellent: vitamin C and manganese

Very good: copper

Good: vitamins B1 and B6, dietary fibre, folate, and pantothenic acid.

Pineapple contains a protein digesting enzyme, bromelain, which is responsible for many of this fruit's health benefits including: aiding digestion; reducing inflammation and swelling; and, possibly, anti-cancer benefits. Bromelain is so beneficial that it is now extracted from pineapples and sold as a dietary supplement.

Additional health benefits of pineapple includes: antioxidant protection and immune support; energy production; and eye-protection.

Plums

Plums are a round, juicy, sweet tasting fruit that come in a range of vibrant colours – the skin can be red, purple, blue-black, red, green, yellow or amber, while the flesh can be yellow, green and pink and orange. There are six different categories: Japanese, American, Damson, Ornamental, Wild and European/Garden (prunes are the dried version of European plums). Plums are available from spring to the end of autumn.

Allergen: no

Introduction: 7 months

Selection: Good quality plums will have a rich colour and should still have a slight whitish bloom (coating), which shows that they have not been over handled. Ripe plums yield to gentle pressure. Plums will continue to ripen after being picked, so you can buy unripe ones and ripen them at home by leaving them at room temperature for a couple of days.

According to the EWG, plums and prunes one of the foods least contaminated with pesticides so buying organic is optional, although always recommended.

When buying prunes, make sure that they have not had a sulphur-based preservative added to them in the drying process.

Storage:

Ripe, raw, uncut ⇢ sealed container/bag ⇢ refrigerator ⇢

3-5 days

ripe, raw, pitted → sealed container/bag → freezer → 6-8 months

Preparation/Use:
Plums can be enjoyed raw or cooked, puréed or cut into little pieces (without the skin) for your little one to gum on. Dehydrated plum slices are also really delicious – they make a great finger food to gnaw on when those teeth are coming out and a mess-free out-and-about food. The best methods of cooking plums are steaming, baking and poaching.

To soften prunes, simply soak in boiled water until they plump up – then add them to purées.

Sulphur-free prune juice is a great remedy for relieving constipation in your little one – but too much may cause cramps.

Nutritional Value:
Very good: vitamin C

Good: vitamin K, copper, dietary fibre, and potassium..

Prunes normalise blood sugar levels; help lower cholesterol; ease and prevent constipation; help maintain a healthy colon; act as a prebiotic.

Pomegranate

The pomegranate is a beautiful, ancient fruit, originally native to the Middle East. They are a symbol of health, fertility, rebirth, prosperity and abundance. The fruit is about the size and shape of an orange, its skin has a pinkish-red colour and a leathery texture. The inside of the pomegranate is filled with bitter, inedible white membranes that hold hundreds of ruby-red seed sacs containing the sweet pulp and juice. They are available in summer.

Allergen: no

Choking hazard: yes

Introduction: 12 months

Selection: Pomegranates are picked when ripe, so when you see them in stores they are ready to eat. When selecting a pomegranate, consider that the heavier the fruit is, the juicier it will be.

Storage:
Whole fruit → cool, dark place → 2 months

Peeled fruit → sealed container → freezer → 6 months

Preparation/Use:
While you may be put off by the manual labour needed to harvest the arils, it can be quite an effortless process:

♥ Cut the pomegranate in half
♥ Hold the cut side over a bowl
♥ Tap the shell firmly with a wooden spoon
♥ The arils will drop out, leaving the inedible membranes behind.

Be warned... Pomegranate juice stains fingers, clothes and carpeting. Sitting outside is the best place to enjoy pomegranates and their delicious mess!

Nutritional Value:
Excellent: vitamins C and K, antioxidant polyphenols (micronutrients)

Good: fibre, copper, potassium, folate, manganese, thiamin and vitamin B5

Pomegranates protect human cells from oxidation, protect the kidneys and protect and regenerate the liver. They boost the immune system; are anti-allergic; have anti-cancer benefits; protect the heart from free radicals; lower cholesterol and they offer direct DNA protection.

Potato

The potato probably needs no introduction! There are about 100 varieties of this popular vegetable and they range in size, shape, colour, starch content and flavour. Potatoes are generally round or oval in shape – although you get finger-shaped ones too. The edible skin of potatoes is generally brown, red or yellow, and may be smooth or rough, while the flesh is yellow or white. The flavour is neutral and they have a creamy rich texture. They belong to the nightshade family (which includes eggplant, tomatoes and bell peppers).

Although potatoes often get labelled as unhealthy – this is largely due to the way they are prepared - deep fried as chips, crisps or French fries, or served - with high fat sauces, cheese and/or bacon etc. Potatoes prepared in a healthy way are actually quite nutritious.

Fried and processed foods made with potatoes contain a potentially toxic and cancer-causing substance known as acrylamide (a by-product of the high-heat cooking methods). It is important to minimize your little one's exposure to these foods.

Allergen: yes

May cause a reaction in people with a latex allergy or those sensitive to nightshade vegetables.

Introduction: 7 months

Selection: Potatoes are one of the EGW's Dirty Dozen so you should only buy organic. Furthermore, a GM potato has recently been approved and without effective labelling to know which potatoes are GM and which aren't you should only buy organic potatoes.

Potatoes should be firm, well shaped and relatively smooth, and should be free of decay that often manifests as wet or dry rot. Potatoes should not be sprouting or have any green on the skin - this indicates that they may contain the toxic alkaloid solanine that has been found to cause a host of different health conditions such as circulatory and respiratory depression, headaches and diarrhoea.

Storage:
Raw, uncut ⇢ unwrapped ⇢ cook, dark place – 2 months

Cooked ⇢ sealed container ⇢ refrigerator ⇢ 7 days

Preparation/Use:
Soak the potatoes in a salt-, vinegar-, or hydrogen peroxide water solution for 20 minutes then rinse under running water.

Most of the nutrients are found in the skin of the potato, so it is preferable not to peel it. If you choose to peel potatoes, do so with a potato peeler to ensure you only take off the thinnest layer. Peeled potatoes tend to discolour quickly - they should be submerged in a bowl of cold water until you are ready to cook them.

Potatoes can be cooked in a variety of ways – steamed, baked, roasted or boiled.

When making mashed potato or potato purée, do not use an electric blender or food processor! The starches respond by becoming glue-like. Simply mash cooked potato with a fork or with a potato masher.

Nutritional Value:
Very good: vitamin B6

Good: potassium, copper, vitamin C, manganese, phosphorus, niacin, dietary fibre, and pantothenic acid.

Potato Starch, Potato Starch Flour and Potato Flour

Potato starch and potato flour are not one in the same, although both are gluten-free.

Potato starch (also known as potato starch flour) is made from starch extracted from potatoes that then undergoes a refining process. Potato flour is made from dehydrated cooked potatoes that are ground into a powder. It has a distinct smell of potato whereas the starch does not. Potato flour is heavier than potato starch.

Potato starch

Potato starch is not a nutritionally dense food although current research suggests that potato starch is a good source of resistant starch which acts as a prebiotic. It is used as a thickening agent and is a good substitute for other thickeners such as corn-starch. Dishes in which it has been added as a thickening agent should not be boiled. It can be used for flouring before frying (it browns well), and can be used in cakes and biscuits if blended with other flours.

Potato starch can be fully substituted for tapioca starch. Potato starch and corn-starch are interchangeable as well, but that works better for quantities of a ¼ cup or less.

Potato flour

Potato flour has a strong potato flavour and is a heavy flour so a little goes a long way. It is high in many vitamins including vitamin C and vitamin B6; it is also a good source of potassium, calcium, and dietary fibre, and contains some protein, as well.

Since potato flour attracts and holds water, it is great for producing moist baked goods such as breads, pancakes, and waffles. Potato flour is good for batter or coating meats and fish before deep-frying as well as adding texture and flavour to flour blends used for baking.

Allergen: no

Introduction: 6 months

Storage:: Sealed container ⇢ cool, dry place ⇢ 6 months

Pumpkin Seeds (Pepitas)

Pumpkin seeds are flat, dark green seeds found in the centre of the pumpkins. Pumpkin seeds have a chewy texture and a subtly sweet, nutty flavour. Pumpkin seeds are available in a variety of forms including: raw and shelled, raw and unshelled, roasted and shelled, roasted and unshelled.

Allergen: no

Introduction: 12 months

Selection: When choosing pumpkin seeds make sure there is no evidence of moisture or insect damage and that they are not shrivelled. It is best to purchase certified organic raw pumpkin seeds to avoid unnecessary exposure to potential contaminants. By purchasing raw, you will be able to soak the seeds and control the roasting time and temperature thereby avoiding unnecessary damage to the good fats in the seeds.

Glossary of Ingredients

You can, of course, buy a whole pumpkin, scoop out the seeds, rinse and prepare (as below) and use the flesh for purées, roasted vegetables or soup.

Storage:: airtight container ⇢ refrigerator ⇢ 1-2 months

Preparation/Use:
Seeds contain anti-nutrients: enzyme inhibitors and phytic acid so it is important to prepare them it such a way that reduces the phytic acid, neutralises the enzyme inhibitors and increases the bio-availability of the nutrients.

Cover the seeds with warm water and add sea salt. The ratio of seeds to salt should be ½ tablespoon salt for every 2 cups of seeds. Soak for six to eight hours (or overnight), then drain, rinse and dehydrate or roast.

Dehydrate the seeds by placing them in a warm oven (no warmer than 65°C/150°F) or dehydrator for 12- 24 hours. Alternatively, roast them at 75°C/170°F for 15 -20 minutes.

Pumpkin seeds can be ground in a coffee grinder and sprinkled on vegetables and fruit or added to smoothies.

Nutritional Value:
Very good: phosphorus, magnesium, manganese, and copper

Good: vitamin E, vitamin B's, zinc, iron, essential fatty acids (omega 3) and protein

Additional: the amino acid tryptophan – a nutrient which relaxes the body, calms the nerves, improves sleep, and transmits signals between neurons.

Pumpkin seeds have anti-oxidant, antiviral, antifungal and antimicrobial benefits.

Quinoa

Quinoa, pronounced "keen wah", is a member of the same food family as spinach, Swiss chard, and beets and originates from South America. All parts of the plant could be eaten but we commonly find it as whole seeds or flour. The gluten-free seeds come in a variety of colours: red, orange, pink, purple, tan, and black. Cooked quinoa seeds are slightly crunchy, fluffy and creamy, with a delicate slightly nutty flavour.

Allergen: no

Introduction: 12 months

Quinoa is easier to digest than other grains and is more nutritious – it would be a great one to start with.

Selection: When buying quinoa make sure there is no evidence of moisture in the packet. Quinoa expands to several times its original size during the cooking process – so there is no need to buy too much at once.

Storage:
Uncooked ⇢ airtight container ⇢ cool, dark place ⇢ 4 months

Cooked ⇢ sealed container ⇢ refrigerator ⇢ 3-5 days

Cooked ⇢ sealed container ⇢ freezer ⇢ 2 months

Preparation/Use:
Seeds contain anti-nutrients: enzyme inhibitors and phytic acid so it is important to prepare them it such a way that reduces the phytic acid, neutralises the enzyme inhibitors and increases the bio-availability of the nutrients.

Cover the quinoa with warm water and add an acid medium (whey, lemon juice or apple cider vinegar). The ratio of quinoa to acid should be ½ tablespoon acid for every 2 cups of seeds. Soak for twelve to twenty-four hours (or overnight), then drain, rinse and cook or dehydrate.

To cook: Add one-part quinoa to two parts boiling water or broth. After the liquid has returned to a boil, turn down the heat, cover and simmer for about 15 minutes or until the grains are translucent have what looks like a white-spiralled tail.

Porridge
When cooking soaked, dehydrated and ground quinoa seeds for homemade baby porridge, use ¼ cup of ground seeds per 1-2 cups of water, broth or coconut milk – more or less as you see fit. The key is to whisk continuously as you are cooking to avoid clumping.

Nutritional Value:
Quinoa is a nutrient dense food and a complete, high-quality protein (a source of all the essential amino acids).

Very good: manganese

Good: copper, magnesium, fibre, folate and zinc

Additionally: calcium, vitamins E and B, and iron.

Quinoa has anti-inflammatory and antioxidant benefits.

Quinoa Flour

Quinoa flour is made by grinding quinoa seeds. It is one of the most nutritious gluten-free flours. It has a nutty and earthy flavour that pairs well with fruits, nuts, spices like cinnamon, cardamom, cumin and coriander, as well as herbs like rosemary.

Allergen: no

Introduction: 12 months

Storage:: Quinoa flour can be stored for up to 6 months if kept in the fridge or freezer.

Preparation/Use:: For each recipe using flour, you could soak the flour in the cooking liquid overnight and continue cooking or baking the next day. This may be completely inconvenient and the recipe might have to be adjusted. Where possible make your own flours from soaked and dehydrated whole grains/seeds.
How to make quinoa flour:

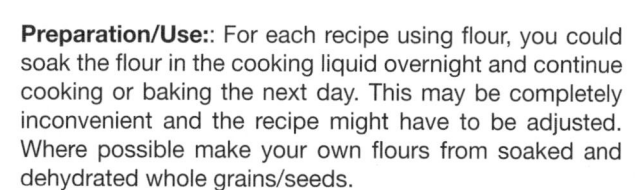

Soak and dehydrate your quinoa as described above. Once dry, grind the kernels in a coffee grinder or food processor. Store extra flour in a sealed container in the fridge.

Use: You can substitute this flour for half of the all-purpose gluten-free flour in many recipes to add a nutritional punch. It works well as a thickening agent, in bread, muffin, pastry and cookie recipes and can be added to smoothies as a protein powder.

Raisins

Raisins are made from dehydrating grapes in a process that either involves the heat of the sun or a mechanical process of oven drying. Among the most popular types of raisins are Sultana, Malaga, Monukka, Zante Currant, Muscat, and Thompson seedless.

The dehydration process results in the grapes' concentration of sugars increasing as well as some loss of their **Nutritional Value:**. For every gram of raisins, you get four times the amount of sugar that you would be getting in a gram of grapes, even though you are not getting any more vitamins and minerals.
That said, raisins do make a healthy contribution to snacks, muesli, and other recipes and are a very convenient, no-mess out-and-about food for your little one once they are old enough to gum their food.

Allergen: no

Introduction: 10 months (**Choking hazard**)

Selection: Raisins are made from grapes, and grapes are listed by the EWG as one of the Dirty Dozen. It is best to choose organic raisins and ensure that they are free of sulphur, sulphites and vegetable oils. Commercially grown raisins are usually treated with sulphur dioxide gas during processing. They may also be treated with sulphites to extend their shelf life. The vegetable oil used is often genetically modified canola oil. (The same applies for all dried fruit.)

Storage:: Sealed container ↝ cool, dark place ↝ 6-12 months

Use: Add raisins to purées, or soak them to soften and plump them up as a finger food.

Nutritional Value:
Raisins are one of the richest sources of the mineral boron and provide concentrated amounts of phytonutrients. They also have a significant amount of iron, calcium, potassium and fibre.

Raspberries

Raspberries are brightly coloured, sweet, juicy berries with a hollow structure – great for slipping onto the tips of little fingers! As an aggregate fruit they are composed of many small individual fruits (drupelets) that make up the structure of the raspberry. There are three basic groups of raspberries: red-, purple-, and black raspberries. Black raspberries may actually be dark enough to be indistinguishable from blackberries in terms of colour (blackberries, however, do not have a hollow centre). Raspberries are in season in Summer.

Allergen: no

Introduction: 8 months

Selection: Choose berries that are firm, plump, and deep in colour, while avoiding those that are soft, mushy, or mouldy.

Storage:
Sealed container ↝ refrigerator ↝ 2 days

Sealed container ↝ freezer ↝ 1 year

They can be added to smoothies directly from the freezer.

Preparation/Use:: Soak the raspberries in a salt-, vinegar-, or hydrogen peroxide water solution for 20 minutes then rinse under running water.
Raspberries are best eaten raw – purée them, mash them, add them to smoothies or use as a first finger food.

Nutritional Value:
Excellent: phytonutrients, vitamin C, manganese, and dietary fibre

Very good: copper

Good: vitamins E and K, pantothenic acid, biotin, magnesium, folate, omega-3 fatty acids, and potassium.

Raspberries have exceptionally diverse anti-inflammatory and antioxidant benefits; obesity and blood sugar benefits; as well as anti-cancer benefits.

Red Pepper (Bell Pepper)

See Bell Pepper

Rice

Rice is the seed of a grass but is classified as a gluten-free grain in the food world. It is one of the most widely consumed staple foods for a large part of the world's population. There are over 8000 varieties of rice!

It is often categorised by its size – being either short grain, medium grain or long grain. Short grain, which has the highest starch content, makes the stickiest rice, while long grain is lighter and tends to remain separate when cooked.

Rice can also be categorised according to the way or degree to which it is milled. This is what makes brown rice different to white rice. Brown rice, often referred to as whole rice, is the whole grain with only its inedible outer hull removed. Brown rice still retains its nutrient-rich bran and germ. White rice is both milled and polished, which removes the bran and germ along with all the nutrients contained within these important layers. Fully milled and polished white rice is required to be enriched with vitamins B1, B3 and iron.

Some of the most popular varieties of rice include:

- **Short-grain brown rice:** A nutty flavoured rice ideal for pilaffs, risotto and your little one. It is the easiest rice to digest and the best one to start with.
- **Arborio:** A round grain, starchy white rice, traditionally used to make the Italian dish risotto.
- **Basmati:** An aromatic rice that has a nutlike fragrance, delicate flavour and light texture.
- **Sweet rice:** Almost translucent when cooked, this very sticky rice is traditionally used to make sushi and mochi.
- **Jasmine:** A soft-textured long grain aromatic rice that is available in both brown and white varieties.

Allergen: no

Introduction: 12 months. Grains require certain digestive enzymes in order to be digested properly. These enzymes are not present in large enough quantities in your little one's immature digestive system until they are a year old – and only really when they are two years' old

Selection: Although not on the EWG's Dirty Dozen list, it is still advisable to buy organic rice wherever possible as genetically modified varieties are currently being tested and may be introduced to the market soon. When buying ice, make sure there is no evidence of moisture in the packet. Always choose brown, or whole, rice.

Storage:
Uncooked rice ⇢ airtight container ⇢ cool, dry place ⇢ 6 months

Cooked rice ⇢ airtight container ⇢ refrigerator ⇢ 1 day

Cooked rice ⇢ airtight container ⇢ freezer ⇢ 1 month

Cooked rice can develop several potential toxins under certain conditions involving time, temperature, and presence of moisture, bacterial spores, or fungi. As such cooked rice should only be kept in the fridge for 1 day. Place cooked rice in a tightly sealed container as soon as you have cooked it. Allow it to cool, then place it in the fridge.

Preparation/Use:: Whole grains contain anti-nutrients: enzyme inhibitors and phytic acid so it is important to prepare them it such a way that reduces the phytic acid, neutralises the enzyme inhibitors and increases the bio-availability of the nutrients.

Cover the rice with warm water and an acid medium (whey, lemon juice or apple cider vinegar). The ratio of rice to acid should be ½ tablespoon acid for every 2 cups of grains. To remove more phytates, you can add a tablespoon of buckwheat grains to the soaking bowl (this increases the phytase necessary for the breaking down of phytate.) Soak for twelve to twenty-four hours (or overnight), then drain, rinse and cook, or dehydrate.

Add one-part rice to two parts boiling water or broth. After the liquid has returned to a boil, turn down the heat, cover and simmer for about 20 - 35 minutes (depending on the variety).

Rice porridge

Use ¼ cup of ground, soaked and dehydrated rice per 1-2 cups of water – more or less as you see fit. The key is to whisk continuously as you are cooking to avoid clumping. Alternatively, simply purée already cooked rice.

Nutritional Value:
Excellent: manganese

Good: selenium, phosphorus, copper, magnesium, and niacin

Additionally: phytonutrients, B vitamins, iron, essential fatty acids, fibre and amino acids.

Whole rice has anti-cancer and anti-oxidant benefits. As with other whole grains, brown rice lowers the risk of Type 2 diabetes; protects against heart disease; and lowers LDL (bad) cholesterol.

Rice Flour

Rice flour is made from finely milled rice, and comes in both white and brown varieties. It is best to use brown rice flour as it still contains the nutritious bran and layers covering the kernel. For most recipes, both brown and white rice flour may be used interchangeably, but brown rice has a nuttier flavour. Rice flour is commonly used in Japanese cuisine to make rice noodles and traditional

Japanese desserts.

Rice flour is best in baked foods such as bread, cookies and cake, it creates a slightly grainy texture with a fine, dry crumb. When used in yeast products it does not rise well – but that is overcome by combining a few different gluten-free flours in a recipe. Rice flour makes a good thickener.

Allergen: no

Introduction: 12 months

Selection: Once brown rice is milled its exposed oils can cause the flour to go rancid. When choosing rice flour, make sure it has not been in the shop for too long. It is preferable to buy organic.

Storage:
Tightly sealed container ⇢ cool, dark place ⇢ 3-6 months

Tightly sealed container ⇢ freezer ⇢ 12 months

Preparation/Use:: For each recipe using rice flour, you could soak the flour in the cooking liquid overnight and continue cooking or baking the next day. This may be completely inconvenient and the recipe might have to be adjusted. Where possible make your own flours from soaked and dehydrated whole grains.
How to make rice flour:

Simply soak and dehydrate your rice as described above in Brown Rice. Once dry, grind the kernels in a coffee grinder or food processor. Pour through a sieve to remove any bigger particles.

Rooibos

Rooibos (pronounced Roy-boss and meaning Red Bush) is a plant indigenous to South Africa where it has been used by the indigenous Bushman for hundreds of years. Its leaves are used for making a naturally caffeine-free tea.

Allergen: no

Introduction: 6 months (start with 30–60 ml)

Selection and Storage:: Choose organic tea in unbleached tea bags. Store tea bags in an airtight container.

Preparation/Use:: Place tea bag in a mug of boiling water and allow to steep for 5 minutes. Allow the tea to cool and serve as is, or with milk. If your baby is older than a year old, you can sweeten it with honey. Alternatively cut some sweet fruit into the tea while it is brewing and allow the sweetness of the fruit to flavour the tea. Rooibos is also often made with a slice of lemon added to it.

Nutritional Value:
Good: copper, iron, magnesium, calcium, zinc and potassium

Rooibos can soothe digestive disorders – such as constipation, diarrhoea, stomach cramps, colic and nausea. It can also be used topically to treat skin conditions such as eczema and sunburn. There are many creams available in South Africa using Rooibos as an ingredient. Alternatively, you can bath in the tea, or use the tea as a wash. If your little one has a nappy rash, simply place an unused teabag in his/her nappy in the area of the rash. Change the teabag with every nappy change. The rash should disappear in a day or two.

Rosemary

Rosemary is a herb with leaves that look like flat pine needles. They are deep green in colour on top and silver-white underneath. Its flavour and unique health benefits makes it an indispensable herb for every kitchen.

Allergen: no

Introduction: 6 months

Selection: Whenever possible, choose fresh rosemary over the dried form of the herb since it has a far better flavour. Fresh rosemary should look vibrant and should have a deep sage green colour, and be free from yellow or dark spots. If you buy dried rosemary, make sure it has not been irradiated (organic dried herbs will not be irradiated).

Storage:
Fresh rosemary, unwashed ⇢ plastic bag ⇢ refrigerator ⇢ 10-14 days

Fresh rosemary, unwashed, chopped ⇢ in ice-cube trays, covered with olive oil, water or stock ⇢ freezer ⇢ 4-6 months. Add a cube to purées, stews or soups.

Dried rosemary ⇢ sealed glass container ⇢ cool, dark place ⇢ 6 months

Alternatively, you can place some sprigs in vase of water on your kitchen counter.

Preparation/Use:
Soak the rosemary in a salt-, vinegar-, or hydrogen peroxide water solution for 20 minutes then rinse under running water. As the rosemary stem is difficult to eat, the leaves should be removed from the stem. Alternatively, add the whole sprig to season soups, stews and meat dishes, then simply remove it before serving. It should be added towards the end of cooking so it can retain its taste, colour and nutritional value (the flavour can become bitter after long cooking).

Rosemary can be added to purées, soups, stews and are a great addition to meat dishes in particular.

As with other herbs, you can make a medicinal tea from

the leaves – place some fresh rosemary into boiling water, steep for at least 10-15 minutes, strain, and sip throughout the day.

You can also make rosemary infused oil. Place a sprig or two of completely dry rosemary leaves into a glass jar, top with olive oil, replace the lid, and shake lightly. Store in a warm, dark place for two weeks, strain, and then simply pour back into the glass jar.

Nutritional Value:
Good: vitamin A (in the form of pro-vitamin A carotenoid phytonutrients).

Rosemary contains substances that are useful for stimulating the immune system, increasing circulation, and improving digestion. Rosemary also contains anti-inflammatory compounds that may make it useful for reducing the severity of asthma attacks. In addition, rosemary has been shown to increase the blood flow to the head and brain, improving concentration. Traditionally it has been used as an antiseptic, antidepressant, analgesic, antiviral, anti-inflammatory, disinfectant, aphrodisiac, and expectorant.

Sage

Sage is a herb with lance-shaped velvety soft leaves which are greyish-green in colour with a silvery bloom covering. It has a soft, yet sweet savoury flavour. Sage has been held in high regard throughout history both for it culinary and medicinal properties.

Allergen: no

Introduction: 6 months

Selection: Whenever possible, choose fresh sage over the dried form of the herb since it has a far better flavour. It should have vibrant green-grey leaves. They should be free from darks spots or yellowing.

If you buy dried sage, make sure it has not been irradiated (organic dried herbs will not be irradiated).

Storage:
Fresh sage, unwashed → plastic bag → refrigerator → 7 days

Dried sage → sealed glass container → cool, dark place → 6 months

Preparation/Use:
Soak the sage leaves in a salt-, vinegar-, or hydrogen peroxide water solution for 20 minutes then rinse under running water.

Sage leaves can be added to purées, soups, stews, mashed potatoes, gnocchi and scrambled eggs. Since the flavour of sage is delicate, it is best to add the herb near the end of the cooking process.

As with other herbs, you can make a medicinal tea from the leaves – place some fresh sage into boiling water, steep for at least 5 - 10 minutes, strain, and sip throughout the day. Traditionally this has been called the "thinker's tea" and helps ease depression, treat sore throats, coughs and infant diarrhoea.

Sage should not be consumed in excess if you are still breastfeeding as it may dry up your milk supply.

Nutritional Value:
Sage contains a variety of healing volatile oils.

Excellent: vitamin K

Good: vitamin A (in the form of pro-vitamin A carotenoid phytonutrients).

Sage has potent antioxidant and anti-inflammatory benefits as well as anti-microbial and anti-bacterial properties making it an excellent natural remedy for fungal, viral, and bacterial infections. It is an excellent memory enhancer and digestive aid.

Salt

Salt is a crystalline mineral made of two elements, sodium (Na) and chloride (Cl). Salt is essential for life — you cannot live without it. Sodium and chloride serve important functions in the body - like helping the brain and nerves send electrical impulses. As with most things, however, too much sodium can hurt you and your little one who's kidneys are still immature.

There is an enormous difference between common, refined table salt and natural, unrefined salt - one is health damaging, and the other is healing.

Natural unrefined salt is 85% sodium chloride while processed, table salt is 98%.

Ordinary table salt undergoes a great deal of processing or chemical cleaning. Besides the much higher concentration of sodium chloride, it also contains chemicals such as artificial iodine and anti-caking agents and is dehydrated at over 650°C (1 200°F). This high heat alters the natural chemical structure of the salt into something that your body does not recognize.

Unrefined salt (such as Himalayan Salt or sea salt) has a lower sodium chloride content and includes up to 84 other naturally occurring beneficial minerals, including many trace minerals like silicon, phosphorous and vanadium. It is minimally processed — hand-mined and hand-washed and its crystalline structure stores vibrational energy, which is restorative to your body. It does not contain iodine (which is added to ordinary table salt). Be sure to add some dulse flakes or other seaweeds to your little one's food to ensure they get this important mineral.

Allergen: no

Introduction: While it is not a good idea to get your little one too used to salty food by adding salt to already cooked food as adults do, there is no reason why you should not add a touch Himalayan or sea salt to the dishes you are cooking for your little one.

Selection: It is important to choose a natural salt free of pollutants and to avoid processed salt and all the processed foods in which it is hidden.

Storage:: Store in a tightly sealed container.

Satsuma (Naartjie / Tangerine)

See Naartjie.

Scallion (Green Onion / Spring Onion)

See Spring Onion.

Seaweed (Sea Vegetables)

Seaweed?! Yes, Western culture is beginning to enjoy the taste and **Nutritional Value:** of sea vegetables, otherwise known as seaweed, which have been a staple of the Japanese diet for centuries. A variety of edible and highly nutritious sea vegetables can now be found in health food shops.

Sea vegetables are neither plants nor animals but classified in a group known as algae. There are both salt water varieties as well as fresh water sea vegetables. There are thousands of types - each of which are classified into categories by colour - either brown, red or green. Each is unique, having a distinct shape, taste and texture. Some of the most common ones are: nori, hijiki, wakame, arame, kombu and dulse.

- ♥ Nori: is a dark purple-black colour that turns phosphorescent green when toasted. It is best known as an ingredient in sushi roll. Nori is 28% protein, more than sunflower seeds or lentils. It is also an excellent source of calcium, iron, manganese, fluoride, copper, and zinc. Of the sea vegetables, nori is one of the highest in vitamins B1, B2, B3, B6, B12 as well as vitamins A, C and E.
- ♥ Kelp: is light brown to dark green in colour. Often sourced from North America and Europe.
- ♥ Kombu: very dark in colour and generally sold in strips or sheets. It is traditionally used as a flavouring for soups. Adding kombu to the cooking water when preparing beans is said to make the bean more digestible.
- ♥ Wakame: is quite similar to kombu. It is most commonly used to make Japanese miso soup.
- ♥ Arame: is a this lacy, wiry sea vegetable which is sweeter and milder in taste than many others
- ♥ Dulse: has a soft, chewy texture and a reddish-brown colour. It is commonly available as a coarse powder or flakes making it easy to shake over food much as you would salt. It is commonly sourced from England and Ireland. Dulse is an excellent source of calcium and potassium - making it a useful addition to any dairy-free diet. Dulse is approximately 22% protein, higher than chickpeas (garbanzo beans), almonds or whole sesame seeds. A handful (about 30g) offers more than 100% RDA of vitamin B6, iron and fluoride, as well as 66% RDA of vitamin B12. Dulse is relatively low in sodium, yet quite high in potassium, phosphorus, manganese, and iodine as well as vitamin A. Dulse is also a highly alkaline vegetable.

Sea vegetables are a good source of iodine for those who do not use conventional table salt (which is fortified with iodine).

Introduction: 8 months

Remember, it is a nutrient dense food – a little goes a long way.

Selection: Many sea vegetables originate in the East and have, as a result, been a topic of ongoing debate and research with regards to heavy metal contamination – especially since the Fukushima incident. It is important to buy organic sea vegetables to ensure you are not exposed to the heavy metals which may be present in sea vegetables which have been sourced from polluted sea waters. Some certified organic sea vegetables have been farmed in a process that's usually referred to as "aquaculture" or "mariculture" and that involves a closely-monitored, contained-water environment for the sea vegetables. Others have been wild-harvested, but are from regions where ocean waters are better protected against contaminants.

Look for sea vegetables that are sold in tightly sealed packages. Avoid those that have evidence of excessive moisture.

Storage:: Sealed glass container ↔ cool, dark place ↔ several years

Preparation/Use:
Many types of sea vegetables require soaking for 5-10 minutes before adding to your dish. It is best to follow the directions on the package. Many of the seaweeds expand up to eight times their original size when soaked. The soak

Glossary of Ingredients

water can be used for soups or to sauté vegetables in.

Sea vegetables can be eaten raw.

Sprinkle flakes into your little one's purées or any other food as a nutritional enhancer or salt replacement. They are a great addition to broths and stews and can be used in the cooking water when preparing any grains to add extra nutrients and flavour.

Nutritional Value:
They are nutritionally unique in their wide variety of minerals – a variety that closely matches that found in human blood and that is simply not found in any other vegetable.

Excellent: iodine, vitamin C, manganese, and vitamin B2

Very Good: vitamins A (in the form of carotenoids) and copper

Good: vitamins B1 and B6, complete protein, pantothenic acid, potassium, iron, zinc, niacin and phosphorus

Additionally: vitamin B12

Sea vegetables have antioxidant, anti-inflammatory, anti-cancer, anticoagulant, antithrombotic, and antiviral benefits.

Sesame Seeds

Sesame seeds are tiny, flat oval seeds with a nutty flavour and a subtle crunch. They come in a variety of different colours, including white, yellow, black and red. Sesame seeds are highly valued for their high content of oil that is very resistant to rancidity. They are also the main ingredients in tahini (sesame seed paste) that is used to make hummus.

Allergen: yes

Sesame seeds can cause a severe allergic reaction in some people. Your little one is at more risk of experiencing an allergic reaction if he/she is under a year old; if there is a family history of food allergy; or, if he/she suffers from atopic dermatitis, or if there is a family history of atopic dermatitis. Research in this area suggests that individuals with food allergy to peanuts, walnuts, hazelnuts, or cashews may also experience an allergic response to sesame seeds.

Introduction: 12 months

Selection: Choose sesame seeds that have no evidence of moisture. Since they have a high oil content and can become rancid, it is preferable to buy the seeds in smaller pre-packaged containers.

Storage:
Unhulled ↦ airtight container ↦ cool, dark place ↦ 6-12 months

Hulled ↦ airtight container ↦ refrigerator or freezer ↦ 1 year

Preparation/Use:
Sesame seeds can be ground in your coffee grinder and added to smoothies or purées. Alternatively, coat fruit and vegetable pieces in them so your little one will be able to get a better grip.

Tahini (or sesame seed paste) can also be added to smoothies or spread on toast.

Nutritional Value:
Excellent: copper

Very good: manganese and protein

Good: calcium, phosphorus, magnesium, iron, zinc, molybdenum, vitamin B1, selenium, and dietary fibre.

Sesame seeds have a cholesterol lowering effect; prevent high blood pressure; provide relief from arthritis; support respiratory health and have some anti-cancer benefits.

They make a useful addition to any dairy-free diet due to their high calcium content (a ¼ cup of sesame seeds provides more calcium than 1 cup of milk) and they are a great source of iron and protein for vegan or vegetarians – and little ones who aren't big meat eaters like Mila.

Sesame Oil

Sesame oil is an edible vegetable oil derived from sesame seeds. It has a strong flavour and a little bit goes a long way. It has a fairly high concentration of inflammatory omega-6 fatty acids, which is another reason to use it sparingly.

Allergen: yes

Sesame seeds can cause a severe allergic reaction in some people. Your little one is at more risk of experiencing an allergic reaction if he/she is under a year old; if there is a family history of food allergy; or, if he/she suffers from atopic dermatitis, or if there is a family history of atopic dermatitis. Research in this area suggests that individuals with food allergy to peanuts, walnuts, hazelnuts, or cashews may also experience an allergic response to sesame seeds.

Introduction: 12 months

Storage:: Sesame oil is exceptionally resistant to rancidity due to the naturally occurring antioxidants. It is not necessary to store it in the fridge.

Use: Light sesame oil has a high smoke point and is suitable for deep-frying, while dark sesame oil (from roasted sesame seeds) has a slightly lower smoke point and is only suitable for stir frying, or sautéing. Sesame oil can of course be drizzled on food after it has been cooked.

Soil

Soil? Yes, soil! While I am not suggesting you add it to tonight's dinner, I do suggest you let your little one eat the handful she puts in her mouth.

Soil is a superfood.

While fermented foods are an excellent source of probiotics (beneficial bacteria), the strains found in organic productive soil are extraordinarily hardy. They can survive heat, shock, and stomach acid, and most importantly they thrive in the environment that makes up the gut. My naturopath recently told me of a new treatment whereby people with chronic digestive issues are being advised to go back to the garden where they lived as a baby and to eat some of the soil from there. You see, your baby's relatively sterile gut is populated with these life forces in the days following birth: from the birth canal, the mother's nipples, the breast milk, and… the environment in which they live – both household dust and the garden soil. It is this initial colony that must survive and thrive for the rest of your little one's life in order to ensure good health.

These days most babies are brought up in overly sterile environments, are not spending enough time getting their hand and feet dirty in good quality soil, and fruits and vegetables are not eaten straight out of the ground – instead they are thoroughly washed to remove pesticides which also washes off the beneficial bacteria. A decrease in exposure to these organisms is being linked to increased rates of asthma and allergies in children. These bacteria are responsible for building a strong immune system and are also known to produce 80 -90% of the body's serotonin – the chemical responsible for mood and social behaviour, appetite and digestion, regular bowel function, sleep, blood clotting, and memory.

An added benefit of your little one eating a bit of soil now and then is the iron and zinc it contains. Since breast milk is designed to be low in iron (as pathogens such as E Coli are known to feed off it) babies are said to need additional iron from around 6 months of age (when their birth supply runs out). This is also the time they are likely to be spending more time on the floor and crawling in the garden. Good quality soil has all the iron and zinc your little one may need to boost his/her intake without needing to get it from the fortified processed foods.

Sorghum Flour (Milo Flour)

Sorghum is an ancient gluten-free cereal grain domesticated in Ethiopia and Sudan. It has long been considered a safe grain alternative for people with celiac disease and gluten insensitivity. It is the fifth most important cereal crop in the world, largely because of its natural drought tolerance and versatility as food, feed and fuel. The sorghum plant is a tall, broad-leafed grass that looks similar to corn. It grows well in dry areas, and can adapt to weather extremes. Sorghum kernels vary in colour from white and pale yellow to deep red, purple, and brown. Its neutral, slightly sweet flavour and light colour make it easily adaptable to a variety of dishes.

Sorghum, which does not have an inedible hull like some other grains, is commonly eaten with all its outer layers, thereby retaining the majority of its nutrients. It can be cooked in the whole grain form similar to rice or barley. Whole grain sorghum takes longer to cook than other grains.

Sorghum flour is produced by grinding the whole sorghum grain kernel. Traditionally this flour has been used create pancakes, fermented and unfermented porridges and flatbreads - such as the jowar roti in India. In the West, it is becoming more common to use sorghum flour in baked goods.

Allergen: no

Introduction: 12 months. Grains require certain digestive enzymes in order to be digested properly. These enzymes are not present in large enough quantities in your little one's immature digestive system until they are a year old – and only really when they are two years old.

Selection: Sorghum flour can be found in many specialty health food stores in the same section as other flours. You might also find it in the gluten-free section, or at ethnic food markets. It may be listed under another name - in India, sorghum flour is referred to as jowar atta.

When buying your sorghum flour make sure there is no moisture in the package.

Storage:
Airtight container ⇢ cool, dark place or fridge ⇢ 2 months

Airtight container ⇢ freezer ⇢ 4 months.

Preparation/Use:
Grain and nut flours have the same anti-nutrients as whole grains and as such should also be soaked to release the phytic acid and enzyme inhibitors. For each recipe using flour, you could soak the flour in the cooking liquid overnight and continue cooking or baking the next day. This may be completely inconvenient and the recipe might have to be adjusted. Where possible make your own flours from soaked and dehydrated whole grains.

It can be added or substituted in any recipe that calls for flour such as cakes, cookies, breads and muffins - although sorghum flour often produces a drier, crumbly final product. Adding extra oil or another fat source and eggs can improve the texture, and adding a leavening agent such as baking powder or baking soda will help the dough rise.

While some gluten free flours, such as rice flour, can add a gritty texture to cookies or bread, sorghum flour has a smoother texture that many people prefer. Add 15% to 20% sorghum flour to your flour mixes to make delicious breads, cakes, and cookies.

Nutritional Value:
Very Good: unsaturated fats, protein, fibre, phosphorus, potassium, calcium, magnesium, copper, iron, thiamin, riboflavin, and vitamin B6 (niacin).

It has more antioxidants than blueberries and pomegranates. In addition, the starch and protein in sorghum take longer than other similar products to digest. This slow digestion is particularly helpful for those with diabetes.

Sorghum has antioxidant and anticancer benefits. It can help control blood sugar levels; boost the immune system; regulate the digestive system; prevent anaemia; provide sustainable energy and promote healthy bone development.

Spanspek (Cantaloupe / Muskmelon)

Spanspek is a round melon with a thick rind covered in a tan-coloured 'netting' – a skin with a raised mosaic-like pattern on it. It has light orange, sweet and juicy flesh surrounding a cavity filled with cream coloured, edible seeds.

Allergen: no

Introduction: 7 months

Selection: A ripe spanspek will feel heavy for its size, have a light floral scent, a tan (not grey or green) coloured rind and yield to gentle pressure on the top (where it was attached to the vine). If your melon is slightly unripe, leave it at room temperature for a couple of days, then place in the fridge.

Although spanspek is listed as one of the EWG's clean 15 foods, they are often contaminated by five of the longest-lasting pesticide chemicals. Dieldrin, a very toxic and carcinogenic insecticide, still gets taken up through the spanspek's roots even though it was banned in 1983 in South Africa (in 1974 in the USA). Finding organic spanspek is advisable.

Storage:
A fully ripe spanspek should be kept in the fridge and for no more than 3 – 4 days.

Preparation/Use:: The risk of bacterial contamination in cut spanspek is significant. As with all melons, the whole, uncut spanspek should be washed with a scrubbing brush and a salt-, vinegar-, or hydrogen peroxide water solution prior to cutting.
Washed spanspek should not be refrigerated - the rind absorbs moisture and this can lead to mould forming. If you are not going to eat the whole fruit, rather remove the entire rind, and store cut melon pieces in a tightly sealed container in the fridge. Do not leave cut spanspek at room temperature for longer than 2 hours as there is a risk of salmonella or E coli contamination.

Cut off the top (stem end, where the vine was attached) of the spanspek and discard - research shows that bacterial contamination is more likely to occur in this spot. Next, scoop out and save the seeds and slice your spanspek in whatever size sections you like. Alternatively, you can scoop out the flesh.

Be sure to wash your hands and utensils thoroughly afterwards.

To prepare the seeds, simply place them in a sieve and rinse under cool running water to remove the pulpy fibres. Shake the sieve to release excess water then place the seeds in a single layer on a cookie sheet and lightly roast them in the oven at 75°C (160-170°F) for 15-20 minutes. By roasting them for a relatively short time at a low temperature you can help minimize damage to their healthy oils. Alternatively, you can dry them in your dehydrator. These are a great addition to smoothies and are a healthy snack when your little one is chewing properly.

Nutritional Value:
Spanspek is a unique fruit in terms of its nutrient diversity (it has over 19 vitamins and minerals). It contains a wide variety of antioxidant and anti-inflammatory phytonutrients.

Excellent: vitamin A (in the form of carotenoids) and vitamin C

Very good: potassium

Good: dietary fibre, vitamins B1, B3 (niacin), B6 and K, folate, magnesium and copper. The seeds are a good source of omega-3 fatty acids.

Spanspek provides anti-inflammatory, anti-anxiety and antioxidant support. It boosts the immune system and hydrates and alkalises the body.

Spinach

Spinach is a nutrient-dense dark green leafy vegetable. It has a delicate texture and a mild slightly sweet, bitter and salty taste which becomes stronger when cooked. It belongs to the same plant family as Swiss Chard and beetroot. There are many different varieties including

Glossary of Ingredients

Savoy, smooth-leaf, semi-Savoy and baby spinach.

Allergen: no

Spinach is high in oxalates and nitrates.

Introduction: 8-12 months

Selection: Spinach is one of the EWG's Dirty Dozen so it is important to buy organic.

Choose spinach that has vibrant deep green leaves and stems with no signs of yellowing. The leaves should not be wilted or bruised. Avoid leaves that have a slimy coating as this is an indication of decay.

Storage:
Fresh, unwashed, raw ⇢ airtight bag ⇢ refrigerator ⇢ 5-7 days

Cooked ⇢ sealed container ⇢ freezer ⇢ 2 months

Cooked spinach does not store well in the fridge.

Preparation/Use:
Soak the spinach in a salt-, vinegar-, or hydrogen peroxide water solution for 20 minutes then rinse under running water.

Boiling is the best way of cooking spinach as this allows some of the oxalates and nitrates to leach out of the vegetable. Only boil for one minute with the lid off the pot.

Baby spinach does not have a high concentration of oxalates and nitrates and can be enjoyed raw by adding it to your vegetable juice or salads.

Nutritional Value:
Excellent: vitamins A (in the form of carotenoids), B2, B6, C, E, and K, manganese, folate, magnesium, iron, copper, calcium, and potassium

Very good: dietary fibre, phosphorus, vitamin B1, zinc, protein, and choline

Good: omega-3 fatty acids, niacin, pantothenic acid, and selenium.

Spinach has an unusual mixture of phytonutrients that makes it a superfood in terms of antioxidant and anti-inflammatory potential. It anti-inflammatory, antioxidant and anti-cancer benefits; and, it helps to build and maintain strong bones and healthy eyes. Raw spinach is a great laxative and maintains a healthy digestive tract.

Spring Onion (Green Onion / Scallion)

Spring onions have hollow green edible leaves (like the common onion) with an under-developed edible root bulb. They are used as a vegetable and can be eaten either raw or cooked. Spring onions have a milder taste than most onions.

Allergen: no

Introduction: 7 months

The concern with spring onions (as with other members of the 'allium' plant family such as onions, shallots, garlic and leeks) is that they may cause gas. This is less likely to happen if they are cooked.

Selection: Choose spring onions that have a crispy stalk, are the size and width of a pencil with well-formed, green leaves. Avoid over-mature, yellow leaves as they have a stronger flavour like that of onions. Avoid those with withered, yellow discoloured or dry tops.

Storage:: Store spring onions in an airtight container in the fridge where they will last for 7 to 10 days.

Preparation/Use:: Soak the spring onions in a salt-, vinegar-, or hydrogen peroxide water solution for 20 minutes then rinse under running water. Trim off the roots and peel off one or two layers of outer thick leaves. Chop into desired sizes. For your little one, spring onions are usually one of many ingredients in a recipe – not served as a stand-alone food.

Nutritional Value:
When eating the leaves and the bulbs, spring onions are a source of vitamins A, B6, C, and K.

Spring onions support the growth, development and maintenance of strong bones. They have antioxidant benefits and support the development of healthy eyes.

Stevia (extract and leaves)

A herb that has been used by South Americans for centuries, stevia is now widely available as a sweetener and sugar substitute. It is extracted from the leaves of the plant species Stevia rebaudiana. It is a member of the sunflower family and grows abundantly throughout South America and other subtropical areas.

Although the leaf itself has sweetness to it, some people experience a bitter after-taste that is somewhat like liquorice. Stevia extract is on average 250 to 300 times sweeter than sugar - but without the calories and no significant effect on glucose levels. Fresh or dried stevia leaves are 30 to 40 times sweeter than sugar.

Stevia is available as a dry powder, tea, as an extract (or liquid), in capsule and pill form.

Allergen: no

Introduction: 10-12 months (use in moderation)

Selection: Take care to find green stevia powder, which

Glossary of Ingredients

is the unprocessed whole form of the stevia leaf unlike the processed white stevia powders and stevia liquids that are popular in supermarkets. Choose stevia that is minimally processed and has no other added ingredients. Brand name stevia products often include things like erythritol and dextrose (both obtained from GMO corn), silica, 'natural flavours (that are anything but natural) and, agave inulin (a highly processed fibre derivative from the blue agave plant).

You can usually find the dried leaves, green leaf powder and pure extract in health shops.

Alternatively, you can purchase a stevia plant and make your own! You can dry and grind the leaves, or steep them in alcohol to make your own extract.

Storage:: Store stevia leaves and extract in a sealed container in cool, dark place and follow the expiry date on the packaging.

Use: Stevia does not work very well in baked goods but it is an excellent sweetener in dressings, smoothies and cold desserts.

Strawberries

Fragrantly sweet, heart-shaped strawberries are the most popular type of berry fruit in the world. They have a bright red flesh with small seeds piercing its surface, and a small, green leafy cap and stem.

Although they have become increasingly available year-round, their peak seasons are spring and summer.

Not only are they delicious, but strawberries are also among the fruits and vegetables ranked highest in health-promoting antioxidants.

Allergen: yes

The most common reaction to strawberries is itching or a rash where the fruit comes into contact with the skin (usually around the mouth). Reactions to strawberries can occasionally be severe and may involve swelling of the throat. Strawberries can also cause hives elsewhere on the body and cause the symptoms of asthma and eczema to worsen. They may also contribute to nappy rash due to the acidity in the fruit.

Introduction: 8 months

Selection: Strawberries are listed by the EWG as one of the Dirty Dozen. It is highly recommended to only buy organic strawberries, or grow your own. They are easy to grow and your little one will have such fun picking them from the garden – Mila is delighted every time she finds a ripe one!

Strawberries do not continue to ripen once they have been picked – so it is important to buy ones that are fully ripe.

Choose berries that are firm, plump, free of mould, and which have a shiny, deep red colour and attached green caps.

Storage:

Unwashed → sealed container → refrigerator → 2-5 days

Washed and towel dried → sealed container → freezer → 1 year

Preparation/Use:

If your strawberries are not organic, soak them in a salt-, vinegar-, or hydrogen peroxide water solution for 20 minutes, rinse under running water and only then cut off the stems and caps (otherwise they will absorb too much moisture during the soaking process). If they are organic, simply rinse them under running water while rubbing gently.

Strawberries are best eaten raw for maximum nutritional benefit. They are an excellent addition to purées and smoothies and make a great finger food when your little one is able to gum foods.

Nutritional Value:

Strawberries provide an outstanding variety of phytonutrients and digestion-aiding enzymes.

Excellent: vitamin C and manganese

Very good: dietary fibre, iodine, and folate

Good: copper, potassium, biotin, phosphorus, magnesium, vitamin B6, and omega-3 fatty acids.

Strawberries have antioxidant-, anti-inflammatory-, cardiovascular-, blood sugar- and anti-cancer benefits. They are helpful in treating inflammatory bowel conditions as well as inflammation-related arthritis.

Recent studies show that when strawberries are consumed with regular sugar, the strawberries were able to decrease the blood sugar elevations caused by the sugar. This could be useful for when your little one has to attend a sugar-laden party!

Sundried Tomatoes

Sun-dried tomatoes are ripe tomatoes that have been dried in the sun. Non-organic sundried tomatoes are usually pre-treated with sulphur dioxide before being placed in the sun in order to improve quality – so be sure to buy organic, or additive-free ones.

After drying, the tomatoes retain their nutritional value.

> Glossary of Ingredients

Sunflower Seeds

Sunflower seeds come from the centre of the beautiful, bright yellow sunflower. The seeds are greyish-green or black and encased in tear-dropped shaped grey or black shells that have black and white stripes.

Allergen: no

Introduction: 12 months

Selection: When buying unshelled seeds, ensure that the shells are firm and not broken or dirty. If you choose shelled seeds, avoid those that are yellowish in colour as they have probably gone rancid.

Storage:
Airtight container ⇢ cool, dark place ⇢ 2-3 months

Airtight container ⇢ fridge/freezer ⇢ 12 months

Preparation/Use:
Seeds contain anti-nutrients: enzyme inhibitors and phytic acid so it is important to prepare them it such a way that reduces the phytic acid, neutralises the enzyme inhibitors and increases the bio-availability of the nutrients.

How to soak seeds

Cover the seeds with warm water and add sea salt. The ratio of seeds to salt should be ½ tablespoon salt for every 2 cups of seeds. Soak for six to eight hours (or overnight), then drain, rinse and dehydrate or roast.

Dehydrate by placing in a warm oven (no warmer than 65°C/150°F) or dehydrator for 12- 24 hours.

Sunflower seeds can be ground in a coffee grinder and sprinkled on vegetables and fruit or added to smoothies.

And what about sunflower oil you may ask? I stay away from vegetable oils such as corn, canola, soybean and sunflower oil due to their overly high concentration on omega-6 fatty acids. Olive oil and coconut oil are, in my opinion, far healthier options.

Nutritional Value:
Excellent: vitamin E

Very good: copper and vitamin B1

Good: manganese, selenium, phosphorus, magnesium, vitamin B6, folate, and niacin.

Additionally: protein, vitamin D, vitamin K, zinc and iron.

Sunflower seeds have powerful anti-inflammatory and anti-oxidant benefits. They have the ability to enhance the immune system and decrease the risk of certain cancers. Their high magnesium content helps build healthy bones, produce energy and lower blood pressure.

Sunshine

Vitamin D is an essential nutrient - it builds bones and muscles, ensures proper hormone development, reduces inflammation, boosts the immune system and protects against cancer (including skin cancer). It is almost impossible to get your vitamin D needs met by food alone. Sunshine is a vital ingredient in you and your little one's daily nourishment!

Like all living things, we need sunshine, and it feels good for a reason. Much as plants harness the sun's rays through photosynthesis, our bodies use sunlight to help the skin produce vitamin D.

Sunshine has been demonized (by the media and western medicine) as a cause of cancer but, much like fat and salt, it is in fact very good for us when consumed wisely and in moderation. UV paranoia and the use of sunscreens (which block vitamin D production) are contributing to an increased incidence of many diseases due to vitamin D deficiency. Vitamin D deficiency is silent and it is deadly – it can lead to cancer, heart disease, high blood pressure, Type I diabetes, multiple sclerosis, osteoporosis and depression. If a pregnant mother is deficient in vitamin D, her child will be born with a deficiency. Infants that are vitamin D deficient at birth can remain deficient for the first several months after birth, which may put them at risk of developing many chronic diseases much later in life.

The best way to optimise vitamin D levels is through safe, sunscreen-free exposure to the sun. Requirements for vitamin D are different according to age, body weight, skin colouration etc. But generally we all need 15 – 30 minutes of unprotected sun exposure two to four times a week – exposing as much of the skin as possible. It is best to be out in the sun (unprotected) before 10 am and after 3pm when the sun's rays are less harsh. After 30 minutes of unprotected time, you will need to apply natural sunscreen, or put a hat and long sleeves on.

Did you know that nutrition can offer safe and effective sun protection? Eating an anti-inflammatory diet high in healthy fats (the building blocks for healthy skin), with lots of fruit and vegetables (high in antioxidants) while avoiding junk food (inflammatory) allows you to spend more time in the sun without burning (sunburn is a type of inflammation).

Carrot juice, when ingested, works from the inside as a natural sunscreen. The orange pigments, powerful anti-oxidants and beta-carotene work on protecting your skin from the inside out by increasing the skin's immunity while protecting and conditioning the skin. So add some to your little one's morning veggie juice in the summer months!

While vitamin D synthesis requires UV light rays, it is just one frequency of (sun)light; there are eight others and each one has its own unique healing power:

♥ The sun's light kills bad bacteria helping to disinfect

457

Glossary of Ingredients

and heal wounds.

- ♥ Sunlight has a beneficial effect on skin disorders, such as psoriasis, acne, eczema and fungal infections of the skin.
- ♥ Sunlight lowers cholesterol. In the absence of sunlight, the opposite happens; substances convert to cholesterol.
- ♥ The sun's rays lower blood pressure.
- ♥ Sunlight penetrates deep into the skin to cleanse the blood and blood vessels.
- ♥ Sunlight increases oxygen content in human blood.
- ♥ It has a whole lot of 'feel-good-factor'!

Note: the body cannot generate vitamin D when sitting behind a glass window, because the UVB rays necessary for vitamin D production are absorbed by glass.

Sweet Corn (Corn / Mielie / Maize)

Sweet corn is a variety of maize with a high sugar content. Sweet corn is the result of a naturally occurring change in the genes of the maize plant. Sweet corn is picked when the fruit is immature (before the kernels dry out) and is prepared and eaten as a vegetable.

Sweet corn is a long cylindrical vegetable that tapers towards one end. It has edible kernels on a central non-edible cob. The kernels are either yellow or white (there are, however, many other colours of maize) and have a deliciously sweet, milky flavour. The corn is wrapped with green paper-like leaves.

The following nutritional information is for corn (maize), not specifically the variety known as sweet corn.

Corn is a very versatile, popular gluten-free food. For some people, corn is a staple food that provides the foundation for tortillas, burritos, polenta, mieliemeal and pap. For others, corn is a snack food that comes in the form of popcorn and corn chips. For your little one – corn-on-the-cob is a great finger food that is particularly useful when he/she is teething!

Allergen: yes

Introduction: 12 months

Selection: Choose corn that is in the refrigerated section of the supermarket or displayed in the shade at a farmer's market as it is susceptible to microbial contamination when stored in warm temperatures. Look for corn with husks that are fresh, green and not dried out. The leaves should wrap the ear tightly. The kernels should be plump and tightly arranged in rows.

It is vitally important to buy certified organic, non-GMO corn (and corn products)! The majority of all corn grown in South Africa (and America) is genetically modified in two different ways. Not only have the genes of the plant been altered with foreign genes - bacteria has been introduced into the plant's DNA - but GMO crops are also sprayed with significantly more pesticides.

There are genetically modified varieties of sweet corn on the market too, although these seem to have been less successful than the GMO maize/corn and, as a result, may not be as prevalent.

Storage:
Airtight container ⇢ refrigerator ⇢ 3 days. It is best to leave the husk on the corn, as this will protect its flavour.

Blanched, corn on the cob ⇢ airtight container ⇢ freezer ⇢ 1 year.

Blanched corn kernels ⇢ airtight container ⇢ freezer ⇢ 2-3 months

Preparation/Use:
Remove the husks from the corn and soak the cobs in a salt-, vinegar-, or hydrogen peroxide water solution for 20 minutes then rinse under running water..

Place the cob in boiling water for 5 – 15 minutes or until the kernels are bright yellow and you can smell the sweet corn smell!

Allow to cool, then cut the kernels off the cob to serve as a finger food. Alternatively, (if your little one is still teething and gumming food), slice only the very outer layer of kernel skin off, leaving the rest of the kernel attached to the cob. This will allow you little one access to the fleshy part of the kernel. Smear the cob with ghee, sprinkle with salt, and serve. Expect your little one to be kept busy for quite a while!

Nutritional Value:
Corn is not a nutrient-dense food but it does contain phytonutrients and is a good source of pantothenic acid, phosphorus, niacin, dietary fibre, manganese, and vitamin B6. It is also a source of many B-complex vitamins and protein.

Corn has antioxidant, digestive and blood sugar benefits.

Sweet Potato

Sweet potatoes are a root vegetable that belong to an entirely different food family than the common potato They considered one of the healthiest vegetables. There are about 400 different varieties. The skin and flesh of the sweet potato may be white, cream, yellow, orange, pink, or deep purple The although cream and orange flesh are the most common. Sweet potatoes can be shaped like a potato - short and oval - or longer with tapered ends.

Allergen: no

Introduction: 6 months (ideal first food)

Selection: Choose sweet potatoes that are firm and do not have any cracks, bruises or soft spots.

Storage:
Whole, uncooked ·· uncovered ·· cool, dark place ·· 10-14 days

Cooked ·· sealed container ·· refrigerator ·· 7 days

Cooked ·· sealed container ·· freezer ·· 4-6 months

Preparation/Use:
If you purchase organically grown sweet potatoes, you do not need to peel them. If you buy conventionally grown ones, you should peel them since the skin is sometimes treated with dye or wax. You can peel them after cooking.

As the flesh of sweet potatoes will darken upon contact with the air, you should cook them immediately after peeling and/or cutting them. If this is not possible, to prevent oxidation, keep them submerged in water until you are ready to cook them.

To cook: cut them into thick slices and steam for 7 minutes - this not only brings out their great flavour but helps to maximize their **Nutritional Value:**. You can add cinnamon, nutmeg, and/or cloves for extra flavour and nutrition. Alternatively, you can bake them at 200°C (400°F) for 45 minutes – wash, poke holes in the skin, then bake.

Nutritional Value:
Excellent: vitamin A (in the form of beta-carotene)

Very good: vitamin C and manganese

Good: copper, dietary fibre, niacin, vitamin B5, and potassium

Tahini

Tahini is a paste made from ground sesame seeds. It is extremely versatile and can be used in cooking sweet and savoury dishes. It has an earthy, nutty flavour.

Allergen: yes

Sesame seeds (and therefore tahini) can cause a severe allergic reaction in some people. Your little one is at more risk of experiencing an allergic reaction if he/she is under a year old; if there is a family history of food allergy; or, if he/she suffers from atopic dermatitis, or if there is a family history of atopic dermatitis. Research in this area suggests that individuals with food allergy to peanuts, walnuts, hazelnuts, or cashews may also experience allergic response to sesame seeds.

Introduction: 12 months

Storage:: Tahini must be stored in the fridge once opened where it will last for up to 5 months.

Use
Besides being one of the main ingredients in hummus, you can use tahini to make Mila's Meals chocolate spread, Mila's Meals chickpea fudge, salad dressing or simply add it to purées and smoothies.

Nutritional Value:
Tahini is a nutritionally dense food and a great way to boost the nutrients in any of your little one's dishes.

Excellent: calcium and protein

Very good: healthy unsaturated fat, fibre, vitamin E, vitamins B1, B2, B3, B5, B15, phosphorus, magnesium, potassium, copper and iron

Good: folate and Methionine, which aids in liver detoxification.

The nutrients in tahini promote healthy cell growth and prevent anaemia as well as having anti-inflammatory and antioxidant benefits.

It makes a useful addition to any dairy-free diet due to its high calcium content and its a great source of iron and protein for vegans or vegetarians – and little ones who are not big meat eaters like Mila.

Tamari

Tamari is a Japanese form of soy sauce, traditionally made as a by-product of miso paste. It is a thicker, darker, less salty, fermented soy sauce that contains less wheat than conventional soy sauce (if any) - be sure to check it says "gluten-free". It is used to add a full, savoury, umami flavour to a meal.

Allergen: yes

Introduction: 12 months

Selection: You can find tamari in most health food shops and Asian markets. Be sure to read the label to ensure that it is wheat-free and that it doesn't contain any additives, such as MSG. Look for the phrase "contains no artificial colours or flavours" on the label, as well as the phrase "naturally brewed."

Since soybeans are one of the most common GMO crops, it is very important to choose organic tamari.

Storage:: Unopened tamari can be kept in a cool, dark place. Once the bottle is opened, it should be stored in the fridge.

Glossary of Ingredients

Nutritional Value:
Tamari contains many different types of antioxidants. It is also a very good source of the amino acid tryptophan, a good source of vitamin B3 (niacin) and manganese and protein.

Tamari has antioxidant and anti-inflammatory benefits. It can boost the immune system.

Tangerine (Naartjie / Satsuma)

See Naartjie.

Tapioca Flour

The cassava (or manioc) plant is native to Brazil, but is now grown in tropical regions around the world. It produces edible green leaves and large, starch-rich tubers. Tapioca flour (also known as tapioca starch) is made from these roots. Some varieties of cassava contain lethal amounts of cyanide that must be cooked out, leaving a dry and nutritious flour. When that flour is further processed into a pure starch, the result is tapioca. It is a slightly sweet, light, soft, fine white flour.

Tapioca flour is an excellent addition to any gluten-free kitchen, but as with other gluten-free flours it must form part of a combination of flours when baking.

Tapioca is not a nutritionally dense food – it predominantly consists of carbohydrates. It is low in saturated fat, protein and sodium; has no significant essential vitamins or dietary minerals and no dietary fibre.

Allergen: no

Introduction: 7 months

Selection: Genetically modified strains of cassava are under development so it would be wise to buy only organic tapioca flour.

Storage:: Tapioca flour is a fairly resilient flour. It can be stored at room temperature in a sealed container.

Use: Tapioca flour helps bind gluten free recipes; improves the texture of baked goods; adds crispness to crusts and chew to baked goods. Tapioca flour is an extremely smooth flour, and makes for a great thickener in sauces, pies and soups since it never discolours and contains no discernible taste or smell. It thickens at a lower temperature than other starches making it a good choice for correcting sauces that are too thin at the last moment. It also freezes and thaws better than corn-starch making it a better choice for pies and pastries that are going to be frozen and then eaten later.

It can also be used to replace corn starch (use 2 T. tapioca flour for each 1 T. corn-starch)

Thyme

Thyme is a delicate looking herb that is indigenous to the Mediterranean. The elliptical-shaped leaves are curled and very small. The upper leaf is green-grey in colour on top, with a whitish colour underneath. It has a strong fragrance and a subtle, slightly minty flavour.

Allergen: no

Introduction: 6 months

Selection: Whenever possible, choose fresh thyme over the dried form of the herb since it has a far better flavour. The leaves of fresh thyme should be a vibrant green-grey in colour. They should be free from dark spots or yellowing.

If you buy dried thyme, make sure it has not been irradiated (organic dried herbs will not be irradiated).

Storage:
Fresh thyme ⇢ wrapped in damp paper towel in a plastic bag ⇢ refrigerator ⇢ 10-14 days

Dried thyme ⇢ sealed glass container ⇢ cool, dark place ⇢ 6 months

Preparation/Use:
Soak the thyme in a salt-, vinegar-, or hydrogen peroxide water solution for 20 minutes then rinse under running water.

Thyme can be added to purées, soups, stews and scrambled eggs. Its flavour complements vegetable-, chicken- and fish dishes particularly well. It should be added towards the end of cooking so it can retain its taste, colour and nutritional value.

As with other herbs, you can make a powerful and very healing medicinal tea from the leaves – place some fresh thyme into boiling water, steep for at least 10 minutes, strain, and sip throughout the day. Honey or lemon can be added.

Nutritional Value:
Excellent: vitamin C

Very good: vitamin A (in the form of pro-vitamin A carotenoid phytonutrients)

Good: iron, manganese, copper, and fibre.

Thyme has a long history of use in natural medicine in connection with chest and respiratory problems including coughs, bronchitis, and chest congestion. Thyme has antiseptic, antiviral, antibacterial and carminative benefits.

Tomato

Tomato is a very popular and versatile food that comes in thousands of different shapes, sizes, flavours and colours. There are small cherry-, bright yellow-, pear-shaped-, green and even a black striped tomato. Although most people consider the tomato to be a vegetable, it is actually a (not-so-sweet) fruit. They have a subtle sweetness and a slightly bitter and acidic taste.

Allergen: yes

Can cause a reaction in people with a latex allergy as well as those sensitive to vegetables of the nightshade family.

Introduction: 10-12 months

Tomatoes can be quite acidic and harsh on your little one's tummy. They can cause nappy rashes and can aggravate reflux, asthma and eczema. Cooked tomatoes will be less acidic.

Selection: Choose tomatoes that have deep, rich colours and smooth skins free from wrinkles, cracks or bruises. Ripe tomatoes will yield to slight pressure and will have a noticeably sweet fragrance.

Cherry tomatoes are one of the EWG's Dirty Dozen so purchasing organic is important.

Since they are so easy to grow, so why not give that a try? One plant keeps producing fruit for a while and will lead to many more as they self-seed very easily. Mila loves picking the bright red fruits from our plant!

Please avoid canned tomatoes - and all canned food! Food cans are lined in order to prevent the metallic taste from the cans transferring to the food. These liners usually contain Bisphenol A (BPA) - a xenoestrogen (it mimics natural oestrogen in the body) and a toxic endocrine disrupting chemical.

If you buy tomato sauce, choose an organic brand (with no added sugars, salts and preservatives) that is packaged in glass.

Storage:
Tomatoes will continue to ripen after picking so if your tomatoes are under-ripe, store them at room temperature, out of direct sunlight until they are fully ripe.

Ripe tomatoes, whole, uncooked ↦ uncovered ↦ cool, dark place ↦ 1 week

Ripe tomatoes, whole, uncooked ↦ sealed bag ↦ refrigerator ↦ 2 weeks

Cooked tomatoes ↦ sealed container ↦ refrigerator ↦ 5 days

Cooked tomatoes ↦ sealed container ↦ freezer ↦ 6 months

Preparation/Use:
Soak the tomatoes in a salt-, vinegar-, or hydrogen peroxide water solution for 20 minutes then rinse under running water.

Tomatoes can be eaten raw or cooked. Cooking tomatoes reduces their acidic and bitter qualities, brings out their sweetness and increases the bio-availability and anti-oxidant activity of the tomatoes nutrients. It is best to steam, sauté or roast them. Adding a healthy fat to them when cooking, or eating them increases the bio-availability of the nutrients.

Some recipes may call for the skin and seeds to be removed – but remember these are the most nutrient-dense part of the fruit. To remove the skin of a tomato, simply drop them into a bowl of boiling hot water and leave them for 10 minutes. Rinse under cold water and peel away the skin. To remove the seeds, cut the tomato in half and scoop the seeds out with a spoon.

Perhaps one of the best (and most enjoyable) ways of introducing tomato to your little one is in the form of homemade ketchup or tomato sauce.

Nutritional Value:
Excellent: vitamins C and K, biotin and molybdenum

Very Good: copper, potassium, manganese, dietary fibre, vitamins A (in the form of beta-carotene), B6 and E, folate, niacin, and phosphorus

Good: chromium, pantothenic acid, protein, choline, zinc, and iron.

Tomatoes provide a unique and vast variety of phytonutrients but, most significantly, they are an amazing source of lycopene - a powerful anti-oxidant. This is the phytonutrient that gives fruits and vegetables like tomatoes and watermelon a pink or red colour.

Tomatoes provide heart and bone support and have anti-cancer benefits.

Turmeric

Turmeric comes from the edible underground root of the Curcuma longa plant. It is native to Indonesia and southern India, where it has been harvested for more than 5,000 years. It resembles ginger and has a tough brown skin and a deep orange flesh. Turmeric has a peppery, warm, slightly bitter flavour and a mild fragrance. It is best known as an ingredient in curry, but it is also used to add a bright yellow colour to various other foods (such as mustard sauce). Once the root is harvested, it is boiled, dried, and ground to prepare distinctive bright yellow spice powder.

Turmeric has been used throughout history as an ingredient,

healing remedy and textile dye (due to its bright yellow-orange colour). Long known as a powerful medicine in China and India, it is currently receiving a lot of attention in the western world for its healing abilities. It is now sold in capsule form to be taken as you would any other supplement! The active healing agent in turmeric is curcumin.

Allergen: no

Introduction: 6 months

Selection: Turmeric can be found whole and raw or as a ready-ground spice.

Always buy spices that have not been irradiated.

When buying fresh turmeric, look for roots that are firm and avoid soft, dried, or shrivelled ones.

Storage:
Fresh turmeric ↔ refrigerator ↔ plastic bag or airtight container ↔ 1-2 weeks

Fresh turmeric ↔ freezer ↔ plastic bag or airtight container ↔ 6 months

Dried turmeric ↔ airtight, glass container ↔ cool dark place ↔ 6 months

Use:
Be careful when cooking with turmeric – it will stain whatever it touches!

Turmeric is a necessary ingredient of curry powder. It is used extensively in Indian and Southeast Asian cooking. Turmeric is also added to mustard blends and relishes. It can be used to provide a bright yellow colour to any meal – or play dough!

Do to its many healing properties, I sneak some into Mila's food whenever possible.

An excellent way to include it in your little one's (or your) diet is by making Golden Milk:

Place 3 cups coconut milk, 1 t. ground turmeric, 1 T. coconut oil and a pinch of pepper into a saucepan and heat for 5 minutes until hot but not boiling. Stir in 1 t. raw honey/maple syrup, cool and serve. A far healthier alternative to conventional hot chocolate!

Nutritional Value:
Excellent: iron and manganese

Good: vitamins B6 and C, dietary fibre, potassium and magnesium

Turmeric is a powerful anti-inflammatory and anti-oxidant and as such is a useful remedy for flatulence, jaundice, menstrual difficulties, toothache, bruises, chest pain, IBS, colic, arthritis, cancer prevention and inhibiting cancer cell growth. It can help detoxify the liver, improve digestion of fats, decrease congestion and improve skin conditions such as eczema, psoriasis and acne.

Vanilla (pods, essence and powder)

The fragrant vanilla beans are the fruits of a tropical climbing orchid – the only fruit-bearing orchid. Unripe vanilla pods are harvested, blanched briefly in boiling water, sweated and sundried until they turn dark-brown and wrinkled.

Allergen: no

Introduction: 6 months (in its natural form)

Selection: Vanilla can be purchased as an extract, a whole pod, or in powder form.

When buying vanilla essence, it is important to find one that is alcohol-, sugar-, colouring-, flavouring- and preservative-free – please check the labels. A far healthier (and more flavourful) option to to buy whole vanilla pods and scrape the seeds directly from them. Another pure form of vanilla is vanilla powder which is made from ground vanilla beans – only! It does not have alcohol, sugar, preservatives, colouring or artificial flavours.

Storage:
Vanilla beans ↔ airtight, glass container ↔ cool, dark place ↔ 2 years

Vanilla powder ↔ airtight, glass container ↔ cool, dark place ↔ 1 year

Vanilla essence ↔ sealed, glass container ↔ cool, dark place ↔ 3 years

Nutritional Value:
Vanilla extract and powder contain small amounts of B-complex groups of vitamins such as niacin, pantothenic acid, thiamin, riboflavin and vitamin B-6. It also contains small traces of minerals such as calcium, magnesium, potassium, manganese, iron and zinc.

Vanilla has antioxidant, anti-depressant and anti-inflammatory properties.

Watermelon

Watermelon is a fruit native to Southern Africa. A watermelon can be can be round, oblong, or spherical in shape and have a smooth hard rind (usually green with dark green stripes or yellow spots) and a juicy, sweet interior flesh with many seeds. While the common variety has a pink to red flesh, there are others that feature orange, yellow, or white flesh. They are in season from spring to autumn. Watermelon has an extremely high water content giving its flesh a juicy and thirst-quenching texture while still being subtly crunchy.

A special note on seedless watermelons: seedless watermelons are not the result of genetic engineering. Seedless watermelons are the result of hybridisation. Seedless watermelons will typically appear to contain some white seeds even though they are labelled as seedless. These white seeds are not actually seeds, but only empty seed coats.

Allergen: no

Introduction: 6 months

Selection: While watermelons are not on the EWG's Dirty Dozen list, it has been reported that growers in China use a synthetic growth stimulator in their cultivation. In order to avoid possible exposure to this, check where the watermelon has been grown or purchase organic ones.

A fully ripened watermelon will feel heavy for its size and have a ground spot (the side that was resting on the ground while it was growing) that has turned creamy yellow in colour.

Storage:
Uncut, whole ↦ cool, dark place ↦ 3 weeks

Cut ↦ sealed container ↦ refrigerator ↦ 1 week

Preparation/Use:
Wash the uncut watermelon well with a salt-, vinegar-, or hydrogen peroxide water solution – especially if you plan on eating or juicing the rind. The flesh can be sliced, cubed, or scooped into balls.

It is important to note that the entire watermelon is edible and nutritious! Try adding the rind to your little one's vegetable juices and the seeds to his/her juices or smoothies. The rind can also be pickled (fermented) and the seeds can be roasted and eaten as a snack.

Nutritional Value:
Watermelon a nutrient-dense food with a high lycopene content and significant amounts of the amino acid citrulline.

Excellent: lycopene

Very Good: vitamin C.

Good: pantothenic acid, copper, biotin, potassium, vitamins A (in the form of carotenoids), B1, and B6 and magnesium.

The watermelon seeds contain magnesium, iron, zinc, protein, monounsaturated and polyunsaturated fatty acids and fibre while the rind is a good source of chlorophyll.

Watermelons provide anti-inflammatory and anti-oxidant support and are an excellent hydrating food.

Whey

The information below relates to whey from goat's milk kefir.

Remember the nursery rhyme about little Miss Muffet eating her curds and whey? "Little Miss Muffet sat on her tuffet eating her curds and whey…". I sang this song many times, but it was not until I began my traditional and whole foods journey that I discovered what whey actually is!

Many people have heard of whey as a protein powder supplement, however the original whey is something quite different.

Whey is the tart, golden liquid remaining after milk has been curdled and strained. Milk is curdled during the cheese, yoghurt or kefir making process. Sweet whey is a natural by-product of the cheese making process. You can make your own 'sour whey' by straining yoghurt or kefir. Liquid whey was known to the founding fathers of medicine as "healing water." In fact, Hippocrates frequently recommended whey to his patients.

Whey from fermented milk (such as that made from kefir or yoghurt) is virtually lactose-free as the cultures digest the lactose during the fermentation process.

Hypoallergenic: According to Dr. Thomas Cooper goat's whey can be used as a hypo**Allergen**ic protein substitute for children and adults who are allergic to cow's milk. Dr. Cooper notes that over 90 percent of children who have an allergy to cow's milk do not show allergy symptoms when using goat's whey. For people who cannot tolerate cow's milk, goat's whey can be a good way to attain the benefits of drinking milk without the symptoms.

Introduction: 8 months

Storage:: Airtight, glass jar ↦ refrigerator ↦ 6 months

Preparation/Use:
To make your own whey is so simple:

Line a sieve with cheesecloth or a coffee filter and place over a bowl. Pour in the kefir/yoghurt. Cover and allow to stand over night. In the morning you will have kefir/yoghurt cheese in the strainer, and whey in the bowl.

Whey can be added to any purée or smoothie for a nutrient boost. It can also be used for fermenting fruit and vegetables or when soaking your nuts, seeds, legumes and grains.

Nutritional Value:
Excellent: probiotics

Very Good: calcium and phosphorus

Good: B vitamins, potassium, zinc and selenium.

Whey has anti-oxidant-, antiseptic- and immune-boosting benefits. It is a complete protein that is

Glossary of Ingredients

easy digested and assimilated by the body. Whey will assist the kidneys and liver in the elimination of toxins. The probiotics in whey aid digestion and assimilation of nutrients and support the immune system.

"Whey is the liquid gold essence of milk that supports our immune system and maintains our protective flora throughout life. This long-forgotten, valuable food should again be made part of our regular diet for good colon health."

- *Nourishing Traditions. Sally Fallon*

Xylitol

Xylitol is a sugar alcohol found naturally in many fruit and vegetables and is produced in small amounts by the human body. The xylitol you find in the shops is a processed sugar – it is just as different to the naturally occurring xylitol as synthetic vitamins are to naturally occurring vitamins in foods.

Xylitol has the same sweetness as sugar but a lower glycaemic index and has therefore become a popular sweetener in food and health products.

But let's look at how is it created…

While xylitol can be sourced from xylan found in the fibres of birch and beech trees, rice, oat, wheat and cotton husks, the main source of xylitol for commercial use is corn cobs – and there is a high chance these are genetically modified. Commercially available xylitol is produced by the industrialised process of sugar hydrogenation. In order to hydrogenate anything, a catalyst is needed, and in the case of xylitol, Raney nickel is used - a powdered nickel-aluminium alloy. Once the xylitol is extracted and processed, you are left with a white, crystalline powder that looks like sugar.

The general consensus is that xylitol can be good for dental health – but that only supports using it as an ingredient in your toothpaste, not so much your food!

Xylitol can have unfavourable effects on the digestive tract especially when eaten in large quantities (causing cramps and diarrhoea). Children (being smaller and with underdeveloped systems) will obviously be much more sensitive to xylitol's effects.

Those who suffer from seizures of any kind should stay away from xylitol as it has been known to increase the frequency of epileptic attacks.

Bottom line: xylitol is a highly processed sugar; it is not a whole food (like honey, maple syrup or stevia); and, it is far from natural. So then, you may be wondering why I have included it in this book?

I have only used xylitol in a couple of recipes – ice-cream and cake icing. Both these items will not form part of your little one's regular diet – treats if you wish. In the case of ice-cream - I actually give it to Mila quite regularly – I use honey and I add kefir, so it becomes a source of probiotics. The xylitol option is for people like her granny (Ouma Miemie) who really does not like the taste of honey!

Special warning: Xylitol is Highly Toxic to Dogs. So if you own a dog, then keep xylitol out of reach (or out of your house altogether). If you believe your dog accidentally ate xylitol, take it to the vet immediately.

Introduction: It is not a common **Allergen** so technically you could introduce it when you start solids. However, for all the reasons mentioned above, it is best left as late as possible and then only in treats.

Selection: If you can, buy xylitol that has not been made from corn.

Storage:: Store xylitol in a sealed container in a cool, dark place.

Yoghurt

Yoghurt is a dairy item that I included in Mila's diet in the early days as she was not strictly dairy intolerant. And oh my goodness how she loved it! I say 'was not strictly dairy intolerant' because now that she is 3 years old she has been taken off all forms of dairy – after struggling with constant colds and a snotty nose for much of this winter, removing any form of dairy has made a remarkable difference.

Yoghurt can be made from either animal or plant foods. Animal-based yoghurt is referred to as 'dairy' yoghurt and plant-based yoghurt as 'non-dairy' yoghurt. Dairy yoghurt can be made from cow's milk, sheep's milk, and goat's milk. Soymilk and coconut milk yogurt are popular non-dairy yoghurts (although I do not advocate the use of any soy products due to it being a GMO crop), and I recently saw a pea yoghurt! Non-dairy yogurt tends to have less protein than dairy yogurt but contain more fibre. Live bacterial cultures can be present in equivalent amounts in both dairy and non-dairy yogurt, depending on the fermentation and production process used by the manufacturer.

Making yoghurt is a fairly simple process involving nothing more than milk, heat, and what is called a 'starter culture'. Starter cultures are lactic acid bacteria's (LAB) and often specifically include Lactobacillus bulgaricus, Bifidobacterium and Streptococcus thermophiles. After the milk is heated to a temperature of approximately 80°C (180°F) and then allowed to cooled to approximately 45°C (110°F), the starter culture is added. The mixture is kept at the same constant temperature for another three to five hours to allow fermentation to occur. The yoghurt is then refrigerated and ready for eating.

Yoghurt is easier to digest than milk since much of the lactose (as well as the milk proteins) are digested during the fermenting (or culturing) process.

Allergen: yes (if made from dairy)

Introduction: 8 months

Selection: Choose grass-fed, organic, plain full-fat yoghurt. Read the label to make sure it is free from sugar, preservatives, flavourings or any other added nasties – the only additives that should be in there are the probiotics or live cultures.

Storage:: Yoghurt must always be kept in the fridge. Follow the expiration date on the package.

Preparation/Use:: You can add your own flavours to plain yoghurt – blend in some fruit, vanilla powder, superfood powders, honey and/or maple syrup.
It is a fairly simple process to make your own yoghurt from scratch too!

Zucchini

See Baby Marrows.

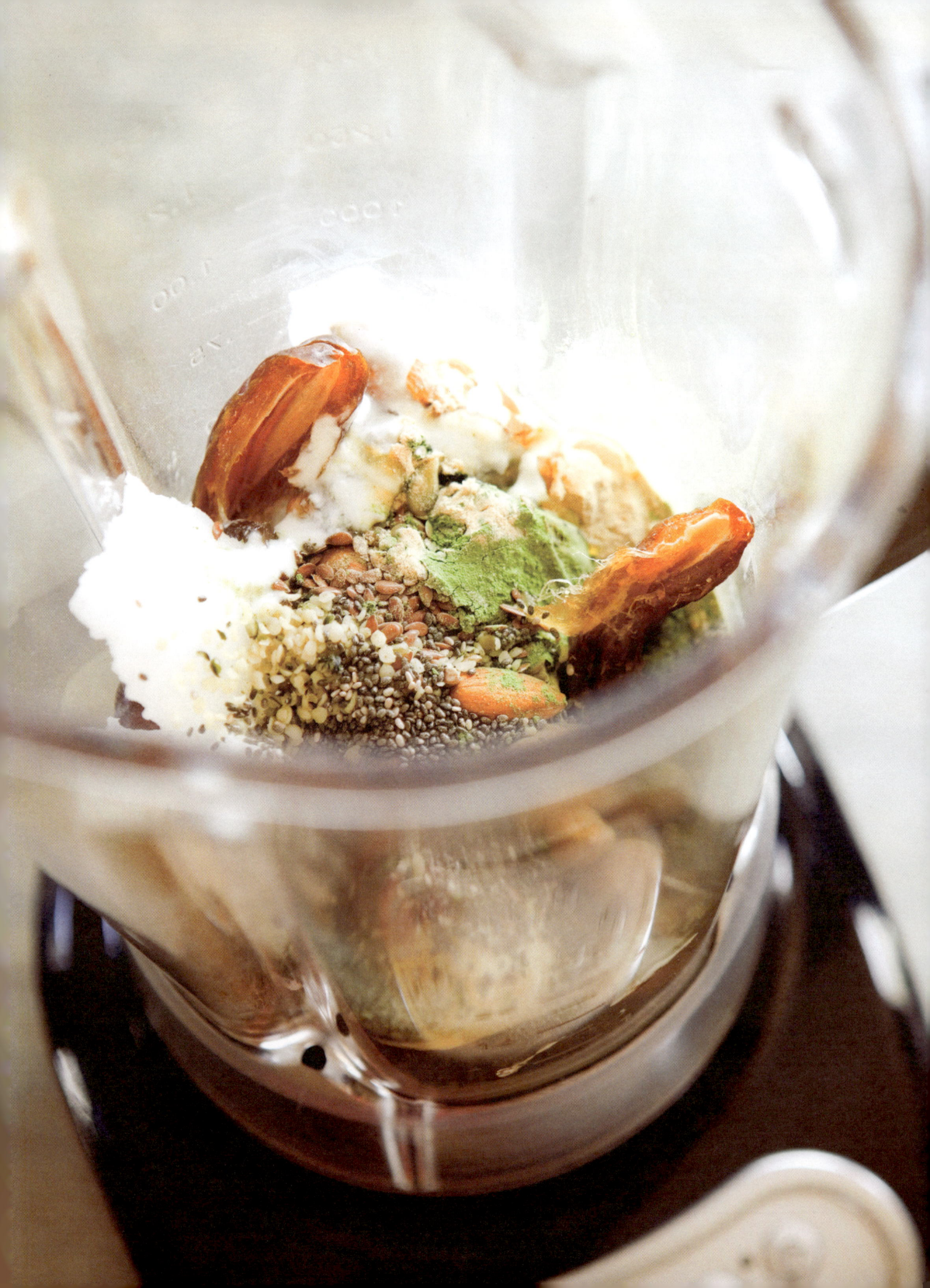

Equipment

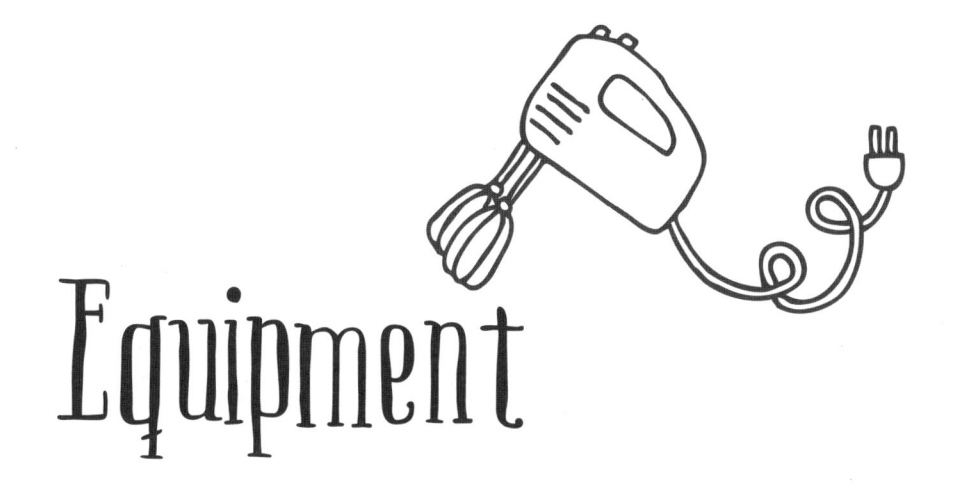

Equipment

The Essentials

Besides the usual forks, spoons, sharp knives, chopping boards, pots and pans that any kitchen would have, you will need the following for preparing baby food:

- **VEGETABLE SCRUBBING BRUSH**
- **VEGETABLE / POTATO PEELER**
- **COFFEE GRINDER:** Useful for grinding grains for porridge as well as seeds, spices etc.
- **STEAMER:** An electric steamer is great as you can set the timer and walk away! There were too many times in the early days when I still had mushy 'mommy-brain' when I put something on the stove to boil, then Mila needed a nappy change or something, and half an hour later the smoke from my kitchen reminded me I had been cooking! Alternatively, a colander or a sieve suspended over a pot of boiling water works well. Perhaps set an egg timer or an alarm clock as a reminder!
- **SLOW COOKER:** I do not know where I would be without my slow cooker! It really is an essential for many reasons, but as a new mom with limited time and energy, a slow cooker can make a really wholesome and highly nutritious one-pot meal for the whole family with very little time invested on your part. I love being able to do the prep in the morning and then having a meal ready to eat in the evening. It even cooks for you while you are sleeping! You can also put grains in before you go to bed and have warm ready-to-eat porridge in the morning. When it comes to making healing broths which need to cook for 24 - 48 hours, it is indispensable.
- **SIEVE:** A metal or plastic sieve for pushing baby food through to purée small to medium quantities in a hassle-free way.
- **FOOD PROCESSOR, MINI-BLENDER OR HAND-HELD BLENDER:** For processing baby food and making smoothies - I have both a large magi-mix (which really became useful after the purée stage) and a mini-processor which was ideal for purées.
- **PLASTIC OR GLASS STORAGE CONTAINERS:** Food safe, BPA-free re-usable plastic containers or ideally, glass containers for storing food. It's a great idea to start saving any glass jars you have left over once the honey or other foods are finished. You can freeze food in these glass jars – as long as there is a gap between the food and the lid to allow for expansion.
- **ICE TRAYS:** Ice trays or specially designed baby food freezing trays are a must have. Food can be frozen into cubes and defrosted and used as meals.
- **ZIPLOC BAGS:** You can transfer the frozen blocks into Ziploc bags - this allows you to re-use the ice trays reducing the need to buy too many.
- **ICE LOLLY MOULDS:** Ice lollies are a great way to soothe teething pain and to get extra nutrients into your little one (if you freeze freshly made fruit and vegetable juices or smoothies).

The oh-so-nice-to-haves!

These items are quite pricey – but I see it as an investment in good health. Perhaps buy them gradually or ask friends to club together for your birthday present.

- ♥ **JUICER:** I was fortunate enough to receive a juicer as a wedding present. It was a centrifugal juicer which produces juice by using a cutting blade to first chop up the produce and then spin the produce at a very high speed. These juicers are the most affordable ones, but they are less efficient at extracting juice so you end up using a lot of produce to make one glass of juice. They also create heat and friction that can oxidize the fresh juice, degrading the taste as well as compromising the quality of nutrients.

  A couple Christmases ago I received my dream machine… An Oscar juicer! I cannot recommend this piece of equipment highly enough! An Oscar juicer is a masticating juicer which crunches the fruit or veggies into a pulp at slow speed, releasing juice in the process. It produces a high juice yield and a very dry pulp – so less wastage, and less produce used to make that same one glass of juice. It also produces little-to-no-heat and thus minimises oxidation. These types of juicers are pricey though! But with a 20-year guarantee, I'm pretty comfortable that I will not have to replace it anytime soon. It can be used to make other things besides juices including purées, nut butters and pasta. Mila and I are having great fun making our own noodles at the moment!

- ♥ **DEHYDRATOR:** this is a real 'nice-to-have' as an oven can be used to similar effect. The benefits of a dehydrator are that: you can set it to very low temperatures which remain accurate; air is efficiently circulated; your oven is not preoccupied for long periods of time when you may need to cook something else; and, dehydrators use less electricity than an oven would for the long drying times required to dehydrate food.

  I LOVE my dehydrator – even though I am not a raw foodie. It has been so useful in making Mila's food – she is a 'pick'" eater in the sense that since graduating from purées, she has refused to eat anything that looks like a vegetable – unless its dehydrated! I will never forget the looks on other mom's faces when Mila happily ate a jar of dehydrated broccoli chips while their kids ate ice cream! Kale chips, beetroot chips, butternut chips soon followed. Now that she's three years old, Mila gets most of her veggies in in the form of 'fruit' leather! Yes, there is fruit in it, but this sneaky mama also adds beetroot, sweet potato and butternut – not to mention a variety of superfood powders!

  The list of delicious (and nutritious) foods you can make in a dehydrator is endless – and they are generally the foods that you would otherwise buy in processed form, loaded with additives, from the supermarket. Things like muesli, crackers, oat bars, dried fruit and fruit leather.

  Since dehydrators are so pricey, and it is not something you generally use everyday, an idea might be for you and some friends to buy one together. They are portable – so each of you could get a once weekly turn to use it.

- ♥ **ICE-CREAM MACHINE:** this definitely is not an essential as a blender or some elbow grease can make a decent ice-cream. But the machines aren't too expensive, they save you a lot of effort and make really smooth and creamy ice-creams.

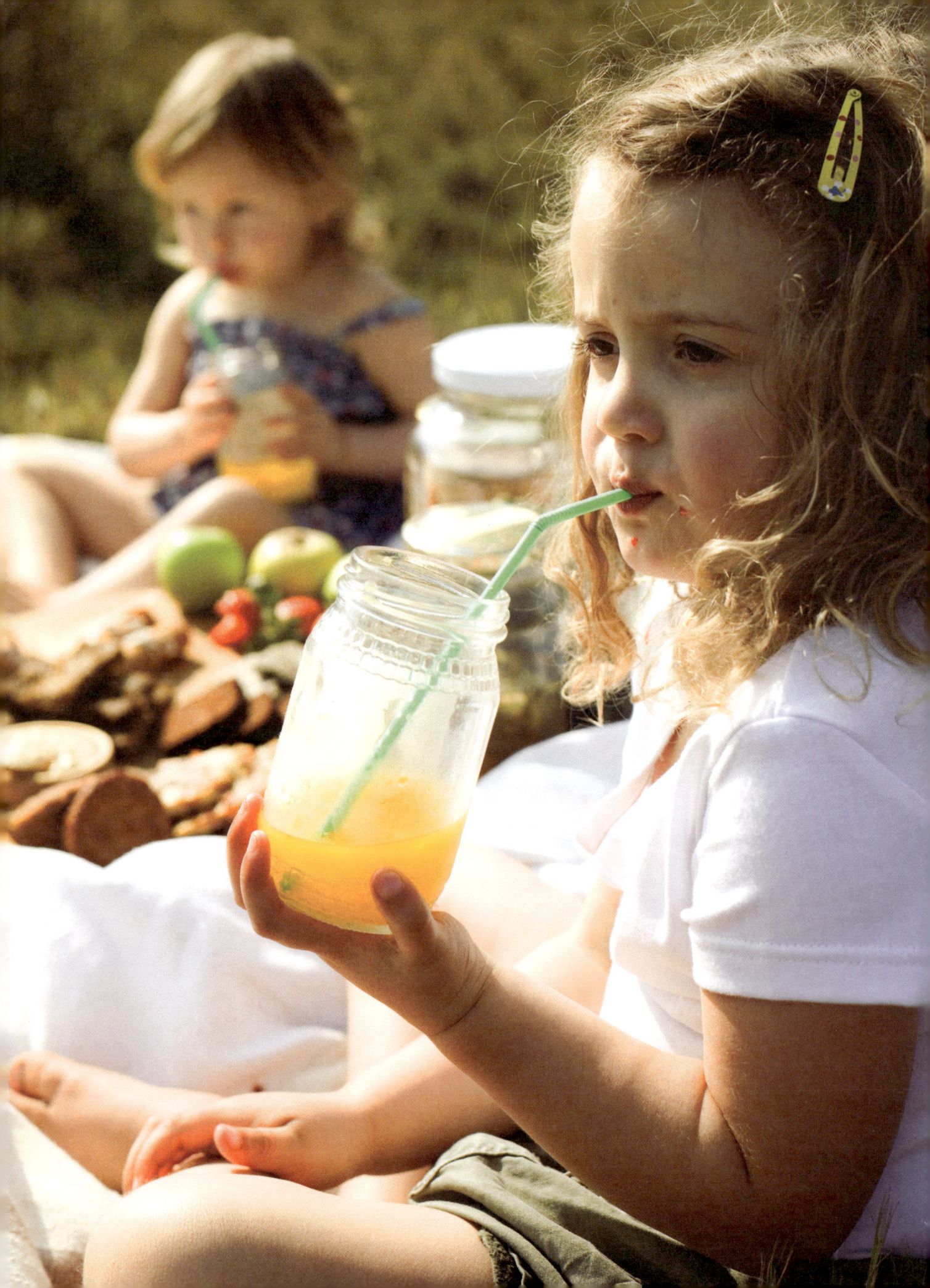

Additional Info:

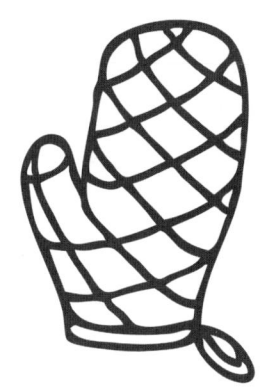

Conversion Charts, Say Who?, Appendix, References, Recipe Index, Index

Conversions Charts

OVEN TEMPERATURES

CELSIUS (°C)	CELSIUS (°C) fan assisted	FAHRENHEIT (°F)	GAS MARK	DESCRIPTION
40°C		105°F		
45°C		110°F		
50°C		120°F		
55°C		130°F		
110°C		225°F	¼	Very cool
120°C	100°C	250°F	½	Very cool
140°C	120°C	275°F	1	Very cool / very slow
150°C	130°C	300°F	2	Cool / slow
160°C	140°C	325°F	3	Warm / moderately slow
180°C	160°C	350°F	4	Moderate
190°C	170°C	375°F	5	Moderately hot
200°C	180°C	400°F	6	Hot
220°C	200°C	425°F	7	Very Hot
230°C	210°C	450°F	8	Very Hot

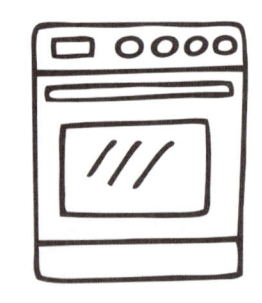

Conversion Charts

Capacity

STANDARD	METRIC	OUNCES	PINTS
¼ teaspoon (1/4t.)	1ml		
½ teaspoon (1/2t.)	2ml		
1 teaspoon (1t.)	5ml		
1 tablespoon (1T.)	15ml		
2 tablespoons (2T.)	30ml	1 fluid ounce (fl. oz.)	
¼ cup	60ml	2 fluid ounce (fl. oz.)	
1/3 cup	80ml	2 2/3 fluid ounce (fl. oz.)	
½ cup	125ml	4 fluid ounce (fl. oz.)	
	150ml	5 fluid ounce (fl. oz.)	¼ pint
2/3 cup	160ml	5 1/3 fluid ounce (fl. oz.)	
¾ cup	200ml	6 fluid ounce (fl. oz.)	
1 cup	250ml	8 fluid ounce (fl. oz.)	½ pint
1 ¼ cup	300ml	10 fluid ounce (fl. oz.)	
1 ½ cup	375ml	12 fluid ounce (fl. oz.)	
1 2/3 cup	400ml	13 fluid ounce (fl. oz.)	
1 ¾ cup	450ml	15 fluid ounce (fl. oz.)	
2 cups	500ml	16 fluid ounce (fl. oz.)	1 pint
2 ½ cups	600ml	20 fluid ounce (fl. oz.)	
3 cups	750ml	25 fluid ounce (fl. oz.)	
4 cups	1 litre (1l)		
(1000ml)	34 fluid ounce (fl. oz.)	1 quart	
	3,87 litres (3,87l) (3785ml)	128 fluid ounce (fl. oz.)	1 gallon

My Shorthand

c = cup	
T. = Tablespoon	
t. = Teaspoon	
fl. oz. = fluid ounce	
°C = degrees Celsius	
°F = degrees Fahrenheit	
ml = millilitre	
l = litre	
g = gram	
kg = kilogram	
cm = centimetre	
mm = millimetre	
a pinch = ½ ml	
" = inch	

Weight

STANDARD	METRIC
½ oz.	15g
1 oz.	30g
2 oz.	60g
3 oz.	90g
4 oz.	125g
6 oz.	175g
8 oz.	250g
10 oz.	300g
12 oz.	375g
13 oz.	400g
14 oz.	425g
1 lb	500g
1 ½ lb	750g
2 lb	1 kg

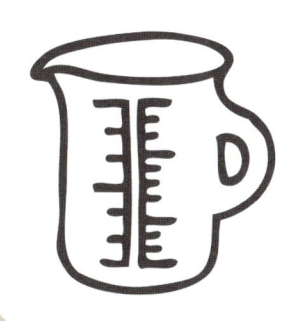

Length

METRIC	IMPERIAL
2.5 cm	1 inch (1")
15 cm	6 inch (6")
30.5 cm	12 inch (12")

473

Say Who?

Deepak Chopra MD, Facp.

Founder of The Chopra Foundation and co-founder of The Chopra Center for Wellbeing, is a world-renowned pioneer in integrative medicine and personal transformation, and is Board Certified in Internal Medicine, Endocrinology and Metabolism. He is a Fellow of the American College of Physicians and a member of the American Association of Clinical Endocrinologists. Chopra is the author of more than 80 books translated into over 43 languages, including numerous New York Times bestsellers.

www.deepakchopra.com

Weston A Price

Weston Andrew Valleau Price (September 6, 1870 – January 23, 1948) was a dentist known primarily for his theories on the relationship between nutrition, dental health, and physical health. In 1939, he published Nutrition and Physical Degeneration, detailing his global travels studying the diets and nutrition of various cultures. The book concludes that aspects of a modern Western diet (particularly flour, sugar, and modern processed vegetable fats) cause nutritional deficiencies that are a cause of many dental issues and health problems.

www.westonaprice.org

Sally Fallon Morell

As author of the best-selling nutritional cookbook series Nourishing Traditions, Sally Fallon Morell is the leading spokesperson for a return to nutrient-dense diets including raw milk, animal fats, organ meats, bone broths and lacto-fermented foods. She is the founding president of the Weston A. Price Foundation and a founder of A Campaign for Real Milk (realmilk.com). She is also president of NewTrends Publishing, which publishes books on diet and healthy, including books in the Nourishing Traditions series.

www.westonaprice.org

Natasha Campbell-Mcbride, MD. MMedSci (neurology), MMedSci (nutrition)

Dr Natasha Campbell-McBride is a medical doctor with two postgraduate degrees: Master of Medical Sciences in Neurology and Master of Medical Sciences in Human Nutrition.

She graduated as a medical doctor in Russia. After practising for five years as a Neurologist and three years as a Neurosurgeon she started a family and moved to the UK, where she got her second postgraduate degree in Human Nutrition.

She is well known for developing a concept of GAPS (Gut And Psychology Syndrome), which she described in her book Gut And Psychology Syndrome - Natural Treatment for Autism, ADHD, Dyslexia, Dyspraxia, Depression and Schizophrenia, now in its second edition. You can learn about GAPS on www.gaps.me

In her clinic Dr Campbell-McBride works as a nutritional consultant with many patients with heart disease, high blood pressure, arrhythmia, stroke and other complications of atherosclerosis. She has become acutely aware of the existing confusion about nutrition and these conditions, which spurred an intensive study into this subject. The result of this study was her book Put Your Heart In Your Mouth! - What Really Is Heart Disease And What We Can Do To Prevent And Even Reverse It.

www.doctor-natasha.com

Joshua Rosenthal

Joshua Rosenthal is a pioneer and visionary in holistic health and wellness. He holds a Master's of Science in Education and has over 30 years of experience in health and wellness including creation of the concept of Health Coach.

Joshua founded the Institute for Integrative Nutrition 25 years ago. IIN started with a small group of students in a rented kitchen in New York City and has grown into an online global phenomenon with over 60,000 students and graduates from over 120 countries.

His vision and leadership have empowered people to reach their personal and professional goals, and continue to exponentially improve the landscape of the health and wellness industry around the world.

David Wolfe

"David 'Avocado' Wolfe is the rock star and Indiana Jones of the superfoods and longevity universe. The world's top CEOs, ambassadors, celebrities, athletes, artists, and the real superheroes of this planet—Moms—all look to David for expert advice in health, beauty, herbalism, nutrition, and chocolate!"

David is a lead educator and presenter at the annual Longevity Conference, Institute of

Integrative Nutrition, and the Body-Mind Institute, where he hosts his own course.

www.davidwolfe.com

Rudolf Steiner

"The soul needs nourishment as well as the body."

Rudolf Steiner was an Austrian philosopher, social reformer, architect, artist and scientist. He founded a spiritual movement called Anthroposophy, which works on the basis that children's creative, spiritual and moral dimensions need as much attention as their intellectual ones. He founded the first Steiner school in Stuttgart, Germany in 1919 after a request from the owner of the Waldorf-Astoria cigarette factory to open a school for the workers' children. Rudolf Steiner was the founder of biodynamic agriculture, and his work in spiritual science, therapeutic medicine, art, architecture and education, continues to influence those working in these fields, providing strong relevance for the 21st century.

Joel Fuhrman, MD.

Joel Fuhrman, M.D. is a family physician, New York Times best-selling author and nutritional researcher who specializes in preventing and reversing disease through nutritional and natural methods. Dr. Fuhrman is an internationally recognized expert on nutrition and natural healing, and has appeared on hundreds of radio and television shows including The Dr. Oz Show, The Today Show, Good Morning America, and Live with Kelly and Michael. Dr. Fuhrman's own hugely successful PBS television shows, 3 Steps to Incredible Health and Dr. Fuhrman's Immunity Solution bring nutritional science to homes all across America. Dr. Fuhrman has worked on several scientific journal publications. Dr. Fuhrman is the Research Director of the Nutritional Research Foundation and a member of the Dr. Oz Show Medical Advisory Board. He is a graduate of the University of Pennsylvania School of Medicine (1988) and has received the St. Joseph's Family Practice Resident's Teaching Award for his contribution to the education of residents.

www.drfuhrman.com

Donna Gates, M.Ed., ABAAHP

Donna Gates, M.Ed., ABAAHP, is an Advanced Fellow with the American Academy of Anti-Aging Medicine, she is on a mission to change the way the world eats. The Body Ecology Diet was the first of its kind—sugar-free, gluten-free, casein-free, and probiotic rich. In 1994, Donna introduced the natural sweetener stevia to the U.S., began teaching about fermented foods, and coined the phrase "inner ecosystem" to describe the network of microbes that maintains our basic physiological processes—from digestion to immunity. Over the past 25 years, Donna has become one of the most respected authorities in the field of digestive health, diet, and nutrition. A recognized radio host of The Body Ecology Hour with Donna Gates on

Hay House radio, Donna regularly contributes to The Huffington Post and The Daily Love, and lectures at the "I Can Do It!" Conference, The Longevity Now Conference, and Women's Wellness Conference.

www.bodyecology.com

Sue Dengate

Sue Dengate is a psychology graduate and former high school teacher who became interested in the effects of food additives after the birth of her first child 20 years ago. Since then, Sue has focused on the effects of food chemicals on children's behaviour, health and learning ability. She is author of the bestselling Fed Up series, published by Random House Australia. In 2001, Sue completed a round the world 'supermarket tour' to compare the use of food additives in 15 countries. Her groundbreaking study about the behavioural effects of a common bread preservative was published in a medical journal in 2002. Sue, helped by her husband Dr Howard Dengate, a food scientist, runs the Food Intolerance Network through the website www.fedup.com.au. Sue was an Australian of the Year finalist in 2009.

Hiromi Shinya

Dr. Hiromi Shinya developed the now standard technique of non-invasive colonoscopic surgery. He is a professor of surgery at Albert Einstein College of Medicine and Head of the Endoscopic Center of Beth Israel Hospital in New York as well as an adviser for Maeda Hospital and Hanzomon Gastrointestinal Clinic in Japan. He is also Vice Chairman of the Japanese Medical Association in the USA.

www.enzymefactor.com/

Hanna Grotepass, MBChB

Dr Hanna Grotepass is a medical doctor, homeopath, spiritual and lifestyle mentor. She brings an enlightened and balanced approach to the art of healing.

Hanna approaches health and healing from a holistic perspective which quite simply is a form of healing that considers the whole person – body, mind, spirit, and emotions – in the quest for optimal health and wellness. The integration of neuroscience, neuroplasticity and meditation hold her current interest.

A mother of three grown children, she raised her own family with the attitude that life is sacred, offering us the opportunity to evolve to our highest divine potential and so make a positive contribution to the greater whole.

She practices in Knysna on the scenically beautiful Garden Route, South Africa.

Appendix

Food Additives

Colours

Colourants add the colour which processed food lacks - they help hide the processed mush that is being sold as food and enhance food's appeal to consumers, especially children.

Colours can either come from natural sources, such as E100, which comes from turmeric, or they can be artificial and man-made – these are the ones you need to avoid.

The colours used in foods and drinks make up the E numbers from 100 to 199.

In red: In the UK, the six artificial colours in red (the so called Southampton Six) were subjected to a 'voluntary phase out' by the end of 2009. In the EU, foods containing the Southampton Six colours have to carry the warning: "may have an adverse effect on activity and attention in children".

Some of the big manufacturers in the UK are extending the voluntary ban to all artificial colours, especially Brilliant Blue 133. In the best known example, when UK Smarties changed to all natural colours in 2006, blue Smarties were withdrawn until a suitable natural alternative could be found. Health concerns about Brilliant Blue were raised by a laboratory study showing that Brilliant Blue may interact with other additives such as MSG to interfere with the development of the nervous system.

In South Africa: all the colours which the European manufacturers have to warn consumers about, remain perfectly legal for use in our food. Only tartrazine has to be identified by name on labels, by law. Do not be fooled into a false sense of health by a food label stating "Tartrazine-free" – tartrazine-free does not mean colour-free. South African food manufacturers have simply swopped tartrazine for Sunset Yellow (E110).

The Southampton Six

Blue #1 and Blue #2   Number: 133*

Also known as: Brilliant Blue FCF

Used in: candy, cereal, soft drinks, sports drinks and pet foods

Reasons to avoid: May cause chromosomal damage

Banned in: Austria, Sweden, Switzerland, France, Germany and Norway, Finland

Red dye # 3 (also Red #40)   Number: 124*
Also known as: Ponceau, Brilliant Scarlet

Used in: fruit cocktail, maraschino cherries, cherry pie mix, ice cream, candy, bakery products, soda, gelatine desserts, pastries, sausage and many more.

Reasons to avoid: Has been proven to cause thyroid cancer and chromosomal damage in laboratory animals, may also interfere with brain-nerve transmission. Banned from use in many foods and cosmetics in 1990 after 8 years of debate. This dye continues to be on the market until supplies run out!

Banned in: UK, EU, USA

Allura Red   Number: 129*
Banned in: UK, EU

Yellow #6   Number: 110; 122
Also known as: Sunset Yellow; Azorubine

Used in: Cheese, macaroni and cheese, candy and carbonated beverages, lemonade, crisps and many more.

Reasons to avoid: Increases the number of kidney and adrenal gland tumours in laboratory animals, may cause chromosomal damage. May cause occasional, but sometimes-severe, hypersensitivity reactions.

Banned in: Sunset Yellow: UK, EU | Azorubine, Carmoisine: UK, EU, USA, Canada, Japan

478

Appendix

Yellow #5 — **Number: 102*; 104; 107**
Also known as: Tartrazine; quinoline yellow; yellow 2G

Used in: Cheese, macaroni and cheese, candy and carbonated beverages, lemonade, gelatin desserts, pet food, baked goods.

Reasons to avoid: The second-most-widely used colouring causes allergy-like hypersensitivity reactions, primarily in aspirin-sensitive persons, and triggers hyperactivity in some children. It may be contaminated with such cancer-causing substances as benzidine and 4-aminobiphenyl (or chemicals that the body converts to those substances).

Banned in: Tartrazine (102) - UK, EU | Quinoline (104) - UK, EU, USA, Japan, Canada

Other colours to avoid:

Amaranth — Number: 123
Banned in: USA, previously banned in Norway

Erythrosine — Number: 127

Indigotine — Number: 132

Green S — Number: 142
Banned in: USA, Japan, Canada

Fast Green FCF — Number: 143
Banned in: UK, EU

Brilliant Black — Number: 151
Banned in: USA, Canada, Japan

Brown HT — Number: 155
Banned in: USA, Canada, Japan

Natural Colour — Number: 160b — **Also known as:** Annatto

Preservatives

Preservatives are added to food to allow the products remain in an edible state for longer. The art of preserving food has existed for centuries - salt and vinegar have traditionally been used to preserve products such as biltong and sauerkraut. Today, salt and vinegar are still used, but are overshadowed by synthetic and manmade preservatives.

E numbers from E200 to E299 fall into the preservative category.

In red: Especially important to keep out of your little one's diet.

Sorbates (Numbers: 200, 201, 202, 203)

Also known as: Sorbic Acid (E200); Potassium Sorbate (E202); Calcium Sorbate (E203)

Used in: Cream cheese, cottage cheese, reduced fat spreads, bread, flat breads, baked goods, pasta, yoghurt, fruits juices and cordials, syrups, spreads and dips. Also widely used in pharmaceuticals and toiletries.

Sorbic acid and potassium sorbate are used in a number of foods describing themselves as 'natural'. Although sorbates occur naturally in some fruits, for commercial use they are manufactured synthetically, so it is misleading to describe them as natural.

Reasons to avoid: Sorbates have been associated with asthma, eczema, contact dermatitis, eye irritation, nasal irritation and burning mouth syndrome and the full range of food intolerance reactions including IBS and children's behaviour problems (ADHD and others).

Benzoates (Numbers: 210, 211, 212, 213)

Also known as: Benzoic acid; Sodium, calcium & potassium benzoates.

Used in: fruit juice, carbonated drinks, cordials, syrups, pickles.

Reasons to avoid: They appear to be safe for most people, though they cause hives, asthma, or other allergic reactions in sensitive individuals.

Another problem occurs when sodium benzoate is used in beverages that also contain ascorbic acid (vitamin C). The two substances, in an acidic solution, can react together to form small amounts of benzene, a chemical that causes leukaemia and other cancers. A lawsuit filed in 2006 by private attorneys ultimately forced Coca-Cola, PepsiCo, and other soft-drink makers in the U.S. to reformulate affected beverages - typically fruit-flavoured products.

Sulphites (Numbers: 220, 221, 222, 223, 224, 225, 226, 227, 228)

Also known as: Sulphur dioxide (E220); Sodium sulphite (E221); Sodium bisulphate (E222); Sodium metabisulphite (E223); Potassium metabisulphite (E224); Potassium sulphite (E225); Potassium bisulphate (E228); sulphites; bisulphites; metabisulphites.

Used in: This list is enormous – far too long to list everything here. Please see www.fedup.com for the itemised list.

The most pertinent foods sulphites can be found in include: Baked goods; fruit juices and cordial; condiments and relishes; canned fish; uncooked shellfish; fresh grapes; dried fruit; pre-cut / processed fruit and vegetables; French Fries; gelatine; deli meats (cold cuts), sausages; molasses; syrups; grain products and pasta; jams and jellies; soup and soup mixes; wine; beer; cider *(mama's and papa's*

Appendix

- stick to your gin and tonic, whisky and soda or vodka!)

The only way to avoid sulphites is to avoid all processed foods.

Reasons to avoid: Sulphites destroy thiamine (vitamin B1) and vitamin E and are also thought to destroy folate (in the food to which they are added, and in your body).

Best known for their effects on asthmatics since the well publicised 'salad bar' deaths of the 1970s and 80s - at least 12 asthmatics died from eating salads that had been sprayed with sulphites in restaurants.

In 1984, Australian researchers found that more than 65% of asthmatic children were sensitive to sulphites, and in 1999 the conservative World Health Organisation (WHO) revised upward their estimate of the number of sulphite-sensitive asthmatic children, from 4% to 20-30%.

Symptoms of sulphite sensitivity: headaches, IBS, behavioural problems (ADHD and others), breathing problems and rashes. In severe cases, sulphites can actually cause death by closing down the airway altogether, leading to cardiac arrest.

Banned in: USA - total prohibition on the use of sulphites in meats since 1959. Sulphited meats are widely eaten in other countries.

Nitrates and Nitrites (Numbers: 249, 250, 251, 252)
Also known as: Sodium Nitrate / Sodium Nitrite

Used as a preservative, colour fixer and flavouring - this chemical just happens to turn meats bright red. It makes processed meats appear fresh and vibrant.

Used in: bacon, ham, hot dogs, deli meats, corned beef, smoked fish and other processed meats.

Levels of nitrates are increasing in our fruit and vegetables as well due to overuse of artificial fertilisers – another reason to purchase organic produce.

Reasons to avoid: These additives have been associated with a range of intolerance symptoms such as headaches, IBS, skin rashes, asthma, children's behaviour problems (ADHD and others), difficulty falling asleep, growing pains, stuttering and frequent night waking,

They are highly carcinogenic once they enter the human digestive system. They form a variety of nitrosamine compounds that enter the bloodstream and wreak havoc with a number of internal organs: the liver and pancreas in particular. Sodium nitrite is widely regarded as a toxic ingredient - the USDA tried to ban this additive in the 1970's but was vetoed by food manufacturers who complained they had no alternative for preserving packaged meat products.

In August 2009, the WCRF (World Cancer Research Fund) issued a warning to parents, suggesting they limit their children's intake to 70 grams of processed meat per week.

Banned in: Not permitted in organic foods.

Propionates (Numbers: 280, 281, 282, 283)

Also known as: Propionic acid (E280); Sodium propionate(E281); Calcium propionate (E282); Potassium propionate (E283); cultured wheat, cultured dextrose or cultured whey - 'natural' preservatives

Used in: commercial breads, crumpets and other baked goods.

Propionates occur naturally in small amounts in natural foods (such as cheese) and are also produced naturally in the human gut as part of the digestion process. In tiny amounts they are not harmful but, as with other additives, the effects are dose related.

You are unlikely to be affected immediately by the amount of propionate preservative in one slice of bread but the effects are cumulative – they build up slowly over days or weeks, varying with the dose.

Reasons to avoid: Like all additives, this preservative was not tested (before approval) for its effects on children's behaviour and learning abilities.

Symptoms: Can contribute to hyperactivity in children (Swain et al); irritability, restlessness, inattention and sleep disturbance – difficulty falling asleep and/or frequent night waking (Dengate and Ruben 2002); neurotoxic to children with propionic academia.

Other reported symptoms include: migraine and headaches; gastrointestinal symptoms such as stomach aches, irritable bowel, diarrhoea; urinary urgency, bedwetting; eczema and other itchy skin rashes; nasal congestion (stuffy or runny nose); depression, unexplained tiredness, foggy brain; speech delay, impairment of memory and concentration; tachycardia (fast heart beat); arrhythmia; seizures; growing pains; loud voice (no volume control); adult acne.

Synthetic Antioxidants

Most people think antioxidants are beneficial, and this is true for natural antioxidants such as vitamin C and vitamin E. However, there are two groups of synthetic antioxidants that can cause nasty side effects - gallates and synthetic antioxidants tBHQ, BHA and BHT.

Antioxidants in food work in a similar way to preservatives - extending the shelf life of food and improving their taste and appearance. They do this by preventing, or slowing down, oxidation – that is, preventing rancidity in fats and

Appendix

oils and the natural browning by enzymes in fruit and vegetables.

The 5% labelling loophole (relevant in some countries)

This states that if the amount of an ingredient (such as vegetable oil) in a product (such as bread) forms less than 5% of the product, a food additive (such as antioxidant BHA E320) in that ingredient does not have to be listed if the additive is no longer "performing a technological function".

Synthetic antioxidants are the most hidden of all additives.

Antioxidants can be natural or synthetic. Natural or safe antioxidants include numbers E300 – E309 (E300 is Vitamin C, also known as ascorbic acid; E306-309 are Vitamins E's)

In red: Especially important to keep out of your little one's diet.

In green: Safe to consume

Ascorbic acid (Number: E300)   Also known as: vitamin C

Found in: soft drinks, condensed milk and jams.

As naturally occurring antioxidants are an essential element of food production, they're in huge demand. To help cope with the demand, they have also been artificially created too. This is what's called nature identical substances. They are identical in structure to the original substances, as their molecular structure has been copied, and are used in the same way.

Tocopherols (Numbers: E306 – E309)   Also known as: vitamin E

Found naturally in products such as nuts, soya, sunflower seeds and maize and they're used in products to help preserve them. They're most commonly found in products such as vegetable oils, cocoa and margarine.

As naturally occurring antioxidants are an essential element of food production, they're in huge demand. To help cope with the demand, they have also been artificially created too. This is what's called nature identical substances. They are identical in structure to the original substances, as their molecular structure has been copied, and are used in the same way.

Gallates (Numbers: 310, 311, 312)

Also known as: Propyl gallate (E310); Octyl gallate (E311); Dodecyl gallate (E312)

Used in: Any food that contains fats or oils may contain these antioxidants and they are not necessarily labelled. Margarines, vegetable oils, fried foods, and any food containing vegetable oil.

Reasons to avoid: Gallates tend to build up from small doses eaten nearly every day. These additives can be associated with the full range of food intolerance reactions such as: irritability, restlessness and difficulty falling asleep; mood swings, anxiety, depression, panic attacks; inattention, difficulty concentrating or debilitating fatigue; eczema, urticaria, contact dermatitis (from cosmetics etc.) and other skin rashes; reflux, sneaky poos, bloating, abdominal pain, stomach aches and other irritable bowel symptoms including constipation; headaches or migraines; frequent colds, flu, bronchitis, tonsillitis, sinusitis; stuffy or runny nose, throat clearing, cough or asthma; joint pain and arthritis.

TBHQ (Number: 319)

Also known as: tBHQ tert-Butylhydroquinone (E319)

Used in: Any food that contains fats or oils may contain these antioxidants and they are not necessarily labelled. Margarines, vegetable oils, fried foods, and any food containing vegetable oil.

Reasons to avoid: build up from small doses eaten nearly every day. These additives can be associated with the full range of food intolerance reactions such as irritability, restlessness and difficulty falling asleep; mood swings, anxiety, depression, panic attacks; inattention, difficulty concentrating or debilitating fatigue; eczema, urticaria, contact dermatitis (from cosmetics etc) and other itchy skin rashes; reflux, sneaky poos, bloating, abdominal pain, stomach aches and other irritable bowel symptoms including constipation; headaches or migraines; frequent colds, flu, bronchitis, tonsillitis, sinusitis; stuffy or runny nose, throat clearing, cough or asthma; joint pain and arthritis.

BHA (Number: 320)

Also known as: butylated hydroxyanisole (E320)

Used in: cereals, chewing gum, potato chips, and vegetable oils, frozen sausages, enriched rice, lard, shortening, candy, jelly, margarines, vegetable oils, fried foods, food containing vegetable oil.

BHT (Number: 321)

Also known as: butylated hydroxytoluene (E321)

Used in: cereals, chewing gum, potato chips, and vegetable oils, frozen sausages, enriched rice, lard, shortening, candy, jello. Any food that contains fats or oils may contain these antioxidants and they are not necessarily labelled. Margarines, vegetable oils, fried foods, food containing vegetable oil.

Reasons to avoid BHA and BHT: They build up from small

Appendix

doses eaten nearly every day. These additives can be associated with the full range of food intolerance reactions such as irritability, restlessness and difficulty falling asleep; mood swings, anxiety, depression, panic attacks; inattention, difficulty concentrating or debilitating fatigue; eczema, urticaria, contact dermatitis (from cosmetics etc.) and other itchy skin rashes; reflux, sneaky poos, bloating, abdominal pain, stomach aches and other irritable bowel symptoms including constipation; headaches or migraines; frequent colds, flu, bronchitis, tonsillitis, sinusitis; stuffy or runny nose, throat clearing, cough or asthma; joint pain and arthritis.

Affects the neurological system of the brain, alters behaviour and has potential to cause cancer. BHA and BHT are oxidants which form cancer-causing reactive compounds in your body.

Banned / restricted in: In Europe, antioxidants BHA (E320) and BHT (E321) have been identified as a possible cause of local skin reactions, for example, contact dermatitis. When these additives are used in medications, the following health warning must appear on the package leaflet: "May cause mild irritation to the skin, eyes and mucous membranes".

Flavour Enhancers

Food manufacturers and processing plants use flavour enhancers and flavourings to add flavour to processed food that would otherwise be bland, tasteless and unappetising (largely due to the production process).

Flavour enhancers are not the same as flavourings.

Flavourings are used to add a flavour to products. They are governed by different laws to food additives (and flavour enhancers) - they do not have eNumbers and precise details do not usually need to be listed in the ingredients – making it difficult for you to know what you are eating. They come in both natural and man-made (synthetic) forms.

Flavour enhancers are designed to enhance the existing flavour of products without adding any new tastes or flavours of their own. They are used widely in food and drinks and come in both natural and manmade or synthetic forms.

Some forms of flavour enhancers have existed for centuries. Take salt, for example. It's been used for hundreds of years to improve the flavour of meat products and is perhaps the world's best known natural flavour enhancer. Similarly, vinegar and sugar have been used for years to pep up flavours in foods.

Flavour enhancers are labelled on food ingredient packets with E numbers from E600 to E699.

Sometimes, especially in South Africa, the manufacturer may choose to use the long chemical name, rather than the shortened E number, which makes it more difficult for consumers to identify the presence of E numbers.

Special Note:

Monosodium glutamate (MSG) is the salt of one of the most abundant naturally-occurring non-essential amino acids. In its natural form it is found in tomatoes, potatoes, mushrooms, and other fruit and vegetables. MSG was first isolated from kombu seaweed in 1908 by a professor at Tokyo University (kombu is known for adding the umami flavour to Asian cuisine). He then became a partner in Ajinomoto, now a multi-billion-dollar company providing more than half the world's MSG. MSG flavour enhancers are now cultured on yeasts in giant factories.

Due to consumer demand for food without nasty additives, the names "MSG" or "monosodium glutamate" or the number 621 are being phased out of our foods. This is not necessarily a reason to celebrate. Instead, many manufacturers are now using glutamate-containing ingredients such as hydrolysed vegetable protein and yeast extracts - and the product can legally claim "No MSG" or "No added MSG"!

Glutamates (Numbers: 620, 621, 622, 623, 624, 625)

Also known as: MSG / Monosodium glutamate / umami (E621); Glutamic acid (E620); Monopotassium glutamate (622); Calcium glutamate (623); Monammonium glutamate (624); Magnesium glutamate (625)

Used in: Chinese food, many flavoured snacks, noodles, chips, cookies, seasonings, soups, sauces, seasoned salt, ready-made or frozen meals, deli meats, pies, sausages, vegetarian burgers and sausages, fast food, restaurant food.

Reasons to avoid: MSG is known as an excitotoxin, a substance which overexcites cells to the point of damage or death. MSG effects the neurological pathways of the brain and disengages the "I'm full" function which in turn leads to weight gain and obesity. Can lead to Chinese Restaurant Syndrome - symptoms included burning, numbness, facial pressure, chest pain and headaches.

Reactions can include: migraines, diarrhoea, nausea, stomach cramps, irritable bowel symptoms, asthma, insomnia, depression, heart palpitations, ventricular fibrillation, AF (arterial fibrillation), anxiety, irritability, sleep disturbance, children's behaviour and attention problems.

Banned / restricted in: Children are more vulnerable to the effects of additives than adults. MSG and other flavour enhancers are not permitted in foods manufactured specifically for infants and young children (12 months or less).

Ribonucleotides (MSG Boosters) (Numbers: 627, 631, 635)

Also known as: Disodium guanylate (E627); Disodium inosinate (E631); Ribonucleotides (E635)

Used in: Chinese food, many flavoured snacks, noodles, chips, cookies, seasonings, soups, sauces, seasoned salt, ready-made or frozen meals, deli meats, pies, sausages, vegetarian burgers and sausages, fast food, restaurant food.

Reasons to avoid: Scientists discovered that these chemicals could boost the flavour enhancing effect of MSG up to 15 times. Not only do they boost the flavouring ability of MSG, they also seem to boost adverse reactions to MSG. These additives were not tested for their effects on consumers before release, and food additive effects are not monitored by food regulators. As well as the usual MSG reactions, rashes called Ribo Rash are often reported.

Hydrolysed Vegetable or Plant Proteins (free glutamates - essentially the same as MSG)
Also known as: HVP; Yeast Extract; HPP

- ♥ The food industry is getting very clever with naming this particular additive. It can be called a variety of names in any combinations of:
    - ♥ Hydrolysed, autolysed, formulated
    - ♥ vegetable, wheat, gluten, soy, maize, plant
    - ♥ protein
    - ♥ yeast (except in baked products like bread), yeast flakes
    - ♥ yeast extracts (Vegemite, Marmite and similar foods such as Promite, Natex savoury spread, Vegespread and Vecon contain free glutamates)

Reasons to avoid: The same as for MSG. Due to consumer demand for food without nasty additives, the names MSG or monosodium glutamate or the number 621 are being phased out of our foods. Instead, many manufacturers are now using these ingredients and the product can legally claim "No MSG" or "No added MSG". Ribonucleotides can also be added to boost the effects of the free glutamate.

Sweeteners

The traditional ingredient for adding sweetness is sugar, but as we become aware of the negative health affects of it, food manufacturers are substituting it with artificial sweeteners (or intense sweeteners) and sugar-free sweeteners (or sugar alcohols). The alternative sweeteners in use today are forms of food additives. While they may be lower in calories, they are not necessarily healthier for us. Besides the numerous side affects reported by consumers, in 2014, a comprehensive study at the prestigious Weizman Institute showed that the three most commonly used artificial sweeteners - aspartame (951), sucralose (Splenda) and saccharin - can cause elevated blood glucose levels by altering the beneficial bacteria in the gut in a way that can promote both obesity and diabetes. This was a surprising finding as these sweeteners have long been promoted as ways of avoiding obesity and managing diabetes.

Artificial sweeteners have E numbers but are often better known by there brand names:

Sucralose (E955), for example, was originally sold under the brand name Splenda, and aspartame (E951), has been marketed under a variety of names, including NutraSweet, Equal and Canderel.

The role of sweeteners in foods and drinks is pretty self-explanatory – they are there to make products taste sweet while allowing food manufacturers to claim their products are "diet" and "sugar-free" – a big marketing plus.

Artificial Sweetener (Numbers: 950, 951, 952, 954, 955, 957, 959)

Also known as: Acesulphame-K (E950); Aspartame (NutraSweet, Equal, Canderel) (E951); Cyclamates (E952); Saccharin (E954); Sucralose (E955); Thaumatin (E957); Neohesperidine dihydrochalcone (E959)

Used in: "diet" and/or "sugar-free" foods, drinks, sweets, and medication.

Reasons to avoid:

Aspartame (E951, Nutrasweet, Equal) - believed to be a neurotoxin and carcinogen and accounts for more reports of adverse reactions than all other foods and food additives combined. Known to erode intelligence and affect short-term memory, it may also lead to a wide variety of ailments including brain tumour, lymphoma, diabetes, multiple sclerosis, Parkinson's, Alzheimer's, fibromyalgia, chronic fatigue, depression, anxiety attacks, dizziness, headaches, nausea, mental confusion, migraines and seizures.

Acesulphame-K (E950) - caused cancer and tumours in animal tests.

Aspartame (E951, Nutrasweet, Equal) - linked to many health problems including headaches, seizures and brain tumours. The FDA has received more complaints about aspartame than any other food additive.

Cyclamates (E952) - suspected carcinogen.

Saccharin (E954) - linked to bladder and reproductive cancers banned in the USA in 1977 but reinstated with strict labelling provisions.

Sucralose (E955) - caused kidney and liver damage in tests, more research needed.

Cyclamates banned in UK and USA in 1970.

High Fructose Corn Syrup

Also known as: HFCS

Used in: Most processed foods, breads, candy, flavoured yoghurts, salad dressings, canned vegetables, and cereals.

Reasons to avoid: A highly refined artificial sweetener made from genetically modified corn. It has become the number one source of calories in America. It is found in almost all processed foods. HFCS leads to weight gain faster than any other ingredient, increases your LDL ("bad") cholesterol levels, and contributes to the development of diabetes and tissue damage, among other harmful effects.

Sugar-free sweeteners (Numbers: 420, 421, 953, 965, 966, 967, 968,1200)

Sugar alcohols also known as Polyols or individually as: Sorbitol (E420); Mannitol (E421); Isomalt (E953); Maltitol or hydrogenated glucose syrup (E965); Lactitol (E966); Xylitol (E967); Erythritol (E968); Polydextrose (E1200)

Used in: Drinks, yoghurts, sweets, toothpaste and medications.

Reasons to avoid: Can have a laxative effect in large doses or in sensitive consumers - diarrhoea, stomach cramps, bloating or gas, misdiagnosis of IBS.

Trans Fats

Vegetable oil, usually a liquid, can be made into a semi-solid shortening by reacting it with hydrogen. This partial hydrogenation process reduces the levels of polyunsaturated oils - and creates trans fats. In doing so these oils become more stable and have a similar texture and flavour to saturated fats. Margarine is an example of a partially hydrogenated oil. Food companies use hydrogenated fat in dough-based foods like doughnuts, pastries, biscuits, cookies and crackers. Since the hydrogenation of oil increases a food's shelf-life, manufacturers use it in many shelf-stable snack foods and baked foods. Fast food restaurants also like trans fats for commercial deep fat frying, since the oil can be used repeatedly.

Also known as: Partially hydrogenated vegetable oils; trans fatty acids

Used in: margarine, chips and crackers, baked goods, fast foods (deep-fried), microwave popcorn, icing.

Reasons to avoid: Trans fat increases LDL ('bad') cholesterol levels while decreasing HDL ('good') cholesterol; increases the risk of heart attacks, heart disease and strokes; and, contributes to increased inflammation, diabetes and other health problems.

The Institute of Medicine has advised consumers to consume as little trans fat as possible, ideally less than about 2 grams a day (that much might come from naturally occurring trans fat in beef and dairy products). The Harvard School of Public Health researchers estimate that trans fat have been causing about 50,000 premature heart attack deaths annually, making partially hydrogenated oil one of the most harmful ingredients in the food supply.

Banned in: Denmark

Individual Concerns:

Potassium Bromate

Potassium Bromate is used to increase volume in bread and bread rolls. Most potassium bromate breaks down during the baking process, but tests have confirmed that trace amounts can remain in finished baked goods.

Reasons to avoid: Potassium bromate is known to cause cancer in animals and is classified as a category 2B carcinogen (possibly carcinogenic to humans) by the International Agency for Research on Cancer (IARC). Even small amounts in bread can create problems for humans.

Banned in: European Union, Argentina, Brazil, Canada, Nigeria, South Korea, Peru, Sri Lanka, China.

Aluminium

Found in the mineral salts, acidity regulators, anti-caking agents category of food additives: eNumbers 500 – 599

Aluminium is one of the eight most abundant elements on earth making up about 8.2 percent of the earth's crust. It is found in all plants and living organisms. All natural food contains trace amounts of aluminium.

However, in nature aluminium exists only combined to other elements – it does not exist as a metal. Metal aluminium, is a human invention and the human body does not need aluminium.

Numbers: 520, 521, 522, 523; 541; 555; 555; 556; 559

Appendix

Also known as: Aluminium sulphate (alum); Aluminium sodium sulphate; Aluminium potassium sulphate; Aluminium ammonium sulphate; sodium aluminium phosphate; Aluminium sodium silicate; Aluminium potassium silicate; Aluminium calcium silicate; aluminium silicate; aluminium nicotinate, aluminium stearate.

Found in: processed cheeses, table salt, baking powders, pickles, bleached flour, prepared dough, cake mixes, non-dairy creamers, vanilla powders and some donuts and waffles, antacids, aspirin, prescription medications such as pain-killers and anti-diarrhoea medicines, toothpastes, nasal sprays, antiperspirants, dental amalgams, and pesticides.

Milk formulas for babies can contain up to four hundred times more aluminium than breast milk.

Cooking foods, especially acidic foods like fruits, tomatoes and wine, in pans made from aluminium can cause aluminium to leach into your food. As does the use of tin foil when cooking.

Reasons to avoid: In animal studies, aluminium has been found to adversely affect the reproductive and nervous systems, as well as having neurological effects such as changes in behaviour, learning and motor response. Some human studies have also suggested a potential association between aluminium and Alzheimer's Disease. Ingesting small amounts of aluminium may not cause harm, but over time aluminium builds up within your body.

References

UNLEARN

Campbell-McBride, N. Gut and Psychology Syndrome: Natural Treatment for Autism, Dyspraxia, A.D.D., Dyslexia, A.D.H.D., Depression, Schizophrenia. Medinform Publishing; Revised & enlarged edition (November 15, 2010)

Fallon Morell, S and Cowan, TS. The Nourishing Traditions Book of Baby & Child Care. Newtrends Publishing, Inc.; 1 edition (March 16, 2013)

Scientific American, December 1995; British J of Nutrition, 2000:84 (Suppl. 1) : S3-S10, S75-S80, S81-S89).

Oski, F. Don't Drink Your Milk. Teach Services Inc; 9 edition (April 1992)

Fallon-Morrell, S. www.realmilk.com

Teicholz, N. The Big Fat Surprise: Why Butter, Meat and Cheese Belong in a Healthy Diet. Simon & Schuster; 1St Edition edition (May 13, 2014)

Shanahan, C. Should You Feed Your Baby Iron Fortified Foods? http://www.foodrenegade.com,

http://healthybabybeans.com/archives/tag/grains

http://www.westonaprice.org/health-topics/the-liver-files/

http://www.westonaprice.org/health-topics/nourishing-a-growing-baby/

http://www.healthychild.com/treating-reflux-and-colic-in-babies/

http://www.westonaprice.org/health-topics/calming-the-cry-of-colic/

http://www.drdeborahmd.com/ear-infections

http://www.consumer-health.com/services/cons_take44.php

http://ahealthierwei.com/category/mcd/

http://www.westonaprice.org/health-topics/nourishing-a-growing-baby/

http://www.askdrsears.com/topics/feeding-eating/family-nutrition/facts-about-fats/smart-fats-growing-brains

http://www.westonaprice.org/health-topics/nourishing-a-growing-baby/

http://wellnessmama.com/8464/healthy-saturated-fat/

http://www.drfranklipman.com/letting-go-of-your-fear-of-fats/

http://www.drfranklipman.com/what-is-your-take-on-cholesterol/

https://www.theconnection.tv/second-brain-gut/

http://www.mommypotamus.com/dirt-the-superfood-that-makes-you-happier-smarter-healthier/

The Healthy Home Economist, http://www.thehealthyhomeeconomist.com

Food Renegade, http://www.foodrenegade.com

ESSENTIAL NUTRIENTS

http://www.westonaprice.org/health-topics/nourishing-a-growing-baby/

http://www.whfoods.com/genpage.php?tname=specialneed&dbid=7

http://raisingchildren.net.au/articles/vitamin_d.html

http://www.drweil.com/drw/u/ART02806/phosphorus

http://www.superfoods.co.za

http://www.thesuperfoods.net/cacao/cacao-nutritional-facts

http://www.herbwisdom.com/herb-maca.html

FEEDING

Fallon Morell, S and Cowan, TS. The Nourishing Traditions Book of Baby & Child Care. Newtrends Publishing, Inc.; 1 edition (March 16, 2013)

Gates, D. and Schatz, L. The Body Ecology Diet: Recovering Your Health and Rebuilding Your Immunity. Hay House; Revised edition (June 15, 2011)

Price, WA. Nutrition and Physical Degeneration. Price Pottenger Nutrition; 8th edition (2009)

Campbell-McBride, N. Gut and Psychology Syndrome: Natural Treatment for Autism, Dyspraxia, A.D.D., Dyslexia, A.D.H.D., Depression, Schizophrenia. Medinform Publishing; Revised & enlarged edition (November 15, 2010)

van Lierop, M and Barron, E. Feeding Your Baby CD

Nourishing Our Children. Baby's First Foods: When and What? https://nourishingourchildren.wordpress.

com/2011/12/14/babys-first-foods-when-and-what/
Nourishing Our Children. Why cereal should NOT be one of baby's first foods. nourishingourchildren.wordpress.com/2012/01/09/how-do-you-define-processed-foods/
Weston A. Price Foundation. Sacred Foods for Exceptionally Healthy Children, www.westonaprice.org/childrens-health/sacred-foods-for-exceptionally-healthy-babies-and-parents-too
Weston A. Price Foundation. Nourishing a Growing Baby. http://www.westonaprice.org/health-topics/nourishing-a-growing-baby/
Cheeseslave. Starting solids at 4-6 months. www.cheeseslave.com/when-to-feed-baby-why-start-solids-at-4-to-6-months/
Homemade Baby Foods Recipes, http://www.homemade-baby-food-recipes.com),
Momtastics's Wholesome Baby Food, http://wholesomebabyfood.momtastic.com)

WHAT TO FEED WHEN

van Lierop, M and Barron, E. Feeding Your Baby CD
Simply Being Well, www.simplybeingwell.com
Nourishing Our Children, www.nourishingourchildren.org
Weston A. Price Foundation, www.westonaprice.org/
Food For Kids Health, www.foodforkidshealth.com
Homemade Baby Foods Recipes, http://www.homemade-baby-food-recipes.com),
Momtastics's Wholesome Baby Food, http://wholesomebabyfood.momtastic.com)

ADDITIVES

Food Intolerance Network, http://www.fedup.com.au
Hungry For Change, http://www.hungryforchange.tv
Explore E Numbers, http://www.exploreenumbers.co.uk
Center for Science in the Public Interest, http://www.cspinet.org
Codex Alimentarius International Food Standards, http://www.codexalimentarius.org/standards/gsfa/
http://education.guardian.co.uk/print/0,3858,5360498-108229,00.html
Suez J et al, Artificial sweeteners induce glucose intolerance by altering the gut microbiota. Nature, 2014; DOI: 10.1038/nature13793
Swithers SE. Artificial sweeteners are not the answer to childhood obesity. Appetite. 2015 Mar 28. pii: S0195-6663(15)00129-4. http://www.ncbi.nlm.nih.gov/pubmed/25828597
? Olney JW, Farber NB, Spitznagel E, Robins LN, J. Increasing brain tumor rates: is there a link to aspartame Neuropathol Exp Neurol. 1996;55(11):1115-23.
Soffritti M, and others Aspartame administered in feed, beginning prenatally through life span, induces cancers of the liver and lung in male Swiss mice. Am J Ind Med. 2010 Dec;53(12):1197-206. Ramazzini Institute
Walton RG and others, Adverse reactions to aspartame: double-blind challenge in patients from a vulnerable population. Biol Psychiatry. 1993 Jul 1-15;34(1-2):13-7.

DIRTY DOZEN

Environmental Working Group (EWG), http://www.ewg.org/foodnews/summary.php

ALLERGENS

Allergy Society of South Africa, Patient Information Brochure. http://www.mm3admin.co.za/documents/docmanager/8e7be0a4-2b8d-453f-875e-cd1e5132b829/00036179.pdf
Food Intolerance Network, http://www.fedup.com.au/factsheets/support-factsheets/allergy-or-intolerance

IRRADIATION

http://www.mercola.com/article/irradiated/irradiation.htm

GMO'S

http://www.responsibletechnology.org/faqs
http://www.nongmoproject.org/learn-more/
http://africabio.com/gmos-in-south-africa/

References

http://www.globalhealingcenter.com/natural-health/what-is-the-bt-toxin/
http://www.enviropaedia.com/topic/default.php?topic_id=116
http://www.gmo-compass.org/eng/database/e-numbers/
African Cente for Biodiversity, http://acbio.org.za

EAT FROM THE RAINBOW

Whole Kids Foundation, https://www.wholekidsfoundation.org
Government of South Australia, Eat A Rainbow Bingo Game. http://www.sahealth.sa.gov.au/wps/wcm/connect/94e177804378fe4db428ffc9302c1003/Eat_a_Rainbow_bingo_game%28comms%29.pdf?MOD=AJPERES&CACHEID=94e177804378fe4db428ffc9302c1003

RAW VS COOKED

http://bodyecology.com/articles/cook_vegetables_maximum_nutrition.php

TOXINS

Cerazy, J. and Cottingham, S. Lead Babies: How Heavy Metals are Causing Children's Autism, ADHD, Learning Disabilities, Low IQ and Behavior Problems. iUniverse (February 26, 2010)
http://permaculturenews.org/2012/11/01/why-glyphosate-should-be-banned-a-review-of-its-hazards-to-health-and-the-environment/
http://www.anh-usa.org/half-of-all-children-will-be-autistic-by-2025-warns-senior-research-scientist-at-mit/
http://ecowatch.com/2015/01/23/health-problems-linked-to-monsanto-roundup/
http://www.webmd.com/children/environmental-exposure-head2toe/bpa
http://www.ewg.org/research/timeline-bpa-invention-phase-out
http://www.saferstates.com/toxic-chemicals/bisphenol-a/
http://www.health24.com/Medical/Cancer/News/SA-bans-BPA-in-baby-bottles-20130409
http://www.pregnancy.org/lead-babies-breaking-cycle-learning-disabilities
http://www.cehn.org/files/trainingmanual/manual-metal.html
http://www.healthychild.org/easy-steps/chemical/
http://www.controlyourimpact.com/articles/deodorants-antiperspirants-parabens-and-breast-cancer/
http://www.healthychild.org/chemicals-to-avoid-in-your-personal-care-products/

ORGANIC

Rauch SA, Braun JM, Barr DB, et al: Associations of prenatal exposure to organophosphate pesticide metabolites with gestational age and birth weight. Environ Health Perspect 2012, 120:1055-1060.
Zhang Y, Han S, Liang D, et al: Prenatal exposure to organophosphate pesticides and neurobehavioral development of neonates: a birth cohort study in Shenyang, China. PLoS One 2014, 9:e88491.
Bouchard MF, Bellinger DC, Wright RO, et al: Attention-Deficit/Hyperactivity Disorder and Urinary Metabolites of Organophosphate Pesticides. Pediatrics 2010, 125:e1270-e1277.
Bouchard MF, Chevrier J, Harley KG, et al: Prenatal exposure to organophosphate pesticides and IQ in 7-year-old children. Environ Health Perspect 2011, 119:1189-1195.
https://www.drfuhrman.com/library/organicvsconventional.aspx
http://ecowatch.com/2015/01/23/health-problems-linked-to-monsanto-roundup/
http://www.anh-usa.org/half-of-all-children-will-be-autistic-by-2025-warns-senior-research-scientist-at-mit/

FACTORY FARMS

https://www.aspca.org/fight-cruelty/farm-animal-cruelty/what-factory-farm
http://foodrevolution.org/blog/tag/factory-farms/
http://www.drfranklipman.com/basics-on-factory-farming/
http://certifiedhumane.org/free-range-and-pasture-raised-officially-defined-by-hfac-for-certified-humane-label/

WHY NOT GLUTEN

Braly, J., Hoggan, R., Wright, J. Dangerous Grains: Why Gluten Cereal Grains May Be Hazardous To Your Health. Avery; Later Edition edition (August 26, 2002)
Perlmutter, D. and Loberg, K. Grain Brain: The Surprising Truth about Wheat, Carbs, and Sugar--Your Brain's

Silent Killers. Little, Brown and Company; 1 edition (September 17, 2013)
http://www.mindbodygreen.com/0-7482/10-signs-youre-gluten-intolerant.html
http://www.foodrenegade.com/the-rise-of-gluten-intolerance/
http://www.cureceliacdisease.org/archives/faq/what-is-the-difference-between-gluten-intolerance-gluten-sensitivity-and-wheat-allergy

WHY NOT DAIRY

Shinya, H. The Enzyme Factor. Millichap Books (April 1, 2010)
http://articles.mercola.com/sites/articles/archive/2013/09/29/dr-perlmutter-gluten.aspx
http://www.whfoods.com/genpage.php?tname=nutrient&dbid=45
http://www.rense.com/general26/milk.htm
http://www.healthline.com/health/allergies/casein
http://www.breakingtheviciouscycle.info/knowledge_base/detail/casein-sensitivity/
http://www.drfranklipman.com/got-tummy-troubles/
http://drhyman.com/blog/2010/06/24/dairy-6-reasons-you-should-avoid-it-at-all-costs-2/
http://www.askdrsears.com/html/3/t032400.asp

WHY NOT SUGAR

Appleton, N. Lick The Sugar Habit. Avery; 2 edition (February 1, 1988)

ALTERNATIVES

http://www.mtcapra.com/benefits-of-goat-milk-vs-cow-milk/
http://bodyecology.com/articles/benefits_of_real_butter.php
http://www.drweil.com/drw/u/QAA401323/Is-Coconut-Sugar-a-Healthier-Sweetener.html

DON'T JUST EAT FOOD

http://www.faithful-to-nature.co.za/natural-organic-blog/2010/07/going-organic/why-go-organic
http://www.keeperofthehome.org/2007/12/what-are-you-putting-onto-your-skin-and-into-your-body.html
http://www.ewg.org/skindeep/
http://www.healthylife.net.au/healthy-you/wellbeing-lifestyle/skin-absorbing-facts-about-the-body-s-largest-organ/
http://www.spotlessliving.info/household-cleaning/kitchen/

SOUL FOOD

The Institute For Integrative Nutrition®
Hamilton, D. Why Kindness is Good for You. Hay House UK (February 15, 2010)
http://drdavidhamilton.com/why-babies-need-love/
http://www.huffingtonpost.com/matthew-melmed/babies-mental-health-matters_b_7213290.html
http://www.wholefamily.com/parent-center/child-development/that-which-is-asleep-will-awaken-rudolph-steiner-on-babies
https://www.psychologytoday.com/blog/moral-landscapes/201111/do-we-need-declaration-the-rights-the-baby
http://raisingchildren.net.au/articles/why_play_is_important.html
http://www.healyourlife.com/7-spiritual-laws-for-kids
http://startingpoint.org/what-does-it-mean-to-be-a-spiritual-person-2/
http://www.purposefairy.com/68155/26-powerful-lessons-to-learn-from-nature/
http://www.bubblesacademy.com/blog/baby-brain-development/
http://www.raisesmartkid.com/3-to-6-years-old/4-articles/35-the-benefits-of-exercise-on-your-kids-brain
http://www.medicaldaily.com/messy-kids-make-better-learners-how-playing-food-helps-toddlers-learn-words-faster-264139

GLOSSARY

http://www.herbwisdom.com/
http://www.whfoods.com

Index

A
additive intolerance   68
adhd   57
agar agar   188
agave nectar   113
allergens   51
allergy vs. intolerance   51
all good tomato sauce   250, 264
all spice   115, 387, 393
almond flour   105, 214, 222, 240, 258, 262, 336, 338, 374, 393
almond milk   109, 376
almond nut butter   322
almonds   105, 110, 142, 158, 186, 228, 240, 276, 286, 324, 374, 376, 393, 436
aluminium   484
amaranth   184, 212, 394
amaranth flour   105
antacid   386
ant deterrent   387
antifungal   383
anti-nutrients   76
antioxidants   66
apple   148, 154, 156, 166, 186, 192, 203, 218, 220, 226, 252, 280, 350, 366, 394
apple cider vinegar   194, 242, 314, 340, 356, 358, 395
apple juice   230
applesauce   212
arrowroot   316, 328, 395
arsenic   58
artichoke (globe artichoke)   395
artificial flavours   66, 70
artificial sweetener   66, 70, 483
athletes foot remedy   387
aubergine   396
autism   57
avocado   152, 164, 294, 326, 342, 396
avocados   342
avoid these additives   70

b
baby marrow   396
baby powder   386
baby tomatoes   310
baking powder   397
baking soda   385, 397
banana   142, 150, 154, 164, 214, 222, 242, 398
banana skin   387
baobab   115, 142, 150, 186, 203, 222, 398
basil   190, 276, 310, 398
bay leaves   194, 314, 356, 358, 399
beef   179, 358, 399

beef stock   312
beetroot   148, 282, 400
beetroot juice   344
bell pepper   400
beneficial bacteria   30
benzoates   479
berries   152, 168
BHA   382, 481
BHT   382, 481
bicarbonate of soda   385
biodynamic   87
Bisphenol-A   56
black cumin   356
black pepper   401
blackstrap molasses   112, 115, 144, 240, 401
blueberries   364, 402
body ecology   163, 360
body lotion   383
bone broth   115, 250, 312, 314, 354
bottled water   138
BPA   56
brain-gut connection   31
brinjal   402
broccoli   170, 402
brown rice   184
brown rice flour   218, 340
buckwheat   186, 403
buckwheat flour   106
bum cream   383
butter   99
butternut   170, 192, 220, 240, 244, 250, 288, 306, 404
butter oil   420

c
cabbage   368, 404
cacao   115, 230, 405
cadmium   58
cage-free   79
calcium   42
cantaloupe   405, 454
caraway   356, 368
carbohydrates   40
cardamom   322, 356, 405
carrots   146, 148, 218, 226, 260, 282, 312, 314, 316, 338, 358, 362, 406
casein   97
cashew nuts   190, 207, 230, 278, 280, 320, 324, 342, 406
cauliflower   172, 407
cayenne pepper   407
celery   148, 250, 314, 356, 358, 408

Index

celiac disease 95
chamomile tea 139
chemical cuisine 66
chemicals 382
chia seeds 142, 186, 203, 300, 326, 408
chicken 175, 252, 262, 264, 316, 356, 409
chicken broth 192, 194, 252, 290, 316
chicken livers 290
chickpea 175, 236, 246, 284, 409
chickpea flour 106, 242, 244, 322, 340, 375, 410
chocolate mousse recipe 326
cholesterol 34, 40
choline 42
Chris Masterjohn 96
chromium 43
cinnamon 115, 184, 186, 192, 194, 212, 214, 216, 218, 220, 240, 324, 338, 350, 366, 387, 410
clarified butter 420
cleaning 384
cleaning and healing wounds 388
cleanliness, food preparation 132
clean tile surfaces, hydrogen peroxide 388
clothes bleach 385
clothes washing powder 386
clove 240, 282, 284, 411
coconut 320, 411
coconut flakes 218
coconut flour 214, 228, 252, 258, 262
coconut milk 110, 142, 150, 152, 154, 184, 188, 216, 220, 234, 244, 272, 312, 316, 328, 336, 344, 371, 376, 411
coconut oil 115, 142, 144, 212, 216, 218, 234, 252, 296, 326, 332, 340, 342, 344, 383, 412
coconut sugar 112, 218, 220, 234, 412
coconut water 371
colic 30, 370
colic remedy 386
constipation 370
constipation remedy 387
convenience vs. conscience 54
conversions charts 472
copper 43
coriander 246, 312, 314, 356, 413
corn 413, 458
corn starch 378
cough and cold remedy 384
courgettes 312
cradle cap 383
cradle cap remedy 384
cranberries 216, 220, 244, 413
create-your-own smoothie 154
cucumber 146, 148, 414
cultured (fermented) foods 360
cumin 194, 246, 284, 312, 368, 414
curry powder 316, 415

d

dairy 97
dairy-free 108
dairy-free milk 310
date jam 214
dates 113, 142, 152, 154, 158, 222, 230, 282, 298, 300, 320, 324, 326, 330, 340, 342, 415
David Wolfe 72, 475
Deepak Chopra 122, 124, 474
deodorant 384, 386
desiccated coconut 262, 324, 415
detox bath 385
dibutyl phthalate 382
digestive enzymes 76
dill 362, 415
dip dips & spreads 274
'dirty dozen' of skin care 382
dirty dozen plus™ 89
dishwashing 388
disinfect toothbrushes 388
Donna Gates 163, 360, 476
drain cleaner 386
drawn butter 420
Dr. Frank Lipman 34, 360
Dr. Hanna Grotepass 13
Dr. Joel Fuhrman 39
Dr. Lipman 35
Dr. Mercola 370
dried coconut 412
dulse 115, 304, 306
dysbiosis 28, 29

e

ear infection 32, 383
eat from the rainbow 74
eating in finger foods 232
eczema 386
egg 182, 240, 246, 250, 258, 270, 304, 306, 308
eggplant 288, 416
eggs 28, 115, 214, 220, 244, 248, 258, 260, 262, 272, 310, 336, 338, 416
e-numbers 67
Environmental Working Group (EWG) 61, 89, 382
enzyme 76, 97
enzyme inhibitors 77
equipment 467
essential nutrients 39
extra virgin olive oil 284

f

factory farms 78
feeding with awareness 51
fennel 356
fibre 40
filtered water 138
fish 260, 417
'fixers' 163
flavour 163
flavour enhancers 66, 70, 482
flaxseed 212, 246
flaxseed oil 115, 418
flaxseeds 142, 214, 220, 224, 226, 228, 234, 242,

491

Index

324, 332, 418
folate 42
food additives 66, 478
food additives to avoid 68
food allergy 53
food combinations 163
food detective 68
food intolerance 53
food introduction chart 48
food is love 120
food is sacred 124
food preparation 131
formaldehyde-releasing preservatives 383
'free-from' 101
free-range 78, 79
freezing food 132
from the fork 302
fruit 164, 203
fruit and vegetable wash 90
fruits and veggies 83

g
gallates 481
garbanzo beans 419
garlic 194, 246, 250, 252, 260, 276, 288, 290, 292, 306, 308, 312, 314, 316, 356, 358, 362, 419
gem squash 419
genetic roulette 83
germs 28
ghee 99, 115, 184, 322, 420
ginger 194, 240, 262, 420
glutamates 482
gluten 94
gluten-free 104
gluten-free blends 106
gluten-free flour 105, 268
gluten intolerance 95
glyphosate 55
GM 84
GMO 55, 78, 83, 84
goat cheese 248, 250, 252, 421
goat milk powder 144
goat's milk 108, 218, 220, 242, 272, 310, 371, 421
good bacteria 360
gooseberry 422
grace 125
grains 184
grapes 422
grass-fed 78, 80
green onion 423, 451, 455
green powder 150, 188, 203, 230, 320, 324, 326, 423
ground beef 312
guar gum 424
gut 28

h
hake 258, 417
Hanna Grotepass 477

happy time 46
hazelnuts 296
healing wounds 388
healthy child 61
healthy fats 40
healthy world 61
heavy metals 57
hemp 115, 424
hemp milk 110, 376, 425
hemp powder 425
hemp seed oil 115, 425
hemp seeds 158, 186, 425
herbs 163
high fructose corn syrup 484
Hiromi Shinya 97, 477
homogenisation 25
honey 142, 150, 152, 186, 188, 216, 230, 240, 264, 296, 322, 324, 328, 332, 336, 338, 340, 342, 344, 364, 384, 426
household disinfectant 388
how gluten works 95
HPP 483
HVP 483
hydrogen peroxide 90, 388
hydrolysed vegetable 483

i
ice cream 328
ice lollies 334
IIN® 119
infant nutrition 39
iodine 43
iron 43
irradiation 91

j
Joel Fuhrman 476
Joe Stout 144
Joshua Rosenthal 18, 119, 475
juice 140

k
Kahlil Gibran 128
kale 154, 173, 206, 228, 426
kefir 115, 142, 188, 328, 370, 427
kefir grains 371
kombu 356, 358
kudu 312

l
lactase 31, 97, 370
lactose 97
lamb 177, 312, 314, 428
lead 58
lemon 146, 148, 264, 284, 385, 428
lemon juice 222, 226, 244, 260, 262, 288, 292, 294, 342
lentils 174, 194, 250, 314, 429
lice 383

Index

liver 27, 115, 180, 182, 430
living water 139
love 119, 430
lucuma 115, 186, 430

m

maca 115, 142
macadamia 190, 431
maca powder 431
macro nutrients 40
magnesium 42
Maha Chohan 12
maize 432, 458
mandarin 434
manganese 43
mango 168, 316, 432
manuka honey 384
maple syrup 112, 144, 150, 152, 184, 188, 212, 322, 332, 336, 338, 340, 342, 344, 433
Masaru Emoto 13
massage oil 384, 387
mayonnaise 280
meat 78
melons 169
mercury 59
mess 118
microbiome 28
micro-organism 28
mielie 433, 458
milk kefir 372
millet 184, 433
minerals 42
moisturiser 384
Monsanto 55
moringa 115, 142, 186, 203, 434
MS 144
Mt. Capra 144
muskmelon 454
mustard powder 434

n

naartjie 148, 434
Nancy Appleton 100
nappy rash 384, 386
nappy rash remedy 384
nappy soak 386
Natasha Campbell-Mcbride 475
natural sweeteners 112
nature 123
nectarine 435
negative consequences of sugar 100
nitrates 480
nitrites 480
non-celiac gluten sensitivity 95
non-GMO 87
nut butter 330, 344, 435
nutmeg 115, 192, 214, 216, 220, 240, 322, 350, 435
nutrient enhancers 115
nutrients 76

nutritional yeast 207, 228, 278, 436

o

oats 142, 216, 220, 230, 242, 246, 436
olive oil 115, 144, 236, 384, 437
olives 236, 436
onion 192, 194, 246, 250, 252, 260, 288, 290, 292, 306, 308, 312, 314, 316, 356, 358, 437
oranges 438
oregano 439
oreganum 236, 439
organic 78, 80, 83, 87
organisation, food preparation 132
ostrich 312, 439
oven cleaning 386
oven temperatures 472

p

pantry items 348
papaya 440
paprika 248, 260, 262, 264, 440
parabens 59, 382
parfum 383
parsley 148, 226, 248, 252, 260, 276, 290, 441
parties 101
party food & 318
pasteurisation 25
pasture-raised 78, 80
pathogens 28
peach 156, 167, 441
pear 167, 218, 442
peas 154, 442
PEG compounds 383
pepitas 445
peppercorns 356
pesticides 55
pesto 270, 304
petrolatum 383
phosphorous 42
physical activity 121
phytic acid 76
phytonutrients 74
pineapple 148, 443
pineapples 146
pink-eye remedy 385
play 126
plums 443
pomegranate 444
potassium 42
potassium bromate 484
potato 238
potato 314, 444
potato flour 105, 244, 378, 445
potato starch 218, 234, 254, 272, 445
potato starch flour 445
prebiotics 44
preparing food 132
preparing purées 162
preservatives 66, 70, 479

493

Index

probiotic   144, 188, 370
probiotics   28, 44, 360
processed food   64, 66
propionates   480
protein   40
pumpkin seeds   186, 224, 445

q

quick look guide   70
quinoa   184, 248, 446
quinoa flour   106, 218, 374, 446
quinoa milk   110, 376

r

rainbow nutrition   74
raisins   186, 218, 220, 230, 242, 447
raspberries   447
raw cacao   296, 320, 326, 330, 336, 340, 342
raw food movement   72
raw milk   25
raw vs. cooked   72
reactions to additives   67
reasons to avoid GMOs   85
red pepper   447
references   486
refined food   63, 64
refined & processed foods   62
reheating food   133
remedy for mosquito bites   387
ribonucleotides   483
rice   308, 448
rice cereal   22
rice flour   105, 212, 234, 254, 272, 374, 378, 448
rice milk   109, 376
rooibos tea   139, 156, 386, 449
rosemary   314, 449
Roundup   55
Rudolf Steiner   119, 476

s

sage   254, 450
Sally Fallon Morell   474
salt   33, 450
satsuma   434, 451
saturated fats   33, 34
sauerkraut   115, 368
scallion   423, 455
sea vegetables   451
seaweed   451
selenium   43
sesame oil   262, 452
sesame seeds   142, 452
shredded coconut   186
siloxanes   383
sinus relief   388
skin   382
smoked snoek   292
snotty noses   32
soaking   77
sodium   44
sodium lauryl sulphate   382

soil   453
sole   256, 417
something sweet   318
sorbates   479
sore throat   384
sorghum flour   106, 216, 218, 220, 242, 453
soul food   119
South Africa   81, 86
soy milk   109
spanspek   454
spices   163
spinach   148, 152, 154, 173, 226, 228, 248, 454
spirituality   122
spiritual lessons   123
spiritually symbolic foods   125
spiritual practice   122
splinter removal   387
spring onion   260, 423, 451, 455
sprouts   148
stevia   112, 342, 455
stock   354
strawberries   300, 456
strawberry jam   300
sucanat   112
Sue Dengate   477
sugar   100
sugar-free   112
sulphites   479
sunburn remedy   386
sundried tomatoes   236, 250, 282, 456
sunflower seeds   142, 186, 214, 224, 226, 324, 332, 457
sunscreen   383
sunshine   457
sweet corn   458
sweeteners   483
sweetness   101
sweet potato   169, 216, 226, 234, 238, 250, 254, 260, 266, 290, 292, 314, 316, 336, 338, 458
symptoms   94, 98
synthetic antioxidants   70, 480

t

tahini   192, 284, 296, 459
tamari   226, 459
tangerine   148, 434
tapioca flour   106, 218, 220, 234, 238, 244, 250, 254, 258, 272, 340, 344, 460
tapioca starch   212
tap water   138
TBHQ   481
tea   139
teething necklace   387
the '3-day wait rule   51
The Clean Fifteen™   89
The Dirty Dozen   88
The Southampton Six   478
The Weston A. Price Foundation (WAPF)   47
thirsty   136
thyme   460
tomato   190, 461

Index

tomato sauce 312
topical treatment 384
toxins 55
trace minerals 43
transfats 34, 66, 70, 484
treats not sweets 102
triclosan 383
tummy soother 387
turmeric 115, 194, 258, 260, 262, 270, 304, 306, 356, 461

V

vanilla 150, 212, 214, 218, 220, 230, 342, 462
vanilla extract 158, 296, 328, 342, 344
vanilla powder 296, 320, 324, 326, 336, 338, 340
vitamin A 27, 41
vitamin B1 41
vitamin B2 41
vitamin B3 41
vitamin B6 41
vitamin B12 41
vitamin C 41
vitamin D 41
vitamin E 42
vitamin K 42
vitamin L 42
vitamins 41

W

wart remedy 387
water 44, 138
watermelon 146, 462
weight 473
Weston A Price 474
what not to eat 46
what's a GMO 83
what to eat when 46
wheat allergy 95
whey 362, 364, 366, 372, 463
whole food 62, 64
whole grains 24
why not gluten 94

X

xenoestrogens 59
xylitol 113, 328, 344, 464

y

yoghurt 188, 464
yoghurt and cheese 372

z

zinc 43
zucchini 210, 218, 260, 288, 316, 465

Recipe Index

Almond Flour   374
Almond Milk   376
Apple Purées   167
Applesauce   350
Avo Purées   164
Banana Purées   166
Beef Bone Broth   358
Beef Purées   180
Breadcrumbs   352
Broccoli Purées   172
Bubbling Berries   364
Buffalo Wings   264
Butternut & Apple Muffins   220
Butternut & Cranberry Fritters   244
Butternut Purées   170
Butternut Soup   192
Carrot Cupcakes   338
Cauliflower Purées   172
Cheesy Crackers   228
Chicken Balls   252
Chicken Bone Broth   356
Chicken Curry   316
Chicken Nuggets   262
Chicken Purées   177
Chickpea Flatbread   236
Chickpea Flour   375
Chickpea Fudge   322
Chickpea Purées   175
Chocolate Spread   296
Choc-Nut Fudge   320
Choc-Nut Spread   296
Chocolate Icing   342
Chocolate (Or Vanilla) Cupcakes   336
Coconut Icing   344
Coconut Milk   376

Cottage Pie   312
Cupcake And Cake Decorations   346
Date Balls   324
Date Jam   298
Dhal   194
Dilly Carrots   362
Dried Fruits   200
Eggs
   Crustless Quiche   310
   Egg Fried Rice   308
   Green Eggs   304
   Immune Booster Eggs   306
   Orange Eggs   306
   Scrambled Eggs   304
Fermented Apple Sauce   366
Fishcakes   260
Flours   374
Fruit Leather   202
Gluten-Free Play Dough   378
Green Yoghurt   188
Guacamole   294
Hemp Milk   376
Homemade Formula   144
Hummus   284
Ice Cream Base   328
Iced Tea   156
Ice Lollies   334
Icings   342
Juice
   Watermelon Cooler   146
   Juices   146
   Beginner's Juice   146
   Everyday Veggie Juice   148
   Weekend Break   148
Kale Chips   206
   Cheesy Kale Chips   207

Index

Herby Kale Chips   206
   Plain Salted Kale Chips   206
Kale Purées   174
Kefir Whey   372
Lamb Casserole   314
Lamb Purées   178
Lentil Purées   174
Liver Purées   180
Mango Purées   168
Maple Syrup Teething Biscuits   212
Milk Kefir   371
Mock Fish Fingers   256
Morning Glory Muffins   218
Muesli   186
Nana Cakes   222
Nana-Choc Ice Cream   330
Nut Butter   286
Nut Butter Icing   344
Nut Milk   158
Oat Bars   230
'Ontbijtkoek' - Spiced Breakfast Cake   240
Peach Purées   168
Pear Purées   167
Pesto   276
Pesto 'Pancake'   270
Pizza   268
Porridge   184
Purées   162
Quinoa Bites   248
Quinoa Flour   374
Quinoa Milk   376
Raisin And Banana Flapjacks   242
Raw Ice Cream Cups   332
Raw Tomato And Basil Soup   190
Real Fish Fingers   258

Real Pancakes   272
Rice Flour   374
Rice Milk   376
Rösti   238
Ruby Red Icing   344
Rusks   214
Sauce
   All Good Tomato Sauce   282
   Egg-Free Mayonnaise   280
   No-Dairy Cheese Sauce   278
Sauerkraut   368
Simple Seed Crackers   224
Boo Boo Smoothie   142
Smoothies   150
   Berry Blaze   152
   Grass Green   154
   Super Smooth   150
Spinach Purées   173
Chicken Liver Pâté   290
Snoek Pâté   292
Sticky Chocolate Layer Cake   340
Sweet Potato Bread   234
Sweet Potato Chips   266
Sweet Potato Gnocchi   254
Sweet Potato Muffins   216
Sweet Potato Purées   169
The First Egg   182
Vanilla Icing   342
Veggie Bites   250
Veggie Crackers   226
Veggie Spread   288
Water Kefir   371
Yoghurt   188
Zucchini Crisps   210

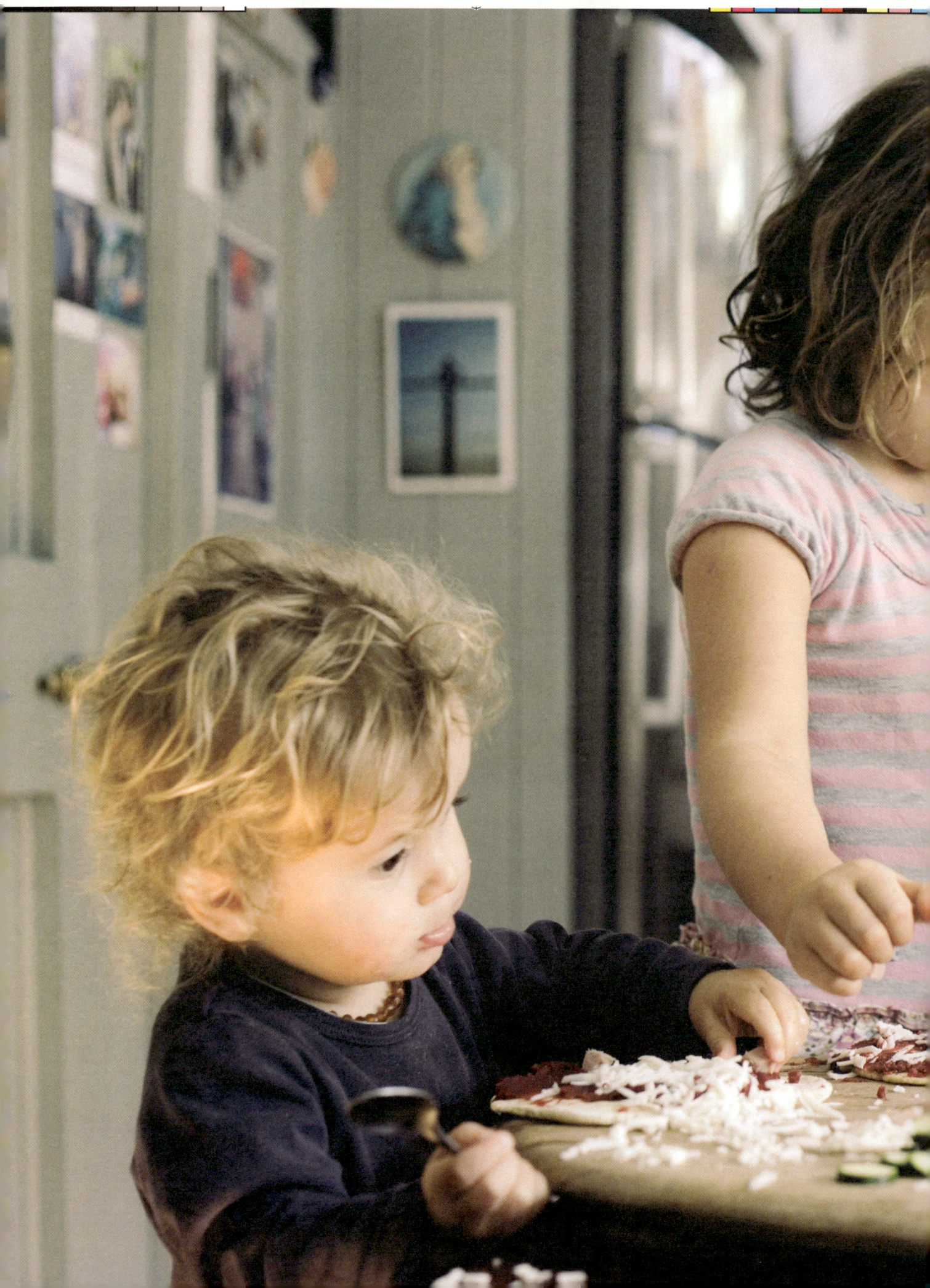

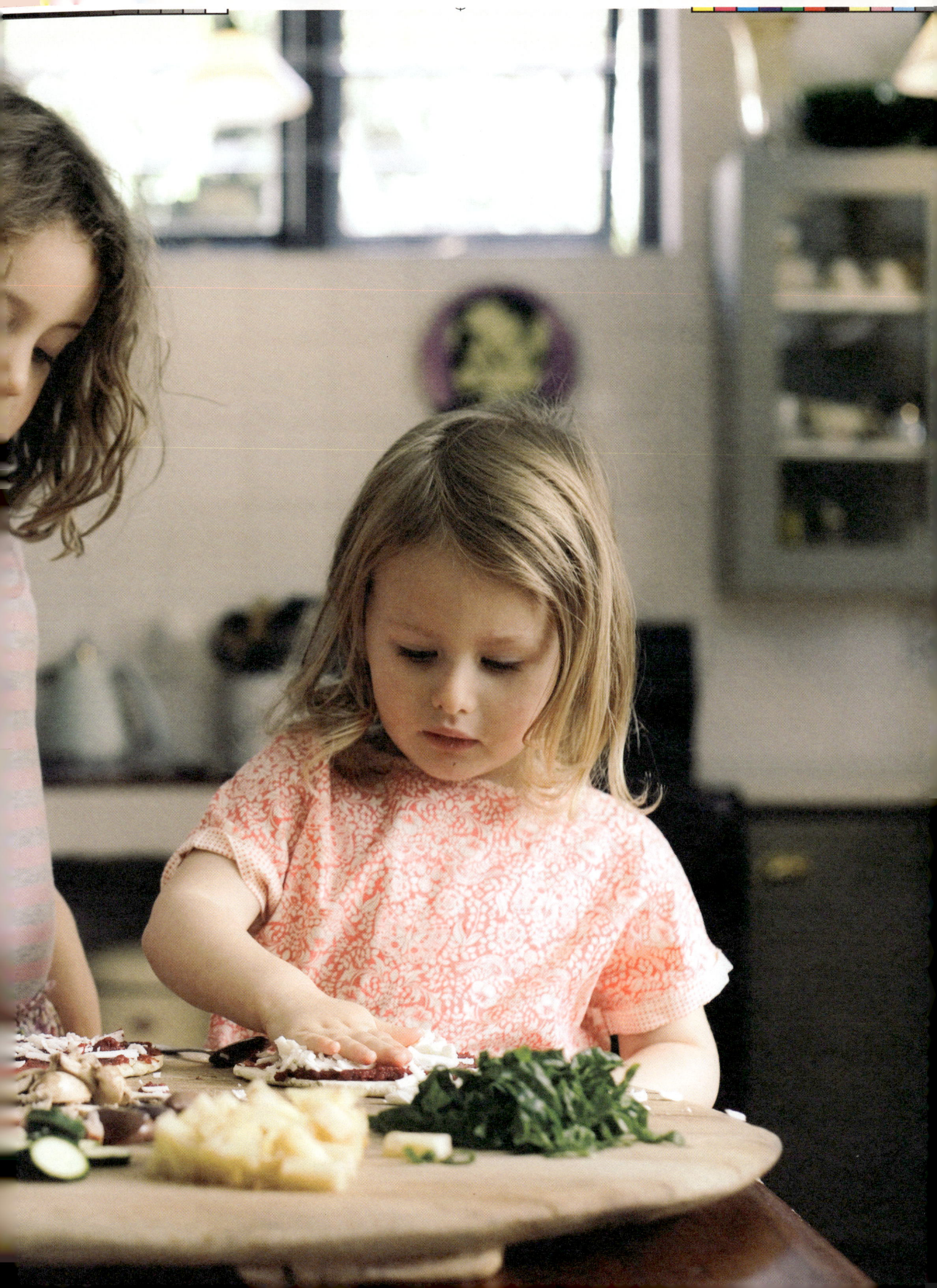